Clinical Medicine
Lecture Notes

Lecture Notes

Welcome to the series home page for the *Lecture Notes* books for medical students and junior doctors.

- The series covers over 35 subjects providing the concise core knowledge required by medical students and junior doctors
- Each book written by an expert teacher in note form, with bullet lists, illustrations, and summary boxes
- A panel of medical students reviews each text to ensure that the coverage is exactly right for its audience
- Ideal as course textbooks or revision aids

Lecture Notes Clinical Biochemistry, 10th Edition
Peter Rae, Mike Crane, Rebecca Pattenden
ISBN: 978-1-119-24868-2
Oct 2017

Lecture Notes: Haematology, 10th Edition
Christian S. R. Hatton, Deborah Hay, David M. Keeling
ISBN: 978-1-119-26425-5
Sep 2017

Lecture Notes: Infectious Diseases, 6th Edition
B. K. Mandal, E. G. L. Wilkins, E. M. Dunbar, Richard Mayon-White
ISBN: 978-1-405-10820-1
Feb 2004

Clinical Medicine
Lecture Notes

John R. Bradley

CBE MA DM FRCP
Consultant Physician and Honorary Professor of Experimental Medicine
University of Cambridge School of Clinical Medicine
Cambridge University Hospitals
Cambridge

Mark Gurnell

MA (MedEd) PhD FAcadMEd FRCP
Clinical SubDean, Senior Lecturer and Honorary Consultant Physician
University of Cambridge School of Clinical Medicine
Cambridge University Hospitals
Cambridge

Diana F. Wood

MA MD FRCP
Director of Medical Education, Clinical Dean and Honorary
Consultant Physician
University of Cambridge School of Clinical Medicine
Cambridge University Hospitals
Cambridge

Eighth Edition

WILEY Blackwell

This edition first published 2019
© 2019 John Wiley & Sons Ltd

Edition History
Blackwell Publishing Ltd (7e, 2012)

The right of John R. Bradley, Mark Gurnell, and Diana F. Wood to be identified as the authors of the editorial material in this work has been asserted in accordance with law.

Registered Office(s)
John Wiley & Sons, Inc., 111 River Street, Hoboken, NJ 07030, USA
John Wiley & Sons Ltd, The Atrium, Southern Gate, Chichester, West Sussex, PO19 8SQ, UK

Editorial Office
9600 Garsington Road, Oxford, OX4 2DQ, UK

For details of our global editorial offices, customer services, and more information about Wiley products visit us at www.wiley.com.

Wiley also publishes its books in a variety of electronic formats and by print-on-demand. Some content that appears in standard print versions of this book may not be available in other formats.

Library of Congress Cataloging-in-Publication Data

Names: Bradley, John R., 1958– author. | Gurnell, Mark, author. | Wood, Diana F., author.
Title: Clinical medicine. Lecture notes / by John R. Bradley, Mark Gurnell, Diana F. Wood.
Other titles: Clinical medicine | Clinical medicine lecture notes
Description: Eighth edition. | Hoboken, NJ : Wiley, 2019. | Includes bibliographical references and index. |
Identifiers: LCCN 2018010565 (print) | LCCN 2018011920 (ebook) | ISBN 9781118973424 (pdf) |
    ISBN 9781118973417 (epub) | ISBN 9781118973431 (pbk.)
Subjects: | MESH: Clinical Medicine | Handbooks
Classification: LCC RC48 (ebook) | LCC RC48 (print) | NLM WB 39 | DDC 616–dc23
LC record available at https://lccn.loc.gov/2018010565

Cover design: Wiley
Cover image: © Thomas Northcut/Getty Images

Set in 8.5/11pt Utopia by SPi Global, Pondicherry, India

Printed in Singapore by C.O.S. Printers Pte Ltd

10 9 8 7 6 5 4 3 2 1

Contents

Preface to the Eighth Edition

History-taking and examination remain the essential tools of clinical examination. However, the environment in which medicine is practised continues to change, with advances in technology and an increasing evidence base to guide decision-making. The eighth edition follows the format of previous editions of this book with two sections: Clinical Examination and Clinical Medicine. Each section has been updated to reflect the more objective methods of assessment that are now used and the increased evidence upon which clinical practice is based.

It is rewarding to discover how many readers have found the text useful for study, for revision, and for clinical practice. Please continue to let us have your views.

John R. Bradley
Mark Gurnell
Diana F. Wood

Acknowledgements

We would like to thank Dr Francesca Crawley, Dr Ellie Gurnell, Dr Jane Sterling and Dr Mark Lillicrap for their contributions, help and advice during the preparation of the manuscript.

Preface to the First Edition

This book is intended primarily for the junior hospital doctor in the period between qualification and the examination for Membership of the Royal Colleges of Physicians. We think that it will also be helpful to final-year medical students and to clinicians reading for higher specialist qualifications in surgery and anaesthetics.

The hospital doctor must not only acquire a large amount of factual information but also use it effectively in the clinical situation. The experienced physician has acquired some clinical perspective through practice: we hope that this book imparts some of this to the relatively inexperienced. The format and contents are designed for the examination candidate but the same approach to problems should help the hospital doctor in his everyday work.

The book as a whole is not suitable as a first reader for the undergraduate because it assumes much basic knowledge and considerable detailed information has had to be omitted. It is not intended to be a complete textbook of medicine and the information it contains must be supplemented by further reading. The contents are intended only as lecture notes and the margins of the pages are intentionally large so that the reader may easily add additional material of his own.

The book is divided into two parts: the *clinical approach* and *essential background information*. In the first part we have considered the situation which a candidate meets in the clinical part of an examination or a physician in the clinic. This part of the book thus resembles a manual on techniques of physical examination, though it is more specifically intended to help the candidate carry out an examiner's request to perform a specific examination. It has been our experience in listening to candidates' performances in examinations and hearing the examiner's subsequent assessment that it is the failure of a candidate to examine cases systematically and his failure to behave as if he were used to doing this every day of his clinical life that leads to adverse comments.

In the second part of the book a summary of basic clinical facts is given in the conventional way. We have included most common diseases but not all, and we have tried to emphasise points which are under stressed in many textbooks. Accounts are given of many conditions which are relatively rare. It is necessary for the clinician to know about these and to be on the lookout for them both in the clinic and in examinations. Supplementary reading is essential to understand their basic pathology, but the information we give is probably all that need be remembered by the non-specialist reader and will provide adequate working knowledge in a clinical situation. It should not be forgotten that some rare diseases are of great importance in practice because they are treatable or preventable, e.g. infective endocarditis, hepatolenticular degeneration, attacks of acute porphyria. Some conditions are important to examination candidates because patients are ambulant and appear commonly in examinations, e.g. neurosyphilis, syringomyelia, atrial and ventricular septal defects.

We have not attempted to cover the whole of medicine, but by cross-referencing between the two sections of the book and giving information in summary form we have completely omitted few subjects. Some highly specialised fields such as the treatment of leukaemia were thought unsuitable for inclusion.

A short account of psychiatry is given in the section on neurology since many patients with mental illness attend general clinics and it is hoped that readers may be warned of gaps in their knowledge of this important field. The section on dermatology is incomplete but should serve for quick revision of common skin disorders.

Wherever possible we have tried to indicate the relative frequency with which various conditions are likely to be seen in hospital practice in this country and have selected those clinical features which in our view are most commonly seen and where possible have listed them in order of importance. The frequency with which a disease is encountered by any individual physician will depend upon its prevalence in the district from which his cases are drawn and also on his known special interests. Nevertheless, rare conditions are rarely seen; at least in the clinic. Examinations, however, are a 'special case'.

We have used many generally accepted abbreviations, e.g. ECG, ESR, and have included them in the index instead of supplying a glossary.

Despite our best efforts, some errors of fact may have been included. As with every book and authority, question and check everything – and please write to us if you wish.

We should like to thank all those who helped us with producing this book and, in particular, Sir Edward Wayne and Sir Graham Bull who have kindly allowed us to benefit from their extensive experience both in medicine and in examining for the Colleges of Physicians.

David Rubenstein
David Wayne
November 1975

Part 1

Clinical Examination

The medical interview

Good communication between doctor and patient forms the basis for excellent patient care and the clinical consultation lies at the heart of medical practice. Good communication skills encompass more than the personality traits of individual doctors – they form an essential core competence for medical practitioners. In essence, good communication skills produce more effective consultations and, together with medical knowledge and physical examination skills, lead to better diagnostic reasoning and therapeutic intervention. The term 'communication skills', when applied to medical practice, describes a set of specific skills that can be taught, learned and assessed. A large evidence base shows that health outcomes for patients and both patient and doctor satisfaction within the therapeutic relationship are enhanced by good communication skills.

In this chapter the medical interview as a whole will be considered and then the way in which communication skills should be approached in different types of assessment encountered by students and trainees is reviewed.

There are a number of different models for learning communication skills in use throughout the world. They are generally similar and all emphasise the importance of patient-centred interview methods. This chapter is based on the Calgary–Cambridge model (Fig. 1.1) which has been widely adopted in Europe and the USA and with which the authors are familiar as a means of teaching and learning and as a framework for assessment (Silverman et al. 2005). Like all clinical skills, communication skills can only be acquired by experiential learning. This may take the form of small group learning with role play, the use of actors in simulated learning environments or, for more experienced learners, in recorded real consultations with subsequent feedback.

Effective consultation

Effective consultations are patient-centred and efficient, taking place within the time and other practical constraints that exist in everyday medical practice. The use of specific communication skills together with a structured approach to the medical interview can enhance this process. Important communication skills can be considered in three categories: content, process and perceptual skills (see Table 1.1); these mirror the essential knowledge, skills and attitudes required for good medical practice. These skills are closely interrelated so that, for example, effective use of process skills can improve the accuracy of information gathered from the patient, thus enhancing the content skills used subsequently in the consultation.

Structure

Providing structure to the consultation is one of the most important features of effective consultation. Process skills should be used to develop a structure that is responsive to the patient and flexible for different consultations. Six groups of skills can be identified and each will be considered in the sections that follow. *Sequential in the consultation:*

- initiating the session
- gathering information (including from physical examination)
- explanation and planning
- closing the session

Throughout the consultation:

- organisation
- relationship building

Clinical Medicine Lecture Notes, Eighth Edition. John R. Bradley, Mark Gurnell, and Diana F. Wood.
© 2019 John Wiley & Sons Ltd. Published 2019 by John Wiley & Sons Ltd.

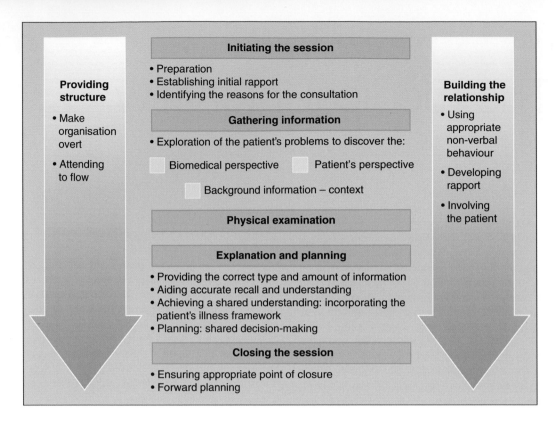

Figure 1.1 The Calgary–Cambridge Guide. Source: Kurtz, S. et al. (2005) *Teaching and Learning Communication Skills in Medicine,* 2nd edn. Oxford: Radcliffe Publishing.

Table 1.1 Categories of communication skills

Skill	Examples
Content skills	
What the doctor communicates	Knowledge-based: appropriate questions and responses; accurate information gathering and explanation to patient; clear discussion of investigation and treatments based on knowledge
Process skills	
How the doctor communicates	Skills-based: verbal and non-verbal communication skills; relationship building; organising and structuring the interview
Perceptual skills	
What the doctor is thinking	Attitude-based: clinical reasoning and problem-solving skills; attitudes towards the patient; feelings and thoughts about the patient; awareness of internal biases

Initiating the session

The initial part of a consultation is essential to form the basis for relationship building and to set objectives for the rest of the interview. Before meeting a patient, the doctor should prepare by focusing him- or herself, trying to avoid distractions and reviewing any available information such as previous notes or referral letters.

Initiating the session

Establish rapport: greet the patient, confirm their name, introduce yourself and explain your role, attend to the patient's comfort.

Identify the reason for the consultation: use an appropriate opening question, listen to the patient, confirm the problem and screen for any other issues that the patient may wish to discuss.

Confirm an agenda for the consultation.

 Physical examination

Ask permission: gain the patient's consent for examination.

Ensure that the patient is comfortable: position them adequately for the examination; if doing a full examination, cover parts of the body not being examined actively.

Be clear and precise: explain what you are going to do in advance.

Be aware: the patient may be embarrassed or in pain.

Gathering information

An accurate clinical history provides about 80% of the information required to make a diagnosis. Traditionally, history-taking focused on questions related to the biomedical aspects of the patient's problems. Recent evidence suggests that better outcomes are obtained by including the patient's perspective of their illness and by taking this into account in subsequent parts of the consultation. The objectives for gathering information should therefore include exploring the history from both the biomedical and patient perspectives, checking that the information gathered is complete and ensuring that the patient feels that the doctor is listening to them.

Further information is gathered from the physical examination. Establishment of a good rapport during the first part of the consultation will facilitate communication during the examination. An appropriate chaperone should be present during the physical examination.

Explanation and planning

Explanation and planning is crucially important to the effective consultation. Establishment of a management plan jointly between the doctor and the patient has important positive effects on patient recall, understanding of their condition, adherence to treatment and overall satisfaction. Patient expectations have changed and many wish to be more

 Explanation and planning

Avoid jargon: use clear concise language; explain any medical terminology.

Find out what the patient knows: establish prior knowledge; find out how much they wish to know at this stage.

'Chunk and check': provide information in small amounts and check understanding; use this to assess how to proceed.

Organise explanation: develop a logical sequence; categorise information; repeat and summarise; signpost what is coming next; use diagrams or charts, written information or instructions.

Relate the information to the patient's perspective.

Respond to patient's cues: verbal and non-verbal; allow patient to ask questions or clarify information.

Involve the patient: share thoughts; reveal rationale for opinions; offer your opinion of what is going on and name it where possible; explore management options; take the patient's lifestyle and cultural background into account in the discussion.

Negotiate a mutually agreeable action plan: check that this meets the patient's expectations and addresses their concerns.

 Gathering information

Ask the patient to tell their own story.

Listen attentively: do not interrupt; leave the patient time and space to think about what they are saying.

Use open and closed questions: clarify issues in the history; use clear, concise and easily understood questions; move from open to closed questions then back again.

Use verbal and non-verbal facilitation: silences, repetition, paraphrasing.

Pick up on patient's verbal and non-verbal clues: acknowledge them by checking.

Summarise at intervals: verify your understanding; allow the patient to correct or add to the history.

Encourage the patient to express their feelings: actively seek their ideas, concerns and expectations.

involved in decision-making about investigation and treatment options. The goals of this part of the consultation are thus to gauge the amount and type of information required by each individual patient, to provide information in a way that the patient can remember and understand and which takes their perspectives into account, to arrive at a shared understanding of the problem and to engage the patient in planning the next moves.

Closing the session

Closing the interview allows the doctor to summarise and clarify the plans that have been made and what the next steps will be. It is also important to ensure that contingency plans are in place in case of unexpected

events and that the patient is clear about follow-up arrangements. Continuing to foster the doctor–patient relationship in this way has positive effects on adherence to treatment and health outcomes.

Two essential parts of effective consultation skills run throughout the interview – organisation and relationship building. The way in which these two are used is shown in Table 1.2.

Organisation allows a flexible but ordered and logical process to occur within an appropriate time-frame. It encourages patient participation and collaboration and facilitates accurate information gathering.

Building a relationship with the patient involves a number of communication skills that enable the doctor to establish rapport and trust between themselves and the patient. It maximises the chances of accurate information gathering, explanation and planning and can form part of the development of a continuing relationship over time. It is vital to patient and doctor satisfaction with the consultation process.

 Closing the session

Summarise: review the consultation and clarify the plan of action; make a contract with the patient about the next steps.

Describe contingency plans: explain any possible unexpected outcomes; how and when to seek help.

Final check: ensure that the patient agrees and has no further questions.

Special circumstances

Certain circumstances demand a special approach to communication skills, such as breaking bad news, dealing with cultural diversity, using an interpreter,

Table 1.2 Skills for organising the consultation and building the relationship

Organising the consultation		Building the relationship	
Summarising	Summarise the end of a specific line of enquiry; confirm your understanding; allow patient to correct; order information; reflect on what to do next.	Non-verbal communication	Includes eye contact, facial expression, posture, proximity, body movement, touch; use of time, your appearance, manner; the environment.
Signposting	Structure the interview overtly; draw attention to what you are about to say; introduce summaries; help patient to understand where the interview is going; ask permission to move on through the interview.	Rapport	Accept patient's views; empathise to show understanding of patient's views and feelings; support by expressing concern, willingness to help, acknowledge efforts to cope; be sensitive towards embarrassing or difficult issues.
Sequencing	Maintain a logical sequence to the interview; use flexible but ordered organisation by signposting and summarising.	Involve the patient	Share your thoughts to encourage patient interaction; explain your rationale for doing things; explain your actions during the physical examination.
Timing	Pace the interview; use other skills to achieve good timing.		

Breaking bad news

Prepare: ensure you have all the clinical details and know the facts; set aside enough time; encourage the patient to bring a relative or friend.

Start the session: review what has happened so far; assess the patient's state of mind; find out what they know and what they are thinking.

Share the information: warn the patient that the news is not good; give the information clearly and in small amounts; relate to the patient's perspective; do not overwhelm with information in the first instance; check repeatedly that the patient understands.

Be sensitive: respond to the patient's emotions – tears, anger, denial; allow time for silences and questions and respond to them honestly; gauge the patient's wishes for information and respond accordingly; be empathic and concerned; check the patient's understanding of what you have said and elicit their concerns and understanding of the situation; do not be afraid to show your own emotions.

Make a plan: explain what will happen next; give hope but be realistic; confirm your role as a partner in care.

Closure: summarise and check the patient's understanding; respond to additional questions; check the patient's support systems and offer to speak to family if requested; make an early follow-up appointment.

 Approach to communication skills assessment

Past papers: the format of the examination should be available for review; look at the communication skills stations; familiarise yourself with the format; are the process and content components weighted and, if so, how?

Be prepared: obtain as much information as possible in advance of the assessment; how long are the stations? Is the station simply an observed communication scenario or is a structured viva involved? In some examinations the clinical scenario is available in advance of the examination to allow preparation of content – if so, read it carefully and be certain of the medical facts.

Read the instructions: in most summative assessments the scenario is presented at the station with a few minutes' reading time. Read the scenario carefully. Think about the content as well as the process skills.

Be clear about the task: are you required to take a history, to give information, gain consent for a procedure, talk to a relative or colleague?

Make a plan: before you enter the station, have a clear plan as to how you will approach the consultation and what you wish to achieve.

Think about what you might encounter: communication skills assessments usually use simulated patients who may respond in a number of ways. For example, how will you deal with an emotional patient, a non-communicative patient or an angry response to breaking bad news?

Listen to the examiner: if you are asked to present and discuss the case, listen carefully to the examiner and present the salient features in a clear and logical manner.

and consultation with the elderly, with mentally ill patients or the parents of a sick child. In essence, the core communication skills described here form the basis for any of the more difficult communication skills scenarios. Complex situations require the doctor to use basic skills to a higher level. Preparation and planning, listening to the patient, delivering information in small amounts with regular checking and allowing time for information to be assimilated and for questioning are paramount. Closure is also important, ensuring the patient knows what is happening and is clear about the next steps.

Assessment of communication skills

Clinical competence is assessed at all levels of medical education. Communication skills are usually assessed in undergraduate examinations by stations in Objective Structured Clinical Examinations (OSCEs). More varied assessments take place for postgraduates, including stations in the Royal College of Physicians MRCP Part 3 examination (Practical Assessment of Clinical Examination Skills; PACES) and mini-CEX assessments as part of ongoing workplace-based assessments for trainees. Students and trainees attempting these assessments should have been through appropriate communication skills

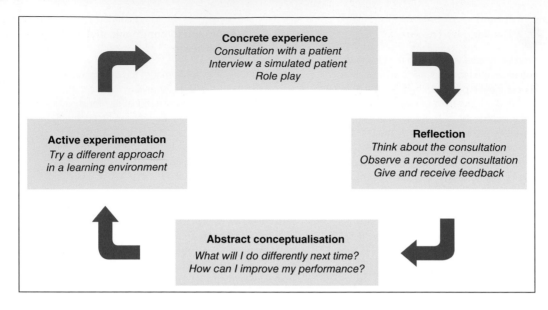

Figure 1.2 Application of the Experiential Learning Cycle to learning communication skills. The learning process may begin with any of the four types of experience. The cycle enables the learner to build on existing knowledge and skills, to take responsibility for their own progress and to use real-life clinical and simulated encounters to promote further learning. Source: Kolb, D.A. (1984) *Experiential Learning: Experience as the Source of Learning and Development.* Englewood Cliffs, NJ: Prentice Hall.

experiential learning programmes allowing them to develop skills in simulated environments and practise them in clinical settings (Fig. 1.2). Whatever the assessment format, a number of factors should be addressed.

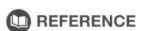 **REFERENCE**

Silverman, J., Kurtz, S. and Draper, J. (2005) *Skills for Communicating with Patients*, 2nd edn. Oxford: Radcliffe Publishing.

2

General examination

Introduction

General examination can reveal abnormalities in a number of systems, which may assist in making an accurate diagnosis.

Disorders of gait, speech and mood should be apparent on first meeting the patient and during the consultation process. Dyspnoea may be observed and abnormal movements, including tremor or paucity of facial expression, should be noted.

During the general examination, obvious features of systemic disease in one site should be correlated with signs elsewhere.

Hands

Note

- joint disorders – arthritis, gout, deformity
- neuromuscular changes – muscle wasting, loss of function
- skin temperature
  - warm, cyanosed hands with bounding pulse in CO_2 retention
  - cold pale hands with arterial disease
- fingers
  - Raynaud's phenomenon, other signs of systemic sclerosis
  - nicotine staining
  - Osler's nodes (endocarditis, vasculitis)
- nails
  - anaemia (pallor, koilonychia)
  - peripheral cyanosis
  - splinter haemorrhages

- clubbing – swelling of the ends of the fingers with increased curvature of the nails and loss of the angle at the nail beds
- palmar erythema
- Dupuytren's contracture
- tremor
  - fine tremor may be exaggerated by placing a piece of paper over the patient's outstretched hands
  - outstretched hands exaggerate the coarse tremor of CO_2 retention
  - flapping tremor in hepatic failure, uraemia – ask the patient to cock their wrists with the hands outstretched
  - resting tremor of Parkinson's disease – hands flexed and showing coarse 'pill-rolling' tremor relieved by intention
  - intention tremor – benign or cerebellar

Face

Check for

- anaemia: examine the insides of the eyelids, look for glossitis (pernicious anaemia) and angular cheilitis
- dental hygiene, tonsillar enlargement, buccal pigmentation inside the mouth

Cardiorespiratory system

- cyanosis: examine the underside of the tongue
- observe pursing of the lips on expiration in obstructive airways disease
- lupus pernio indicates sarcoidosis

Clinical Medicine Lecture Notes, Eighth Edition. John R. Bradley, Mark Gurnell, and Diana F. Wood.
© 2019 John Wiley & Sons Ltd. Published 2019 by John Wiley & Sons Ltd.

Gastrointestinal system

- jaundice – examine the sclera
- spider naevi
- Peutz–Jeghers syndrome – intestinal polyps with skin and oral pigmentation
- hereditary haemorrhagic telangiectasia

Neurological system

- upper motor neuron (UMN) or lower motor neuron (LMN) facial palsy: differentiate stroke from Bell's palsy; examine the external auditory meatus for evidence of herpes zoster
- ptosis and oculomotor palsies
- Parkinsonism
- myopathy: cataract and frontal baldness suggest dystrophia myotonica
- ophthalmic herpes zoster including the conjunctiva

Endocrine system
Observe typical features of

- thyrotoxicosis: including thyroid eye disease in Grave's disease
- hypothyroidism
- Cushing syndrome
- acromegaly
- Paget's disease involving the skull

Autoimmune diseases

- systemic lupus erythematosus – photosensitive 'butterfly rash'
- scleroderma – microstomia, tightening of the skin
- dermatomyositis – 'heliotrope' periorbital rash

Skin diseases

- acne vulgaris
- acne rosacea
- psoriasis: check behind the ears
- port wine stain – capilary malformation

Rheumatological system

- gouty tophi – check the pinnae

Neck

Examine

- the jugular venous pressure (JVP)
- the thyroid gland
- cervical lymph nodes including the occipital group

Axillae

With shoulders relaxed examine

- anterior, posterior and lateral walls and apices of axillae for lymphadenopathy

Breasts (Fig. 2.1)

Examine systematically in women and men where indicated

- nipples
- four quadrants of each breast
- axillary tails of each breast
- axillae

Legs

Cardiorespiratory system

- pitting oedema – note the extent of peripheral oedema
- evidence of peripheral vascular disease – absent foot pulses, delayed capillary filling, ulceration, gangrene
- varicose veins – note and examine formally if present
- ulceration – note whether venous or arterial
- assess the temperature of the dorsum of each foot, noting asymmetry, interdigital infection and loss of hair
- palpate the dorsalis pedis and posterior tibial pulses
- palpate the popliteal and femoral pulses
- auscultate for bruits over femoral pulses

Rheumatological system

- obvious joint deformity consistent with specific arthritides including gout
- bone deformity – Paget's disease in the tibiae

Neurological system

- Charcot joints
- peripheral neuropathy

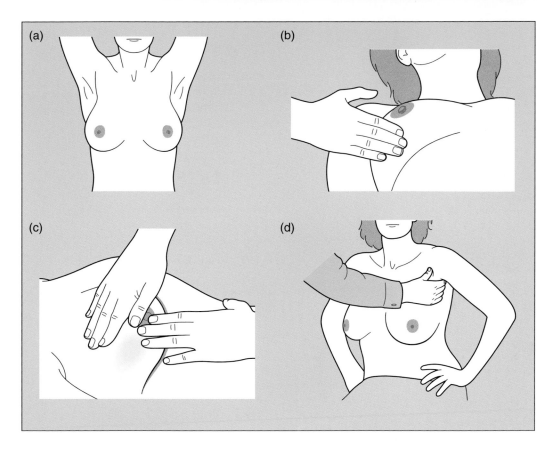

Figure 2.1 Breast examination. (a) Inspection. (b) Palpation. (c) Non-dominant hand stretching the skin. (d) Examination of the axilla.

- effects of chronic neurological lesions – UMN (stroke), multiple sclerosis, polio
- subacute combined degeneration of the cord; hereditary ataxias

Skin

- cellulitis
- varicose eczema with haemosiderosis
- psoriasis
- specific skin lesions – erythema nodosum

Endocrine system

- pretibial myxoedema
- pyoderma gangrenosum

Notes

Lymphadenopathy

A systematic approach to the detection of lymphadenopathy is required. Examine all the major lymph nodes in a logical order:

- cervical
- supraclavicular
- axillary
- inguinal

If lymphadenopathy is detected, examine the abdomen for hepatosplenomegaly.

3

Cardiovascular system

Introduction

Diagnostic accuracy when assessing patients with cardiovascular disease relies heavily on the medical history. A characteristic history of cerebrovascular or peripheral vascular disease may be elicited. Key features in the cardiovascular history are shown in Box 3.1.

Systematic and thorough examination of the cardiovascular system is a core skill for physicians. Accurate assessment of peripheral cardiovascular signs aids the interpretation of auscultatory findings. Patients with ischaemic heart disease may have few physical signs and physicians should be aware of the likely sites and significance of scars from previous surgical or radiological intervention. Cardiac valvular disease and septal defects usually give rise to murmurs, which may be diagnostic. In clinical practice arrival at the final cardiac diagnosis is aided by an electrocardiogram (ECG), chest X-ray (CXR) and echocardiogram (ECHO) and by more complex radiological intervention as appropriate including magnetic resonance imaging (MRI), computerised tomography (CT) and angiography.

General inspection

Note

- peripheral or central cyanosis: central cyanosis is accompanied by peripheral cyanosis by definition
- dyspnoea and orthopnoea

- malar flush
- xanthelasmata

Blood pressure

- Measure the blood pressure lying and standing

Hands

Inspect for

- clubbing
- splinter haemorrhages
- palmar erythema
- nicotine staining

Arterial pulses

Palpate

- radial pulse to assess the rate and rhythm
- radial and brachial pulses in both arms, comparing right and left
- carotid pulses
- radial and femoral pulses simultaneously to assess radiofemoral delay

Rate

- count radial for at least 15 s if rhythm regular, at least 30–60 s if irregular
- check the jugular venous pressure (JVP) whilst counting

Clinical Medicine Lecture Notes, Eighth Edition. John R. Bradley, Mark Gurnell, and Diana F. Wood.
© 2019 John Wiley & Sons Ltd. Published 2019 by John Wiley & Sons Ltd.

Box 3.1 Important features in the cardiovascular history

Chest pain:	onset
	duration
	nature
	precipitating factors
	relieving factors
	distribution and radiation
	previous episodes
	associated symptoms
	(nausea, vomiting, sweating)
Breathlessness:	on exertion
	orthopnoea
	paroxysmal nocturnal
	dyspnoea
Cough:	with or without sputum
	production
Oedema:	ankle swelling
	swelling of lower limbs and
	sacral area
Syncope:	on exertion
	postural
	sudden
Calf pain:	intermittent claudication
Peripheral	cold peripheries with colour/
vascular	sensory changes
disease (PVD):	
Others:	transient hemiparesis
Visual	transient (e.g. amaurosis
disturbance:	fugax)
Risk factors:	smoking
	obesity
	hypertension
	diabetes
	hyperlipidaemia
	oral contraception
Past history:	hypertension
	cerebrovascular disease
	peripheral vascular disease
	congenital heart disease
Medication:	antihypertensives
	anti-anginal therapy
	statins
	oral contraceptives and
	oestrogen replacement
	therapy (HRT)
Family history:	ischaemic heart disease
	diabetes
	hypertension
	hyperlipidaemia

Rhythm

- regular (sinus rhythm)
- regularly irregular (extra or dropped beats)
- irregularly irregular (atrial fibrillation; the pulse rate is different from the heart rate; listen and count at the apex whilst palpating the pulse)

Volume and character (Table 3.1)

- collapsing pulse: raise the patient's arm above the level of the heart whilst holding four fingers over the anterior forearm
- slow – rising, low volume, alternans, bisferiens and paradoxus by palpating the carotid pulse

Jugular venous pressure and pulse (Table 3.2; Fig. 3.1)

The patient should be lying at 45° with the neck relaxed. The JVP is seen welling up between the two heads of sternomastoid in the front of the neck on expiration.

Measure

- the vertical height of the top of the column of blood above the sternal angle.

The sternal angle is about 5 cm above the left atrium when the patient is lying at 45°. The normal central venous pressure (CVP) is 7 cm and therefore the jugular vein is normally just visible.

In the neck, the venous pulse differs from the arterial pulse:

- its height varies with posture, it is impalpable and low pressure means that it is easily abolished by light finger pressure
- it fills from above when light finger pressure is applied to the root of the neck
- the height varies with respiration (fall with inspiration and rise with expiration)
- there are two peaks with each pulsation, 'a' and 'v'.

The JVP is a better guide to right atrial pressure than the superficial external venous pulse which may be tortuous or obstructed by soft tissues in the neck.

If neither is obvious:

- Suspect a low level: unless the liver is tender, press on the abdomen gently but firmly. The

Table 3.1 Abnormalities of the arterial pulse

Type	Character	Seen in
Slow-rising	Low amplitude, slow rise, slow fall	Aortic stenosis
Collapsing	Large amplitude, rapid rise, rapid fall	Aortic incompetence; severe anaemia, hyperthyroidism; arteriovenous shunt, heart block, patent ductus arteriosus
Low volume	Thready	Low cardiac output states; hypovolaemic shock; valvular stenosis; pulmonary hypertension
Alternans	Alternate large- and small-amplitude beats (rarely noted in pulse; usually on taking blood pressure)	Left ventricular failure
Bisferiens	Double-topped ('notched')	Aortic stenosis with aortic incompetence
Paradoxus	Pulse volume decreases excessively with inspiration	Cardiac tamponade, constrictive pericarditis, severe inspiratory airways obstruction
Absent radial		Congenital anomaly (check brachials and blood pressure)
		Tied off at surgery or catheterisation. Arterial embolism

Table 3.2 Raised jugular venous pressure (JVP)

Character	Compression of neck and abdomen	Conclusion
Non-pulsatile	No change in JVP	Superior mediastinal obstruction • carcinoma of bronchus • large goitre • platysmal compression
Pulsatile	Jugular vein fills and empties	Right heart failure Expiratory airways obstruction Fluid overload Cardiac tamponade

'hepato-jugular reflux' (not 'reflex') has no pathophysiological significance; the sole purpose of this manoeuvre is to demonstrate the vein and to show that it can be filled (i.e. that the pressure is not high).

- Suspect a high level: the top of the column may be above the mastoid. Check if the ear lobes move with the cardiac cycle and sit the patient vertically to get a greater length of visible jugular vein above the right atrium.

If the jugular venous pressure is raised (especially if >10cm):

- A large 'a' wave (corresponding with atrial systole) occurs when the right atrial pressure is raised, e.g. tricuspid stenosis, pulmonary hypertension, pulmonary stenosis and mitral stenosis.
- A cannon wave is a massive 'a' wave occurring in complete heart block when the right atrium contracts against a closed tricuspid valve.

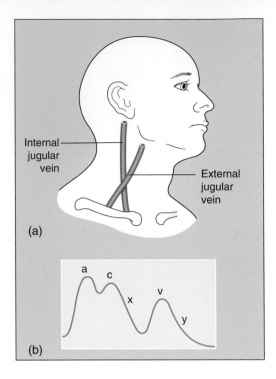

(a)

(b)

Figure 3.1 (a) Surface markings of the internal and external jugular veins. (b) Jugular venous pulse waveform.

- There is no 'a' wave in atrial fibrillation because there is no atrial systole.
- A large 'v' wave (corresponding with ventricular systole) indicates tricuspid incompetence (usually secondary to marked heart failure).

Heart

Observe

- scars of previous surgery
- visible apex beat
- visible parasternal heave

Palpate

- apex beat
- left parasternal area
- apex, base and aortic areas for thrills

The apex beat may be thrusting in left ventricular hypertrophy, displaced by cardiomegaly or left ventricular dilatation or tapping in nature, suggesting the accentuated first sound of mitral stenosis.

A parasternal heave is present when there is right ventricular hypertrophy.

Thrills are palpable murmurs felt over the relevant area in systole or diastole.

Auscultate the precordium (Fig. 3.2)

- Use the bell of the stethoscope to examine low-pitched noises, especially diastolic murmurs at the apex, and the diaphragm to examine high-pitched noises and the precordium generally.
- Palpate the right carotid artery when auscultating to identify the stages of the cardiac cycle.
- Ask the patient to roll onto their left side and listen over the apex to accentuate mitral murmurs and check their radiation.
- Ask the patient to sit up, lean forward and hold their breath in expiration to listen for aortic diastolic murmurs.
- Check for radiation of aortic stenotic murmurs to the carotid area.

Identify

- first and second heart sounds
- additional heart sounds
- murmurs and their radiation
- pericardial friction rub

First heart sound (S1): occurs at the onset of systole when mitral and tricuspid valves close; loud in hyperdynamic circulation and mitral stenosis, soft in heart failure and mitral regurgitation.

Second heart sound (S2): occurs at the end of systole when aortic and pulmonary valves close; split on inspiration (A2 then P2); fixed splitting in atrial septal defect; variable splitting with bundle branch blocks.

Third heart sound (S3): occurs immediately after S2 in early diastole; normal in young people and pregnancy; presents as 'gallop rhythm' in left ventricular failure.

Fourth heart sound (S4): occurs at the end of diastole before S1; present in severe left ventricular hypertrophy and aortic stenosis.

Systolic clicks: occur in early or mid-systole; indicate aortic or pulmonary stenosis, mitral valve prolapse and prosthetic heart valves.

Opening snap (OS): occurs in early diastole; indicates mitral stenosis with mobile valve leaflets and prosthetic valves; absent in calcific mitral stenosis.

Cardiac murmurs: auscultatory features are shown in Table 3.3.

Pericardial friction rub: low-pitched and scratchy; heard over the lower sternum; varies with posture and breathing.

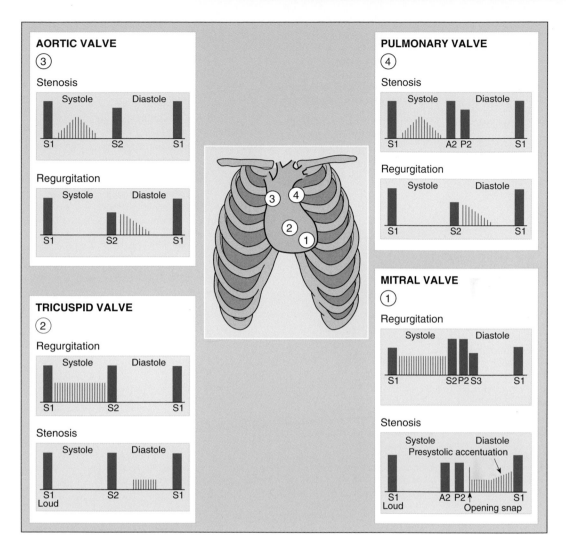

Figure 3.2 Suggested stethoscopic route (1–4) for listening to heart valves. 1, apex; 2, lower left sternal edge; 3, left second intercostal space; 4, right second intercostal space.

Complete the examination

- auscultate the carotids for bruits
- examine for ankle oedema
- sit the patient up and examine the lung bases for crackles and pleural effusions and check for sacral oedema
- examine the abdomen for hepatomegaly (which may be pulsatile) and abdominal aortic aneurysm
- dipstick the urine

Notes

Heart failure

A full cardiovascular history should be taken, focusing on evidence of chronic ischaemia or hypertension.

Left ventricular failure (LVF)

Signs

- dyspnoea on exertion or at rest
- tachycardia

Table 3.3 Characteristics of cardiac murmurs

Lesion	Murmur and position	Radiation and notes
Aortic stenosis	Harsh ejection systolic, maximal in second RICS; often loud with thrill. Possible ejection click	Radiates into neck
Aortic regurgitation	Blowing early diastolic decrescendo murmur maximal in third LICS, occasionally in second RICS. Best heard with patient sitting forwards in expiration	Radiates between right carotid and cardiac apex. Look for signs of coexistent connective tissue or other disorders
Mitral stenosis	Mid or late rumbling diastolic murmur at apex; presystolic accentuation if sinus rhythm. Loud mitral first sound. Opening snap if valve pliable	Turn patient on left side (and exercise) to accentuate murmur. Often atrial fibrillation
Mitral incompetence	Pansystolic at apex	Radiation to axilla; often heard parasternally
Mitral prolapse	Midsystolic at apex. High-pitched with click	Usually benign. Rarely associated connective tissue disease
Tricuspid incompetence Pulmonary stenosis	Pansystolic; maximal lower sternum Midsystolic; maximal in second LICS. Click if stenosis is valvular	'V' wave in neck and pulsatile liver increase on inspiration. Pulmonary component of second sound quiet and delayed
Pulmonary incompetence	Blowing early diastolic murmur, maximal in second and third LICS	Very rare
Ventricular septal defect	Loud, rough, pansystolic; maximal at third to fourth LICS parasternally	Small VSDs common
Atrial septal defect	Pulmonary systolic murmur with fixed split second sound	Possible tricuspid diastolic murmur if atrial septal defect flow is large
Patent ductus arteriosus	Machinery murmur, maximal in late systole, extending into diastole. Maximal in second to third LICS in mid-clavicular line	Also audible posteriorly
Coarctation of the aorta	Loud rough systolic, maximum over apex of left lung both posteriorly and anteriorly	Murmurs of scapular and internal mammary shunt collaterals. Radial femoral delay. Hypertension in arms

RICS, right intercostal space; LICS, left intercostal space; VSD, ventricular septal defect.

- gallop rhythm
- fine bi-basal crackles of pulmonary oedema
- pleural effusions

Right ventricular failure (RVF)

Signs

Signs of LVF plus

- raised JVP
- ankle oedema
- sacral oedema
- hepatomegaly
- ascites

If RVF is secondary to chronic lung disease (cor pulmonale) there is clinical evidence to suggest chronic obstructive pulmonary disease, pulmonary embolism or other forms of chronic lung disease.

Hypertension

A full cardiovascular history should be taken. Specific features in the history of a patient with hypertension are shown in Box 3.2.

Mild or moderate hypertension usually produces no abnormalities on physical examination other than raised blood pressure. Physical signs suggest long-standing or severe hypertension.

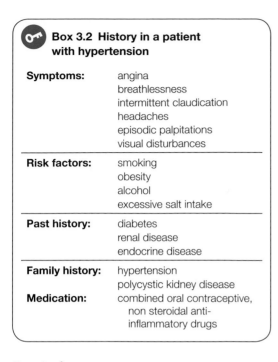

Box 3.2 History in a patient with hypertension

Symptoms:	angina
	breathlessness
	intermittent claudication
	headaches
	episodic palpitations
	visual disturbances
Risk factors:	smoking
	obesity
	alcohol
	excessive salt intake
Past history:	diabetes
	renal disease
	endocrine disease
Family history:	hypertension
	polycystic kidney disease
Medication:	combined oral contraceptive, non steroidal anti-inflammatory drugs

Examine for

- left ventricular hypertrophy
- loud A2 second heart sound
- heart failure

- cerebrovascular disease
- hypertensive retinopathy
- renal failure

Consider secondary causes of hypertension.

Look for evidence of

- renal artery stenosis: renal artery bruit in the epigastrium
- polycystic kidney disease
- other forms of chronic kidney disease
- coarctation of the aorta: radial-femoral arterial pulse delay, weak femoral pulses, bruits of the coarctation and of the scapular anastomoses, visible pulsation of the anastomoses
- Cushing syndrome
- acromegaly

Phaeochromocytoma and primary hyperaldosteronism (Conn syndrome) have no specific features on physical examination.

The ECG

A normal ECG is shown in Fig. 3.3.

Aide mémoire

- horizontally one little square is 0.04 s; one big square is 0.2 s

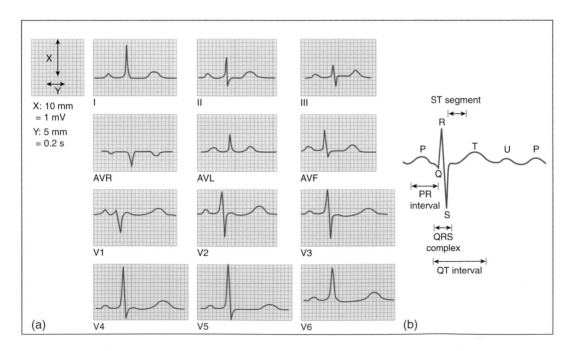

Figure 3.3 (a) Normal 12-lead electrocardiogram (ECG). (b) Waves of the normal ECG.

- vertically one little square is 0.1 mV
- normal PR interval is 0.12–0.2 s
- normal QRS duration is up to 0.12 s

The QT interval varies with rate. Upper limits of normal are approximately:

- rate 60/min QT 0.43 s
- rate 75/min QT 0.39 s
- rate 100/min QT 0.34 s.

Rate

- Count the large squares between two QRS complexes and divide into 300 (i.e. if two squares, the rate is 150/min).
- If the rate is less than 60/min the patient has a bradycardia; if greater than 100/min, a tachycardia.

Regularity

- Use the edge of a piece of paper to mark off a series of R waves, and then shift the paper along one or more complexes.
- The marks on the paper will still correspond with the R waves if the rhythm is regular. Total irregularity usually indicates atrial fibrillation.

Estimate the mean frontal QRS axis (Fig. 3.4)

- To gain a rough idea of the axis, find the limb lead with the maximum net positive deflection (sum of the positive R wave and negative Q and S waves); the axis lies close to this.
- Calculate the total deflection (R wave minus Q and S waves) in leads I and AVF which are perpendicular to each other (at 0 and 90°, respectively).
- Add these together as vectors (use the squares on the ECG paper); the net vector is the axis (see Fig. 3.4).
- The normal range is 0–90°.

Check individual waves and intervals

- for their presence, shape and duration.

P wave (atrial depolarisation)

- is most easily seen in V1 and V2
- is peaked in right atrial hypertrophy and bifid in left atrial hypertrophy (left atrial depolarisation occurs slightly later than right, giving a second peak)
- may be 'lost' (in the QRS complex) in nodal rhythm.

PR interval

- PR interval measured from the beginning of the P wave to the beginning of the QRS complex is usually 0.12–0.2 s.

- If the PR interval is prolonged or a normal 1 : 1 ratio of PQRS complexes is lost heart block is present (Fig. 10.14, Chapter 10).
- A short PR interval occurs in atrioventricular re-entrant tachycardias.

QRS complex

- The QRS complex is caused by the rapid depolarisation of the right and left ventricles.
- If the QRS complex is longer than 0.12 s bundle branch block exists.
- Pathological (broad, deep) Q waves are greater than 0.04 s (one small square wide) and greater than 0.2 mV. They may be normal in AVR or V1.

ST segment

- The ventricles are depolarised during the ST segment, which is normally isoelectric.
  T wave
- The T wave is caused by repolarisation of the ventricles.

QT interval

- The QT interval is measured from the beginning of the QRS complex to the end of the T wave. It varies with heart rate, and the corrected QT (QTc) is calculated by dividing the QT interval by the square root of the preceding R–R interval. QTc values between 0.35 and 0.45 s are considered normal. Prolongation is associated with ventricular arrhythmias.

U wave

- occurs after the T wave and can be a normal finding.

Peripheral vascular system

Patients with peripheral vascular disease may complain of:

- transient motor or sensory loss in transient ischaemic attacks (TIAs)
- intermittent claudication
- intermittent visual loss.

General examination

Compare and assess

- temperature of the dorsum of each foot
- haemosiderosis, lipodermatosclerosis
- loss of hair over lower limbs and feet
- arterial ulceration
- venous ulceration

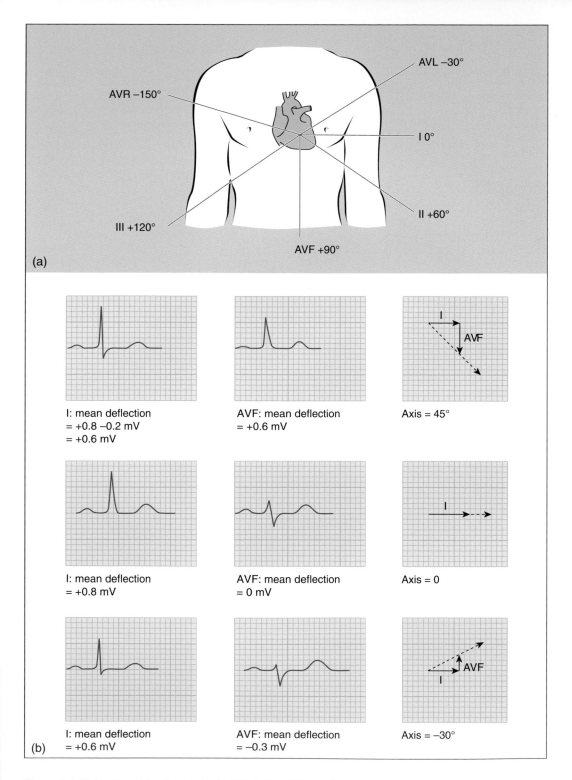

(a)

(b)

I: mean deflection
= +0.8 −0.2 mV
= +0.6 mV

AVF: mean deflection
= +0.6 mV

Axis = 45°

I: mean deflection
= +0.8 mV

AVF: mean deflection
= 0 mV

Axis = 0

I: mean deflection
= +0.6 mV

AVF: mean deflection
= −0.3 mV

Axis = −30°

Figure 3.4 (a) Position of the limb leads. (b) Calculation of the cardiac axis.

Check

- capillary return in the great toe

Examine the arterial pulses

- radial
- brachial
- carotid
- femoral
- popliteal
- posterior tibial
- dorsalis pedis

Palpate

- the abdomen for evidence of abdominal aortic aneurysm

Auscultate for bruits

- carotid arteries
- epigastrium (renal artery stenosis)
- femoral arteries

Examine

- varicose veins where present

4

Respiratory system

Clinical assessment of the respiratory system is essential for accurate diagnosis, particularly in the context of acute respiratory disease where speedy clinical decision-making is of the essence. Whilst simple radiography, measurement of oxygen saturation and blood gas analysis are available in the majority of emergency clinical settings, the mainstay of diagnosis remains the clinical assessment. In chronic lung disease, the availability of sophisticated radiology and respiratory physiology can be used to confirm the diagnosis and monitor disease progress.

History

Key features of the history in a patient with respiratory disease are shown in Table 4.1.

Examination

Key abnormalities detected on examination of the chest are shown in Table 4.2.

General observation: note

- dyspnoea
- cyanosis
- evidence of loss of weight

Examine the hands for

- clubbing
- tobacco staining
- coarse tremor of outstretched hands
- bounding radial pulse

Check

- the pulse rate
- the height of the jugular venous pressure
- the tongue for cyanosis

Observe

- the shape of the chest and spine
- scars
- chest movements for symmetry and expansion
- the use of accessory muscles in the neck and shoulders
- visibly enlarged cervical lymph nodes

Count

- the respiratory rate

Examine the front and back of the chest in a logical manner, usually by palpating, percussing and auscultating the front of the chest first, followed by the rear. When examining the back of the chest, ask the patient to put their hands on their hips to facilitate examination of the lung bases laterally.

Palpation

The anterior surface markings of the lungs are shown in Fig. 4.1.

Palpate for

- chest expansion, comparing the movements of the two sides
- the trachea in the suprasternal notch to assess mediastinal shift with the patient's neck partially extended. (Local anatomical and pathological variants may produce tracheal deviation in the absence of lung disease, e.g. a goitre or spinal asymmetry.

Clinical Medicine Lecture Notes, Eighth Edition. John R. Bradley, Mark Gurnell, and Diana F. Wood.
© 2019 John Wiley & Sons Ltd. Published 2019 by John Wiley & Sons Ltd.

Table 4.1 Key features of the history in respiratory disease

Feature	Details	Rationale
Basic details	Age, sex, current and previous occupations	Identify risk of occupational lung disease
Symptoms	Dyspnoea, chest pain, wheeze, cough, sputum and haemoptysis	Establish pattern of symptoms and their likely causes
Past medical history	Previous episodes or other lung disease	Suggestive of chronic or relapsing symptoms, i.e. asthma, COPD
Allergies	Identify known allergies in patient or family	Potential for allergic lung diseases
Smoking	Establish accurate smoking history	Increased risk of chronic lung disease and cancer

Table 4.2 Physical findings in common chest diseases

Pathology	Reduced chest wall movement	Mediastinal shift	Percussion note	Breath sounds	Vocal resonance	Added sounds
Pleural effusion	Affected side	Away from lesion (if large effusion)	Stony dull	Reduced or absent	Reduced or absent	Possibility of crackles above the effusion
Pneumothorax	Affected side	Away from lesion (if tension)	Normal or hyper-resonant	Reduced or absent	Reduced or absent	None
Consolidation	Affected side	None	Dull	Bronchial breathing	Increased	Crackles
Generalised fibrosis	Both sides	None	Normal	Vesicular	Increased	Fine, end-inspiratory crackles
Localised fibrosis	Affected side	Towards lesion	Dull	Bronchial breathing	Increased	Coarse crackles
Chronic obstructive pulmonary disease	None or both sides	None	Normal	Vesicular with prolonged expiration	Normal	Coarse crackles, expiratory wheezes
Asthma	Both sides	None	Normal	Vesicular with prolonged expiration	Normal	Expiratory wheezes

The position of the heart apex beat is of no help in assessing lung disease except if there is marked mediastinal shift.)
- cervical lymphadenopathy

Percussion

- examine the apices by percussing the clavicles
- move down the chest alternating right and left to compare both sides

Auscultation
Listen for

- bronchial breathing
- diminished breath sounds
- added sounds
  - wheezes
  - crackles
  - pleural rubs
- vocal resonance

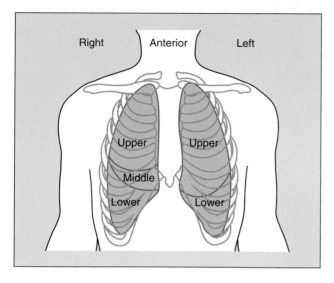

Figure 4.1 Surface markings of the lungs. Oblique fissures run along the line of the fifth/sixth rib; a horizontal fissure runs from the fourth costal cartilage to the sixth rib in the mid-axillary line. Note: On auscultation posteriorly you are listening mainly to lower lobes. Anteriorly you are listening mainly to upper lobes and on the right the middle lobe.

Notes

Haemoptysis

Aetiology: common

- lung cancer
- tuberculosis
- pulmonary embolism with infarction
- infection (e.g. pneumococcal pneumonia, lung abscess and *Klebsiella pneumoniae*)

Aetiology: uncommon

- foreign body – history of general anaesthetic, visit to dentist or inhalation of food
- coagulation disorders
- bronchiectatic cavities
- mitral stenosis
- Wegener's granulomatosis
- Goodpasture syndrome
- intrapulmonary vascular tumours

Investigation of haemoptysis

The usual clinical problem is to exclude carcinoma and tuberculosis. A full history and clinical examination will usually identify pulmonary infarction, foreign body, bronchiectasis, mitral stenosis and pulmonary oedema.

Perform

- sputum microscopy and culture, including for acid-fast bacilli

- sputum cytology for malignant cells
- chest X-ray
- CT or MRI scan to define the site and nature of the lesions seen on chest X-ray
- bronchoscopy with biopsy for cytology and culture
- CT-guided biopsy of mass lesions
- isotope (V/Q) lung scan +/– CT pulmonary angiogram if embolism is suspected

About 40% of patients with haemoptysis have no demonstrable cause. In patients who have had a single small haemoptysis, no other symptoms and a normal chest X-ray a follow-up chest X-ray after 1–2 months may be sufficient. Patients who have more than one small haemoptysis should be referred for further investigation.

Clubbing

Finger clubbing is associated with a range of respiratory diseases, but also with disease in the cardiovascular and gastrointestinal systems. Rarely, clubbing may be familial and innocent.

Respiratory causes

- carcinoma of bronchus
- chronic suppurative lung disease: empyema, lung abscess, bronchiectasis, cystic fibrosis
- fibrosing alveolitis
- asbestosis
- mesothelioma

Cardiac causes

- cyanotic congenital heart disease
- subacute bacterial endocarditis

Gastrointestinal causes

- Crohn's disease
- ulcerative colitis
- hepatic cirrhosis

Cyanosis

Cyanosis is a clinical description that refers to the blue-ish colour of a patient's lips and tongue (central) or fingers (peripheral). Central cyanosis is always accompanied by peripheral cyanosis.

Cyanosis is an unreliable guide to the degree of hypoxaemia. Central cyanosis is usually caused by the presence of an excess of reduced haemoglobin in the capillaries. Thus, in anaemia, severe hypoxaemia may be present without cyanosis.

Examine

- the underside of the patient's tongue and their finger nail beds (compare nail beds with your own)

If the tongue is cyanosed, the cyanosis is central in origin and secondary to:

- chronic bronchitis and emphysema, often with cor pulmonale
- congenital heart disease (cyanosis may be present only after exercise)
- polycythaemia
- massive pulmonary embolism.

If the tongue is not cyanosed but the finger nail beds are, the cyanosis is peripheral and secondary to:

- physiological causes (cold)
- pathology in peripheral vascular disease (the cyanosed parts feel cold).

Left ventricular failure may produce cyanosis that is partly central (pulmonary) and partly peripheral (poor peripheral circulation).

A rare cause of cyanosis, not caused by increased circulating reduced haemoglobin, is the presence of methaemoglobin (and/or sulphaemoglobin). The patient is relatively well and not necessarily dyspnoeic. Methaemoglobinaemia is usually drug-induced, e.g. sulphonamides, primaquine or nitrites.

Investigation of the respiratory system

Chest radiology

Normal chest X-rays are shown in Fig. 4.2 (postero-anterior) and Fig. 4.3 (lateral). Fig. 4.4 is a radiological chest diagram of lobar collapse. CT chest scans are shown in Fig. 4.5.

CT scanning is more sensitive than plain CXR and may be useful in detecting interstitial lung disease, cavitation and empyema.

Blood gases

The normal arterial values are:

- PaO_2 10–13 kPa (values fall with age)
- $PaCO_2$ 4.7–6.0 kPa
- pH 7.35–7.45
- Standard HCO_3^- 23–27 mmol/l

The pH indicates acidosis or alkalosis.

$PaCO_2$ reflects alveolar ventilation.

PaO_2 reflects ventilation/perfusion imbalance, gas transfer or venous-to-arterial shunts.

$PaCO_2$

- raised may account for an acidosis of respiratory origin, e.g. respiratory failure
- reduced may account for an alkalosis as a result of hyperventilation

PaO_2

- raised suggests the patient is on added oxygen
- reduced indicates lung disease (the $PaCO_2$ is usually high) or a right-to-left shunt

HCO_3^-

- raised standard HCO_3^- accounts for a metabolic alkalosis
- reduced accounts for a metabolic acidosis (usually renal or diabetic ketoacidosis)

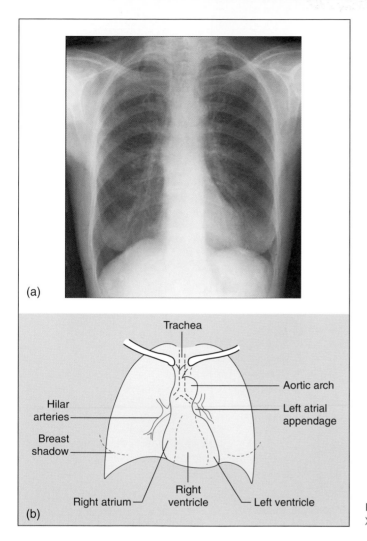

(a)

(b)

Trachea

Aortic arch

Left atrial
appendage

Hilar
arteries

Breast
shadow

Right atrium

Right
ventricle

Left ventricle

Figure 4.2 (a) Postero-anterior chest
X-ray. (b) Diagrammatic representation.

Also seen with venous admixture from right-to-left shunts
- Low $PaCO_2$, normal PaO_2: usually hyperventilation.

Interpretation of blood gases

Arterial gas patterns

- High $PaCO_2$, low PaO_2: respiratory failure resulting from chronic obstructive pulmonary disease, asthma or chest wall disease (e.g. ankylosing spondylitis, neuromuscular disorders).
- Normal or low $PaCO_2$, low PaO_2: hypoxia as a result of parenchymal lung disease with normal airways. Hyperventilation due to hypoxia lowers the $PaCO_2$ (e.g. pulmonary embolism, fibrosing alveolitis.

Causes of hypoxaemia

- *Hypoventilation*: sedative drugs, central nervous system disease, neuromuscular disease, chest trauma, obstructive sleep apnoea. The arterial $PaCO_2$ is characteristically high.
- *Ventilation/perfusion imbalance*: hyperventilation of some alveoli cannot compensate for the hypoxaemia resulting from the hypoventilation of other alveoli. Transfer factor is reduced.
- *Physiological shunt (venous admixture)*: deoxygenated blood passes straight to the left heart without

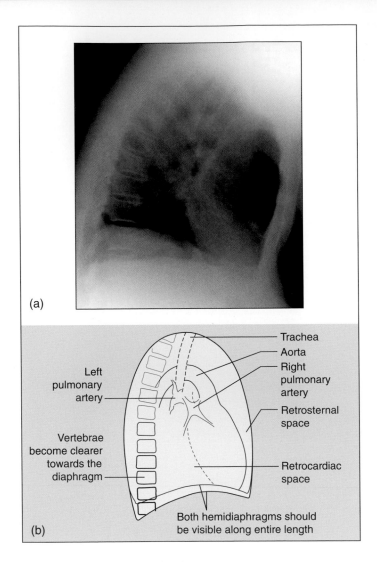

(a)

(b)

Trachea
Aorta
Right pulmonary artery
Retrosternal space
Retrocardiac space
Both hemidiaphragms should be visible along entire length
Left pulmonary artery
Vertebrae become clearer towards the diaphragm

Figure 4.3 (a) Lateral chest X-ray. (b) Diagrammatic representation.

perfusing ventilated alveoli. This occurs in cyanotic congenital heart disease. The arterial PaO_2 is not significantly improved by the administration of oxygen.

- Low inspired oxygen concentration because of altitude or faulty apparatus.

Type 1 respiratory failure (low PaO_2, normal/low $PaCO_2$)

Patients with lung disease causing hypoxaemia with hyperventilation, e.g. pulmonary oedema, pneumonia, asthma, pulmonary fibrosis and pulmonary thromboembolism.

Type 2 respiratory failure (low PaO_2, high $PaCO_2$)

Patients with hypoxaemia and a high $PaCO_2$ due to defective ventilation caused by airways obstruction, reduced chest wall compliance or central nervous system disease.

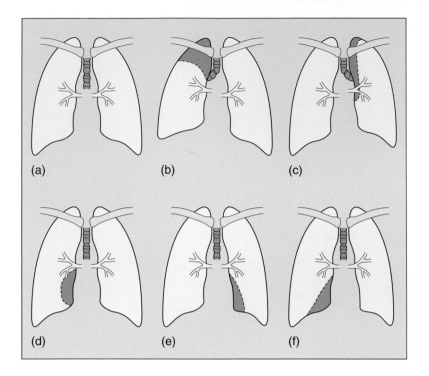

Figure 4.4 Diagrammatic representation of radiological appearance of lobar collapse. (a) Normal. (b) Right upper lobe: trachea deviated to right, right diaphragm and hilium elevated. (c) Left upper lobe: trachea deviated to left, left hilium and diaphragm elevated. (d) Right middle lobe: right heart border lost. (e) Left lower lobe: trachea may deviate to left, shadow behind heart. (f) Right lower lobe: trachea may deviate to right, outline of right diaphragm lost.

Pulmonary function tests

Spirometry (Fig. 4.6)

Subject exhales as fast and as long as possible from full inspiration into a spirometer, before and after bronchodilatation.

Interpretation

- Volume expired in the first second is the forced expiratory volume in 1 s (FEV1).
- Total expired is the forced vital capacity (FVC). Relaxed (slow) vital capacity may provide a better measure of trapped gas volume in chronic airways obstruction.
- Constriction of the major airways reduces the FEV1 more than the FVC.
- Restriction of the lungs reduces the FVC and, to a lesser degree, the FEV1.
- FEV1 : FVC (FEV%) ratio is low in obstructive airways disease (e.g. chronic bronchitis and asthma)

and normal or high in fibrosing alveolitis and other interstitial lung diseases.
- Peak expiratory flow rate (PEFR) measures the rate of flow of exhaled air at the start of a forced expiration.

Normal values for all these tests vary with age, sex and size and appropriate nomograms should be consulted.

Transfer factor

- measures the transfer of a small concentration of carbon monoxide in the inspired air on to haemoglobin
- vital capacity must be over 1 litre and subject able to hold the breath for 15 s
- reduced in diseases that reduce ventilation or perfusion or alter the balance between them
- increased in pulmonary haemorrhage.

Correction must be made for haemoglobin concentration, because transfer factor varies directly with haemoglobin. Its chief value is for monitoring progression in interstitial disease and in confirming a diagnosis of pulmonary haemorrhage.

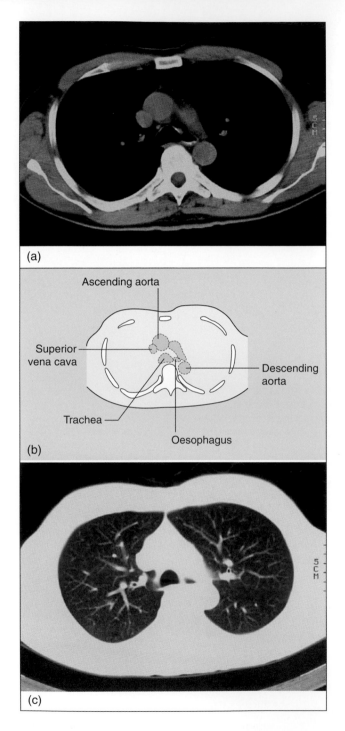

Figure 4.5 (a) CT of chest at the level of T4 vertebra. (b) Diagrammatic representation. (c) The same CT in which a different window setting has been used to visualise the lung markings (the window settings determine the range of densities displayed).

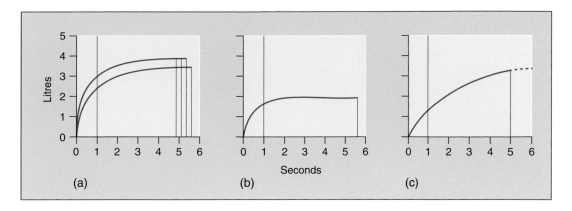

Figure 4.6 Spirometric patterns. (a) Normal (elderly man) forced expiratory volume/forced vital capacity (FEV/FVC) = 3.0/4.0 = 75%. (b) Restrictive, FEV/FVC = 1.8/2.0 = 90%. (c) Obstructive, FEV/FVC = 1.4/3.5 = 40%.

5

The abdomen

Examination of the abdomen may reveal abnormalities in a number of different systems including gastrointestinal, renal, haematological and cardiovascular disorders. Metabolic abnormalities including acute diabetic ketoacidosis and chronic hypercalcaemia may present with abdominal pain. In a patient with an acute abdomen, careful history-taking and examination forms a vital part of the initial management. In individuals with chronic disease, the history should dictate appropriate further investigations.

Key features in the history relating to gastrointestinal disease are shown in Table 5.1.

Examination of the abdomen

General observation: note

- is the patient in pain?
- evidence of weight loss

Inspect

- tongue, mouth, teeth and throat
- limbs for evidence of IV drug use

Examine the hands for

- clubbing
- leukonychia, koilonychia
- palmar erythema
- spider naevi
- Dupuytren's contracture

Inspect the eyes and conjunctivae for

- anaemia
- jaundice
- xanthelasmata

Palpate for lymphadenopathy

- neck
- supraclavicular fossae
- axillae
- groins

A scheme for examination of the abdomen is shown in Fig. 5.1. Lie the patient flat (one pillow) with arms by the sides. Look before palpation, have warm hands and palpate gently so as to gain the patient's confidence and to avoid hurting them. Ask the patient to let you know if you are hurting them. Check this by looking at the patient's face periodically during palpation, especially if you elicit guarding or rebound tenderness.

Observe the abdomen for

- general swelling with eversion of the umbilicus in ascites
- visible enlargement of internal organs: liver, spleen, kidneys, gall bladder, stomach, urinary bladder and pelvic organs
- abnormally distended veins: usually in cirrhosis with the direction of flow away from the umbilicus (portal hypertension). The flow is upwards from the groin in inferior vena cava obstruction (Fig. 5.2)
- scars of previous operations, striae, skin rashes and purpura
- pigmentation
- visible peristalsis

Clinical Medicine Lecture Notes, Eighth Edition. John R. Bradley, Mark Gurnell, and Diana F. Wood.

Table 5.1 Key features of the history in gastrointestinal disease

Feature	Details	Rationale
Basic details	Age, sex, occupation	Identify age-related and occupational risks
Symptoms	Dysphagia, dyspepsia, vomiting, haematemesis, abdominal pain, weight loss, diarrhoea, constipation, lower GI bleeding, symptoms of malabsorption including steatorrhoea, jaundice, pale stools, dark urine	Establish pattern of symptoms and their likely causes. Length of history important in aetiology of diarrhoea and jaundice
Past medical history	Previous episodes or other GI disease; blood transfusions; recent anaesthesia	May suggest recurrent or chronic GI disorder; hepatitis
Social history	Contacts with jaundiced patients; recent travel; residence abroad	Risk of infectious hepatitis; infectious diarrhoea
Family history	Family history of jaundice	Consider Gilbert's syndrome
Alcohol, smoking, drug abuse	Establish alcohol and smoking history; enquire after IV drug abuse	Important in aetiology of a number of GI and hepatic diseases
Medication	Careful history, in particular aspirin and NSAIDs, steroids; phenothiazines, oral contraception, antibiotics	Many drugs with GI/hepatic side effects

NSAIDs, non-steroidal anti-inflammatory drugs.

Palpate and percuss

- For internal organs and masses: start palpation in the right iliac fossa and work upwards towards the hepatic and splenic areas, first superficially and then deeper.
- Percuss the liver and spleen areas to avoid missing the lower border of a very large liver or spleen.

Liver

- The upper border is in the fourth to fifth intercostal space on percussion.
- The liver moves down on inspiration.
- Percussion over the liver is dull.
- If enlarged, the liver edge may be tender, regular or irregular, hard, firm or soft.
- Pulsatility suggests tricuspid incompetence.
- The liver may be of normal size but low because of hyperinflated lungs in chronic obstructive airway disease.

Spleen

- Smooth rounded swelling in left subcostal region, usually with a distinct lower edge.
- The spleen enlarges diagonally downward and across the abdomen in line with the ninth rib.

- The examining hand cannot get above the swelling.
- Percussion over the spleen is dull.
- There is a notch on the lower border of the spleen
- The spleen may be more easily palpated with the patient lying on the right side with the left leg flexed and abducted.

Kidneys

- Palpated in the loins bimanually, i.e. most easily felt by pushing the kidney forwards from behind on to the anterior palpating hand.
- They move slightly downwards on inspiration.
- The examining hand can easily get between the swelling and the costal margin.
- Percussion is resonant over the kidneys.
- The lower pole of the right kidney can often be felt in thin normal persons.

Abnormal masses

- Palpate for abnormal masses particularly in the epigastrium (gastric carcinoma) and suprapubic region (bladder distension, ovarian and uterine masses). Describe in terms of their size and margins.
- Note colonic masses. The descending colon is commonly palpable in the left iliac fossa.

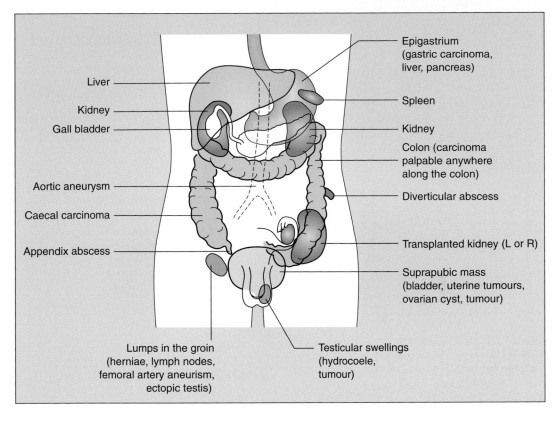

Liver

Kidney

Gall bladder

Aortic aneurysm

Caecal carcinoma

Appendix abscess

Epigastrium
(gastric carcinoma,
liver, pancreas)

Spleen

Kidney

Colon (carcinoma
palpable anywhere
along the colon)

Diverticular abscess

Transplanted kidney (L or R)

Suprapubic mass
(bladder, uterine tumours,
ovarian cyst, tumour)

Lumps in the groin
(herniae, lymph nodes,
femoral artery aneurism,
ectopic testis)

Testicular swellings
(hydrocoele,
tumour)

Figure 5.1 Examination of the abdomen: (1) gently palpate all quadrants for tenderness and masses; (2) feel for enlarged liver, spleen or kidneys, and for masses arising from the bowel (in the left and right iliac fossae), the epigastrium (stomach and pancreas), the aorta (aneurysm), or the pelvis (uterus, bladder and ovaries); (3) percuss and auscultate over enlarged organs or masses; (4) examine hernial orifices and external genitalia in men; and (5) perform a rectal examination.

- The abdominal aorta is pulsatile, bifurcates at the level of the umbilicus and is easily palpable in thin and lordotic patients. Abdominal aortic aneurysms are expansile.
- Check for ascites: examine for shifting dullness by noting a change in percussion note with the patient supine and lying on their left side. A fluid thrill may be demonstrable in large, tense effusions.

Complete the examination

- femoral pulses
- hernial orifices
- leg oedema
- external genitalia
- digital rectal examination

Auscultate for

- bowel sounds
- renal and femoral bruits

Notes

Splenomegaly

The major causes of splenomegaly are haematological and infectious (Table 5.2).

Hepatomegaly

The causes of hepatomegaly are shown in Table 5.3.

Hepatosplenomegaly

The causes are similar to those for splenomegaly alone:

- chronic leukaemias
- cirrhosis with portal hypertension
- lymphoproliferative disorders
- myelofibrosis

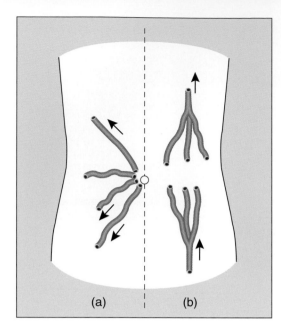

Figure 5.2 Blood flow through dilated anterior abdominal wall veins. Portal vein and inferior vena caval occlusion can be distinguished by the different directions of flow below the umbilicus. (a) Direction of flow in portal vein occlusion. (b) Direction of flow in inferior vena caval occlusion.

Palpable kidneys

The left kidney is nearly always impalpable, but the lower pole of a normal right kidney may be felt in thin people.

Unilateral enlargement

- renal cell carcinoma
- hydronephrosis
- cysts
- hypertrophy of a single functioning kidney

Bilateral enlargement

- polycystic kidney disease
- bilateral hydronephrosis
- amyloidosis

Following *renal transplantation* a kidney may be palpable in one iliac fossa and the patient may appear cushingoid as a result of steroid therapy. Look for scars of previous surgery and forearm arteriovenous shunts.

Mass in right subcostal region

Consider

- liver (including Riedel's lobe)
- colon
- kidney
- gall bladder (rarely)

Investigations

- ultrasound: identifies solid or cystic masses
- abdominal CT scan
- liver function tests
- urine for haematuria and proteinuria
- stool for occult bleeding

As appropriate

- sigmoidoscopy, barium enema and colonoscopy
- CT or MRI scan

Suprapubic mass

Consider

- bladder distension
- pregnancy
- uterine masses (usually benign fibroid tumours, rarely malignancy)
- ovarian tumours

Ascites

Clinical features

- abdominal distension
- dullness to percussion in the flanks
- shifting dullness
- fluid thrill

Causes

- intra-abdominal neoplasia including gynaecological pathology
- hepatic cirrhosis with portal hypertension
- congestive cardiac failure
- constrictive pericarditis
- nephrotic syndrome
- low albumin states
- tuberculous peritonitis

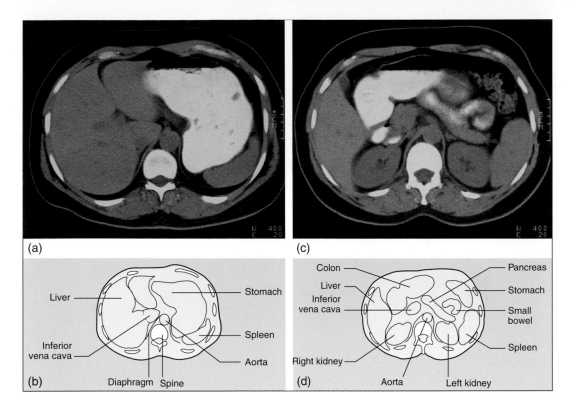

Figure 5.3 (a) CT and (b) diagrammatic representation at the level of T11 vertebra. (c) CT and (d) diagrammatic representation at the level of L1 vertebra.

Diagnostic paracentesis should be performed and examined for:

- protein content (>30 g/l suggests an exudate, <30 g/l suggests a transudate)
- microscopy and bacterial culture (including acid-fast bacilli)
- cytology.

Paracentesis may occasionally be required for the relief of severe symptoms; repeated paracentesis leads to excessive protein loss and should be avoided if possible.

Dysphagia

Dysphagia includes both difficulty with swallowing and pain on swallowing. The former symptom is more prominent in obstruction and the latter with inflammatory lesions.

Causes
Common

- carcinoma of the oesophagus
- carcinoma of the gastric fundus
- peptic oesophagitis (with pain) proceeds to stricture with difficulty in swallowing

Rare

- achalasia of the cardia
- external pressure: carcinoma of the bronchus, retrosternal goitre
- dysmotility syndrome
- neurological disease: myasthenia gravis, bulbar palsies
- Plummer–Vinson syndrome – iron deficiency anaemia, koilonychia and glossitis with a post-cricoid oesophageal web

Investigations

- haemoglobin, serum iron and ferritin
- barium swallow (Fig. 5.4)

Table 5.2 Causes of splenomegaly

Massive splenomegaly	Chronic myeloid leukaemia Myelofibrosis Malaria Visceral Leishmaniasis (Kala–Azar)			
Other causes: Infectious	**Bacterial** Brucellosis Salmonella Septicaemia Bacterial endocarditis TB		**Viral** Glandular fever Viral hepatitis CMV	**Protozoal** Trypanosomiasis
Haematological	Megaloblastic anaemia Idiopathic thrombocytopenia Congenital spherocytosis Autoimmune haemolytic anaemias Polycythaemia rubra vera Hodgkin's disease Lymphomas Chronic lymphatic leukaemia			
Inflammatory/ granulomatous disease	Sarcoidosis Felty syndrome SLE			
Congestive	Hepatic cirrhosis Extrahepatic portal hypertension			
Storage diseases	Niemann–Pick, Gaucher's			
Others	Amyloidosis			

Table 5.3 Causes of hepatomegaly

Common	Congestive cardiac failure Secondary carcinomatous deposits Cirrhosis
Other causes: Infectious	Glandular fever Viral hepatitis HIV/AIDS Amoebic cysts Hydatid cysts
Haematological	Leukaemia Lymphoma
Malignant	Hepatoma
Granulomatous disease	Sarcoidosis
Storage diseases	Gaucher's
Others	Primary biliary cirrhosis Haemochromatosis Amyloidosis

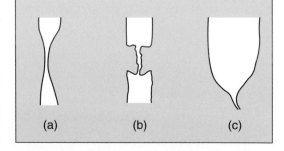

(a) (b) (c)

Figure 5.4 Barium swallow X-ray. (a) Benign peptic stricture. Smooth narrowing, usually at lower end of oesophagus in association with reflux or hiatus hernia. (b) Malignant stricture irregular narrowing with shouldered edges. (c) Achalasia. Smooth narrowing of the lower end of the oesophagus with dilatation above.

- upper GI endoscopy with biopsy to differentiate between benign peptic stricture and carcinoma
- signs of bowel obstruction
- hepatomegaly
- findings from digital rectal examination and sigmoidoscopy

Diarrhoea

Acute gastroenteritis with diarrhoea and vomiting is the second most common group of disorders affecting the whole community (second to acute respiratory infections). *Specific features on examination in a patient with diarrhoea include*

- evidence of weight loss, anaemia and clubbing
- abnormal abdominal masses
- signs of bowel obstruction
- hepatomegaly
- findings from digital rectal examination and sigmoidoscopy.

Infectious diarrhoea

Non-specific

- generally acute and viral in origin
- infant diarrhoea is usually caused by a rotavirus
- treatment of infectious diarrhoea is generally symptomatic

Food poisoning

- *Salmonella typhimurium* uncommon in Western countries
- *Salmonella enteritidis* infection from eggs and poultry
- *E. coli* serotypes generally from processed meat
- staphylococcal food poisoning, produced by the bacterial toxin, from precooked meats and dairy foods

Campylobacter *infection*

- common cause of bacterial gastroenteritis
- carried and communicated by cattle (milk), also common in poultry
- incubation takes up to a week, followed by fever, myalgia and cramping diarrhoea, occasionally bloody

Clostridium difficile *infection ('pseudomembranous colitis')*

- follows antibiotic therapy; generally in hospital inpatients

Dysentery

- bacillary dysentery caused by *Shigella* organisms
- consider amoebic dysentry and giardiasis in individuals recently returned from endemic areas

Enteric fevers

- consider typhoid and paratyphoid in individuals recently returned from endemic areas

Cryptosporidium

- causes severe and sometimes intractable diarrhoea in HIV/AIDS

Non-infectious diarrhoea

Consider

- drugs
- diverticular disease
- colon cancer: alternating with constipation
- irritable bowel syndrome
- inflammatory bowel disease: ulcerative colitis and Crohn's disease
- malabsorption syndromes
- thyrotoxicosis

Investigation
Acute diarrhoea

- full blood count for anaemia, liver and renal function tests
- blood cultures for *E. coli, Salmonella typhi, S. paratyphi* and *S. enteritidis* where indicated in the history
- stool examination for cysts, ova and parasites
- stool culture
- sigmoidoscopy: biopsy and histology may be diagnostic

Chronic diarrhoea

- full blood count for anaemia, liver and renal function tests
- sigmoidoscopy with biopsy
- barium enema
- endoscopic duodenal biopsy if the history suggests malabsorption
- small-bowel barium studies if Crohn's disease suspected

Bloody diarrhoea

- colon cancer
- diverticular disease
- ulcerative colitis
- dysentery
- ischaemic colitis
- *Campylobacter* enteritis

Rectal bleeding

- commonly caused by haemorrhoids and fissures
- other causes require investigation with sigmoidoscopy, barium enema and colonoscopy

Dysentery (bacillary and amoebic), typhoid, paratyphoid and cholera are notifiable to the public health authorities in the UK.

Jaundice

General

- Yellow colouration of the skin and sclerae is usually only apparent when the serum bilirubin is over 35 mmol/l.
- Hepatic jaundice causes deep yellow jaundice progressing to a greenish tinge.
- Haemolytic jaundice causes lemon-yellow skin colouration.
- The sclerae are not coloured in those with yellow skin caused by hypercarotinaemia.

Specific features on examination of the abdomen in a jaundiced patient include

- recent operation scars suggesting cholecystectomy or surgery for intra-abdominal carcinoma
- hepatomegaly: irregular when infiltrated with carcinoma or in early cirrhosis, tender in infectious and acute alcoholic hepatitis and occasionally in congestive heart failure
- splenomegaly in portal hypertension, spherocytosis and infectious mononucleosis
- palpable enlarged gall bladder suggesting bile duct obstruction caused by carcinoma of the pancreas (rather than gallstones)
- ascites.

Causes
Common

- viral hepatitis
- biliary obstruction from gallstones or carcinoma of the head of the pancreas
- drugs
- metastases
- intrahepatic cholestasis (including ascending cholangitis and primary biliary cirrhosis)
- infectious mononucleosis
- Gilbert's syndrome

Uncommon

- haemolytic anaemia

- congenital hyperbilirubinaemia
- stricture or carcinoma of the major bile ducts or ampulla

Investigation aims to

- discover the site of any biliary outflow obstruction
- determine the degree of impairment of liver cell function and its cause
- eliminate rare causes such as haemolysis
- establish potential for treatment.

Haematology

Check

- full blood count, reticulocyte count and Coombs' test

A normal reticulocyte count virtually excludes haemolytic jaundice. Leukocytosis may suggest infection or carcinoma. Abnormal mononuclear cells suggest infectious mononucleosis or viral hepatitis.

Liver function tests

- Measure the ability of the liver to perform normal functions (e.g. serum albumin is a measure of protein synthesis; prothrombin time is a measure of synthetic function; bilirubin is a measure of bile salt conjugation and excretion).
- Liver enzymes (alkaline phosphatase, transaminases) are indicators of ductal or liver cell damage.
- In obstructive jaundice the alkaline phosphatase is greatly elevated compared with transaminases; in hepatocellular disease transaminases are predominantly raised.

Bilirubin

- Bilirubin derived from red cell breakdown is transported to the liver where it is conjugated to glucuronic acid. Conjugated bilirubin is secreted in the bile and degraded in the gut by bacteria to form urobilinogen. Urobilinogen is either excreted in the stool or reabsorbed from the gut and excreted by the kidneys.
- Serum bilirubin is predominantly unconjugated in haemolytic jaundice and the other liver function tests are usually normal. It is mainly conjugated in obstructive jaundice.

Causes of increased bilirubin

- hepatocellular failure
- biliary obstruction
- haemolysis
- Gilbert's syndrome

Alkaline phosphatase

Alkaline phosphatase is found in high levels in biliary canaliculi, osteoblasts, intestinal mucosa and placenta.

Elevated in

- obstructive jaundice
- hepatocellular jaundice
- growth in adolescence
- pregnancy

Normal in

- Gilbert's syndrome (page 42, Chapter 5)
- myeloma

A raised level in the absence of other signs of liver disease or abnormal liver function tests suggests the presence of malignant secondary deposits in the bone or Paget's disease. Consider measuring isoenzymes if there is doubt.

Causes of increased hepatic alkaline phosphatase

- extrahepatic cholestasis
- obstructive jaundice
- intrahepatic cholestasis (e.g. cirrhosis, drugs, cholangitis, primary biliary cirrhosis)
- obstructive phase of hepatitis

Causes of increased bone alkaline phosphatase (osteoblastic activity)

- Paget's disease
- bone metastases
- osteomalacia
- hyperparathyroidism
- normal growth in puberty
- fractures

Transaminases

Elevated serum transaminases (alanine aminotransferase, aspartate aminotransferase and gamma glutamyl transferase) indicate hepatocellular damage. Slight elevation is consistent with obstructive jaundice.

Causes of elevated alanine aminotransferase

- active liver cell damage, including drugs, hepatitis and metastatic infiltration
- acute myocardial infarction (peaks at 24–48 h, may fall to normal by 72 h); the degree of elevation reflects the amount of muscle damage
- acute pancreatitis
- haemolysis

Elevated aspartate aminotransferase levels parallel alanine aminotransferase.

γ-glutamyl transferase

- inducible microsomal enzyme
- may be most sensitive index of alcohol ingestion
- raised in most forms of liver disease including acute and chronic hepatitis, cirrhosis and following drugs that induce microsomal enzymes

Urinalysis

- Conjugated bilirubin renders the urine dark yellow.
- Urobilinogen is colourless but on standing the urine turns brown as urobilinogen is converted to urobilin by oxidation.
- Haemolytic jaundice is acholuric (no bilirubin in the urine) but the urine contains excess urobilinogen because excess bilirubin reaches the intestine and is re-excreted as urobilinogen.
- Obstructive jaundice produces dark brown urine with excess bilirubin but a reduction of urinary urobilinogen (little or no bilirubin reaches the gut because of the obstruction and therefore cannot be reabsorbed and re-excreted).

In the early stages of acute viral hepatitis, excess urobilinogen may sometimes be present before clinical jaundice becomes apparent. This is a result of failure of the liver to take up the excess urobilinogen absorbed from the gut. With increasing severity, biliary obstruction develops and as conjugated bilirubin appears in the urine it disappears from the gut and urobilinogen disappears from the urine. The reciprocal effect also occurs during recovery.

Serology

Check

- viral hepatitis serology – hepatitis A–E, cytomegalovirus (CMV) and Epstein–Barr virus (EBV)
- anti-mitochondrial antibodies (primary biliary cirrhosis)
- anti-nuclear factor and smooth-muscle antibodies (chronic active hepatitis)

Abdominal radiology in jaundice

- Plain X-ray and ultrasound may show gallstones.
- Ultrasound, CT (Fig. 5.3) and MRI may show primary or secondary tumours, pancreatic carcinoma, stones in the gall bladder and dilated biliary ducts in obstruction.

Needle liver biopsy

Biliary obstruction is a relative contraindication because of the potential danger of biliary peritonitis. Ultrasound and CT-guided biopsy may provide the histological diagnosis in focal lesions. Check the pro-thrombin time and platelet counts are normal. Fresh frozen plasma will quickly reverse the prothrombin time for the duration of the procedure.

Other investigations

- Endoscopic retrograde cholangiopancreatography (ERCP) is valuable to define obstruction of the pancreaticoduodenal tree, for sphincterotomy, to release stones and to relieve obstruction by insertion of a stent.
- Alpha-fetoprotein is raised in hepatocellular carcinoma.

Congenital non-haemolytic hyperbilirubinaemias

These may explain persistent jaundice in the young after viral hepatitis or slight jaundice in the healthy.

Gilbert's syndrome (autosomal dominant)

- Common congenital hyperbilirubinaemia (1–2% of the population). There is impaired glucuronidation of bilirubin (reduced uridine diphosphate glucuronyl transferase [UDPGT]) resulting in raised unconjugated plasma bilirubin and acholuria. About 40% of cases have a reduced red cell survival with a consequent increase in bilirubin production.
- The plasma bilirubin is usually <35 mmol/l.
- Diagnosis is by exclusion: there is no haemolysis and the other liver function tests are normal.
- Fasting and intercurrent illness produce a rise in plasma bilirubin.
- The liver is histologically normal.
- The prognosis is excellent and treatment unnecessary.

Dubin–Johnson syndrome (autosomal recessive)

- Rare benign disorder of failure to excrete conjugated bilirubin.

- Plasma bilirubin is conjugated.
- Histologically the liver is stained black by centrilobular melanin.

Renal disease

Key features in the history of a patient with renal disease are shown in Table 5.4.

Specific features on examination in a patient with renal disease include:

- uraemic pallor (pale, brownish-yellow appearance of skin)
- bruising
- hypertension and its consequences
- postural hypotension
- signs of dehydration
- hyperventilation from acidosis
- palpable bladder in outflow obstruction
- palpable kidneys: polycystic disease and hydronephrosis

Table 5.4 Key features of the history in renal disease

Renal failure	Thirst Polyuria Nocturia Anorexia Nausea Vomiting Fatigue Itching
Urinary tract infection	Dysuria Frequency Nocturia Haematuria Prostatism Renal stone disease
Medication	Analgesics especially NSAIDs
Past history	Nephritis Diabetes Hypertension Pelvic surgery Pre-eclampsia
Family history	Hypertension Polycystic kidneys Familial nephritis Gout

- ankle or sacral oedema suggesting nephrotic syndrome or fluid overload
- renal artery bruits
- signs of dialysis: arteriovenous fistula, peritoneal dialysis (PD) catheter
- transplanted kidney
- peripheral neuropathy
- pericarditis
- muscular twitching, hiccup, fall in blood pressure and uraemic frost in severe untreated renal failure
- digital rectal examination will reveal prostatic hypertrophy or carcinoma.

Basic investigations

- bloods: urea, creatinine, potassium and bicarbonate. Calculate estimated glomerular filtration rate (eGFR) using recognised equations (e.g. MDRD formula; https://www.kidney.org/professionals/kdoqi/gfr_calculator)
- urinalysis: microscopy, protein and glucose
- ultrasonography: renal outflow obstruction and renal size

Urea and creatinine

Production rate of urea varies, making it a less useful measure of renal function than creatinine, which is produced at a roughly constant rate proportional to skeletal muscle mass.

Increased serum urea

- decreased excretion: renal failure especially dehydration and pre-renal failure
- increased protein catabolism: steroids, surgery, cytotoxic therapy, trauma, infection
- increased protein intake: dietary, gastrointestinal haemorrhage

Decreased serum urea

- decreased synthesis: extensive liver disease, low protein intake (malnutrition or malabsorption)
- increased excretion: increased GFR in pregnancy
- dilution: syndrome of inappropriate ADH secretion (SIADH), excess intravenous fluids

Increased serum creatinine

Impaired renal function: creatinine rises above the normal range when there is ~50% loss of renal function.

Creatinine clearance

- patient performs a 24-h collection of urine and a single measurement of plasma creatinine is made during this time. Creatinine clearance (millilitres per minute) is measured as:

$$\text{urine creatinine concentration (mmol/l)} \times \text{vol(ml)} / \text{plasma creatinine(mmol/l)} \times \text{time(min)}$$

Small quantities of creatinine are excreted by the renal tubules. The creatinine clearance therefore slightly overestimates the GFR. Chromium-51 ethylenediamine tetra-acetic acid (^{51}Cr EDTA) clearance more accurately reflects the GFR. It is calculated from the rate of disappearance of a bolus injection of ^{51}Cr EDTA from the blood.

Decreased serum creatinine

- loss of muscle mass

6

Neurological system

Disorders of the neurological system present with a wide range of symptoms and signs, reflecting numerous pathological mechanisms. For the non-specialist student, trainee or physician, it is important to develop a logical and systematic approach to the clinical history and examination based on knowledge of the underlying anatomy and physiology. Neurological diagnosis has been transformed by advances in radiology and other imaging techniques, including developments in functional imaging. Appropriate use and interpretation of modern investigative techniques rely upon accurate clinical assessment.

History

Key features of the history in a patient with neurological disease are shown in Table 6.1.

Examination of the nervous system

It is important to develop a technique for examination of the nervous system that is rapid and accurate. Analysis of clinical signs is facilitated by knowledge of underlying neuroanatomy shown in the simplified diagrams in this chapter (Fig. 6.1 and Figs. 6.2 to 6.7). Examination of the nervous system also requires clear communication with the patient to promote understanding of the sometimes unfamiliar instructions to be given.

Mental state and higher cerebral function

General observation: note
- general appearance and behaviour
- speech
- mood
- abnormal beliefs and/or perceptions

Cognitive function

Loss of memory for recent events more than for distant events is a feature of organic cerebral disease and an early feature of dementia.

- Use the Mini-Mental State Examination (MME).
- MME consists of 12 questions. Maximum score is 30 and a normal score is 26–30. A score of less than 24 indicates cognitive impairment: 21–25 suggests dementia (likelihood ratio=5), and 20 or less is highly suggestive of cognitive impairment (likelihood ratio=8).

Other tests of cognitive function

Concentration: serial sevens

Ask the patient:

- to subtract 7 from 100, then seven from the answer and so on
- to remember a series of numbers forward and backward: most people can remember five or more forward and four or more backward

Clinical Medicine Lecture Notes, Eighth Edition. John R. Bradley, Mark Gurnell, and Diana F. Wood.
© 2019 John Wiley & Sons Ltd. Published 2019 by John Wiley & Sons Ltd.

Table 6.1 Features of the history in neurological disease

Feature	Details	Rationale
Basic details	Age, sex, handedness, current and previous occupations	CNS orientation; identify risk of occupational disease
Symptoms	Headaches; facial pain; disordered consciousness ('fits, faints and funny turns'); vertigo; sensory symptoms including numbness, paraesthesiae and pain; motor symptoms including weakness, incoordination, involuntary movements and gait disorders; acute confusional states; memory disorders and symptoms of dementia; speech and language problems; visual disturbances; perceptual problems; sphincter disturbance	Establish pattern of symptoms and their likely causes including relapsing and remitting pattern or progressive problems; establish details of symptoms particularly related to their location and nature, precipitating and relieving factors
Past medical history	Cardiovascular disease; diabetes; trauma; inflammatory/immunological disease; infections including HIV/AIDS	Potential causes of neurological disorders
Social and family history	Alcohol; smoking; recreational drug use; family history of similar neurological disorders	Potential causes of neurological disease or vascular impairment; potential genetic syndromes
Medication	Review all medication	Neurological side effects for many medications
Mental state	Assess mental state	Depression is a common feature of chronic neurological syndromes including chronic pain, movement disorders and early dementia

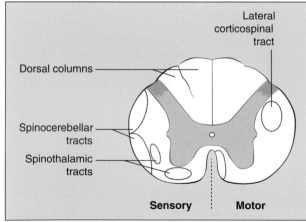

Figure 6.1 Cross-section through the spinal cord.

• to repeat a complex sentence, e.g.: '*The one thing a nation requires to be rich and famous is a large, secure supply of wood.*'

Orientation

Ask the patient, for example:

• their name, date of birth, address
• the date and the place of the interview

• to name the monarch, prime minister, members of favourite sports teams, famous places and capitals.

Mood

Observe:
• facial expression, posture, movement.

Ask the patient:
'*Do you feel sad or depressed, are you anxious or worried, does your mood change rapidly and, if so, what happens?*'

Speech disorders

Dysarthria

Observe:

- slow or slurred speech in conversation
- local lesions in the mouth
- features of pseudobulbar palsy
- generalised motor or myopathic disorders.

Test articulation; ask the patient to repeat: *'Baby hippopotamus'* and *'West Register Street'.*

Expressive (motor) dysphasia and aphasia

Observe:

- patient's understanding is intact
- word finding is difficult
- speech is absent in aphasia.

Nominal dysphasia describes a specific expressive dysphasia in which the patient knows what an object is but cannot name it.

Hold up an object, e.g. a pen.

Ask the patient:

- *'What is this?'*
- *Pause*
- *'Is it a watch?' 'No'*
- *'Is it a key?' 'No'*
- *'Is it a pen?' 'Yes'*

Check for associated spatial problems:

- dressing apraxia: observe the patient
- constructional apraxia: ask the patient to copy your drawing of a house or simple shape.

Receptive (sensory) dysphasia

Observe:

- failure to understand the meaning of words
- fluency: no problem with motor speech but meaningless responses to questions.

Tactile agnosia

This indicates damage to the contralateral sensory lobe. Ask the patient:

- to recognise and distinguish objects placed in the hand (failure known as astereognosis)
- to recognise figures drawn on the palm with the eyes closed (failure known as dysgraphaesthesia).

Cranial nerves

Remember diagrams of cross-sections of the brainstem and of the floor of the fourth ventricle (Figs. 6.2, 6.3) because these may greatly improve the analysis of a cranial nerve lesion. The following paragraphs outline a system for examination of the cranial nerves that recognises the need to examine parts of the head and neck in a logical order rather than by following the order of the cranial nerves directly.

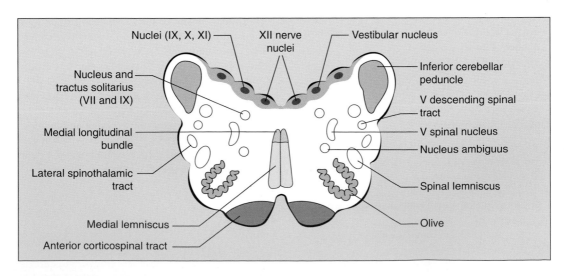

Figure 6.2 Cross-section through the open medulla.

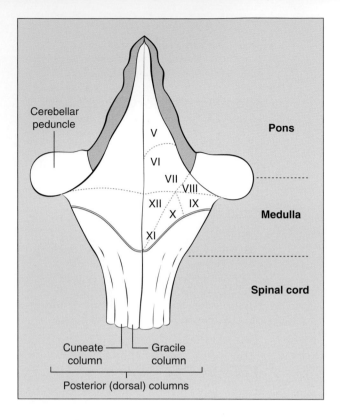

Figure 6.3 Floor of the fourth ventricle showing cranial nerve nuclei.

Sense of smell

Ask the patient:
'Has there been any recent change in your sense of smell?'
If yes:

- assess informally with easily available substances (coffee granules, oranges)
- test formally with fresh 'smell bottles'.

Eyes

Observe and examine:

- *visual acuity,* either quickly with available literature, formally with Snellen charts or by counting fingers if vision is very poor
- *visual fields* to confrontation
  - compare the patient's visual fields with your own
  - the patient's head should be level with yours and at arm's length away
  - when testing the right eye, ask the patient to look straight into your left eye and vice versa for the patient's left eye.

Ask the patient to:
'Keep looking at my eye and tell me when you first see my finger out of the corner of your eye.'

- preferably using a red-headed hatpin, or otherwise your finger, bring the target towards the centre of the field of vision from the four diagonals (upper right, upper left, lower right, lower left)
- the nasal and superior fields are limited by the nose and eyebrow, respectively
- move the pin across the centre of each eye to examine for a central scotoma
- test for visual inattention (extinction and hemineglect) by asking the patient to identify which fingers you are moving with your hands held at the outer edges of the patient's visual fields.

Ptosis

- third nerve lesion (complete ptosis)
- sympathetic lesion (partial ptosis) or as part of Horner syndrome
- generalised muscle weakness (myasthenia gravis, dystrophia myotonica, facioscapulohumeral dystrophy, congenital lesions)

Pupillary reflexes and accommodation

- examine the pupillary reflexes in subdued light
- inspect the pupil for irregularity
- flash a pentorch twice at each eye, once for direct and once for consensual responses; move the torch in from the side so as to avoid an accommodation–convergence reflex
- ask the patient to focus on your finger held at arm's length and then move your finger to the patient's focal point, observing convergence and pupillary constriction

External ocular movements (3rd, 4th and 6th nerve)

Ask the patient:
'Do you have any double vision?'
If the patient has not noticed diplopia:

- test the eye movements formally by asking the patient to follow your finger with their eyes, moving your finger slowly through the gaze regions
- examine upwards and downwards gaze for each eye in full abduction and adduction
- note any nystagmus.

Diplopia is maximal when looking in the direction of action of the paralysed muscle. The image further from the midline arises from the paralysed eye.

If the patient has noticed diplopia:

- ask in which direction it is worst
- move your forefinger in that direction and then ask if the two fingers that the patient sees are parallel to each other (lateral rectus palsy: 6th nerve) or at an angle (superior oblique palsy: 4th nerve)
- cover up each eye in turn and ask which image has disappeared.

Nystagmus

Ask the patient:
'Look at my finger'

- hold the patient's gaze in full abduction in each direction for a few seconds
- examine for nystagmus
- repeat with the eyes in upgaze

Perform fundoscopy

Ask the patient to:
'Focus on a point at a distance ahead and slightly

upwards'
Using the ophthalmoscope:

- check the red reflex
- focus through the lens and vitreous
- assess the optic disc, noting colour, cupping, margins and vessels
- examine the retina in all four quadrants
- observe the macula and major vessels.

Face

Facial expression (7th nerve, motor)

Ask the patient to:
'Screw up your eyes very tightly'

- compare how deeply the eyelashes are buried on the two sides

'Raise your eyebrows'

- compare right and left sides

'Show your teeth'

- compare the nasolabial grooves.

Facial sensation (5th nerve, sensory)

Test the three divisions on both sides:

- light touch with cotton wool
- corneal reflexes.

Mouth

Ask the patient to:
'Clench your teeth' (masseters, 5th nerve, motor)

- palpate the masseters
- test the jaw jerk: place one finger horizontally across the front of the jaw and tap the finger with a tendon hammer with the jaw relaxed and the mouth just open

'Open your mouth and keep it open' (pterygoids, 5th nerve, motor)

- attempt to force it closed
- in a unilateral lesion, the jaw deviates towards the weaker side

'Say aaah' (9th and 10th nerves: both mixed)

- observe the movement of the uvula and soft palate: normally they move upwards and remain central and the posterior pharyngeal wall moves little
- in a unilateral lesion the soft palate is pulled away from the weaker side
- test the gag reflex (9th nerve sensory, 10th nerve motor)

'Put your tongue out' (12th nerve)

Look for:

- wasting
- fasciculation
- protrusion towards the weaker side indicates a unilateral lesion

Neck (11th nerve)

Observe:
- muscle wasting

Ask the patient to:
'Lift your head off the pillows'
'Put your chin on your right (or left) shoulder'

- resist the movement
- observe and palpate the sternomastoids

'Shrug your shoulders'

- attempt to push them down
- observe and palpate the bulk of trapezius

Hearing and vestibular function (8th nerve)

Test hearing:

- whisper a number in each ear in turn, obstructing the contralateral ear
- perform Weber and Rinne tests (see later)
- inspect eardrums with an auriscope if indicated

Test vestibular function if indicated:

- perform the Hallpike manoeuvre (supine lateral head turn against a fixed gaze to determine the cause of vertigo)
- request caloric tests (instillation of hot or cold water into the external auditory canal to test the vestibulo-ocular reflex)

The limbs

Figs. 6.4 and 6.5 give an overview of the motor and sensory systems.

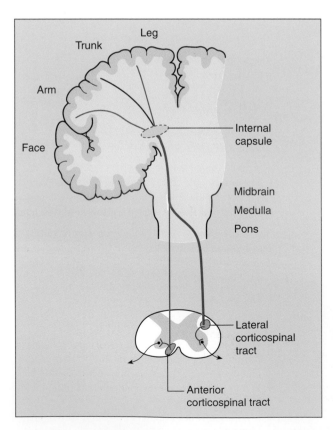

Figure 6.4 Motor pathways.

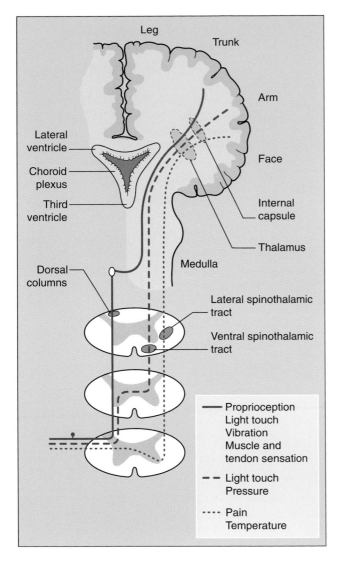

Figure 6.5 Sensory pathways.

Arms: motor system

Observe:

- obvious muscle wasting
- fasciculation or tremor
- wasting of the small muscles of the hand, noting whether ulnar or thenar

Test muscle tone:

- holding the arm, ask the patient to relax and move the arm gently at the elbow and wrist using an irregular rhythm to discourage resistance. Ask the patient to relax and, holding the thigh, shake the leg gently

- note cogwheel rigidity, which may be more obvious at the wrist

Test muscle power in groups. Explain what you are doing to the patient:

'*I am going to test the strength of some of your muscles*'

Shoulder (C5):

'*Hold both arms out in front of you and close your eyes*'

Observe drifting of one arm indicating:

- weakness of the muscles at the shoulder
- loss of position sense with no evidence of weakness
- lesions of the cerebral cortex (when the patient will not be aware of the drift, sometimes even with open eyes)

Shoulder abduction:
'Bend your elbows and lift your arms up to the side; don't let me push them down'

- resist the action

Shoulder adduction:
'Now pull them in towards your chest; don't let me stop you'

- resist the action

Observe:

- winging of the scapula (nerve to serratus anterior, C5, 6, 7)

Elbow:
Flexion: C5, 6, 7 (biceps):
'Bend your elbow, bring your hand to your shoulder; don't let me straighten it'

Extension: C7: (triceps):
'Now straighten your elbows and push me away'

Wrist:
Extension: C7:
'Hold your arms out straight, cock up your wrists; don't let me straighten them'

Hand grip: C8, T1:
'Squeeze my fingers hard and stop me pulling them out of your grip'

Finger abduction: ulnar nerve:
'Spread your fingers apart; don't let me push them together'

- push against 1st and 5th fingers

Finger adduction: ulnar nerve:
Place a piece of paper between straight fingers
'Don't let me pull it out'

- attempt to pull the paper from between the patient's fingers

Abduction of thumb: median nerve:
'Place your hand down flat with the palm upward and the thumb overlying the forefinger. Lift the thumb vertically and don't let me push it down'

Opposition of thumb: median nerve:
'Put your thumb and little finger together and stop me pulling them apart with your forefinger'

Reflexes (Box 6.1)

Tendon reflexes:

- when testing reflexes, it is essential that the muscle involved is completely relaxed
- watch the muscle for contraction

Box 6.1 A simple aide-mémoire for reflexes

A simple *aide-mémoire* for reflexes and controlling muscle groups is 12345678
    Ankle jerk S1, 2
    Knee jerk L3, 4
    Biceps jerk C5, 6
    Triceps jerk C7, 8

Biceps:

- ask the patient to rest their arm across their abdomen with the elbows partially flexed
- place a finger over the flexor tendon and tap your finger

Triceps:

- rest the patient's forearm on yours and tap the triceps tendon directly

Supinator:

- ask the patient to rest their arm across their abdomen with the elbows partially flexed
- hold the patient's hand loosely
- tap the supinator tendon directly above the wrist

If a reflex is difficult to elicit or absent, demonstrate reinforcement:

- ask the patient to concentrate on contracting muscles at a distant site when instructed (e.g. *'Grip your hands together'* or *'Clench your teeth'*).

Coordination

Finger–nose test:

Hold your forefinger at arm's length from the patient:
'Touch my finger, then your nose, then my finger, going backwards and forwards as quickly and accurately as you can'

- intention tremor is more marked when the patient has to stretch to reach your finger
- the tremor is not altered by closing the eyes
- keep your finger still and then ask the patient to repeat the test to establish past-pointing – deviation of the patient's finger consistently to one side of your own indicates the side of a cerebellar lesion

Dysdiadochokinesia:

Demonstrate to the patient:
'Tap rapidly on the back of your hand like this....and now alternate the front and back of your hand like this'

- rapid repetitive alternating movements of the wrists are irregular in both force and rate in cerebellar disease

Muscular weakness alone may make the patient unsteady in all these tests, and this may resemble an intention tremor.

Sensation

The sensory dermatomes are shown in Fig. 6.6. When testing sensation:

- Ensure that the patient understands what sensations you are testing and what is an appropriate response.
- Demonstrate the normal response in an area not thought to be affected (usually over the sternum).
- In all modalities use a single touch; moving a stimulus induces two-point discrimination.
- Always check from side to side, comparing right with left and work systematically.

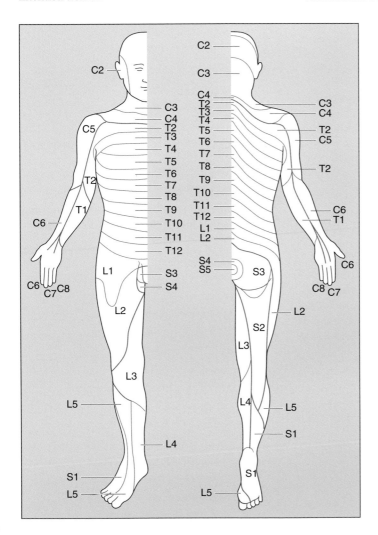

Figure 6.6 Sensory dermatomes. C4 and T2 are the neighbouring dermatomes over the front of the chest at the level of the first and second ribs; C5, 6, 7, 8 and T1 supply the upper limb; C7 supplies the middle finger front and back; T7 supplies the lower ribs; T10 supplies the umbilical region; T12 is the lowest nerve of the anterior abdominal wall; L1 supplies the inguinal region; L2 and 3 supply the anterior thigh (lateral and medial); L4 and 5 supply the anterior shin (medial and lateral); and S1 supplies the lateral border of the foot and sole, and the back of the calf up to the knee.

Joint position sense (proprioception), vibration sense and accurate sensation (pin-prick, two-point discrimination) are relayed in the dorsal spinal tracts. Poorly localised diffuse touch, pain and temperature sensation are carried in the lateral spinothalamic tracts.

Diffuse touch (cotton wool) and accurate touch (pin-prick):

- Establish the normal response by touching cotton wool or neurotips pin onto the sternum and checking the patient's recognition of the sensation.

'*Close your eyes and say "Now" every time you feel the touch*'

- Examine the arms systematically along the distribution of the dermatomes.

Vibration sensation:

- Ensure during testing that the tuning fork is vibrating but not making a loud noise.
- Establish the normal response by placing the tuning fork onto the sternum and checking the patient's recognition of the vibration sensation. Stop the vibration to allow the patient to recognise the difference.

'*With your eyes closed say "Yes" if you can feel the vibration and tell me when it stops*'

- Work distally to proximally, checking over bony prominences in the fingers, wrists and elbows.

Joint position sense (proprioception):

- Establish the normal response: with the patient looking, hold a finger by its sides (holding the top and bottom introduces diffuse touch sensations). Move the finger up and down, explaining what you are doing.

'*Now with your eyes closed tell me whether I move your finger up or down*'

Temperature sensation:

- Use readily available stimuli such as a warm finger and cold tuning fork handle.

'*Now with your eyes closed tell me whether this is cold or warm*'

- Work distally to proximally.

Legs: motor system

Observe:

- obvious muscle wasting
- fasciculation or tremor

Test muscle tone:

- lift the knee off the bed briskly while the patient is relaxed and see if the heel is lifted. Let it drop; observe how stiffly it falls
- roll the leg to and fro, and see if the foot is rigid at the ankle or normally loose
- bend the knee to and fro using an irregular rhythm to discourage resistance

Test muscle power in groups.
Explain what you are doing to the patient:
'*I am going to test the strength of some of your muscles in your legs*'

Hip flexion (L1, L2):
'*Lift your leg up straight and don't let me push it down*'

- push down on the patient's knee

Hip extension (L5, S1):
'*Lift your leg up straight: push my hand down to the bed*'

- place your hand under the ankle and push up to resist this
- do not place your hand under the knee as the patient will move the pelvis to press down

Knee flexion (L5, S1, S2):
'*Bend your knee and bring your heel up to your bottom: don't let me straighten it*'

- put your hand behind the ankle and resist the movement

Knee extension (L3, L4):
'*Now straighten your leg*'

- put your hand on the patient's shin and resist the movement

Ankle plantar flexion (S1):
'*Push your foot down: don't let me push it up*'

- place your hand under the patient's foot and resist the movement

Ankle dorsiflexion (L4, L5):
'*Bend your foot upwards and don't let me pull it down*'

- place your hand on the dorsum of the foot and resist the movement

Reflexes (Box 6.1)

When testing reflexes it is essential that the muscle involved is completely relaxed and watch the muscle for contraction.

Patellar reflexes:

- ensure the knee joint is relaxed and held in flexion
- right knee – place your arm under the knee and rest your hand on the patient's left knee
- left knee – rest your arm over the right knee and support the underside of the left knee
- tap the patellar tendon with reinforcement if necessary

Ankle reflexes:

- externally rotate the patient's ipsilateral hip and partially flex the knee
- place your hand under the foot and gently flex the ankle; do not hold the ankle in extreme flexion
- tap the Achilles tendon with reinforcement if necessary

Clonus:
If the reflexes are brisk examine for ankle clonus:

- with the leg held in the position for examination of the ankle reflexes flex the ankle and sustain the flexion to observe rhythmic contraction of the muscles

Plantar reflexes:

- gently but firmly draw an orange stick up the outer border of the sole and across the heads of the metatarsals
- observe the flexion (normal) or extension (UMN lesion) of the big toe

Coordination

Heel–shin test: this is primarily a test for intention tremor.
Instruct the patient, demonstrating what you mean: *'Put your heel on your knee and slide it down your shin. Move it up and down as quickly and accurately as you can'*

Sensation

The sensory dermatomes are shown in Fig. 6.6.
 Note the caveats given above for examination of the arms.
 Diffuse touch (cotton wool) and accurate touch (pin-prick):

- Establish the normal response by touching cotton wool or neurotips pin onto the sternum and checking the patient's recognition of the sensation.

'Close your eyes and say "Now" every time you feel the touch'

- Examine the legs systematically along the distribution of the dermatomes.

Vibration sensation:

- Ensure during testing that the tuning fork is vibrating but not making a loud noise.
- Establish the normal response by placing the tuning fork onto the sternum and checking the patient's recognition of the vibration sensation. Stop the vibration to allow the patient to recognise the difference.

'With your eyes closed say "Yes" if you can feel the vibration, and tell me when it stops'

- Work distally to proximally, checking over bony prominences in the toes, ankles and knees.

Joint position sense (proprioception):

- Establish the normal response: with the patient looking, hold the big toe by its sides (holding the top and bottom introduces diffuse touch sensations). Move the toe up and down, explaining what you are doing.

'Now with your eyes closed tell me whether I move your toe up or down'

- If abnormal joint position sense is detected, move proximally and test in larger joints (ankle, knee).

Temperature sensation:

- Use readily available stimuli such as a warm finger and cold tuning fork handle.

'Now with your eyes closed, tell me whether this is cold or warm'

- work distally to proximally

If there is evidence of a symmetrical peripheral neuropathy establish the upper border by testing sensation from the foot towards the knee.

Gait

Ask the patient to walk a few steps:

- observe obvious patterns of gait disturbance (see later)

Perform Romberg's test

Ask the patient to stand with feet close together. Stand close and be prepared to support them if you suspect a sensory abnormality.
'Close your eyes'

- observe if the patient is more unsteady with the eyes closed (positive test)
- a positive Romberg's test indicates loss of joint position sense (posterior column lesion)

Truncal ataxia

Ask the patient to stand with feet together:

- swaying suggests truncal ataxia in a cerebellar lesion

Notes

Visual field defects

Field defects (Fig. 6.7) are described by the side of the visual field that is lost; thus 'temporal field loss' indicates loss of the temporal field of vision and denotes damage to the nasal retina or its connections to the visual cortex. Formal perimetry will accurately define defects.

- *Temporal hemianopia* in one eye alone or in both eyes (*bitemporal hemianopia*) suggests a chiasmal compression, usually from a pituitary tumour.
- *Homonymous hemianopia* (loss of nasal field in one eye and temporal field in the other) may occur with any postchiasmal lesion, most commonly following a vascular lesion affecting the occipital cortex (usually with macular sparing, because of the dual blood supply to the occipital cortex from the posterior and middle cerebral arteries). The side of the field loss is opposite to the side of the damaged cortex (i.e. a right-sided cerebral lesion produces a left homonymous hemianopia).
- *Upper quadrantic field loss* suggests a temporal lesion of the opposite cortex or optic radiation or, if bilateral, early chiasmal compression due to pituitary expansion. A lower quadrantic field loss suggests a parietal lesion.
- *Central scotoma*. Loss of vision in the centre of the visual field occurs in acute retrobulbar neuritis, most commonly caused by multiple sclerosis.
- *Hemi-inattention* suggests a contralateral posterior parietal lesion.

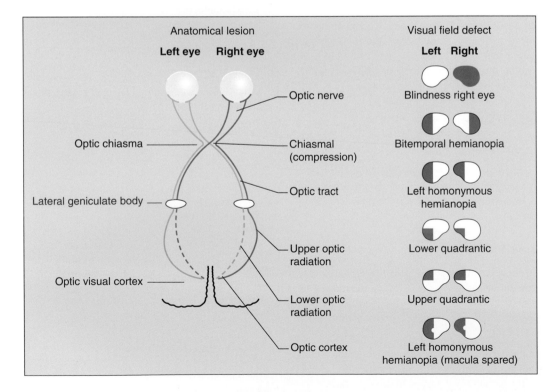

Figure 6.7 Lesions of the optic nerve and tract and effects on visual fields. 'Macular sparing': the macula has extensive cortical representation and may be spared by lesions of the visual cortex.

Pupillary reflexes

Pupil size is controlled by the balance between parasympathetic (constrictor) and sympathetic (dilator) tone.

- *Constriction of the pupil in response to light:* this is relayed via the optic nerve, optic tract, lateral geniculate nuclei, the Edinger–Westphal nucleus of the 3rd nerve and the ciliary ganglion. The cortex is not involved.
- *Constriction of the pupil with accommodation:* convergence originates within the cortex and is relayed to the pupil via the 3rd nerve nuclei. The optic nerve and tract and the lateral geniculate nucleus are not involved.

Therefore:

- If the direct light reflex is absent and the convergence reflex is present, a local lesion in the brainstem or ciliary ganglion is implied, possibly as a result of degeneration in the ciliary ganglia, e.g. the Argyll Robertson pupil.
- If the convergence reflex is absent and the light reflex is present, a lesion of the cerebral cortex is implied, e.g. cortical blindness.

If the pupil is constricted consider:

- Horner syndrome (see later)
- opiates, pilocarpine
- pontine haemorrhage
- Argyll Robertson pupil (irregular, no light reflex)
- normal old age.

If the pupil is dilated consider:

- mydriatics (e.g. homatropine, tropicamide or cyclopentolate)
- 3rd-nerve lesion
- Holmes–Adie syndrome (pupils constrict sluggishly to light, associated with absent tendon reflexes)
- congenital defect.

In the unconscious patient a fixed dilated pupil (3rd-nerve lesion) may indicate temporal lobe herniation on the same side caused by raised intracranial pressure, intracranial bleeding, tumour or abscess.

Horner syndrome

Horner syndrome comprises unilateral:

- partial ptosis (sympathetic)
- miosis (constricted pupil) with normal reactions
- anhidrosis (decreased sweating over face)
- enophthalmos (indrawing of orbital contents).

The syndrome results from lesions of the sympathetic nerves to the eye, anywhere from the hypothalamus downwards through the sympathetic nucleus of the brainstem and during their passage through the cervical and upper thoracic cord, the anterior spinal first thoracic root, the sympathetic chain, stellate ganglion and carotid sympathetic plexus.

Look for evidence of a T1 lesion and scars of previous cervical sympathectomy, palpate the neck and supraclavicular fossae for lymphadenopathy and examine for signs of cardiovascular disease and syringomyelia where indicated.

Eye movements

These are controlled by the 3rd, 4th and 6th nerves. Conjugate movement is integrated by the medial longitudinal bundle, which connects the above nerve nuclei together and to the cerebellum and vestibular nuclei.

Squint (strabismus)

Congenital concomitant squints are present from childhood and are caused by a defect of one eye. The angle between the longitudinal axes of the eyes remains constant on testing extraocular movements, and there is no diplopia.

Paralytic squint is acquired and results from paralysis of one or more of the muscles that move the eye, or paralysis from proptosis.

Lateral rectus palsy (6th nerve)

- produces failure of lateral movement with convergent strabismus
- diplopia is maximal on looking to the affected side
- images are parallel and separated horizontally
- the outermost image comes from the affected eye and disappears when that eye is covered
- 6th nerve palsy may be a false localising sign in raised intracranial pressure

Superior oblique palsy (4th nerve)

- diplopia is maximal on downward gaze
- images are at an angle to each other when the palsied eye is abducted and one above the other when the eye is adducted
- diplopia is noticed most on reading or descending stairs

Third nerve palsy

- may not present with diplopia in the presence of complete ptosis
- when the lid is lifted the eye is seen to be 'down and out' (divergent strabismus)
- there is severe (angulated) diplopia
- the pupil may be dilated
- it may be painful if caused by aneurysm of the posterior communicating artery

Myopathic conditions may cause diplopia in myasthenia gravis, thyroid eye disease and dystrophia myotonica.

Nystagmus

Nystagmus is the repetitive to and fro movement required when the fixed gaze drifts off target ('drift-correction-drift'). Usually the correction is faster than the drift and the direction of the fast phase is the direction of the nystagmus; it is usually more pronounced when the patient looks in the direction of the fast phase. Nystagmus is usually horizontal and conjugate but may be vertical or rotational.

Horizontal nystagmus

- *Vestibular nystagmus* occurs following damage to the inner ear, the 8th nerve or its brainstem connections and is present only in the first few weeks after the damage because central compensation occurs. It is greater on looking *away* from the side of a destructive lesion.
- *Cerebellar nystagmus* occurs usually with lateral lobe lesions; central (vermis) lesions causing severe truncal ataxia may cause no ophthalmic nystagmus. As cerebellar disease is frequently bilateral, nystagmus may occur to both sides. If it is unilateral it is greater *towards* the side of the destructive lesion.

Vertical nystagmus

The direction of jerks is vertical and vertical gaze usually makes it more pronounced.

Rotatory nystagmus

The phases of the nystagmus are equal in duration. It is secondary to an inability to fix objects and focus with one or both eyes because of partial blindness.

Facial palsy

In unilateral UMN lesions, e.g. following a cerebrovascular accident (CVA), movements of the upper face are retained because it is represented on both sides of the cerebral cortex.

Absence of forehead grooves and a sagging lower eyelid are seen in complete LMN lesions (e.g. Bell's palsy).

Taste sensation over the anterior two-thirds of the tongue is supplied by the sensory component of the 7th nerve (chorda tympani) which divides from the motor nerve in the middle ear. Absent taste sensation in this distribution indicates that a facial nerve paresis must be caused by a lesion above this level. Thus this may be observed in herpes zoster of the geniculate ganglion (Ramsay Hunt syndrome) but not in facial palsies associated with tumour of the parotid gland.

Hearing

The anatomy of the ear is shown in Fig. 6.8.

Air conduction is normally better than bone conduction.

Rinne test

Place a vibrating tuning fork behind the ear on the mastoid process and then rapidly move its prongs in line with the external meatus.

Ask the patient:

'*Is it louder behind* (with the tuning fork on the mastoid) *or in front* (with the tuning fork in line with the external meatus)?'

Normally it is louder in front – this is termed Rinne-positive. Negative is abnormal and implies conductive (air) deafness in that ear.

Weber test

Place a vibrating tuning fork on the middle of the patient's forehead.

Ask the patient:

'*In which ear is the noise loudest?*'

In the absence of nerve deafness, the sound is louder in the ear where air conduction is impaired.

Dizziness and giddiness

Dizziness and giddiness are common neurological presenting features. True vertigo suggests a disorder of the brainstem (vascular disease or demyelination), labyrinthitis or Ménière's disease. Dizziness or unsteadiness without vertigo, particularly if intermittent, suggests postural hypotension, a cardiovascular

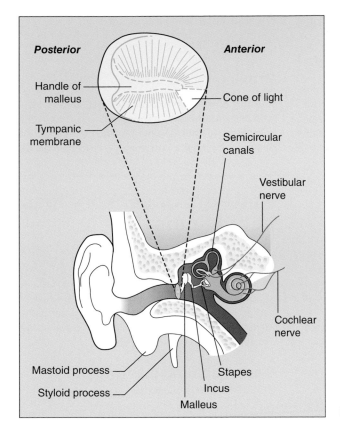

Figure 6.8 Anatomy of the ear.

disorder such as transient cardiac arrhythmias, aortic stenosis or carotid emboli. Transient dizziness is rarely associated with temporal lobe epilepsy. Often no organic cause is found.

Vertigo

Vertigo refers to unsteadiness with a subjective sensation of rotation of the environment around the patient. Vertigo results from disease of the inner ear, 8th nerve or its connections in the brainstem.

Dysarthria

In dysarthria there is an inability to articulate properly because of local lesions in the mouth or disorders of the muscles of speech. There is no abnormality of the content of speech. Certain neurological disorders produce typical dysarthric features such as the scanning speech of cerebellar dysfunction or the monotonous high-pitched tones observed in pseudobulbar palsy.

Dysphasia and aphasia

These are disorders of the symbolic aspects of language, both written and spoken. In right-handed people and 50% of left-handed people, the left hemisphere is dominant for speech. Dysphasia and aphasia are common following stroke.

Pure expressive (motor) dysphasia results from lesions in the postero-inferior part of the frontal lobe (Broca's area). Word finding is difficult in expressive dysphasia and speech absent in aphasia. In nominal dysphasia there is a specific defect in recognition and naming of objects, which may be associated with spatial problems such as dressing and constructional apraxias.

Receptive (sensory) dysphasia results from lesions of the dominant temporo-parietal lobe (Wernicke's area). There is failure to understand the meaning of words although the motor aspects of speech are preserved. This can produce 'fluent dysphasia' when the patient responds to questions with meaningless responses.

Bulbar and pseudobulbar palsies

The symptoms of dysarthria, dysphagia and nasal regurgitation result from paralysis of the 9th, 10th and 12th cranial nerves.

Pseudobulbar palsy (UMN) is the more common disorder and is caused by bilateral lesions of the internal capsule, usually following sequential, bilateral CVAs but also seen in multiple sclerosis. Bulbar (LMN) palsy is rare and usually caused by motor neuron disease or Guillain–Barré syndrome.

Acquired dyslexia (difficulty in reading), dysgraphia (difficulty in writing) and dyscalculia (difficulty in calculating) are features of lesions in the posterior parietal lobe. Agnosia denotes damage to the contralateral sensory cortex and is the inability to understand or recognise objects and forms in the presence of normal peripheral sensation. Tactile agnosia is most common. Visual agnosia describes the inability to recognise objects when viewed and denotes a lesion of the occipital cortex.

Apraxia is the inability to perform complex and sequential actions to command in the presence of normal coordination, sensation and motor power. It occurs with lesions of the parietal cortices connected by the corpus callosum.

Patterns of motor loss in the limbs

Lower motor neuron lesions

There is reduced or absent power with marked muscle wasting. The muscles are flaccid and the reflexes absent. The lesion affects the motor distribution of the spinal root or peripheral nerve.

Upper motor neuron lesion

There is reduced or absent power, with wasting in long-established lesions. The muscle tone and reflexes are increased and clonus may be present. The plantar response is upgoing.

There is a characteristic distribution of weakness:

- in the arms, weakness is more marked in elbow extension than flexion and wrist dorsiflexion than palmar flexion
- in the legs, weakness is more marked in hip flexion, knee flexion and ankle dorsiflexion than in their antagonist movements.

Consequently a hemiplegic person tends to walk with a stiff extended affected lower limb and stiff flexed affected upper limb.

Proximal myopathy

Proximal muscle wasting and weakness seen in myopathic disorders causes a typical rolling gait with difficulty standing from the sitting position, climbing stairs or lifting the arms to comb hair or reach to high shelves.

Patterns of sensory loss in the limbs

Peripheral neuropathy

Reduction or absence of vibration and position senses not only suggest dorsal column loss but also may be part of a mixed sensorimotor peripheral neuropathy. All modalities are reduced, with a 'glove and stocking' distribution of loss being characteristic.

Dorsal column loss without spinothalamic loss

This occurs in both legs in vitamin B_{12} deficiency and in the ipsilateral leg in hemisection of the cord (Brown–Séquard syndrome).

Spinothalamic loss without dorsal column loss (dissociated anaesthesia)

This occurs in syringomyelia, usually in the arms.

Spinal cord lesions

Dissociated sensory loss is a feature of spinal cord lesions.

Cerebral cortical lesions

Astereognosis and dysgraphaesthesia occur with parietal sensory loss.

Isolated peripheral nerve lesions

Median nerve lesion (carpal tunnel syndrome)

Patients with carpal tunnel syndrome complain of tingling and numbness of the fingers and/or weakness of the thumb, which are at their worst on waking and relieved by hanging the arm downwards. It is usually unilateral at the time of presentation and remains so if idiopathic. Pain at the flexor aspect of the wrist may occasionally radiate up to the elbow and, exceptionally, as far as the shoulder. Examination demonstrates:

- *motor loss:* thenar wasting and weakness of thumb abduction and opposition
- *sensory loss:* palmar surface only, on the thumb and two-and-a-half fingers (i.e. index, middle and half of the ring finger)
- *positive Tinel's sign:* percussion over the flexor retinaculum elicits tingling in the same sensory area.

Ulnar nerve lesion

The ulnar nerve supplies all the small muscles of the hand except three of the four muscles of the thenar eminence. It may be compressed in the ulnar tunnel at the wrist or in the ulnar groove at the elbow. Patients may complain of tingling or deadness and/or weakness of the ring and little fingers.

Examination demonstrates:

- *motor loss* with flattening of the contours of the hand caused by muscle wasting. The ring and little fingers are held slightly flexed, and there is loss of power in abduction and adduction of the fingers (claw hand)
- *sensory loss,* back and front, over the one-and-a-half ulnar fingers (i.e. little finger and half the ring finger)
- 'filling in' of the ulnar groove at the elbow and limitation of movement at the elbow.

In 2–3% of people, the ulnar nerve supplies all the hand muscles.

Radial nerve lesion

This is rare and usually results from prolonged local pressure to the nerve (e.g. an arm over the back of a chair). It causes wrist-drop. Sensory loss may be very limited because the median and ulnar nerve territories overlap the radial territory.

Lateral cutaneous nerve of the thigh

Compression causes meralgia paraesthetica, a syndrome characterised by hyperalgesia, burning pain and numbness in the lateral aspect of the thigh.

Lateral popliteal lesion

The lateral popliteal (common peroneal) nerve supplies the peroneal muscles which dorsiflex and evert the foot. The nerve may be damaged as it passes over the head of the fibula, resulting in foot-drop. There may be sensory loss over the outer aspect of the leg and foot.

Abnormalities of coordination

Incoordination is usually caused by one of two abnormalities – cerebellar or proprioceptive dysfunction. Cerebellar dysfunction reflects a failure in controlling accurate limb movements whereas proprioceptive dysfunction is characterised by ignorance of limb position when visual and cutaneous clues are excluded.

Cerebellar incoordination

Cerebellar incoordination is characterised by ipsilateral intention tremor, past-pointing and failure of rapid repetitive coordinated movements (dysdiadochokinesia). It is associated with truncal ataxia, 'scanning' speech and characteristic wide-based gait.

Proprioceptive incoordination (dorsal column loss)

When there is loss of proprioception the patient can still place the limbs accurately by looking at them; tests are performed with the eyes open and the eyes closed. When the patient's coordination is worse with the eyes closed than with them open they are said to have loss of position sense. If there is dorsal column loss but no spinothalamic loss there is said to be a dissociated sensory loss. Dissociated sensory loss is evidence of spinal cord disease. Finger–nose and heel–shin tests are normal when the patient can see but incoordinate when they cannot. Romberg's test is positive. The gait is ataxic and the patient walks on a wide base with high steps. Muscle tone and the tendon reflexes may be diminished.

Combined lower and upper motor neuron lesions

Rarely, combined upper and lower motor neuron lesions are observed. Classically this is seen in subacute combined degeneration of the cord (severe vitamin B_{12}

deficiency) and hereditary ataxias such as the hereditary spinomuscular ataxias (including Friedrich's ataxia). Increased muscle tone and spasticity is associated with absent reflexes, peripheral dorsal column neuropathy and cerebellar signs in the case of the hereditary syndromes. Examination of the feet reveals *pes cavus* due to the combined motor neuron effects.

Abnormal gait

Hemiplegia

The affected leg is rigid and describes a semicircle with the toe scraping the floor (circumduction).

Paraplegia

'Scissors' gait – both paralysed legs are held stiffly in extension and describe a semicircle in turn.

Festinant gait: Parkinson's disease

The footsteps are small in amplitude and tend to accelerate as the patient moves forward towards an obstruction ('*marche au petit pas*'). There is difficulty stopping and turning. The arms tend to be held flexed and characteristically do not swing.

Cerebellar gait

The patient walks on a wide base with the arms held wide with ataxia and veering and staggering towards the side of the disease.

Sensory (dorsal column) ataxia

A high stepping gait. The patient walks on a wide base and looks at the ground.

Steppage (drop-foot) gait

There is no dorsiflexion of the foot as it leaves the ground and the affected leg (or legs) are lifted high to avoid scraping the toe.

'Rolling' gait

The pelvis drops on each side as the leg leaves the ground due to myopathic changes in the pelvic muscles.

Tremors

A tremor is a rhythmic oscillating movement of a limb or part of a limb and may be seen at rest or in action.

Physiological tremor

This is best seen with the arms outstretched and is reproduced by laying a piece of paper across the outstretched hands. It is seen in:

- normal people
- anxiety
- fatigue.

Exaggerated physiological tremor

This is seen in:

- thyrotoxicosis
- hypoglycaemia
- illicit drug ingestion
- excess caffeine intake
- and with prescribed drugs, including:
  - β-agonists
  - theophylline
  - tricyclic antidepressants
  - phenothiazines
  - amphetamines.

Essential tremor

This is similar to physiological tremor but of slower oscillation. It:

- is familial
- increases with age
- is exaggerated by β-agonists, caffeine, anxiety
- is relieved by alcohol, β-blockers.

Resting tremor

This is characteristic of Parkinson's disease. Resting tremor is:

- maximal at rest and with emotion
- inhibited by movement
- demonstrated by passive, slow flexion–extension movements at the wrist
- mainly distal and asymmetrical

- when combined with cogwheel rigidity and flexion comprises the typical 'pill-rolling' tremor of Parkinson's disease.

Intention tremor

This is the oscillation exaggerated at the end of a movement. It is:

- characteristic of cerebellar disease
- reduced or absent at rest
- associated with past-pointing, nystagmus, dysarthria and ataxia, including truncal ataxia.

Asterixis

This is the flapping tremor associated with metabolic disorders. It occurs in:

- end-stage renal failure
- hepatic failure
- hypercapnia
- drug toxicity.

Chorea, athetosis and ballismus

These are rare, non-rhythmic combinations of purposeful movements and abnormal postures caused by disorders of the basal ganglia and their connections. Choreiform movements:

- are non-repetitive, involuntary, abrupt, jerky movements of the face, tongue and limbs
- may be localised or generalised
- occur in lesions of the extrapyramidal system and with phenothiazine toxicity
- are seen in Huntington's disease.

Dramatic jerking (ballismic) movements occur following lesions in the subthalamic structures and slower writhing movements are called athetosis.

Dystonia refers to slow sinuous writhing movements of the face and limbs, especially the distal parts.

In torsion spasm (dystonia) the movements are similar but slower and affect the proximal parts of the limbs. The movements are purposeless.

7

Endocrinology and metabolism

Patients with endocrine and metabolic disorders present with a wide range of symptoms and signs, or with none, the diagnosis being discovered by routine biochemical testing. Diabetes mellitus, thyroid disease and polycystic ovary syndrome are common, most other endocrinopathies are rare and present with classical endocrine syndromes. If the possibility of endocrine disease is raised, then a careful history and examination will establish the likely causes. The diagnosis must be confirmed by appropriate biochemistry, including dynamic testing, and by relevant imaging techniques.

History

Key features of the history in a patient with endocrine and metabolic disease are shown in Table 7.1.

Examination

General observation: note

- height and weight – calculate body mass index (BMI – weight/height^2)
- evidence of weight loss
- obesity and pattern of fat distribution
- loss of secondary sexual characteristics
- evidence of virilisation in women – male pattern hair distribution, altered muscle bulk and body habitus, deep voice and cliteromegaly

Where indicated, e.g. by delayed growth or lack of consonance of pubertal development, make a formal assessment of pubertal status.

Observe

Obvious features of classical endocrine and metabolic syndromes

- Graves' disease
- hypothyroidism
- hyperlipidaemias
- polycystic ovary syndrome
- Cushing syndrome
- acromegaly
- altered mood

Speech and voice disorders

- hoarseness
- virilised – deep voice in women
- slow slurred speech in hypothyroidism
- pressure of speech in thyrotoxicosis

The emphasis of the examination of the endocrine system should be dictated by the particular organ system that appears to be involved.

Hands

Observe

- palmar erythema
- temperature and sweating
- fine tremor of outstretched hands
- thyroid acropachy (swelling and clubbing)
- onycholysis
- orange-yellow discolouration (carotenaemia)
- small muscle wasting
- extensor tendon xanthomas
- increased pigmentation of palmar creases
- soft tissue enlargement and arthropathy

Clinical Medicine Lecture Notes, Eighth Edition. John R. Bradley, Mark Gurnell, and Diana F. Wood.
© 2019 John Wiley & Sons Ltd. Published 2019 by John Wiley & Sons Ltd.

Table 7.1 Key features of the history in a patient with endocrine and metabolic disease

Feature	Details	Rationale
Basic details	Age, sex, height, weight, reproductive status	Establish body mass index; consider growth and development disorders; subfertility
Symptoms	Weight changes; thirst and polyuria; heat intolerance; palpitations; tremor; pruritis; insomnia and irritability; lethargy; depression; diarrhoea or constipation; dry hair; hoarseness; swelling of the neck; dysphagia; periorbital swelling; change in nail beds; menstrual dysfunction; hirsutism; headaches; visual disturbance; muscle weakness; arthralgia; galactorrhoea; loss of libido; loss of secondary sexual characteristics; changes in facial appearance; xanthelasma; renal colic; tetany; skin changes – dry skin, acne, vitiligo, rashes, striae, foot ulcers; symptoms of specific lesions – acanthosis nigricans, pretibial myxoedema, necrobiosis lipoidica	Identify significant symptoms and patterns of change including relapsing patterns
Past medical history	Previous episodes of similar symptoms; other endocrine disorders; autoimmune disease; ischaemic heart disease; hypertension; bone fractures	Consider associated endocrine disorders or autoimmunity; effects of endocrine disease on cardiac dysfunction; hyperlipidaemia; secondary hypertension; endocrine manifestations of malignancy
Social and family history	Alcohol; smoking; diet; number of children and/or desire for pregnancy; family history of autoimmune endocrine disease or genetic cancers	Potential causes of endocrine disease; potential genetic syndromes or cancers
Medication	Review all medication including complementary therapies	Endocrine/metabolic side effects especially with corticosteroids, amiodarone, thiazides

Examine for

- Dupuytren's contracture
- carpal tunnel syndrome: thenar wasting; appropriate sensory changes; perform Tinel's test
- poor joint mobility: the 'prayer sign' will demonstrate impaired metacarpophalangeal (MCP) or interphalangeal (IP) joint extension

Arterial pulse

- bradycardia
- sinus tachycardia
- atrial fibrillation

Blood pressure

- lying and standing blood pressure: note postural hypotension

- Trousseau's sign – maintaining the cuff at above systolic pressure for 3 min induces carpal spasm of the hand and wrist in the presence of hypocalcaemia

Skin

Observe

- hirsutism
- loss of body hair
- greasy skin and acne
- dry skin
- vitiligo
- bruising
- abdominal striae
- folliculitis
- eruptive xanthomatosis

Examine for

- lipodystrophy at insulin injection sites
- acanthosis nigricans

Face

Observe

- cranial nerve palsies
- xanthelasmata
- hypothyroid facies
  - dry, thickened skin
  - hoarse voice
  - periorbital puffiness
  - macroglossia, pallor and 'lemon-yellow' tinge when severe, causing anaemia and carotenaemia
- features of acromegaly
  - increased supraorbital ridges
  - protrusion of lower jaw (prognathism with malocclusion)
  - soft tissue overgrowth
  - macroglossia
  - increased spacing of the teeth
  - deafness
- features of Cushing syndrome
  - moon face
  - acne
  - plethora
  - hirsutism with thinning of scalp hair
- hirsutism
- acne
- frontal alopecia
- mucocutaneous candidiasis

Perform

- Chvostek's sign – tapping over the facial nerve anterior to the ear induces ipsilateral twitching of the facial muscles in the presence of hypocalcaemia

Eyes

Note

- cataracts
- thyroid eye disease
  signs of hyperthyroidism
  - lid retraction
  - lid lag
  signs of Graves' disease
  - exophthalmos
  - proptosis
  - lid retraction
  - lid lag
  - periorbital oedema
  - chemosis
  - conjunctival injection
  - conjunctival ulceration
  - diplopia on upgaze
  - external ophthalmoplegia

Examine

- visual acuity
- visual fields

Perform

- fundoscopy
  - diabetic retinopathy, laser scarring
  - papilloedema

Neck

Examine

- carotid pulses
- carotid bruits
- thyroid gland
- cervical lymphadenopathy

Breasts

Note

- galactorrhoea; spontaneous or expressible
- gynaecomastia

External genitalia

Confirm

- pubertal stage where appropriate

Examine for

- testicular volume, penile length in men
- cliteromegaly in women
- evidence of intersex disorders

Legs

Examine for

- peripheral vascular disease
- proximal myopathy
- peripheral neuropathy
- ischaemic signs in feet

- foot ulceration
- Charcot joints
- necrobiosis lipoidica
- Achilles' tendon xanthomata
- pretibial myxoedema

Notes

The diabetic foot

Examination of the feet in patients with diabetes is essential and should be performed on a regular basis, at least at the annual review and more frequently where there are problems.

Observe

- colour and temperature
  - pale and cool in ischaemia
  - blueish-pink and warm in neuropathy
- callus formation over weight-bearing areas or dorsum of toes
- fungal infection of the toes and toenails
- ulceration
  - establish whether arterial or neuropathic
  - make accurate notes of size, depth, margins, infection
- loss of the plantar arch
- clawing of the toes
- Charcot joints

Palpate

- peripheral pulses

Test

- capillary refill
- sensation formally
  - establish stocking sensory neuropathy if appropriate
- reflexes

Assessment of thyroid status

Assessment of thyroid status involves examination of the thyroid gland and clinical evaluation to establish whether the patient is euthyroid, hyperthyroid or hypothyroid.

Examination of the thyroid gland (Fig. 7.1)

In normal men the thyroid gland is impalpable. A small soft symmetrical enlargement may be present in normal women.

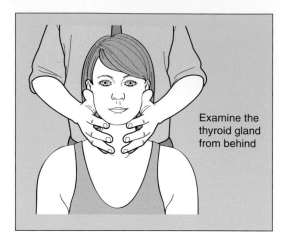

Examine the thyroid gland from behind

Figure 7.1 How to examine a patient's thyroid. Examine the patient from behind.

Patients with multinodular goitres are usually euthyroid but commonly develop subclinical or frank hyperthyroidism after many years. Often the clinical problem relates to their size, which may produce compression of the trachea, oesophagus or laryngeal nerve and sometimes causes distress from the cosmetic appearance.

Single nodules, particularly if the patient is euthyroid, should be regarded as malignant and immediate investigation including ultrasound, fine needle aspiration cytology (+/– radionuclide uptake scanning) should be performed. Rapid expansion in size and the presence of pain suggest malignancy.

During examination of the thyroid gland the patient's chin should be slightly flexed to relax the tissues. The thyroid gland moves upwards on swallowing. To demonstrate this, the patient should be given a sip of water to hold in the mouth and then swallow when asked.

Inspect

- the neck from the front and sides

Observe

- size of the thyroid gland
- obvious asymmetry
- upward movement on swallowing
- scars from previous thyroid surgery

Palpate

- the thyroid from behind both at rest and during swallowing

Assess

- character
  - diffuse, symmetrical enlargement
  - multinodular, usually asymmetrical
  - unilateral solitary nodules
- mobility
- tenderness
- retrosternal extension: feel in the suprasternal notch and percuss over the upper sternum for dullness
- tracheal displacement
- cervical lymphadenopathy

Auscultate

- over a diffusely enlarged gland for a systolic bruit which occurs in thyrotoxicosis

Assessment of thyroid status

Thyrotoxicosis has a number of causes and examination aims to distinguish Graves' disease from non-autoimmune causes of hyperthyroidism.

Signs of hyperthyroidism

General

- evidence of weight loss

Hands

- palmar erythema
- warm, sweaty palms
- fine tremor of outstretched hands – place a piece of paper over the outstretched hands to demonstrate
- onycholysis

Arterial pulse

- sinus tachycardia
- atrial fibrillation

Blood pressure

- systolic hypertension, increased pulse pressure

Hair

- generalised alopecia

Eyes

- lid retraction
- lid lag – ask the patient to fix their gaze on your finger held slightly in front and above their head and to follow your finger with their eyes as you move it slowly downwards in a forwards arc

Neck

- goitre – examine as earlier

Cardiovascular system

- signs of heart failure

Neuromuscular

- hyper-reflexia
- clonus
- proximal myopathy

Signs of G raves' disease (hyperthyroidism plus)

Eyes

- exophthalmos
- proptosis
- periorbital oedema
- chemosis
- conjunctival injection
- conjunctival ulceration
- diplopia on upgaze
- external ophthalmoplegia

Other signs (rarely)

- pretibial myxoedema
- thyroid acropachy
- vitiligo

Signs of hypothyroidism

General

- evidence of weight gain
- hoarse voice
- vitiligo

Hands

- cool hands, dry skin
- myxoedema – examine dorsum of hands
- carotenaemia – orange-yellow discolouration of palms

Arterial pulse

- sinus bradycardia

Blood pressure

- hypertension

Hair

- dry coarse hair
- generalised alopecia
- thinning of eyebrows (rarely outer third)

Eyes

- anaemia
- periorbital myxoedema

Neck

- goitre – examine as earlier
- commonly impalpable thyroid in primary autoimmune hypothyroidism

Cardiovascular system

- pericardial effusion

Respiratory system

- bilateral pleural effusions

Neuromuscular

- delayed relaxation phase of reflexes
- cerebellar signs

8

Musculoskeletal system

Disorders of the musculoskeletal system are common, accounting for around 25% of consultations in general practice in the UK and forming the major causes of physical disability in the elderly population. There are a wide range of underlying pathologies, but non-inflammatory conditions far outweigh inflammatory disorders. The major symptoms of musculoskeletal disorders are pain, stiffness, swelling and immobility; systematic examination is generally regional and attempts should be made to establish the source of pain, which may lie in muscles, tendons and periarticular structures. Diagnosis should be confirmed by appropriate imaging including plain X-rays, CT/MRI scans and radionuclide scans if indicated, together with blood tests for inflammatory markers, haematology and immunology.

History

Key features of the history in a patient with musculoskeletal disease are shown in Table 8.1.

Examination

Before examining the musculoskeletal system it is essential to enquire about painful joints and to examine with care so as not to exacerbate pre-existing pain. Position the relevant joints or region carefully, observe the patient's face during the examination and keep checking for pain.

A rapid, general assessment of the musculoskeletal system is shown in Table 8.2 – the GALS screen. The GALS screen aims to establish:

- if there are any abnormal joints
- the nature of the joint abnormality
- the distribution of joint abnormalities
- whether or not there are associated diagnostic features.

If the GALS screen is normal then further examination is not required during a general medical assessment. Any abnormalities identified should lead to detailed examination of the musculoskeletal system.

Detailed examination of the musculoskeletal system should be performed regionally, involving observation, palpation and manipulation ('Look, Feel and Move'). Always make a quick survey of the patient and their surroundings prior to starting a regional examination routine. Look for obvious clues including evidence of joint replacements, mobility aids and hand warmers.

For each region or affected joint(s):

Observe at rest

- skin changes
- swelling
- muscle wasting
- deformity

Palpate for

- tenderness
  - joint line, periarticular
- warmth
- swelling
  - fluid, soft tissue, bony

Clinical Medicine Lecture Notes, Eighth Edition. John R. Bradley, Mark Gurnell, and Diana F. Wood.
© 2019 John Wiley & Sons Ltd. Published 2019 by John Wiley & Sons Ltd.

Table 8.1 Key features of the history in a patient with musculoskeletal disease

Feature	Details	Rationale
Basic details	Age, sex, height, weight	Establish body mass index; musculoskeletal disorders more common in the elderly and in women
Symptoms	Pain – may be worse on usage (mechanical), after rest (inflammatory) or at night Stiffness – early morning or disuse stiffness (inflammation); may be associated weakness and deformity Swelling, deformity Symptoms of systemic illness – weight loss, fatigue	Identify significant symptom patterns including site, duration and aggravating/relieving factors
Past medical history	Previous episodes of similar symptoms; autoimmune disease; dermatological disease	Consider associated autoimmunity
Social and family history	Occupation; hobbies – sport, gardening; household environment; activities of daily living	Potential causes of injury; inability to cope at home
Medication	Review all medication including complementary therapies	Side effects – NSAIDs, corticosteroids

- crepitus
  - loud and palpable with joint damage
- joint stability

During movement observe

- restriction
- hypermobility
- pain on usage

Notes

Examination of the hands

Careful examination of the hands will reveal musculoskeletal disorders and accompanying general medical or neurological deficits.

Preparation and positioning
With the patient seated, ask them to

- expose their upper limbs to above the elbows
- bend elbows
  - observe extensor surface for rheumatoid nodules, psoriatic plaques, scars, gouty tophi, deformity
- rest their hands, palms downwards on a pillow.

Observe
Dorsum of hand
Skin

- rash
  - psoriasis, Gottron's patches in dermatomyositis (page 323, chapter 18), vasculitis
- atrophy ± purpura
  - rheumatoid arthritis, steroid usage
- rheumatoid nodules
- gouty tophi
- evidence of Raynaud's phenomenon
- sclerodactyly

Nails

- psoriatic pitting
- onycholysis
  - psoriasis
  - thyrotoxicosis
- splinter haemorrhages
  - vasculitis
  - bacterial endocarditis
- clubbing: consider general medical causes of clubbing, especially those associated with rheumatological disease, e.g. pulmonary fibrosis

Table 8.2 The GALS screen

Preliminary questions

Have you any pain or stiffness in your muscles, joints or back?

Can you dress yourself completely without difficulty?

Can you walk up and down stairs without difficulty?

Gait	Symmetry and smoothness of movement
	Normal stride length
	Ability to turn normally
Arms (sitting)	Inspect for wrist/finger swelling/deformity
Hands	Squeeze across 2nd–5th metacarpals (tenderness indicates synovitis of MCP joints)
Grip strength	Turn hands over (inspect for muscle wasting, normal forearm supination/pronation)
Elbows	Power grip (*'Make a tight fist'*)
Shoulders	Precision grip (*'Touch your thumb to individual fingers in turn'*)
	Full extension (*'Put your arms out straight'*)
	Abduction and external rotation (*'Put your hands behind your head'*)
Legs (lying)	
Knees	Inspect for swelling/deformity/quadriceps bulk
	Check for knee effusion
	Check for knee crepitus whilst passively flexing the knee
Hips	Check internal rotation of hips
Feet	Squeeze across metatarsals (tenderness indicates synovitis of MTP joints)
	Inspect for callosities on soles of feet
Spine (standing)	
Inspection from behind	Scoliosis
	Symmetrical muscle bulk
	Level iliac crest
	No popliteal swelling
	Normal hind foot alignment
Trigger points	Pressure over mid-supraspinatus
Inspection from in side	Kyphosis
Inspection from in front	Normal flexion (*'Lean down and touch your toes'*)
	Lateral cervical flexion (*'Touch your ear on your shoulder'*)

Source: Adapted from Doherty, M., Dacre, J., Dieppe, P. and Snaith, M. (1992) The 'GALS' locomotor screen. *Annals of the Rheumatic Diseases* 51: 1165–1169.

Muscles

- wasting dorsal interossei
  - disuse atrophy
  - T1 lesion

Joints

Rheumatoid arthritis

- wrist: subluxation of carpus/distal radio-ulnar joint
- metacarpophalangeal (MCP) joints: swelling ± subluxation; ulnar deviation
- interphalangeal (IP) joints: swelling of proximal interphalangeal (PIP) joints

- Swan neck, Boutonnière deformities of fingers
- Z deformity of thumb

Osteoarthritis

- Heberden's nodes
- Bouchard's nodes

Psoriasis

- dactylitis
- PIP and/or distal interphalangeal (DIP) joint swelling

Gout

- asymmetrical PIP and/or DIP joint swelling

Palmar surface of hand

Skin

- palmar erythema: rheumatoid arthritis
- anaemia
- calcinosis: localised systemic sclerosis
- vasculitis

Muscles

- wasting of all intrinsic muscles
  - disuse atrophy in painful arthritis
  - spinal cord T1 lesion
- disproportionate wasting of thenar eminence
  - carpal tunnel syndrome
- disproportionate wasting of hypothenar eminence
  - ulnar nerve lesion

Palpate (working from proximal to distal)
Joints: establish

- the nature of the swelling
  - synovitis: boggy
  - fluid: fluctuant
  - bone: hard
- whether there is active synovitis
  - warmth over swollen wrist or MCP joints
  - tenderness
- palpate over dorsal wrist joint line
- depress distal ulna
- perform
  - metacarpal squeeze
  - bimanual palpation of IP joints

Skin

- nodules – consistency
- sclerodactyly

Movement
Ask the patient to:

- make a fist and 'bury fingers' (forearm supinated)
  - function of MCP and IP joints
- turn clenched fists over (pronate forearm)
  - function of radio-ulnar joints
- extend little finger alone (rest of fist clenched)
  - integrity of extensor digiti minimi
- extend all fingers
  - integrity of extensor communis
- place palms together
  - flexion contractures of digits
- with palms together, bend wrists back
  - wrist extension
- with hands back-to-back, bend wrists forward
  - wrist flexion.

Patients with wrist synovitis are at risk of extensor tendon rupture. The first tendon to rupture is usually the extensor digiti minimi. Although rarely important functionally, it provides a warning that other extensor tendons are endangered.

Function
Impaired joint movement does not invariably correlate with poor hand function and vice versa.

Test

- power grip
- precision grip
- if relevant, ask the patient to demonstrate doing up buttons or writing

To complete the examination of the hands, an assessment of peripheral neurological function and vascular status should be made.

Sensory examination
Assess sensation in the following areas:

- radial border of index finger
  - median nerve or C6
- ulnar border of little finger
  - ulnar nerve or C8
- over 1st dorsal interosseus muscle
  - radial nerve
- distal middle finger
  - C7
- qualitative change in sensation
  - glove distribution neuropathy moving from distal to proximal

Motor examination
Test

- abduction or adduction of fingers
  - ulnar nerve or T1
- abduction of thumb – the plane of movement is at 90° to the palm
  - median nerve or T1
- extension of fingers or wrist
  - radial nerve or C6/7
- hook grip
  - C8

Perform

- Tinel's test (see Chap. 6, Isolated peripheral nerve lesions) in suspected carpal tunnel syndrome

Vascular examination
Observe

- colour and temperature of hand/individual digits

Palpate

- radial and ulnar pulses
- for capillary return in finger pulps

9

Assessment

Medical students and postgraduate trainees should be aware of some of the basic principles of assessment. An understanding of the way in which examinations are designed, implemented and scored ensures better preparation for the range of assessment formats that may be encountered during medical education and training programmes. In this chapter some important characteristics of assessment will be described briefly followed by a focus on the assessment of clinical competence.

Summative assessments measure the achievement of learning goals at the end of a course or programme of study. Summative assessments are formal and used to determine progression to the next stage of a course, to signify the need for remediation, for graduation purposes or registration with a national professional body. Little feedback is provided to learners. 'High-stakes assessments' are summative assessments with implications for professional progression such as Finals examinations in medical school, membership of Royal Colleges or Specialty Board Examinations in North America.

Formative assessments are designed specifically to provide feedback to learners about their progress. Formative assessments should be ongoing, frequent, non-judgemental and carried out in informal settings. They allow learners to engage with the educational process, offering them the opportunity to identify strengths and weaknesses and take appropriate action. Feedback is central to formative assessment and should encourage learners towards deep learning and understanding. Formative assessments may be in a number of different formats, including Objective Structured Clinical Examinations (OSCEs), mini-Clinical Examinations (mini-CEX), Direct Observation of Procedural Skills (DOPS), Cased-Based Discussions (CBD) or written work.

 Key features of assessment tools

Reliability: reflects the reproducibility of the assessment tool and the accuracy with which a score is being measured. It is higher in written assessments such as multiple choice and extended matching question formats, and lower in clinical competency-based assessments where there are more uncontrolled variables. Reliability is quantitative and reflected by the statistic known as *Cronbach's alpha*. Evaluation using *generalisability theory* can be performed to account for complex variables.

Validity: reflects the accuracy with which a test measures what it is purported to measure. It is a qualitative factor that evaluates the authenticity of an assessment and its fitness for purpose. A number of categories of validity are described; for example, the *content validity* reflects the way in which the test items relate to the curriculum content being assessed, *face validity* refers to the 'real life' nature of the assessment and high *construct validity* suggests that the test discriminates well between the abilities of candidates.

Educational impact: assessment is an important driver of learning; appropriate assessment tools encourage learners to acquire the desired knowledge, skills and attitudes.

Cost-effectiveness: reflects the practical aspects of assessment and helps determine the choice of assessment tool.

Acceptability: successful assessment formats must be acceptable to the teaching faculty and the learners.

Blueprinting: ensures the assessment tool samples content across the full range of learning objectives for the curriculum.

Clinical Medicine Lecture Notes, Eighth Edition. John R. Bradley, Mark Gurnell, and Diana F. Wood.
© 2019 John Wiley & Sons Ltd. Published 2019 by John Wiley & Sons Ltd.

Standard setting

Numerous methods to determine pass marks for different assessment formats are available.

Norm-referencing: in norm-referenced assessments the pass mark is determined by examiners using comparison within the cohort of examinees and thus the pass mark varies at each sitting. A percentage of candidates will pass the assessment on each occasion (*Fixed Percentage Method*). Norm-referencing does not take account of the content of the assessment or the competence of the candidates.

Criterion-referencing: in criterion-referenced assessments the pass mark is set in advance by a team of experienced examiners using their judgement about the degree of difficulty of the assessment and the minimum score expected of a candidate who just reaches the acceptable standard. A number of criterion-referenced standard setting methods are described including the *Angoff* and *Ebel* procedures.

Good practice for summative assessments in medical education demands that a minimum competence (safety) level should be set – the assessment should identify the Pass/Fail border and all candidates who reach the required standard should pass the examination. Assessments should thus be criterion-referenced by experienced examiners who recognise the standard required of the candidates at whatever level of undergraduate or postgraduate experience. Norm-referencing is not acceptable for high-stakes professional examinations.

Borderline group methods: these methods have been developed specifically for use in OSCE and similar formats where an experienced, trained clinician examiner is present at every station to score each candidate. In essence, each examiner scores the candidate using the station checklist – this constitutes the candidate's score for that station. In addition, the examiner awards the candidate a global score, based on an overall judgement of performance. Global rating scales include a spread of judgements such as 'fail – borderline fail – borderline pass – clear pass – outstanding'. The mean score of all candidates marked borderline becomes the pass mark for that station and the mean of all the stations' borderline scores becomes the pass mark for the assessment. These methods have gained credibility as they allow experienced clinicians to make judgements about professional competence and they are currently the gold-standard methods for assessments of clinical competence.

Assessments in medical education fall into three main categories – those that measure knowledge, competence and performance. 'Miller's Triangle' (Fig. 9.1) illustrates the relationship between these categories.

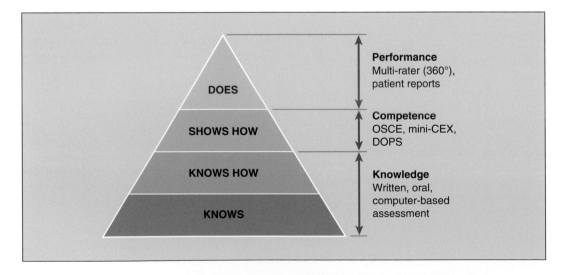

Figure 9.1 Miller's Triangle: categories of assessment methods. Source: Adapted from Miller, G.E. (1990) The assessment of clinical skills/competence/performance. *Academic Medicine* **65** (Suppl.): S63–S7.

Knowledge: this underpins all forms of assessment. Basic and applied knowledge can be tested in a variety of ways, commonly by written, oral or computer-based assessment formats such as multiple choice (MCQ), extended matching (EMQ) and structured essay (SEQ) questions, structured vivas and case-based discussions (CBD).

Competence: tests of competence assess a learner's ability to demonstrate applied knowledge in a controlled environment in which they know they are being assessed. Typically these take the form of skills-based assessments such as OSCEs and variants of the OSCE format, or workplace-based assessments such as mini-clinical examinations (mini-CEX) or direct observations of clinical practice (DOPS).

Performance: performance-based assessments aim to assess the application of knowledge and competence in daily clinical practice. They are more difficult to design and implement and few are in widespread use; these include the multi-rater (or 360°) assessment, observed consultations and patient reports on practice.

Assessment of clinical competence

Objective structured clinical examinations (OSCEs)

Summative assessment of clinical competence generally involves an OSCE or similar format such as the Royal College of Physicians MRCP Part 3 Practical Assessment of Clinical Examination Skills (PACES) examination. In these types of assessment, candidates rotate through a series of stations which may address clinical, communication or practical skills in a series of tasks. Each station is designed individually and marked by an assessor who may be a doctor, another clinician, a non-clinical medical teacher or a simulated patient. Marking schemes are designed in advance and piloted to ensure practicality and efficacy. The time for each station varies according to the task, so that simple practical skills may be allowed 5 minutes whereas more complex communication scenarios will have a longer time allocation. A wide range of skills may be assessed in this way, including simulated practical skills scenarios using manikins or models, communication skills stations with simulated patients and clinical examination of real patients. The range of OSCE stations has increased with improved simulation technology, so that candidates may be faced, for example, with emergency scenarios combining practical skills with simulated patients trained to provide appropriate responses to the ongoing scenario.

OSCEs are more 'fair' than traditional clinical examinations in which candidates were taken to see a varying (often small) number of short cases by one or two examiners and each asked a different set of questions. In an OSCE all candidates experience the same number of stations and perform the same tasks. Reliability is increased as each candidate is scored by a greater number of trained assessors using predetermined criteria, reducing the chance of examiner bias, increasing consistency and resulting in a clearer view of the candidate's overall abilities. The greater the number of stations, the more reliable the assessment and generalisable the results. Reliability is balanced against validity, cost-effectiveness and acceptability – thus examiners may choose to sacrifice a degree of reliability (obtained with simulation) for validity and acceptability (increasing the number of real patients).

OSCE stations are generally marked using a checklist such as the one shown in Fig. 9.2.

Checklists are designed in advance and take into account the learning objectives for the curriculum and the level at which the examination is set. For example, a clinical examination station for a junior medical student might focus on correct physical examination process skills whereas a similar station for postgraduates may include an evaluation of the candidate's overall approach to the patient and their ability to elicit and interpret physical signs correctly.

Mini-clinical examinations (mini-CEX)

The mini-CEX allows a clinical tutor to observe a trainee's interaction with a patient in a clinical setting. Developed for use in postgraduate settings, mini-CEX assessments are increasingly used in the assessment of senior medical students.

The mini-CEX format involves observation of a clinical activity such as taking a focused history, examining a system or giving information. The learner presents the salient features and offers a diagnosis and management plan. The tutor completes a pre-designed checklist and records areas of good practice and new training needs (Fig. 9.3).

Clinical Exam

Centre: Centre 1	**Circuit:** Circuit 2	**Candidate:** Candidate number
Session: Session 1	**Station:** 2	Candidate name

Neurological (PNS) Examination

Key to marking: **G** = good, **A** = adequate, **I** = Inadequate or not done

This station asesses the candidate's ability to examine the peripheral nervous system in upper and lower limb and make a diagnosis

THIS IS A 15 MINUTE STATION

1. Introduction and orientation (name and role and confirms patient's agreement)	G	A	I
2. Rapport (shows interest, respect and concern, appropriate body language)	G	A	I
3. Appropriately exposes the upper and lower limbs	G	A	I
4. Inspects the limb for wasting, involuntary movements and fasciculations as well as scars including the neck and lumbar spine for arm and leg respectively	G	A	I
5. Assesses the muscle tone, including clonus in lower limbs	G	A	I
6. Checks the power of movements at all joints starting proximally – using MRC grading scale and any weakness – including shoulder abduction, elbow flexion/extension, wrist extension, finger extension and abduction and thumb abduction	G	A	I
7. Checks coordination (finger–nose in arm, heel–shin in leg)	G	A	I
8. Checks reflexes +/– with reinforcement biceps, triceps, supinator in upper limb and knee and ankle in lower limb	G	A	I
9. Checks plantar repsonses in lower limb examination (if upper limb case)	G	A	I
10. Checks sensation starting distally with joint position sense, then light touch, pin prick	G	A	I
11. Checks for walking in lower limb examination and prontor drift in upper limb examination	G	A	I
12. Communicates with patient appropriately during examination (explains what he/she is doing, gains patient's co-operation)	G	A	I
13. Examines patient in a professional manner (gentle, watches for pain, maintains dignity and privacy)	G	A	I
14. Closure (thanks patient, leaves patient comfortable)	G	A	I

Examiner to ask:
"Please summarise your key findings"

15. Candidate presents key findings	G	A	I
16. Candidate presents summary in a fluent, logical manner	G	A	I

"What do you think is the most likely diagnosis?"

17. Candidate makes a reasonable attempt at a diagnosis	G	A	I

Figure 9.2 Example of a score sheet for an OSCE station testing the candidate's ability to examine the neurological system. Source: University of Cambridge School of Clinical Medicine 2005.

Approach to the OSCE: prepare, practise and perform

Prepare: study information about the examination available in advance; be clear about what is being examined; familiarise yourself with the format; study sample station checklists and any other information provided. Is there a minimum number of stations you must pass to be successful? What skills are covered in the OSCE? Does it include practical, communication and clinical skills stations or just one of these? How long are the stations? Does the examination use real or simulated patients? Is a structured viva involved at any or all of the stations? Are there data interpretation stations such as radiology or clinical pathology? Think about the stations you are likely to encounter and prepare for each one.

Practise: practise for the exam specifically; attend a course with practice OSCE circuits (usually for postgraduates); see as many patients as possible and practise physical examination skills with a colleague for feedback. Can you examine each of the major systems accurately and efficiently within the allotted time? Practise 'set piece' examinations (for example 'this patient has some difficulty walking – please examine his legs'; 'this lady has some pain in her joints – please examine her hands'). Consider likely communication skills scenarios and practise your approach. Are you

able to perform all the required practical skills? If not, arrange additional training in a skills centre. Practise for the data interpretation stations.

Perform: OSCEs test your clinical competence in a simulated environment – you need to perform! Carefully read the scenario and instructions at each station; be clear about the task. Are you required to take a history, to give information, gain consent for a procedure or talk to a relative or colleague? In a clinical station are you expected to examine a whole system, part of a system or to comment more widely? Plan how you will approach the station before entering it. Listen to the examiner – do they wish you to talk as you examine or present your findings at the end? Watch the clock – ensure that you will finish the station in the allotted time. Answer questions clearly and concisely; do not make up physical signs! If you didn't find anything, say so. Allow the examiner to understand your clinical reasoning and why you would choose a particular course of management.

Finally – move on: try to forget any mistakes you think you have made – the OSCE format means that an atypical poor performance in one station will be compensated by good performance elsewhere.

The clinical encounter should last about 15 min and feedback is provided at the end. Generally during an educational programme several mini-CEX assessments are required, allowing trainee and tutor to monitor progress. Records of mini-CEX assessments form part of a portfolio of clinical training and ensure that the trainee's development of clinical skills has been evaluated and recorded. Although not designed for high-stakes assessment, adequate completion of the required number of mini-CEX assessments may be necessary to ensure progression through a training programme.

Direct observation of procedural skills (DOPS)

The DOPS assessment is a variant of the mini-CEX designed to evaluate a student or trainee's ability to perform practical clinical skills. Trainees choose a skill from the approved list for their stage of training and generally should perform several DOPS at each stage of their educational programmes. The encounters are short and feedback is provided at the end (see Fig. 9.4).

RCP MINI CLINICAL EVALUATION EXERCISE

Assessor's GMC Number

SpR's GMC Number

Date (DD/MM/YY)

☐ ☐ / ☐ ☐ / ☐ ☐

Year of SpR training

○ 1 ○ 2 ○ 3 ○ 4 ○ 5 ○ 6

Patient problem/Diagnosis:

Case Setting   ○ Out-patient   ○ In-patient   ○ A&E   Is the patient: ○ New   ○ Follow-up?

Case Complexity: ○ Low   ○ Moderate   ○ High

Focus of mini-CEX: (more than one may be selected) ○ Data Gathering   ○ Diagnosis   ○ Management   ○ Counselling

What type of consultation was this?   ○ Good news   ○ Bad news ○ Neither

Please mark one of the circles for each component of the exercise on a scale of 1 (extremely poor) to 9 (extremely good). A score of 1–3 is considered unsatisfactory, 4–6 satisfactory and 7–9 is considered above that expected, for a trainee at the same stage of training and level of experience. Please note that your scoring should reflect the performance of the SpR against that which you would reasonably expect at their stage of training and level of experience. You must justify each score of 1–3 with at least one explanation/example in the comments box, failure to do so will invalidate the assessment. Please feel free to add any other relevant opinions about this doctor's strengths and weaknesses.

1. Medical Interviewing Skills
○ Not observed or applicable ○ 1   ○ 2   ○ 3   ○ 4 ○ 5 ○ 6   ○ 7 ○ 8 ○ 9
                                  UNSATISFACTORY   SATISFACTORY   ABOVE EXPECTED

2. Physical Examination Skills
○ Not observed or applicable ○ 1   ○ 2   ○ 3   ○ 4 ○ 5 ○ 6   ○ 7 ○ 8 ○ 9

3. Consideration for Patient/Professionalism
○ Not observed or applicable ○ 1   ○ 2   ○ 3   ○ 4 ○ 5 ○ 6   ○ 7 ○ 8 ○ 9

4. Clinical Judgement
○ Not observed or applicable ○ 1   ○ 2   ○ 3   ○ 4 ○ 5 ○ 6   ○ 7 ○ 8 ○ 9

5. Counselling and Communication skills
○ Not observed or applicable ○ 1   ○ 2   ○ 3   ○ 4 ○ 5 ○ 6   ○ 7 ○ 8 ○ 9

6. Organisation/Efficiency
○ Not observed or applicable ○ 1   ○ 2   ○ 3   ○ 4 ○ 5 ○ 6   ○ 7 ○ 8 ○ 9

7. OVERALL CLINICAL COMPETENCE
                             ○ 1   ○ 2   ○ 3   ○ 4 ○ 5 ○ 6   ○ 7 ○ 8 ○ 9

Assessor's comments on trainee's performance on this occasion (BLOCK CAPITALS PLEASE)

Trainee's comments on their performance on this occasion (BLOCK CAPITALS PLEASE)

Trainee's signature

Assessor's signature

Figure 9.3 Example of mini-CEX assessment: mini-CEX evaluation form. Source: Reproduced by kind permission of Joint Royal Colleges of Physicians Training Board; www.rcplondon.ac.uk/education.

Direct Observation of Procedural Skills (DOPS) – Anaesthesia

Please complete the questions using a cross (x). Please use black ink and CAPITAL LETTERS.

Trainee's surname: ☐☐☐☐☐☐☐☐☐☐☐☐☐☐☐☐☐☐☐☐☐☐☐☐☐☐

Trainee's forename(s): ☐☐☐☐☐☐☐☐☐☐☐☐☐☐☐☐☐☐☐☐☐☐☐☐☐

GMC number: ☐☐☐☐☐☐☐ **GMC NUMBER MUST BE COMPLETED**

Clinical setting:

Theatre	ICU	A&E	Delivery suite	Pain clinic	Other
☐	☐	☐	☐	☐	☐

Procedure:

Case category:

Elective	Scheduled	Urgent	Emergency	Other	ASA Class: 1 2 3 4 5
☐	☐	☐	☐	☐	☐☐☐☐☐

Assessor's position:

Consultant	SASG	SpR	Nurse	Other
☐	☐	☐	☐	☐

Number of times previous DOPS observed by assessor with **any** trainee:

0	1	2–5	5–9	>9
☐	☐	☐	☐	☐

Number of times procedure performed by trainee:

0	1–4	5–9	>10
☐	☐	☐	☐

	Please grade the following areas using the scale below:	Below expectations		Borderline	Meets expectations	Above expectations		U/C*
		1	2	3	4	5	6	
1	Demonstrates understanding of indications, relevant anatomy, technique of procedure							
2	Obtains informed consent							
3	Demonstrates appropriate pre-procedure preparation							
4	Demonstrates situation awareness							
5	Aseptic technique							
6	Technical ability							
7	Seeks help where appropriate							
8	Post procedure management							
9	Communication skills							
10	Consideration for patient							
11	Overall performance							

*U/C Please mark this if you have not observed the behaviour and therefore feel unable to comment.

Please use this space to record areas of strength or any suggestions for development.

Not at all ——— Highly

Trainee satisfaction with DOPS: 1 ☐ 2 ☐ 3 ☐ 4 ☐ 5 ☐ 6 ☐ 7 ☐ 8 ☐ 9 ☐ 10 ☐

Assessor satisfaction with DOPS: 1 ☐ 2 ☐ 3 ☐ 4 ☐ 5 ☐ 6 ☐ 7 ☐ 8 ☐ 9 ☐ 10 ☐

What training have you had in the use of this assessment tool? Face-to-face ☐ Have read guidelines ☐ Web/CDROM ☐

Assessor's signature: . . . . Date: . . . .

Time taken for observation (in minutes): ☐☐ Time taken for feedback (in minutes): ☐☐

Assessor's name: ☐☐☐☐☐☐☐☐☐☐☐☐☐☐☐☐☐☐☐☐☐☐☐☐☐

Assessor's GMC number: ☐☐☐☐☐☐☐ *Acknowledgement: Adapted with permission from the American Board of Internal Medicine.*

PLEASE NOTE: failure to return all completed forms to your administrator is a probity issue.

Figure 9.4 Example of DOPS assessment: DOPS evaluation form. Source: Reproduced with permission of the Royal College of Anaesthetists.

Part 2

Clinical Medicine

10

Cardiovascular disease

Ischaemic heart disease

This typically presents as the tight or crushing central chest pain of angina or myocardial infarction, or the fatigue and breathlessness of heart failure. Less commonly, it presents as an arrhythmia or conduction defect.

Myocardial ischaemia is normally caused by atherosclerosis, but cardiac pain is also produced by:

- aortic dissection
- paroxysmal tachycardias
- severe anaemia, cardiomyopathy, coronary artery embolism and vasculitis – all rare causes.

Coronary artery disease

Lipoprotein-driven atheromatous plaque formation involves inflammation, necrosis, fibrosis and calcification. Thrombi can form on the plaque surface, and rupture of plaques with a thin fibrous cap exposes thrombogenic necrotic core material, leading to thrombosis.

Factors associated with coronary artery disease include:

- *Sex*: it is more common in men than women, particularly before the menopause.
- *Age*: there is a steady increase with age.
- *Smoking*: is a powerful risk factor for coronary heart disease (CHD). Cessation is associated with significant reduction in risk, which can approach that of never-smokers after several years.
- *Hypertension*: the risk of coronary heart disease rises progressively with increasing blood pressure. Although most antihypertensive trials have shown a lower than expected reduction in risk, this may reflect the short duration of the trials.
- *Obesity*: central adiposity is a better marker for CHD risk than the overall level of obesity.
- *Hyperlipidaemia*: CHD is associated with raised total cholesterol and high ratio of total cholesterol to high-density lipoprotein (HDL) cholesterol. Hypertriglyceridaemia appears to be associated more with risk of myocardial infarction than coronary atherosclerosis, possibly because it affects coagulation.
- *Diabetes mellitus*: diabetes approximately doubles the risk of CHD, although the relative risk of myocardial infarction in patients with diabetes is declining.
- *Alcohol*: heavy drinking increases risk of cardiovascular disease, although the association between mortality and alcohol is J-shaped low (see Trials Box 13.1)

Angina pectoris

Diagnosis

The diagnosis of angina is clinical, based on the characteristic history:

- *site*: central chest
- *character*: usually tight, heavy, crushing
- *radiation*: to arms, epigastrium, jaw or back
- *precipitation*: by effort or emotion, particularly after meals or in the cold
- *relief*: within minutes by rest or sublingual or buccal glyceryl trinitrate

There are no specific physical signs. A non-cardiac cause is favoured by continuation for several days, precipitation by changes in posture or deep breathing, the ability to continue normal activities, and lack

Clinical Medicine Lecture Notes, Eighth Edition. John R. Bradley, Mark Gurnell, and Diana F. Wood.
© 2019 John Wiley & Sons Ltd. Published 2019 by John Wiley & Sons Ltd.

of relief by rest. The more common alternatives in the differential diagnosis are oesophageal pain and musculoskeletal pain.

Unstable angina refers to:

- angina of effort of recent onset with no previous history
- increased frequency and/or severity of pre-existing angina
- angina at rest.

Investigation

Electrocardiogram

The electrocardiogram (ECG) is usually normal between attacks, but may show evidence of old myocardial infarction, T-wave flattening or inversion, bundle branch block or signs of left ventricular hypertrophy. ST segment depression is usually seen during attacks and may be provoked by exercise testing. A negative exercise test, in which there is no chest pain, no ST depression, no arrhythmia and no sustained fall in blood pressure, indicates a good prognosis. Radionuclide studies can be performed if the patient is physically unable to exercise. Images at rest are compared with images obtained after pharmacological stimulation of coronary flow to evaluate the presence of local ischaemia or infarction.

In unstable angina there is ST depression or T-wave change during typical anginal pain but without diagnostic elevation in cardiac enzymes. Nitrates can reverse ST segment elevation.

Coronary arteriography may provide unequivocal evidence of arterial narrowing and define its site to guide revascularisation procedures.

Management of stable and unstable angina

Risk factors should be identified and advice given about stopping smoking, losing weight and taking regular exercise. Treat hypertension and hyperlipidaemia. Anaemia should be investigated and treated.

Sublingual glyceryl trinitrate remains the mainstay of symptomatic treatment for acute attacks. The major side effect is headache. It should be taken for pain, and prophylactically before known precipitating events. Long-acting nitrates such as isosorbide-5 mononitrate in a 60-mg sustained release formulation given once daily in the morning can give therapeutic plasma nitrate concentrations during the day, and allow a gradual fall during the night to prevent nitrate tolerance without a pre-dose rebound in angina. Beta-blockers reduce morbidity as well as control symptoms in stable angina. If necessary a dihydropyridine calcium channel blocker such as amlodipine can be added. If a β-blocker is contraindicated or not tolerated, diltiazem or verapamil can be used. Nicorandil, a potassium-channel activator, can also be beneficial. ACE inhibitors should be used in patients who also have left ventricular dysfunction or diabetes, unless there are contraindications. Low-dose aspirin (75 mg/day) reduces the risk of acute coronary events and myocardial infarction in patients with stable angina. Clopidogrel, an adenosine diphosphatase (ADP) receptor antagonist, may confer additional benefits but increases the risk of bleeding (see Trials Box 10.1). Diet and statins should be used to reduce LDL cholesterol with a target of <2.0 mmol/l.

Patients with unstable angina (evidence of ongoing myocardial ischaemia without evidence of infarction) should be admitted to hospital and precipitating factors (e.g. anaemia, arrhythmia) identified and treated. Non-ST segment elevation myocardial infarction (NSTEMI) is a closely related condition in which there is sufficient myocardial damage to release a marker of cardiac injury such as troponin or the MB isoenzyme of creatine phosphokinase (creatine phosphokinase has two subunits, which are either B [brain] or M [muscle] types; CK-MB containing B and M subunits is found in cardiac muscle – see page 91, Chapter 10). Treatment involves bed rest with ECG monitoring whilst pain is ongoing, and escalation of anti-ischaemic therapy. This should include low-dose aspirin, intravenous unfractionated or subcutaneous low-molecular-weight heparin (see Trials Box 10.1) and sublingual nitroglycerin, followed by intravenous nitrates. Beta-blockade can be added if there is ongoing pain and no contraindication. If β-blockers are contraindicated a non-dihydropyridine calcium antagonist (e.g. verapamil or diltiazem) can be used in the absence of severe left ventricular dysfunction or other contraindications. An ACE inhibitor can be added if hypertension persists despite the above measures. Pain should be controlled with morphine if not relieved, and supplemental oxygen administered if needed to maintain $SaO_2 > 90\%$.

Coronary angiography and revascularisation

Indications for coronary angiography differ between units, but angiography with a view to percutaneous coronary intervention or cardiopulmonary bypass surgery should be considered in all patients with evidence of recurrent ischaemia (angina or ST-segment

TRIALS BOX 10.1 Antiplatelet and anticoagulant agents in ischaemic heart disease and myocardial infarction

The **CHARISMA investigators** randomly assigned 15 603 patients with either clinically evident cardio-vascular disease or multiple risk factors to receive clopidogrel (75 mg/day) plus low-dose aspirin (75–162 mg/day) or placebo plus low-dose aspirin and followed them for a median of 28 months. Overall, clopidogrel plus aspirin was not significantly more effective than aspirin alone in reducing the rate of myocardial infarction, stroke or death from cardiovascular causes. There was a suggestion of benefit with clopidogrel treatment in patients with symptomatic atherothrombosis and a suggestion of harm in patients with multiple risk factors. Source: *New England Journal of Medicine* 2006; **354**: 1706–1717.

The **thrombolysis in myocardial infarction (TIMI) IIB trial** randomised 3910 patients with angina/non-Q-wave myocardial infarction to intravenous unfractionated heparin for ≥3 days followed by subcutaneous placebo injections or uninterrupted antithrombin therapy with enoxaparin during both the acute phase and outpatient phase. Enoxaparin was superior to unfractionated heparin for reducing a composite of death and serious cardiac ischaemic events without causing a significant increase in the rate of major haemorrhage. No further relative decrease in events occurred with outpatient enoxaparin treatment, but there was an increase in the rate of major haemorrhage. Source: *Circulation* 1999; **100**: 1593–1601.

 TRIALS BOX 10.2 Revascularisation for coronary artery disease

The **Bypass Angioplasty Revascularisation Investigation (BARI) investigators** compared angioplasty with coronary artery bypass surgery as initial treatment in 1829 patients with multi-vessel disease. Initial treatment by angioplasty did not compromise 5-year survival, although subsequent revascularisation was required more often than in patients treated by surgery in the first instance. In those with diabetes 5-year survival was better in patients treated initially by surgery. Source: *New England Journal of*

Medicine 1996; **335**: 217–225. In an analysis of 10-year clinical outcomes there was no significant long-term disadvantage regarding mortality or myocardial infarction associated with an initial strategy of PTCA compared with CABG. Among patients with treated diabetes, CABG conferred long-term survival benefit, whereas the two initial strategies were equivalent regarding survival for patients without diabetes. Source: *Journal of the American College of Cardiology* 2007; **49**(15): 1600–1606.

changes at rest or with minimal activity) or a strongly positive stress test despite medical therapy.

Coronary revascularisation can be achieved by coronary artery bypass grafting (CABG) or percutaneous coronary intervention (PCI) using catheter-borne devices (usually a balloon or laser) to open stenotic areas within coronary arteries (see Trials Box 10.2). CABG tends to be recommended in patients with three-vessel disease, significant left main coronary artery disease or two-vessel disease with significant proximal left anterior descending coronary artery disease and abnormal left ventricular function. PCI was initially only used for more proximal one-vessel disease. Improved techniques, the advent of drug-eluting stents and improved pharmacological therapies following PCI have reduced the risk of restenosis or

occlusion, and PCI is now used in more complex situations (Trials Box 10.3). Patients should receive dual antiplatelet treatment with aspirin and clopidogrel following PCI with stent placement. The recommended duration of clopidogrel therapy depends on the type of stent.

Myocardial infarction

The European Society of Cardiology, the American College of Cardiology Foundation, the American Heart Association and the World Heart Federation published a universal definition of myocardial infarction in 2007 (Thygesen et al. 2007).

TRIALS BOX 10.3 Revascularisation versus medical treatment in patients with stable coronary artery disease

A network meta-analysis of randomised trials comparing medical treatment with revascularisation found that among patients with stable coronary artery disease, coronary artery bypass grafting reduced the risk of death, myocardial infarction, and subsequent revascularisation compared with medical treatment. All stent-based coronary revascularisation technologies reduced the need for revascularisation to a variable degree. There was evidence for improved survival with new generation drug-eluting stents but no other percutaneous revascularisation technology compared with medical treatment. Source: *BMJ* 2014; **348**: g3859.

The criteria for diagnosis of acute myocardial infarction are met if there is a rise in biomarkers of cardiac injury (preferably troponin) together with at least one of the following:

- symptoms of myocardial ischaemia
- ECG changes indicative of new ischaemia – new ST segment or T-wave changes, or new LBBB (Fig. 10.8)
- development of pathological Q waves (page 20, Chapter 3; and Figs. 10.2 and 10.3)
- evidence of new loss of viable myocardium or new regional wall motion abnormality on imaging
- identification of intracoronary thrombus by angiography or autopsy.

Aetiology

The most common cause is thrombosis in association with an atheromatous plaque that has ruptured. Necrosis of cardiac muscle is followed by scarring.

Rare causes (consider in young patients without risk factors) are:

- coronary artery embolism: from thrombus in left atrium or ventricle, or mitral or aortic valve lesions
- congenital abnormalities, such as anomalous origin of coronary artery from pulmonary artery
- coronary artery vasculitis: consider Kawasaki disease in children (page 329, Chapter 18)
- dissecting aneurysm with coronary artery occlusion.

The size and location of the infarct depend on which artery is involved (Fig. 10.1) and the presence of any collateral supply. Occlusion of:

- left anterior descending affects the anterior wall of the left ventricle, and sometimes the septum
- right coronary artery involves the inferior part of the left ventricle, as well as part of the septum and right ventricle
- left circumflex involves the lateral or posterior walls of the left ventricle.

The infarct may extend from endocardium to epicardium (transmural) or involve only the subendocardial region.

There may be a

- past history of hypertension, stroke, intermittent claudication, diabetes mellitus, hyperlipidaemia, smoking
- family history of cardiovascular disease, hyperlipidaemia.

Symptoms

- Pain: onset, duration (usually over 20 min), character (often tight or compressing), site and radiation (usually chest going to arms or neck). Associated sweating, breathlessness, nausea and vomiting are common. There may be a previous history of angina or myocardial infarction.

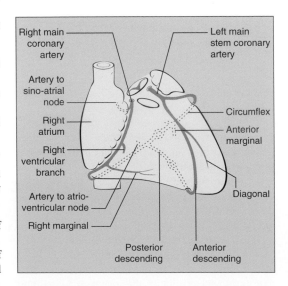

Figure 10.1 Anatomy of the coronary arteries. Note that the right coronary artery supplies both the SA and AV nodes.

NB: Intensity is no guide to the extent of the infarct, especially in the elderly and in diabetics where pain may be absent. If there is interscapular pain associated with a 'myocardial infarction' syndrome, consider dissection of the thoracic aorta.

Examination

Once any distress has been alleviated by pain control there may be no signs. Examine:

- for associated diseases:
  - xanthelasmata and xanthomata of hyperlipidaemia
  - evidence of diabetes, thyroid disease, diabetes mellitus, gout, cigarette smoking (smell and finger staining)
- pulse for small volume (low cardiac output), arrhythmia
- blood pressure (hypotension usually indicates low cardiac output; hypertension may not be long-standing)
- jugular venous pressure (JVP) is usually normal – elevation suggests heart failure
- listen to heart for:
  - fourth heart sound (common); third heart sound if there is heart failure
  - pericardial friction rub
  - mitral regurgitation (papillary muscle dysfunction or ventricular dilatation)
  - ventricular septal defect (VSD) caused by a ruptured septum (rare)
- listen to lungs for basal crackles of heart failure.

Investigations

ECG (see Figs. 10.2, 10.3 and Box 10.1)

Serial ECGs typically show ST segment elevation and T-wave inversion, with the development of Q waves indicating full-thickness myocardial necrosis. Changes occur in the anterior chest (V) leads in anterior myocardial infarction (Fig. 10.2) and in leads II, III and augmented voltage foot (AVF) in inferior myocardial infarction (Fig. 10.3).

Subendocardial myocardial infarction leads to ST segment and T-wave changes, but not Q waves. A normal ECG does not exclude myocardial infarction. Posterior infarction is rare and does not produce Q waves, but gives a tall R wave in V1.

Right ventricular infarction is usually associated with inferior infarction, and produces ST elevation, which can be detected if right ventricular leads (V3R and V4R) are recorded by placing chest electrodes on the right side of the chest in positions equivalent to V3 and V4.

Cardiac biomarkers

Troponin T, from cardiac muscle breakdown, is cardiac specific and the marker of choice.

Creatine kinase (CK) is formed by dimerisation of two polypeptide chains, B and M, giving rise to three different isoenzymes. The predominant isoenzyme in skeletal muscle is MM, whereas in brain it is BB. Cardiac muscle contains both MM and MB, and the MB isoenzyme is used in diagnosis of myocardial infarction, although it is also elevated in skeletal muscle disease and by muscle trauma.

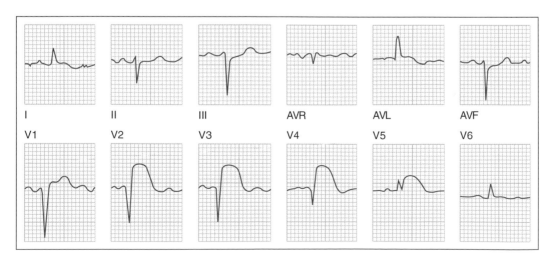

Figure 10.2 Anterior myocardial infarction.

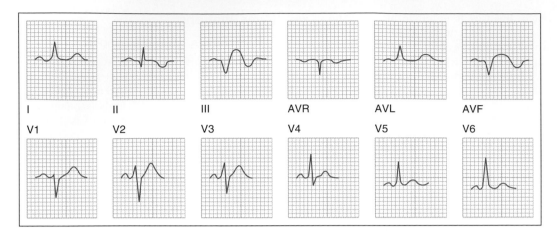

| I | II | III | AVR | AVL | AVF |
| V1 | V2 | V3 | V4 | V5 | V6 |

Figure 10.3 Inferior myocardial infarction.

 Box 10.1 ECG patterns in common clinical conditions

Myocardial infarction

A characteristic pattern of ECG changes typically evolves:

- First few minutes – peaked T waves.
- First few hours – ST segment elevation, inversion of T waves, development of Q waves.
- After a few days the ST segment returns to normal (persistent elevation raises the possibility of left ventricular aneurysm).
- The T waves may eventually become upright, but in full thickness untreated myocardial infarction Q waves persist indefinitely.
- Rhythm abnormalities are common.
- Left bundle branch block (Fig. 10.8) may occur at any stage, making further interpretation of the site, timing or extent of an infarct impossible.

Pulmonary embolism (Fig. 10.4)

- Tachycardia and transient arrhythmias (particularly AF).
- Right axis deviation.
- Right ventricular strain pattern – dominant R wave and inverted T waves in V1–4.
- RBBB.
- Occasionally S1, Q3, T3 pattern (S wave in lead I, Q and inverted T in III).

Ventricular hypertrophy

Large R waves occur over the appropriate ventricle in the chest leads (V1–2 for right ventricular hypertrophy and V5–6 for left ventricular hypertrophy). There tend to be large negative S waves in reciprocal leads (e.g. large S in V1 in left ventricular hypertrophy). A number of voltage criteria for left ventricular hypertrophy have been identified; for example, with normal QRS complexes if the sum of the S in V1 plus the R in V5 is greater than 35 mm, left ventricular hypertrophy is present on voltage criteria.

Digoxin

Sagging (reverse tick) ST segments, T-wave inversion.

Metabolic abnormalities

Hyperkalaemia (Fig. 10.5). Flattened P wave, broad QRS complex, peaked T wave.
Hypokalaemia (Fig. 10.6). Prolonged PR, depressed ST, flattened T wave and prominent U wave.
Hypocalcaemia (Fig. 10.7). Prolonged QT interval.

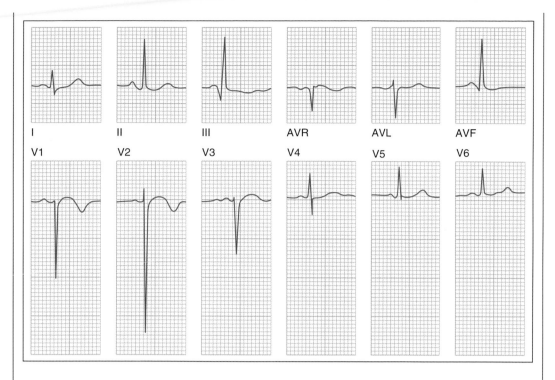

Figure 10.4 Acute pulmonary embolism with S1, Q3, T3 pattern, a mean frontal QRS axis towards the right (+90°) and right ventricular (RV) strain pattern in leads V1–3.

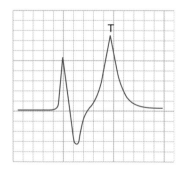

Figure 10.5 Hyperkalaemia.

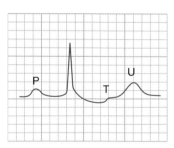

Figure 10.6 Hypokalaemia.

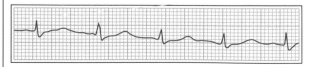

Figure 10.7 Hypocalcaemia. Normal complexes apart from a prolonged QT_c (QT interval corrected for heart rate). Rate 95/min, QT 0.4, QT_c 0.5.

Bundle branch block

- The QRS complex is greater than 0.12 s.
- In left bundle branch block (LBBB) the complex is negative (V- or W-shaped) in V1 (Fig. 10.8). Causes include ischaemic heart disease, myocardial infarction, cardiomyopathy, hypertension and aortic stenosis.
- In right bundle branch block (RBBB) the complex is positive (M-shaped) in V1 (Fig. 10.9). In addition to occurring in conditions associated with LBBB, RBBB occurs in conditions that put a strain on the right ventricle (e.g. COPD, pulmonary embolism). RBBB can occur in an otherwise normal heart.

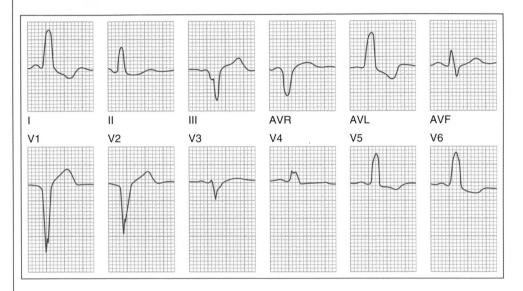

Figure 10.8 Left bundle branch block. RSR (M-shaped QRS complex) is visible in some of the left ventricular leads, I, AVL and V4–6, and notched QS complexes in the right ventricular leads, V1–2.

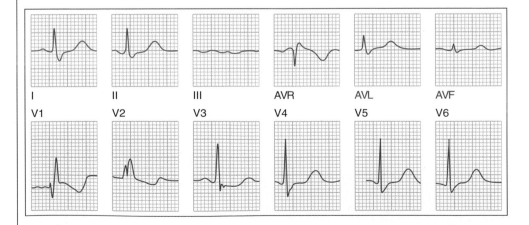

Figure 10.9 Right bundle branch block. RSR in the right ventricular leads V1–2 and slurred S waves in the left ventricular leads I, AVL and V4–6.

Fascicular block
There are three fascicles to the bundle of His: right, left anterior and left posterior. Block of one of the left bundles (unifascicular block) produces the following patterns with QRS complexes of normal width:

- In left anterior hemiblock there is left axis deviation.
- In left posterior hemiblock there is right axis deviation.

Sinoatrial disease (sick sinus syndrome)
This is a chronic disorder often associated with ischaemic heart disease in which sinus bradycardia and/or episodic sinus arrest can alternate with episodes of rapid supraventricular arrhythmia. Symptoms include dizziness, syncope, palpitations and dyspnoea. Permanent pacing may be necessary. Diagnosis is most easily made using 24-h ambulatory ECG monitoring.

Management

Early mortality (within 4 weeks) is chiefly within the first 2 h and usually from ventricular fibrillation. Any patient suspected of having a myocardial infarction requires:

- pain relief – usually in the form of opiates plus anti-emetics
- oxygen to alleviate breathlessness or hypoxia
- aspirin 300 mg to chew immediately
- nitrates should be administered for relief of ongoing ischaemic pain and can be used to control blood pressure and treat heart failure
- transfer to specialist facilities for reperfusion therapy.

Reperfusion therapies

Shortening the time between recognition of symptoms and seeking medical help, and initiation of reperfusion treatment with thrombolysis or primary percutaneous coronary intervention is a key element of management (see Trials Box 10.4).

Several studies in the late 1980s showed that intravenous streptokinase reduced mortality in patients reaching hospital with myocardial infarction from just over 10% to around 8%. ISIS-2 (Second International Study of Infarct Survival) showed that aspirin gives additional benefit, and subsequent trials showed that alteplase had similar effects.

Streptokinase 1 500 000 units is given by intravenous infusion over 1 h. It is cheaper than alternatives

 TRIALS BOX 10.4 Myocardial infarction

In the **Comparison of Angioplasty and Prehospital Thrombolysis in Acute Myocardial Infarction** study, 840 patients who presented within 6 h of acute myocardial infarction with ST-segment elevation were assigned to prehospital fibrinolysis ($n = 419$) with alteplase or primary angioplasty ($n = 421$) and all were transferred to a centre with access to emergency angioplasty. The median delay between onset of symptoms and treatment was 130 min in the prehospital-fibrinolysis group and 190 min (time to first balloon inflation) in the primary-angioplasty group. There was no difference in primary endpoint, which was a composite of death, non-fatal reinfarction and non-fatal disabling stroke at 30 days between the two groups. Source: *Lancet* 2002; **360**(9336): 825–829. Further analysis of the data indicated that prehospital thrombolysis may be preferable to primary PCI for patients treated within the first 2 h after symptom onset. Source: *Circulation* 2003; **108**(23): 2851–2856.

The **PRAGUE-2** study randomised 850 patients with acute ST elevation myocardial infarction presenting within <12 h to the nearest community hospital without a catheter laboratory to either thrombolysis in that hospital (TL group, $n = 421$) or immediate transport for primary percutaneous coronary intervention (PCI group, $n = 429$). The study showed that long-distance transport from a community hospital to a tertiary PCI centre in the acute phase of myocardial infarction was safe. The strategy markedly decreased mortality in patients presenting >3 h after symptom onset. For patients presenting within <3 h of symptoms, thrombolysis results were similar to those subjected to long-distance transport for PCI. Source: *European Heart Journal* 2003; **24**(1): 94–104. The early benefit from the PCI strategy over thrombolysis was sustained during 5 years' follow-up. Source: *European Heart Journal* 2007; **28**(6): 679–684.

Immediate angioplasty was compared with standard therapy with rescue angioplasty after thrombolysis in the **Combined Abciximab REteplase Stent Study in Acute Myocardial Infarction (CARESS-in-AMI)**. Immediate transfer for PCI improved outcome in high-risk patients with ST elevation myocardial infarction treated at a non-interventional centre with half-dose reteplase and abciximab. Source: *Lancet* 2008; **16**(371): 559–568.

Keeley et al. performed a meta-analysis of 23 trials, which together randomly assigned 7739 thrombolytic-eligible patients with ST-segment elevation AMI to primary PTCA ($n = 3872$) or thrombolytic therapy ($n = 3867$). Primary PTCA was better than thrombolytic therapy at reducing overall short-term death, non-fatal reinfarction, stroke and the combined endpoint of death, non-fatal reinfarction and stroke. The results seen with primary PTCA remained better than those seen with thrombolytic therapy during long-term follow-up, and were independent of both the type of thrombolytic agent used and whether or not the patient was transferred for primary PTCA. Source: *Lancet* 2003; **361**(9351): 13–20.

but can cause allergic reactions. Its potential for repeated use is limited by antibody formation. Alteplase (recombinant tissue plasminogen activator, rtPA) is not antigenic but is expensive. It is critically important to start thrombolysis within 12 h of myocardial infarction; additional benefit is obtained if started within 6 h.

Contraindications to thrombolysis are recent bleeding, severe hypertension (blood pressure >200/120 mmHg), active peptic ulceration, recent stroke (within the last 2 months), proliferative diabetic retinopathy, severe liver or renal disease, pregnancy/lactation, bacterial endocarditis and acute pancreatitis.

Primary percutaneous coronary intervention (PCI) is the preferred treatment if it is rapidly available (Trials Box 10.4). The European Society of Cardiology and the American College of Cardiology/American Heart Association Task Forces all recommend a target for the time from arrival in the emergency department to angioplasty (door-to-balloon time) of 90 min.

Beta-blockade

ISIS-1 (First International Study of Infarct Survival) showed that intravenous β-blockade in the early stages of myocardial infarction may confer benefit, but is contraindicated if there is bradycardia, hypotension, heart failure, asthma, sick-sinus syndrome or heart block (second- or third-degree or bifascicular). Long-term β-blockade post-infarction is routine in the absence of contraindications.

Angiotensin-converting enzyme inhibitors

Angiotensin-converting enzyme (ACE) inhibitors are beneficial, particularly in patients with anterior myocardial infarction, but their use may be limited by hypotension.

Anticoagulant and antiplatelet therapy

Guidelines recommend dual antiplatelet therapy with aspirin and an adenosine diphosphate (ADP)-receptor antagonist after ST elevation myocardial infarction and non-ST elevation acute coronary syndrome. Prasugrel and ticagrelor lead to faster and more potent ADP-receptor inhibition, compared with clopidogrel (Trials Box 10.5).

Anticoagulant options include unfractionated heparin, enoxaparin and bivalirudin. NICE Technology Appraisal 230 recommends the thrombin inhibitor bivalirudin in combination with aspirin and clopidogrel for the treatment of adults with ST-segment-elevation myocardial infarction (STEMI) undergoing primary percutaneous coronary intervention (PCI).

Complications

- *Heart failure* (page 103).
- *Shock:* the patient is hypotensive, pale, cold, sweaty and cyanosed. Arrhythmias are common. Treatment is with:
  - oxygen
  - diuretics if pulmonary oedema
  - vasodilators – ACE inhibitors (arterial and venous) or nitrates (venous) if blood pressure allows
  - inotropes – dopamine and dobutamine increase cardiac contractility by stimulating β_1-receptors in cardiac muscle. Low doses of dopamine (<5 mcg/kg/min) induce vasodilatation and increase renal perfusion, whereas higher doses cause vasoconstriction and may exacerbate heart failure.

TRIALS BOX 10.5 Anti-thrombotic therapy

The CURRENT-OASIS 7 trial compared double-dose (600 mg on day 1, 150 mg on days 2–7, then 75 mg daily) versus standard-dose (300 mg on day 1 then 75 mg daily) clopidogrel and high-dose (300–325 mg daily) versus low-dose (75–100 mg daily) aspirin in individuals undergoing percutaneous coronary intervention for acute coronary syndromes. The double-dose clopidogrel regimen was associated with a reduction in cardiovascular events and stent thrombosis compared with the standard dose, whereas efficacy and safety did not differ between high-dose and low-dose aspirin. Source: *Lancet* 2010; **376**: 1233–1243.

TRITON-TIMI 38 compared prasugrel with clopidogrel in patients undergoing percutaneous coronary intervention for ST-elevation myocardial infarction, and found prasugrel was more effective than clopidogrel for prevention of ischaemic events, without an apparent excess in bleeding. Source: *Lancet* 2009; *373*: 723–231.

A double-blind randomized trial comparing ticagrelor and clopidogrel in patients admitted to the hospital with an acute coronary syndrome, with or without ST-segment elevation, found that ticagrelor reduced death from vascular causes, myocardial infarction, or stroke without an increase in the rate of overall major bleeding but with an increase in the rate of non-procedure-related bleeding. *New England Journal of Medicine* 2009; **361**: 1045–1057.

- *Arrhythmias* (see page 100, Table 10.1).
- *Sinus tachycardia*: usually requires no treatment.
- *Supraventricular extrasystoles:* common, but rarely requires treatment.
- *Supraventricular tachycardia:* arise from the atria or atrioventricular junction. Management depends on the nature of the tachycardia.
- *Sinus or nodal bradycardia:* may be caused by sedation, particularly with opiates. If the rate is <50 beats/min and the patient is hypotensive, give atropine 0.6 mg intravenously and repeat twice if necessary. If unsuccessful, consider cardiac pacing.
- *Heart block:* all degrees of heart block are more serious if they complicate anterior rather than inferior infarcts.
  - first-degree: requires no therapy
  - second-degree: monitor and consider atropine. Many physicians would consider cardiac pacing for Mobitz type II with anterior infarcts (page 102)
  - third-degree (complete heart block): atropine and isoprenaline may be helpful while awaiting cardiac pacing.

NB: Complete heart block is more common in inferior myocardial infarctions because the atrioventricular nodal artery is a branch of the right coronary artery; complete heart block complicating anterior infarction is ominous because it implies a large muscle infarction.

- *Ventricular tachycardia:* this can respond to intravenous amiodarone, but proceed to direct current (DC) cardioversion without delay if no success or there is haemodynamic collapse.
- *Ventricular fibrillation:* this is frequently within 6 h of myocardial infarction (see Cardiorespiratory arrest, Figs. 10.15 and 10.16).
- *Electromechanical dissociation* (complexes on ECG with no pulse – see Cardiorespiratory arrest, Figs. 10.15 and 10.16).

Late complications

Ventricular aneurysm can cause heart failure, angina, arrhythmias and emboli from thrombi within the aneurysm. There may be cardiac enlargement and abnormal cardiac pulsation (e.g. an impulse at the left sternal border). Its presence is suggested by ST-segment elevation persisting in convalescence. The aneurysm may be demonstrated by echocardiography, radionuclide studies or left ventriculography. Surgical removal is indicated for heart failure or arrhythmias. Anticoagulants reduce the risk of emboli.

Papillary muscle dysfunction or rupture may cause heart failure. There is a pansystolic or late systolic mitral regurgitant murmur. Echocardiography confirms the diagnosis. Surgery may be indicated.

Ruptured ventricular septum is rare. Urgent surgical repair may be required for severe heart failure.

Myocardial rupture leads to death from tamponade (unless immediate surgery is available). Dressler (post-myocardial infarction) syndrome occurs weeks or months after myocardial infarction or cardiac surgery. It is characterised by fever, pleurisy and pericarditis, and the presence of antibodies to heart muscle.

Table 10.1 Cardiac arrhythmias

Rhythm	Rate Atrial	Ventricular	Diagnosis	Underlying diseases	Therapy
Regular	100+	100+	Sinus tachycardia	Anxiety, cardiac failure, thyrotoxicosis, fever, anaemia	Treat underlying disease
	100–200	100–200	Supraventricular tachycardia	None (60%), thyrotoxicosis, digoxin, tobacco, caffeine, Wolff–Parkinson–White syndrome	Vagal stimulation (pressure on the carotid sinus), β-blocker or verapamil surgical ablation of accessory pathway
	300	70–200	Atrial flutter with block	Ischaemic heart disease, thyrotoxicosis, digoxin	Rate control – β-blocker, calcium antagonist, digoxin; Rhythm control – DC cardioversion, amiodarone, sotalol, verapamil
	60+	15–50	Complete heart block with cannon 'a' waves in jugular vein pulse, variable intensity first sound, wide pulse pressure	Post-infarction, idiopathic, digoxin, cardiomyopathy	Nil if asymptomatic; atropine or cardiac pacemaker
	40–60	40–60	Sinus bradycardia	Athletes, myocardial infarction, myxoedema, hypothermia, sino-atrial disease	As heart block if following myocardial infarction
Irregular			Multiple ectopics (including coupled beats), ECG basically regular	Ischaemia, digoxin, thyrotoxicosis, cardiomyopathy	Stop digoxin and correct hypokalaemia if necessary.
		60–100	Atrial flutter with varying block	Ischaemia, rheumatic heart disease	Rate control – β-blocker, calcium antagonist, digoxin; Rhythm control – DC cardioversion, amiodarone, sotalol
		<100 treated 100+ untreated	Atrial fibrillation (apex rate is only guide to true heart rate; ECG essential)	Ischaemic and rheumatic heart disease, thyrotoxicosis, pulmonary embolism, constructive pericarditis, cardiomyopathy or bronchial carcinoma	Rate control – β-blocker, calcium antagonist, digoxin; Rhythm control – DC cardioversion, amiodarone, sotalol
Cardiac arrest		120–200 No peripheral pulse	Ventricular tachycardia Ventricular fibrillation and sometimes ventricular tachycardia Ventricular asystole	Myocardial infarction and ischaemia	See Figs. 10.15 and 10.16

DC, direct current; ECG, electrocardiogram

Invasive and non-invasive assessment post-myocardial infarction

Patients with ongoing angina (or other evidence of ischaemia) at rest or on minimal exertion or left ventricular dysfunction who have not undergone coronary angiography should undergo angiography to evaluate the need for coronary revascularisation. Patients in whom angiography is not planned should undergo exercise testing towards the end of the hospital admission or early after discharge to assess functional capacity and look for evidence of inducible ischaemia. Echocardiography should be performed to assess left ventricular function. Dipyridamole or adenosine stress myocardial perfusion imaging can be used in patients unable to exercise or if baseline abnormalities compromise ECG interpretation during exercise testing.

Rehabilitation

Cardiac rehabilitation programmes reinforce the importance of secondary prevention and promote adoption of a healthy lifestyle. Dietary education is given to achieve normal BMI and reduce dietary cholesterol and saturated fat. Active involvement in self-rehabilitation should be encouraged. The importance of stopping smoking must be stressed and strategies to help smokers used.

Patients should be encouraged to increase activity gradually over 1–2 months, when return to work can be considered. Patients should be advised about driving restrictions (page 103, Chapter 10).

Long-term pharmacological treatments

Unless contraindicated, aspirin, β-blockade, angiotensin blockade and statins (Trials Box 10.6) should

---

 TRIALS BOX 10.6 Statins

The **Incremental Decrease in Endpoints through Aggressive Lipid lowering (IDEAL)** study enrolled 8888 patients aged 80 years or younger with a history of acute MI: 4439 patients were randomly assigned to receive a high dose of atorvastatin (80 mg/day) and 4449 patients were randomised to usual-dose simvastatin (20 mg/day). During treatment, mean LDL cholesterol levels were 104 mg/dl in the simvastatin group and 81 mg/dl in the atorvastatin group. More intensive lowering of LDL cholesterol did not result in a significant reduction in the primary outcome of major coronary events, but did reduce the risk of other composite secondary endpoints and non-fatal acute MI. There were no differences in cardiovascular or all-cause mortality. Source: *JAMA* 2005; **294**(19): 2437–2445.

In the **Treating to New Targets (TNT)** study, 10 001 patients with coronary heart disease and LDL cholesterol levels of less than 3.4 mmol/l were randomly assigned to receive either 10 mg or 80 mg of atorvastatin per day. The mean LDL cholesterol levels were 2.0 mmol/l during treatment with 80 mg of atorvastatin, and 2.6 mmol/l during treatment with 10 mg of atorvastatin. There was an absolute reduction in the rate of major cardiovascular events of 2.2% and a 22% relative reduction in risk in patients receiving more intensive lipid-lowering therapy.

This occurred with a greater incidence of elevated aminotransferase levels. Source: *New England Journal of Medicine* 2005; **352**: 1425–1435.

The **Pravastatin or Atorvastatin Evaluation and Infection Therapy – Thrombolysis in Myocardial Infarction-22 (PROVE IT TIMI-22)** study enrolled 4162 patients who had been hospitalised for an acute coronary syndrome within the preceding 10 days and compared 40 mg of pravastatin daily (standard therapy) with 80 mg of atorvastatin daily (intensive therapy). The intensive lipid-lowering statin regimen provided greater protection against death or major cardiovascular events than the standard regimen. Source: *New England Journal of Medicine* 2004; **350**: 1495–1504.

The prospective studies collaboration performed a meta-analysis of 61 prospective observational studies consisting of almost 900 000 adults without previous disease and with baseline measurements of total cholesterol and blood pressure. During nearly 12 million person-years at risk between the ages of 40 and 89 years, there were more than 55 000 vascular deaths (34 000 ischaemic heart disease, 12 000 stroke, 10 000 other); 1 mmol/l lower total cholesterol was associated with about a half, a third and a sixth lower ischaemic heart disease mortality in both sexes at ages 40–49, 50–69 and 70–89 years, respectively, with no apparent threshold. Source: *Lancet* 2007; **370**: 1829–1839.

be started in all patients and continued indefinitely. Target LDL cholesterol should be less than 2.0 mmol/l.

Arrhythmias

(See Table 10.1.)

Supraventricular tachycardias

Supraventricular tachycardias arise from the atria or atrioventricular junction. QRS complex is normal unless there is also bundle branch block.

Sinus tachycardia

In sinus tachycardia the rate is >100 beats/min. An underlying cause (anxiety, exercise, fever, anaemia, heart failure, thyrotoxicosis) can usually be identified.

Atrial fibrillation

Atrial fibrillation (AF) is predominantly a disease of the elderly, occurring in >10% of the population aged over 70. Paroxysmal AF terminates spontaneously or with intervention within 7 days of onset. Persistent AF is sustained for more than 7 days. It is considered permanent when a decision to cease attempts to restore or maintain sinus rhythm has been made.

The common causes of AF are:

- ischaemic heart disease
- thyrotoxicosis
- mitral valve disease
- cardiomyopathy.

Management

ECG to confirm diagnosis. Twenty-four-hour ambulatory ECG monitoring if paroxysmal AF is suspected. Indications for echocardiography include high risk of underlying structural or functional heart disease, consideration of cardioversion, and risk stratification for antithrombotic therapy.

Check serum potassium and thyroid function. The aims are to restore sinus rhythm or control the ventricular rate and minimise the risk of embolisation.

A β-blocker or rate-limiting calcium-channel blocker can be used as monotherapy to control rate. If monotherapy does not control symptoms dual combination therapy with a β-blocker, diltiazem or digoxin can be considered.

Rhythm control should be considered if AF is new onset, has a reversible cause, or is thought to be causing heart failure. Direct current (DC) cardioversion can often establish sinus rhythm, but relapse is common. Long-term amiodarone reduces the frequency of relapse, although side effects can limit its use. If AF has been present for >48 h therapeutic anticoagulation is recommended for at least 3 weeks before cardioversion.

NB: Side effects of amiodarone are reversible corneal microdeposits, photosensitivity, skin discolouration, hypothyroidism, hyperthyroidism, diffuse pulmonary alveolitis and fibrosis, peripheral neuropathy and myopathy.

Dronedarone is a second-line treatment option to maintain sinus rhythm in selected patients who have a known cardiovascular risk factor (hypertension requiring at least two agents, diabetes, previous transient ischaemic attack, stroke or embolism, left atrial diameter >50 mm, or age >70) without left ventricular systolic dysfunction or a history of heart failure.

The fivefold increased risk of stroke is reduced by anticoagulation, which should be offered according to stroke and bleeding risks (Box 10.2).

Stroke risk should be reviewed in patients with AF not taking an anticoagulant when they reach age 65 or develop diabetes, heart failure, peripheral arterial disease, coronary artery disease, stroke, transient ischaemic attack or systemic thromboembolism.

 Box 10.2 Antithrombotic therapy in patients with atrial fibrillation

NICE clinical guideline 180 recommends offering anticoagulation with apixaban, dabigatran, etexilate, rivaroxaban or a vitamin K antagonist to people with AF or atrial flutter and a CHA_2DS_2-VASc score of 2 or above, and considering anticoagulation for men with a CHA_2DS_2-VASc score of 1, taking bleeding risk into account. Bleeding risk is increased by uncontrolled hypertension, concurrent medication (e.g. aspirin or non-steroidal anti-inflammatory drugs), harmful alcohol consumption or poor anticoagulant control.

CHA_2DS_2-VASc allocates a score of 1 or 2 for the risk factors **C**ongestive heart failure/LV dysfunction (1), **H**ypertension (1), **A**ge ≥ 75 y (2), **D**iabetes mellitus (1), **S**troke/Transient Ischaemic Attack/Thromboembolism (2), **V**ascular disease (1), **A**ge 65–74 y (1), **S**ex **c**ategory (female gender) (1). Source: *Chest* 2010; **137**: 263–272.

Atrial flutter

The atria discharge at around 300/min, giving the characteristic 'saw-tooth' baseline on ECG (see Fig. 10.10). There is usually atrioventricular block, leading to a ventricular rate of 150/min (2 : 1) or 100/min (3 : 1). The rate is basically regular but is affected by 2 : 1, 3 : 1 and variable block. The causes are similar to AF, although atrial flutter is less common.

Management

Drugs such as sotalol, amiodarone, propafenone and flecainide can be effective in restoring sinus rhythm. DC cardioversion can also be used to terminate atrial flutter.

For patients with AF of ≥48 h or of unknown duration for whom pharmacologic or electrical cardioversion is planned, anticoagulation with warfarin for 3 weeks before elective cardioversion and for at least 4 weeks after sinus rhythm has been maintained is recommended.

Atrial tachycardia

The atrial rate is slower than in atrial flutter, being between 120 and 200/min. The ECG shows abnormally shaped P waves (see Fig. 10.11). There is often a degree of atrioventricular (AV) block.

Management

Terminating an episode of atrial tachycardia

- First try unilateral carotid sinus massage or Valsalva manoeuvre.
- Adenosine (3 mg by rapid injection into central or large peripheral vein) usually causes rapid reversion to sinus rhythm. Its short half-life (10 s) means that side effects (facial flushing, bronchospasm, bradycardia) are usually short-lived.

- Verapamil may be preferable in asthmatics but should be avoided if hypotension or heart failure are present. Verapamil is contraindicated in patients taking β-blockers.
- Amiodarone may be useful in resistant supraventricular tachycardia. Disopyramide can be effective, but it impairs cardiac contractility and has antimuscarinic effects.
- Cardioversion under short-acting general anaesthesia is used when rapid results are required and other procedures have failed.

Preventing atrial tachycardia

If the above fail, sodium-channel blockers (propafenone, procainamide or flecainide) may be indicated. Sotalol, a non-selective β-blocker that also blocks potassium channels, represents an alternative therapy.

Pre-excitation syndromes

In addition to the AV node, an additional connection (accessory pathway) between the atria and ventricles allows atrial impulse to be transmitted more quickly to the ventricles – hence the term pre-excitation syndrome. The main types are Wolff–Parkinson–White and Lown–Ganong–Levine syndromes.

Wolff–Parkinson–White syndrome is caused by an accessory pathway (bundle of Kent) that bypasses the AV junction. It is characterised by a short PR interval and a widened QRS complex because of the presence of a δ wave (see Fig. 10.12). In type A, the ventricular complex is positive in lead V1; in type B, it is negative. Two main arrhythmias occur:

- In *re-entrant tachycardia* the normal (AV node) conduction pathway and the accessory pathway form a circuit through which impulses repeatedly circulate. The δ wave is lost. Drugs that block the AV node (e.g. adenosine, verapamil) usually restore sinus rhythm.

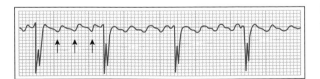

Figure 10.10 Atrial flutter with 'saw-tooth' atrial waves (arrows) and 4 : 1 block.

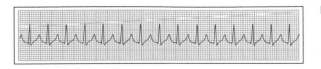

Figure 10.11 Atrial tachycardia.

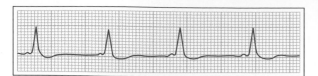

Figure 10.12 Wolff–Parkinson–White (WPS) syndrome. Short PR interval and broad ventricular complex due to δ waves.

- In *atrial fibrillation* most ventricular complexes are broad because of the presence of δ waves on the upstroke. AV nodal blocking drugs may increase the ventricular rate and should be avoided. DC cardioversion usually terminates AF. Amiodarone may be used to slow conduction in the accessory pathway.

Lown–Ganong–Levine is also characterised by a short PR interval but has a normal QRS, i.e. without a δ wave. It is also complicated by paroxysmal tachycardia.

Ventricular tachycardia

The ventricular rate is usually 120–200/min. It usually reflects serious underlying myocardial disease. It is often self-limiting, but if sustained may cause hypotension and shock. The ECG shows a broad-complex tachycardia, and P waves dissociated from the ventricular activity may be seen (see Fig. 10.13). The axis is often bizarre.

Management

Amiodarone can be used, but DC cardioversion should be performed if there is shock.

In *torsade de pointes* the QRS axis progressively changes so that the complexes appear to twist continuously. There is QT prolongation in sinus rhythm. Underlying causes should be identified and treated (anti-arrhythmic drugs, hypokalaemia, hypomagnesaemia, tricyclic antidepressants). Anti-arrhythmic agents may aggravate the condition. DC cardioversion or pacing is often effective in terminating attacks, which if left untreated may degenerate into ventricular fibrillation. Intravenous infusion of magnesium sulphate is also often effective.

Ventricular fibrillation

See Cardiorespiratory arrest, page 103.

Heart block (see Fig. 10.14)

In *first-degree block* the PR interval is prolonged. In *second-degree block* the normal 1: 1 ratio of P : QRS complexes is lost but a relationship between P waves and QRS complexes still exists. The relationship may be either progressive lengthening of the PR interval until one QRS complex is dropped (Mobitz type I or Wenckebach) or dropped QRS complexes without a change in the PR interval (Mobitz type II).

If there is complete dissociation between P waves and QRS complexes *third-degree heart block* exists. The QRS complex rate (and hence ventricular rate) is usually slow (15–50/min) and regular. Cardiac pacing is often required.

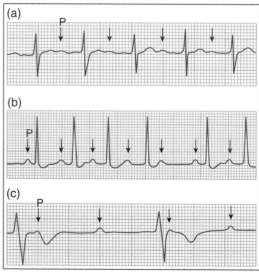

Figure 10.14 (a) First-degree heart block. PR interval 0.3 s. (b) Second-degree heart block (Wenckebach or Mobitz type I). (c) Third-degree heart block with complete atrioventricular dissociation.

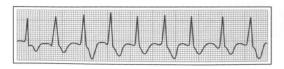

Figure 10.13 Ventricular tachycardia with slightly irregular ventricular QRS complexes and variable T waves because of dissociated superimposed P waves.

Cardiorespiratory arrest

Clinical features

- sudden loss of consciousness
- absent carotid and femoral pulses
- respiratory arrest follows shortly after

Aetiology

- almost invariably cardiac arrhythmia (ventricular fibrillation [VF], ventricular tachycardia [VT] or asystole)
- rarely, the primary event is respiratory arrest (e.g. severe asthmatic attack)

Management

The Resuscitation Council UK Guidelines (https://www.resus.org.uk/resuscitation-guidelines/) contain information about basic and advanced life support, including algorithms for in-hospital resuscitation (Fig. 10.15) and advanced life support (Fig. 10.16).

Cardiovascular disorders and driving

Full details of the DVLA's current medical standards of fitness to drive can be found at https://www.gov.uk/guidance/assessing-fitness-to-drive-a-guide-for-medical-professionals.

Group 1 entitlement

- Angina: driving must cease when symptoms occur at rest, with emotion or at the wheel.
- Acute coronary syndromes: if successfully treated by coronary angioplasty, driving may recommence after 1 week provided no other urgent revascularisation is planned, left ventricular ejection fraction is at least 40% prior to hospital discharge and there is no other disqualifying condition. If not successfully treated by coronary angioplasty, driving may recommence after 4 weeks provided there is no other disqualifying condition.
- Aortic stenosis: disqualified if symptomatic.

- Pacemaker insertion: driving must cease for at least 1 week.
- Arrhythmia: driving must cease if the arrhythmia has caused or is likely to cause incapacity.
- Thoracic and abdominal aortic aneurysm: DVLA should be notified of any aneurysm 6 cm or more in diameter. An aortic diameter of 6.5 cm or more disqualifies the person from driving.

Heart failure

Heart failure has a prevalence in the UK, Scandinavia and the USA of about 1% overall and 10% in the elderly.

New York Heart Association classification

Class I. Patients with cardiac disease but without resulting limitation of physical activity. Ordinary physical activity does not cause undue fatigue, palpitation, dyspnoea or anginal pain.

Class II. Patients with cardiac disease resulting in slight limitation of physical activity. They are comfortable at rest. Ordinary physical activity results in fatigue, palpitation, dyspnoea or anginal pain.

Class III. Patients with cardiac disease resulting in marked limitation of physical activity. They are comfortable at rest. Less than ordinary activity causes fatigue, palpitation, dyspnoea or anginal pain.

Class IV. Patients with cardiac disease resulting in inability to carry on any physical activity without discomfort. Symptoms of heart failure or the anginal syndrome may be present even at rest. If any physical activity is undertaken, discomfort is increased.

Pathophysiology

- *Cardiac size* increases as a result of dilatation or muscle fibre hypertrophy. In response to increased volume load, ventricular volume increases (the heart dilates). This is initially beneficial as the strength of contraction increases as the cardiac muscle is stretched (Starling's law). However, contraction declines as stretch becomes extreme.
- *Cardiac output* is diminished by definition, resulting in reduced perfusion to vital organs.
- *Sympathetic nervous activity* and plasma noradrenaline (norepinephrine) levels increase, leading to increased heart rate, myocardial contractility and arterial and venous tone.

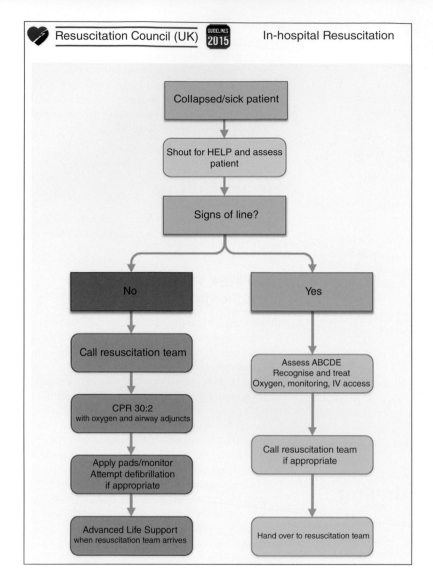

Figure 10.15 In-hospital resuscitation algorithm. Source: Reproduced with the kind permission of the Resuscitation Council (UK). ABCDE, Airway Breathing Circulation Disability Exposure. https://www.resus.org.uk/resuscitation-guidelines/in-hospital-resuscitation/.

- Renal blood flow is reduced, leading to activation of the renin–angiotensin system (see 'Hypertension' page 107, Chapter 10). *Angiotensin II* causes vasoconstriction and, by stimulating aldosterone, sodium and water retention. These mechanisms increase both pre- and afterload.
- *Preload* is the extent to which cardiac muscle is stretched prior to contraction; it is reflected by the ventricular volume at the end of diastole – the *end diastolic volume*.
- *Afterload* is the load the ventricle contracts against during systole, which is produced by the aortic valve and the arterial tree.

Heart failure is therefore associated with vasoconstriction through angiotensin II and sympathetic nervous activity, and salt and water retention. These mechanisms initially increase cardiac output (Starling's law) and blood pressure, but do so at the expense of reduced peripheral blood flow and circulatory congestion.

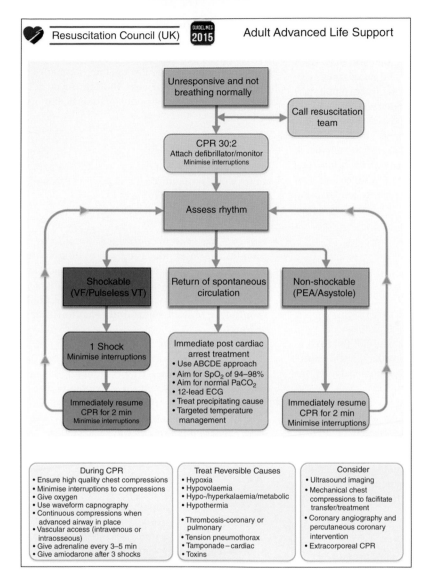

Figure 10.16 Advanced life support algorithm. Source: Reproduced with the kind permission of the Resuscitation Council (UK). PEA, pulseless electrical activity. https://www.resus.org.uk/resuscitation-guidelines/adult-advanced-life-support/#algorithm.

Aetiology

It is important to identify the underlying cause:

- ischaemic heart disease with left ventricular dysfunction (the most common cause)
- hypertension
- cardiomyopathy
- valvular heart disease
- congenital heart disease (ASD, VSD)
- pericardial disease

- in high-output heart failure excessive cardiac workload may result from anaemia, Paget's disease and thyrotoxicosis.

There may also be precipitating factors:

- anaemia
- fluid retention (NSAIDs, renal disease)
- infection (especially of the lungs with reduced PaO_2; endocarditis)
- drugs with negative inotropism (most anti-arrhythmic drugs except digoxin).

Clinical features

In *left heart failure* left ventricular end-diastolic pressure (LVEDP) is increased. Pulmonary congestion causes dyspnoea, orthopnoea and paroxysmal nocturnal dyspnoea, and leads to acute pulmonary oedema. Fatigue results from reduced muscle blood flow. Signs are tachycardia, third heart sound, crackles at the lung bases and pulmonary effusions.

Right heart failure is usually caused by pulmonary congestion of left heart failure. It also complicates lung disease (cor pulmonale), pulmonary hypertension, right ventricular infarction, and pulmonary and tricuspid valve disease. Signs are raised JVP, hepatomegaly (cardiac cirrhosis may occur if chronic), oedema and ascites.

Investigation

All patients with newly diagnosed heart failure require the following:

- full blood count to exclude anaemia
- creatinine and electrolytes to look for evidence of impaired renal function as a cause of fluid retention or a consequence of reduced renal perfusion
- chest X-ray for evidence of cardiomegaly, venous hypertension or pulmonary oedema
- ECG for evidence of myocardial ischaemia or infarction, left ventricular hypertrophy, arrhythmia
- echocardiography to exclude valvular or pericardial disease and assess left ventricular function.

Further investigations, including cardiac radionuclide studies, exercise testing and coronary angiography, may be indicated.

Echocardiography

Thickening of stenotic valves, often with calcification, gives rise to intense echoes with limited movement of the valve leaflets. Doppler can be used to assess pressure gradients across stenosed valves and is extremely sensitive in detecting valve regurgitation. In dilated cardiomyopathy both end-diastolic and end-systolic dimensions are increased, and shortening fraction reduced.

Hypertrophic cardiomyopathy is suggested by thickening of the left and/or right ventricle or interventricular septum in the absence of aortic stenosis or hypertension. There is typically anterior motion of the mitral valve during systole, and mid-systolic closure of the aortic valve. Doppler can be used to detect a pressure gradient across the left ventricular outflow tract.

Pericardial effusion appears as an echo-free space around the heart. If tamponade develops ventricular wall movement is reduced.

Radionuclide studies

Ejection fraction is reduced and there may be dilatation of the heart. A fall in ejection fraction on exercise is a poor prognostic sign. Regional abnormalities of the ventricular muscle usually indicate myocardial ischaemia or infarction. Regional paradoxical movement suggests an aneurysm.

Coronary angiography

Coronary revascularisation is recommended in patients with hypoperfused but viable myocardium.

Treatment

- *Diuretics* are used to control sodium and water retention. Furosemide 40 mg/day or bumetanide 1 mg/day are usually effective. Higher doses may be required and synergism between thiazide and loop diuretics can be exploited. Careful monitoring of fluid status and renal function is required.
- *ACE inhibitors* have beneficial effects on all classes of heart failure. They should be considered in all patients, even if asymptomatic, because they reduce afterload and may enable remodelling of the left ventricle muscle. Use may be limited by side effects, which include hypotension, renal impairment, hyperkalaemia and cough (when angiotensin II receptor antagonists can be substituted).
- *Beta-blockade* with bisoprolol, carvedilol, or metoprolol, titrated from small doses, inhibits the adverse effects of sympathetic activity, outweighing their negative inotropic effects.
- *Low-dose aldosterone antagonists* (e.g. spironolactone or eplerenone) should be considered, but carry the risk of hyperkalaemia.

A *combination of hydralazine and a nitrate* should be considered in patients who are symptomatic despite angiotensin and β-blockade or who are unable to tolerate these treatments.

- *Digoxin* is useful for control of concomitant atrial fibrillation. Recent studies have also shown a benefit in patients with heart failure in sinus rhythm.

Atrial-synchronised biventricular pacemakers (cardiac resynchronisation therapy) eliminate the delay in activation of the left ventricle seen in many patients with left ventricular systolic dysfunction, which can increase left ventricular filling time, reduce mitral regurgitation and reduce septal dyskinesis (see Trials Box 10.7).

TRIALS BOX 10.7 **Cardiac resynchronisation therapy (CRT)**

A systematic review found that cardiac resynchronisation reduces morbidity and mortality in patients with left ventricular systolic dysfunction, prolonged QRS duration and NYHA class 3 or 4 symptoms when combined with optimal pharmacotherapy. Source: *JAMA* 2007; **297**(22): 2502–2514.

A meta-analysis on the effects of cardiac resynchronisation therapy in heart failure patients with narrow QRS complex found that in patients with baseline mechanical asynchrony, who underwent CRT after optimal medical management, there was a significant reduction in NYHA class, improvement in LVEF and increase in 6-min walk distance during follow-up. Source: *Cardiology Journal* 2008; **15**(3): 230–236.

The RESPOND study compared CRT with optimal pharmacological therapy in patients with heart failure and a normal QRS duration, and found that CRT led to an improvement in symptoms, exercise capacity and quality of life. Source: *Heart* 2011; **97**: 1041–1047.

Ventricular arrhythmias and sudden death

Patients with previous cardiac arrest or ventricular arrhythmias are at highest risk of sudden death and should be considered for placement of an implantable cardioverter-defibrillator.

Hypertension

Aetiology

In over 90% of cases no specific cause is found and the hypertension is known as essential. The aetiology is probably multifactorial. Predisposing factors include:

- increasing age
- obesity
- excessive alcohol intake.

Hypertension may be secondary to:

- renal disease
- endocrine disease – Cushing syndrome, Conn syndrome, phaeochromocytoma, acromegaly
- oral contraceptive pill
- eclampsia
- coarctation of the aorta.

Genetic factors

Blood pressure levels show a strong familial aggregation that cannot be accounted for by shared environment alone. However, the genetic and environmental factors contributing to hypertension are likely to be extremely diverse, confounding the search for responsible genes. Attention has principally been directed towards the identification of candidate genes. These include genes involved in the renin–angiotensin system, together with a number of important vasoconstrictor and vasodilator substances that have recently been identified.

Renin–angiotensin–aldosterone system

A number of factors, including hypotension, hypovolaemia and hyponatraemia, stimulate renin release from the juxtaglomerular apparatus. Renin converts angiotensinogen to angiotensin I, which is then converted by ACE to angiotensin II. Angiotensin II causes arteriolar vasoconstriction, activation of the sympathetic nervous system, and antidiuretic hormone (ADH) and aldosterone secretion. In the kidney angiotensin II causes a relatively greater increase in efferent (post-glomerular) compared to afferent (pre-glomerular) arteriolar constriction, thereby maintaining glomerular filtration in the face of reduced renal perfusion.

Endothelins, prostacyclins and nitric oxide

These are derived from the vascular endothelium. They regulate vascular contraction and relaxation, particularly in the coronary circulation. *Endothelins* are a family of structurally related 21-amino-acid peptides and the most potent vasoconstrictors. At least three different isoforms exist. Endothelin-1 (ET-1) is the predominant peptide generated by vascular endothelial cells. It is generated from proendothelin-1 by the action of endothelin-converting enzyme, a metalloprotease. Two distinct endothelin receptors have been identified. ET-1 has been implicated in the pathophysiology of a number of conditions involving vasoconstriction, including heart failure, pulmonary hypertension, subarachnoid haemorrhage, Raynaud's phenomenon and Prinzmetal angina.

Prostacyclin is produced by endothelial cells, platelets and monocytes via a phospholipase A$_2$ (PLA$_2$)-dependent pathway, and causes smooth-muscle cell relaxation and also inhibition of platelet aggregation, via intracellular increases in cyclic 3′,5′-adenosine monophosphate (cAMP). Prostacyclin is synthesised in response to the same inflammatory mediators that raise cytoplasmic-free calcium as nitric oxide. Interleukin-1 (IL-1) and tumour necrosis factor increase the activity of the enzymes mediating prostacyclin generation.

Nitric oxide (NO, originally named endothelial-derived relaxing factor) is produced by oxidation of the guanidine-nitrogen terminal of L-arginine, forming NO and citrulline. Production of NO is regulated via activity of NO synthase, a predominantly cytosolic calcium-calmodulin-requiring enzyme which is similar in structure to cytochrome P450 enzymes. Two distinct types of the enzyme have been identified, designated constitutive and inducible.

Constitutive NO synthase is a calcium-calmodulin-requiring enzyme that is responsible for the transient release of small (picomolar) quantities of NO from vascular endothelium, platelets, mast cells, adrenal medulla and some neurons. Enzyme activity is increased by:

- inflammatory mediators, such as thrombin, histamine, bradykinin, serotonin and leukotriene C$_4$, which raise intracellular calcium
- mechanical forces, such as shear stress
- acetylcholine.

Inducible NO synthase is not dependent on calcium-calmodulin and causes a sustained release of larger (nanomolar) amounts of NO from activated macrophages, neutrophils, vascular endothelium and microglial cells. It is induced by bacterial endotoxin, IL-1, tumour necrosis factor and interferon-γ.

Pharmacology of nitric oxide

NO mediates the action of some commonly used vasodilators. Glyceryl trinitrate and organic nitrate esters react with thiols such as cysteine and glutathione to yield unstable intermediates which release NO. Sodium nitroprusside spontaneously releases NO.

Pathophysiology

In its early stages hypertension is thought to be characterised by increased cardiac output with normal peripheral resistance. As hypertension progresses peripheral resistance increases and cardiac output returns to normal.

Left ventricular hypertrophy (LVH) may be present even in mild hypertension and is associated with increased risk of cardiac dysfunction, atherosclerosis, arrhythmias and sudden death.

Diagnosis of LVH

- ECG: S wave in V1 and R wave in V5 or V6 ≥ 35 mm. May be associated with ST-segment depression or T-wave inversion ('strain pattern').
- Echo: much more sensitive than ECG. The left ventricular mass index (LVMI) is calculated from left ventricular wall thickness and left ventricular internal diameters in systole and diastole, and body surface area.
- Severe LVH present if LVMI > 110 g/m^2 in women or >131 g/m^2 in men.

There is good evidence that treatment of hypertension results in regression of LVH.

Symptoms

There are usually no symptoms of hypertension. Headaches or visual disturbance occur in severe or accelerated hypertension.

Examination

The blood pressure is measured at rest. If high (systolic >140 mmHg, diastolic >90 mmHg), check in both arms, and unless very severe recheck on at least three separate occasions before considering treatment. A large cuff should be used in the 10% of the population with arm circumference over 33 cm. Phase V diastolic (disappearance) should be recorded together with the patient's posture and the arm used.

Mild or moderate hypertension usually gives no other abnormalities on examination. In long-standing or severe hypertension look for evidence of LVH with an aortic ejection murmur and loud aortic second sound. The optic fundi may show evidence of retinopathy with arterial narrowing and arteriovenous nipping (indicating atherosclerosis), haemorrhages and exudates. Papilloedema indicates the presence of malignant hypertension.

Ten percent of cases have an underlying definable cause: it is essential to think of these less common causes.

- Observe the face for evidence of Cushing syndrome – usually caused by corticosteroid administration.
- Examine for aortic coarctation – feel both radials and measure blood pressure in both arms. Look for radial–femoral delay, weak femoral pulses, bruits

of the coarctation and scapular anastomoses, which may produce visible pulsations.

- Listen for an epigastric or para-umbilical bruit of renal artery stenosis.
- Feel for polycystic kidneys.
- Think of chronic kidney disease, phaeochromocytoma (rare) and primary hyperaldosteronism (rare).

Investigation

Routine investigation of hypertension is aimed at detecting treatable disease (usually renal) and assessing cardiac and renal function. All patients require:

- ECG to assess left ventricular size, and if abnormal a chest X-ray
- urinalysis for blood and protein – if abnormal a midstream specimen of urine for cells, casts, proteinuria and evidence of infection, and for albumin to creatinine ratio
- blood, creatinine and electrolytes to assess renal function and look for hypokalaemic alkalosis of Conn or Cushing syndromes (or diuretic therapy)
- plasma metanephrines or 24-h urine collections (×2) for urine fractionated metanephrines (phaeochromocytoma).

Investigate renovascular disease (page 111), Cushing syndrome (page 247, Chapter 16), Conn syndrome (page 250, Chapter 16), phaeochromocytoma (page 253, Chapter 16) or aortic coarctation (page 119).

Management

NICE guideline CG127 on the clinical management of primary hypertension in adults uses the following definitions:

Stage 1 hypertension Clinic blood pressure is 140/90 mmHg or higher **and** subsequent ambulatory blood pressure monitoring (ABPM) daytime average or home blood pressure monitoring (HBPM) average blood pressure is 135/85 mmHg or higher.

Stage 2 hypertension Clinic blood pressure is 160/100 mmHg or higher **and** subsequent ABPM daytime average or HBPM average blood pressure is 150/95 mmHg or higher.

Severe hypertension Clinic systolic blood pressure is 180 mmHg or higher **or** clinic diastolic blood pressure is 110 mmHg or higher.

Treatment (Trials Box 10.8)

Patients should attempt to achieve an ideal weight, avoid excessive alcohol, caffeine and salt and take regular exercise. The NICE guidelines (http://www.nice.org.uk/CG034) recommend offering treatment to:

- people aged under 80 years with stage 1 hypertension who have one or more of the following:
  - target organ damage
  - established cardiovascular disease
  - renal disease
  - diabetes
  - a 10-year cardiovascular risk equivalent to 20% or greater
- people of any age with stage 2 hypertension.

Aim for a target treated clinic blood pressure below 140/90 mmHg in people aged under 80 years, and below 150/90 mmHg in people aged 80 years and over.

Initial drug therapy:
Aged <55 y – angiotensin-converting enzyme (ACE) inhibitor or an angiotensin-II receptor blocker (ARB).

 TRIALS BOX 10.8 Hypertension

The earliest studies showing beneficial effects of antihypertensives used diuretics or β-blockers, but more recent trials have shown benefits from calcium-channel blockers and ACE inhibitors.

A meta-analysis of 147 randomised trials of blood pressure-lowering drugs in the prevention of cardiovascular disease found that the five main classes of blood pressure-lowering drugs (thiazides, β-blockers, angiotensin-converting enzyme inhibitors, angiotensin receptor blockers and calcium-channel blockers) were similarly effective in preventing coronary heart disease events and strokes, with the exception that calcium-channel blockers had a greater preventive effect on stroke and β-blockers had an additional protective effect in preventing coronary heart disease events when given shortly after a myocardial infarction. The authors concluded that with the exception of the extra protective effect of β-blockers given shortly after a myocardial infarction and the minor additional effect of calcium-channel blockers in preventing stroke, all the classes of blood pressure-lowering drugs had a similar effect in reducing CHD events and stroke for a given reduction in blood pressure. Source: *BMJ* 2009; **338**: b1665.

Aged >55 y and black people of African or Caribbean family origin of any age – calcium-channel blocker. If a calcium-channel blocker is not tolerated, or there is evidence or a high risk of heart failure, a thiazide-like diuretic, such as chlorthalidone or indapamide can be used.

Beta-blockers may be considered in younger people if ACE inhibitors or ARBs cannot be used, there is evidence of increased sympathetic drive, or women of child-bearing potential. Avoid combining a β-blocker and thiazide-like diuretic to reduce the risk of diabetes.

For most patients, a combination of an ACE inhibitor or angiotensin II receptor blocker, calcium-channel blocker and thiazide-like diuretic is required to achieve target blood pressure.

Clinic blood pressure that remains higher than 140/90 on three drugs is regarded as resistant hypertension, and addition of low-dose spironolactone (if potassium 4.5 mmol/l or lower); higher dose thiazide (if potassium >4.5 mmol/l), or an α- or β-blocker may be of benefit.

Other drugs that reduce cardiovascular risk must also be considered. These include aspirin and statins for secondary prevention of cardiovascular disease, and primary prevention in treated hypertensive subjects according to risk of cardiovascular disease and local guidelines. Glycaemic control should also be optimised in diabetic subjects.

Thiazide-like diuretics inhibit distal tubular sodium reabsorption. Low doses (e.g. chlorthalidone 25 mg/day) have maximal antihypertensive effect. Higher doses confer little additional antihypertensive effect, but cause more marked adverse metabolic effects, including hypokalaemia, hyponatraemia, hypochloraemic alkalosis, hyperuricaemia, hyperglycaemia and hyperlipidaemia.

Calcium-channel blockers inhibit inward movement of calcium ions through slow channels in cell membranes. They influence the function of cardiac myocytes, the specialised conducting cells of the heart, and vascular smooth-muscle cells. Three classes, which differ in their relative effects on the heart and blood vessels, are available:

- The phenylalkylamine, verapamil, slows conduction in the sino-atrial and atrioventricular nodes and depresses myocardial contraction, but is less potent as a vasodilator.
- The benzothiazepine, diltiazem, slows conduction in the sino-atrial and atrioventricular nodes, but causes less myocardial depression and vasodilatation.

- The dihydropyridines (e.g. nifedipine, nicardipine, amlodipine, felodipine, isradipine, lacidipine) have little effect on cardiac contraction or conduction, but are more potent arterial vasodilators. Dihydropyridines vary in their effects on different vascular beds. Nimodipine acts preferentially on cerebral arteries and is used to prevent vascular spasm following subarachnoid haemorrhage.

ACE inhibitors (e.g. captopril, lisinopril, ramipril) inhibit conversion of angiotensin I to II, which is a vasoconstrictor and stimulates aldosterone production. They should be considered for treatment of hypertension when β-blockers or thiazides are contraindicated or ineffective. They may cause excessive hypotension, particularly in the presence of sodium depletion. In heart failure, first doses are usually given at bedtime, and where possible diuretic therapy should be stopped for a few days before initiating treatment. Side effects include hyperkalaemia (particularly in the presence of renal disease), persistent dry cough, blood dyscrasias, rashes and angioedema. ACE inhibitors should be used with caution in renal disease (see later).

Angiotensin-II receptor antagonists (e.g. losartan, valsartan) are similar in effect to the ACE inhibitors but, because they do not inhibit the breakdown of bradykinin and other kinins, avoid the dry cough that can prohibit the use of an ACE inhibitor.

Beta-blockers reduce blood pressure and cardiac output, block peripheral adrenoceptors and alter baroreceptor reflex sensitivity. Beta-blockers with intrinsic sympathomimetic activity (e.g. acebutalol, pindolol) stimulate as well as block adrenergic receptors, and may cause less bradycardia and coldness of the extremities. Water-soluble β-blockers (e.g. atenolol, nadolol) are less likely to cross the blood–brain barrier and cause sleep disturbance. Some β-blockers have less effect on beta$_2$-(bronchial) receptors (e.g. atenolol, bisoprolol, metoprolol). They are therefore relatively cardioselective, and less likely to provoke bronchospasm. However, all β-blockers should be avoided in patients with asthma or chronic obstructive airways disease.

Beta-blockers are no longer recommended as first-line therapy because of evidence that they perform less well than other drugs, particularly in the elderly, and increasing evidence that they carry an unacceptable risk of provoking type 2 diabetes.

The *aldosterone* antagonist spironolactone may be of value in resistant hypertension.

Moxonidine, methyldopa and *clonidine* are centrally acting antihypertensive drugs. *Aliskiren* inhibits the action of renin.

Severe hypertension

Very severe hypertension (diastolic > 140 mmHg) or malignant hypertension (with papilloedema) should be treated in hospital. BP should be reduced gradually with a calcium-channel blocker. Rapid falls in BP can precipitate myocardial ischaemia and reduce cerebral and renal perfusion, leading to stroke and deteriorating renal function. Intravenous vasodilators, e.g. hydrallazine and sodium nitroprusside, are rarely required.

Hypertension in relation to other conditions

Diabetes

Hypertension is more common in patients with diabetes mellitus. Possible reasons include:

- obesity
- increased sympathetic nervous stimulation and catecholamine production
- diabetic nephropathy
- insulin resistance and the associated hyperinsulinaemia.

Treatment

ACE inhibitors or angiotensin receptor blockers with or without a thiazide diuretic (which may provoke hyperglycaemia) are usually the preferred initial therapy. Calcium-channel blockers, α-blockers and β-blockers are also useful. BP control should be combined with aggressive management of dyslipidaemia and hyperglycaemia.

Renal disease

Hypertension is an important cause and consequence of renal disease.

Hypertension as a cause of renal disease

Estimates of the prevalence of chronic kidney disease because of hypertension vary widely. Renal failure caused by hypertension is more common in black than white people, and there appears to be familial clustering of hypertensive renal disease within the black population, raising the possibility of a genetic susceptibility to hypertensive renal damage.

Renal failure is an invariable feature of *accelerated hypertension* in which acute, severe hypertension is associated with gross intimal hyperplasia leading to occlusion of the lumen of small arteries and arterioles within the kidney. Renal failure is a rapid consequence if the BP is not gradually reduced.

Renal disease as a cause of hypertension

Hypertension may occur in renal disease as a result of:

- activation of the renin–angiotensin–aldosterone system
- retention of salt and water
- altered production or excretion of vasoactive substances (e.g. endothelin)
- alterations in the structure and function of resistance vessels.

Renovascular hypertension

The presence of an abdominal bruit, atherosclerosis elsewhere, hypokalaemia or deteriorating renal function following treatment with ACE inhibitors are all suggestive of renovascular hypertension.

Atherosclerotic renal disease accounts for most cases, is bilateral in 25% of cases, is most common in the elderly and often results from a plaque in the first part of the renal artery. Fibromuscular renal artery disease occurs predominantly in young women, is frequently bilateral and often involves the distal portion of the artery, giving rise to a beaded appearance on arteriography.

Diagnosis

Renal arteriography remains the principal method, although duplex ultrasonography and differential isotope renography before and after captopril may also provide useful information. Contrast-enhanced magnetic resonance angiography provides accurate imaging, but its use is limited because in patients with renal dysfunction exposure to gadolinium contrast agents is associated with nephrogenic systemic fibrosis, a systemic fibrosing disorder that principally affects the skin.

Treatment

Medical treatment is aimed at reducing cardiovascular risk with aspirin, statins and antihypertensive

TRIALS BOX 10.9 Revascularisation in renovascular disease

In the ASTRAL (Angioplasty and STent for Renal Artery Lesions) trial 806 patients with atherosclerotic renovascular disease were randomised either to undergo revascularisation in addition to receiving medical therapy or to receive medical therapy alone.

The investigators found substantial risks but no evidence of a worthwhile clinical benefit from revascularisation in patients with atherosclerotic renovascular disease. Source: *New England Journal of Medicine* 2009; **361**(20): 1953–1962.

agents (ACE inhibitors should be used with caution as renal perfusion in the presence of renal artery stenosis is dependent on angiotensin II). The benefits of revascularisation are unclear (see Trials Box 10.9).

Pregnancy

Stroke volume and heart rate increase during pregnancy, leading to increased cardiac output. BP usually falls during early pregnancy as a result of reduced peripheral resistance, but rises towards non-pregnant values by term.

Gestational hypertension occurs in women who develop hypertension without proteinuria after 20 weeks of gestation. Hypertension before 20 weeks suggests chronic hypertension, which is confirmed if hypertension persists after delivery.

Pre-eclampsia is defined by pregnancy-induced hypertension (systolic blood pressure of 140 mmHg or more or a diastolic blood pressure of 90 mmHg or more on two occasions at least 6 h apart) and proteinuria greater than 300 mg/24 h or urinary protein to creatinine ratio >30 mg/mmol. Serum uric acid is usually raised. It may lead, often rapidly, to haemolysis, epileptic seizures, abnormal liver function tests and low platelet count (HELP syndrome). Pre-eclampsia affects about 5% of primiparae, but is less common in subsequent pregnancies by the same father.

Treatment

Mild pre-eclampsia is treated with bed rest and close maternal and fetal monitoring. NICE guidance (www.nice.org.uk/CG107) recommends treatment for moderate hypertension (150/100–159/109 mmHg) or severe hypertension (≥160/110 mmHg) with labetalol as first line. Calcium-channel blockers do not appear to be teratogenic but can inhibit labour. ACE inhibitors are associated with fetal abnormalities and are contraindicated. Diuretics interfere with physiological plasma volume expansion. Parenteral hydralazine or α-blockers can be used for control of severe hypertension. Seizures (eclampsia) are managed with intravenous magnesium sulphate. Delivery cures both eclampsia and pre-eclampsia. Low-dose aspirin (75–81 mg/day) is effective at preventing pre-eclampsia in women at increased risk.

Valvular heart disease

See Chapter 3, Fig. 3.2.

Aortic stenosis

Aetiology

Valvular stenosis

Valvular stenosis is caused by calcification of an otherwise normal valve. It occurs earlier (5th to 6th decades) in congenital bicuspid valves. Rheumatic valve disease is now rare.

Congenital aortic stenosis (very rare)

Congenital aortic stenosis can be due to subvalvular stenosis (with fibromuscular hypertrophy or hypertrophic obstructive cardiomyopathy) or supravalvular stenosis (with elfin facies and infantile hypercalcaemia; Williams syndrome).

Symptoms

There may be no symptoms initially. Later angina, dyspnoea and syncope (which may be a result of the low cardiac output) occur.

Signs

- Regular slow-rising, slow-falling (plateau) pulse.
- Small pulse pressure (e.g. BP 105/90 mmHg).
- Left ventricular hypertrophy (sustained and heaving apex).
- There may be an aortic thrill in systole.
  - Auscultation: an aortic systolic ejection murmur occurs, maximal in the right second intercostal space radiating to the neck, with

a quiet delayed or absent second sound. An ejection click indicates valvular stenosis. The murmur becomes less marked when the stenosis is very tight because the flow falls as the heart pump fails.

NB: Neither supravalvular nor subvalvular stenosis has an ejection click. Post-stenotic dilatation is uncommon in subvalvular stenosis (see later).

Investigations

- ECG shows LVH and usually left atrial hypertrophy. Severe stenosis in adults is unlikely if LVH is not present.
- Chest X-ray: left ventricular enlargement may not be present, even in the presence of a prominent apex beat. The aortic valve may be calcified (best seen on lateral chest X-ray).
- Echocardiography defines the size of the orifice and degree of thickening and the gradient across the valve, which may be bicuspid, and LV size and function.
- The pressure gradient across the valve can be measured by cardiac catheterisation, when coronary arteriography can also be performed.

Complications

- left ventricular failure
- infective endocarditis
- syncope
- sudden death (probably caused by ventricular arrhythmia)

Management

Valve replacement is indicated for asymptomatic severe stenosis (gradient > 50 mmHg), or for symptomatic deterioration including syncope. Balloon aortic valvuloplasty can be used when valve replacement is not possible.

Aortic regurgitation

Aetiology

Congenital bicuspid valve and infective endocarditis are the most common identifiable causes. Rheumatic valve disease is now a rare cause. Less common associations include seronegative arthritis (ankylosing spondylitis, Reiter syndrome, colitic and psoriatic arthropathy), congenital lesions (coarctation of the aorta, Marfan syndrome), traumatic rupture and syphilis.

Symptoms

There are usually none until dyspnoea from pulmonary oedema occurs. Angina is not common.

Signs

The pulse has a sharp rise and fall ('water-hammer' or 'collapsing') and there is a wide pulse pressure. There may be marked carotid pulsation in the neck (Corrigan's sign). The left ventricle is enlarged and the apex displaced laterally.

There is an early blowing diastolic murmur at the left sternal edge maximal in the left third and fourth intercostal spaces, heard best with the patient leaning forward and with the breath held in expiration. The second sound is quiet. There is usually a systolic flow murmur, which does not necessarily indicate aortic stenosis. There may be a diastolic murmur at the apex, which sounds like mitral stenosis, as the regurgitant aortic jet strikes the mitral valve (Austin Flint murmur).

Investigations

- ECG shows left ventricular hypertrophy.
- Chest X-ray shows cardiac enlargement.
- Echocardiography will demonstrate dilatation of the aortic root and the separation of the cusps. Left ventricular function and dimension can be assessed. The mitral valve can be affected with fluttering of the anterior leaflet and premature closure if the regurgitation is severe.

Management

- *Surgical.* Valve replacement should be considered for symptomatic deterioration if the heart size increases rapidly or if the left ventricular internal diameter is >55 mm on echocardiography in a young patient, even if asymptomatic.

Dominance of the lesion in combined rheumatic aortic stenosis/aortic regurgitation

Aortic regurgitation is dominant if the pulse volume is high, the pulse pressure collapsing and the left ventricle enlarged and displaced. Aortic stenosis is dominant if the pulse is of small volume ('plateau pulse') and the pulse pressure low. The ventricular apex of a hypertrophied ventricle is not necessarily displaced.

Mitral stenosis

Aetiology

This is almost invariably a late consequence of rheumatic fever, and now rare.

Symptoms

- Dyspnoea occurs at night and on exertion and is caused by pulmonary oedema.
- Palpitation is caused by atrial fibrillation. There is a high risk of embolism.
- Haemoptysis is caused by pulmonary hypertension, pulmonary oedema or pulmonary embolism.
- Fatigue and cold extremities are caused by a low cardiac output. Angina may rarely occur.

Signs

- Mitral facies. This is a dusky purple flush of the cheeks with dilated capillaries (malar flush).
- Arterial pulse is of small volume caused by obstruction to flow at the mitral valve. It may be irregular because of atrial fibrillation.
- The apex beat is tapping. This represents a palpable first sound.
- If pulmonary hypertension has developed, there is a left parasternal heave of right ventricular hypertrophy. A diastolic thrill can be present in severe disease.

Auscultation

The mitral first sound is loud because the mitral valve is held wide open by high atrial pressure until ventricular systole slams it shut.

The length of the murmur is proportional to the degree of stenosis. The murmur is easier to hear with the patient lying on the left side. The presence of an opening snap and a loud first sound suggest a pliable valve.

NB: Some of the signs of mitral stenosis can be given by the Austin Flint murmur of aortic regurgitation (the regurgitant aortic jet strikes the normal mitral valve) and very rarely by a left atrial myxoma.

Assessment

- *ECG*: in early disease, the P mitrale of left atrial hypertrophy develops. This disappears with the onset of atrial fibrillation. Right ventricular hypertrophy may be present.
- *Chest X-ray*: characteristically, there is left atrial enlargement and enlargement of the pulmonary arteries. The mitral valve may be calcified. There may be features of pulmonary oedema.
- *Echocardiogram* demonstrates valve thickening and calcification (a mitral valve area of $<1.5\,cm^2$ indicates critical stenosis) and gives an assessment of ventricular function.
- *Pulmonary hypertension*: fatigue and symptoms of right heart failure indicate raised pulmonary vascular resistance. The development of pulmonary hypertension is indicated by a dominant 'a' wave in the jugular venous pulse (unless in atrial fibrillation), a loud pulmonary second sound, right ventricular hypertrophy, rarely pulmonary incompetence and low-volume peripheral arterial pulse (mnemonic: April).
- *Presence of other lesions:* mitral regurgitation and other valve lesions must be noted and assessed, particularly if symptoms indicate surgical intervention.

Complications

- pulmonary oedema
- right heart failure
- atrial fibrillation
- systemic embolisation
- infective endocarditis

Management

Anticoagulation and rate control is indicated when atrial fibrillation develops or there is left atrial enlargement (Box 10.2).

Valvotomy (trans-septal balloon or open valvotomy) is indicated in patients who are symptomatic or have pulmonary hypertension. Valve replacement is indicated if the valve morphology is not suitable for valvotomy or there is left atrial thrombus despite anticoagulation or concomitant moderate to severe regurgitation.

Mitral regurgitation

Aetiology

- floppy (prolapsing) mitral valve leaflets
- ischaemic papillary muscle dysfunction, particularly after inferior myocardial infarction
- severe left ventricular failure with dilatation of the mitral ring
- rheumatic fever
- rarely, cardiomyopathy, congenital malformation (Marfan syndrome), infective endocarditis and rupture of the chordae tendinae

Symptoms

Progressive dyspnoea develops as a result of pulmonary congestion and this is followed by right heart failure. Fatigue and palpitation are common.

Signs

- *Palpitation*: LVH and a systolic thrill are characteristic. A left parasternal heave may be present.
- *Auscultation*: there is an apical pansystolic murmur radiating to the left axilla. The mitral sound is soft. There may be a third sound caused by rapid ventricular filling. A short mid-diastolic murmur in severe mitral regurgitation does not necessarily indicate valve stenosis.
- *Mitral valve prolapse* produces a late systolic click and murmur. It is late because the posterior leaflet of the valve only starts to leak when the ventricular pressure is at its highest. In the middle-aged and elderly it is associated with a wear and tear disorder of the leaflet, chordae or papillary muscles (particularly after myocardial infarction). A floppy valve can be detected in up to 5% of young people by echocardiography. The prognosis is usually excellent, although it has been associated with arrhythmias, syncope, atypical chest pain and bacterial endocarditis.

Investigations

- *ECG* may show LVH and the P mitrale of left atrial hypertrophy. Atrial fibrillation is less common than in mitral stenosis.
- *Chest X-ray*: the left atrium and ventricle are enlarged, the former sometimes being enormous.
- *Echocardiography* helps to distinguish between the various causes and to assess left ventricular function.
- *Assessment of the dominance of the lesions in combined mitral stenosis/mitral regurgitation*: mitral stenosis is more likely to be the dominant lesion if the pulse volume is small (in the absence of failure) and if there is no LVH.

Complications

These are similar to those in mitral stenosis except that infective endocarditis is more common and embolism less common.

Management

Valve repair or replacement is indicated if the symptoms are severe and uncontrolled by medical therapy, or if pulmonary hypertension develops. Indications for anticoagulation are atrial fibrillation, systemic embolism and prosthetic valves.

Other valve disease

Tricuspid regurgitation

Tricuspid regurgitation may be caused by *dilatation of the tricuspid valve ring* in right ventricular failure from any cause, *rheumatic fever* (where it is invariably associated with disease of mitral and/or aortic valves), *endocarditis* in drug addicts, or carcinoid heart disease. The signs include:

- giant 'v' waves in the jugular venous pulse and systolic pulsation of an enlarged liver (both caused by the transmission of ventricular filling through the open tricuspid valve)
- right ventricular enlargement causing marked pulsation at the lower left sternal edge and a pansystolic murmur, loudest in inspiration, heard at the lower end of the sternum.

There is often ankle and sacral oedema, ascites and jaundice from hepatic congestion.

Pulmonary stenosis

Pulmonary stenosis is usually congenital but may follow maternal rubella. Rarely, it is associated with Noonan syndrome (Turner's phenotype affecting males and females with normal chromosome number). Rheumatic fever and carcinoid are extremely rare causes. Fatigue and syncope occur if the stenosis is severe. Patients may show peripheral cyanosis, a low-volume pulse and a large 'a' wave in the jugular venous pulse wave. Right ventricular hypertrophy causes a parasternal heave. There is a systolic thrill and murmur in the pulmonary area (second left intercostal space) and an ejection click. The pulmonary component of the second sound is quiet and late.

Atrial myxoma

Atrial myxoma may mimic valve disease. It is very rare. It usually occurs in the left atrium and presents with features of mitral stenosis, systemic emboli and constitutional upset with fever. It can mimic bacterial endocarditis. It is best diagnosed by echocardiography where the tumour produces characteristic echoes as it moves between the mitral valve leaflets in ventricular diastole and in the atrium in systole. Rarely, it is a manifestation of the autosomal dominant Carney complex.

Congenital heart disease

Congenital heart disease may present as an isolated cardiac abnormality or as part of a systemic syndrome.

Maternal rubella

Maternal rubella infection is dangerous in the first 3 months of pregnancy (particularly the first month when 50% of fetuses are affected). The cardiac lesions are in three groups:

- patent ductus arteriosus
- septal defects: atrial septal defect, ventricular septal defect, Fallot's tetralogy
- right-sided outflow obstruction: pulmonary valve, artery or branch stenoses.

The systemic syndrome includes cataract, nerve deafness and mental retardation. All children are offered rubella vaccine at the age of 12 years. Boys are included to reduce transmission. Fertile women given vaccine must not become pregnant in the immediate future.

If a pregnant woman is in contact with rubella, serum should be taken for antibody levels to rubella if these are not known. If raised, this is evidence of previous infection and there is little or no risk to the fetus. If the titre is not raised, a repeat sample is measured 3–4 weeks later (or if symptoms appear in the mother) and if the titre has risen significantly, this is evidence of recent infection. The earlier that this occurs in the pregnancy, the greater the risk to the fetus.

Down syndrome (usually 21-trisomy)

This is associated with septal defects, particularly ventricular.

Turner syndrome (XO)

This is associated with coarctation of the aorta. Affected females are short and the neck may appear webbed. Ovaries fail to develop properly, leading to primary amenorrhoea. Hearing loss, renal anomalies and hypothyroidism are recognised associations.

Marfan syndrome (arachnodactyly)

This is an autosomal dominant disorder which is caused by the misfolding of fibrillin-1 and affects the aortic media, eyes and limb skeleton. The prevalence is approximately 1 in 5000.

It is characterised by disproportionate length of the long bones, which results in span exceeding height and long fingers and toes. Joints tend to be hyperextensible. There is frequently a high arched palate, pectus excavatum, scoliosis, little subcutaneous fat and lens dislocation with myopia. Aortic valve regurgitation and dissection of the aorta are common, and mitral regurgitation may develop.

Working classification

An asterisk denotes the most frequent.

Stenosis

- semilunar valves: aortic stenosis (supra- and subvalvular and valve stenoses), pulmonary stenosis
- atrioventricular valves: mitral stenosis, tricuspid stenosis
- major arteries: coarctation of aorta*, pulmonary artery stenosis

Regurgitation

- semilunar valves: aortic regurgitation, pulmonary regurgitation (very rare)
- atrioventricular valves: mitral regurgitation, tricuspid regurgitation, Ebstein's anomaly

Shunts

- left-to-right: ASD*, VSD*, patent ductus arteriosus
- (PDA)*, aortopulmonary window
- right-to-left (cyanotic): transposition of the great vessels, Fallot's tetralogy*, Eisenmenger syndrome

Atrial septal defect (ASD)

This accounts for 10% of all cases of congenital heart disease. It occasionally occurs in Marfan syndrome.

- *Ostium secundum* is usually uncomplicated. Compared with other congenital heart defects, there is a high (and late) incidence of atrial fibrillation and an extremely low incidence of endocarditis.

- *Ostium primum* often involves the atrioventricular valves to produce mitral and tricuspid regurgitation and may even have an associated VSD. In most respects (embryology, cardiodynamics, complications and prognosis) it is quite different from ostium secundum ASD.

Symptoms

In simple lesions there are usually no symptoms, although dyspnoea can occur, usually for the first time in middle age. It is usually detected at routine chest X-ray.

Signs

Characteristically, there is fixed, wide splitting of the second sound. Flow through the defect does not itself produce a murmur, but increased right heart output gives a pulmonary flow murmur and large shunts may produce a tricuspid diastolic flow murmur. In ostium primum there may be signs of the associated lesions and mitral (plus occasional tricuspid) regurgitation. The precordium may be deformed and the pulse volume small. A left parasternal lift of right ventricular hypertrophy may be present.

Assessment

ECG

- *Ostium secundum*: there is partial right bundle branch block with right axis deviation and right ventricular hypertrophy. Atrial fibrillation may occur.
- *Ostium primum*: usually, there is left axis deviation with evidence of right ventricular hypertrophy. Conduction defects and junctional dysrhythmias occur.

Chest X-ray

This shows enlargement of the right atrium and ventricle with enlarged pulmonary arteries and plethoric lung fields (evidence of increased right-sided flow). The aorta appears small (evidence of decreased left-sided blood flow).

Cardiac catheterisation

This reveals a step up in oxygen saturation in the right atrium.

Complications

- Eisenmenger syndrome. If the left-to-right shunt through the defect results in pulmonary hypertension with pressure above systemic level, a reversed shunt develops.
- Atrial fibrillation.
- Tricuspid regurgitation (from right ventricular enlargement).
- Infective endocarditis occurs in ostium primum, but
- rarely in ostium secundum defects.

Management

Surgical repair has been largely replaced by endovascular closure.

Patent ductus arteriosus

This represents 15% of all cases of congenital heart disease. It is associated with the rubella syndrome. It is more common in females.

Symptoms

Usually there are none. Bronchitis and dyspnoea on exertion occur later and with severe lesions.

Signs

The pulse may be collapsing (water hammer) and the left ventricle hypertrophied. There is a continuous (machinery) murmur with systolic accentuation, maximal in the second left intercostal space and posteriorly.

Assessment

- The *ECG* is normal or there may be left ventricular hypertrophy.
- *Chest X-ray*: the aorta and left ventricle may be enlarged. The pulmonary artery is enlarged and there is pulmonary plethora.
- *Echocardiography* shows a dilated left atrium and left ventricle.

Complications

- endarteritis (of the ductus)
- heart failure (Eisenmenger syndrome, page 119, Chapter 10, as a result of pulmonary hypertension and shunt reversal)

Management

Indometacin is given within 1–3 weeks of birth to close the duct, possibly by blocking prostaglandin E production in the duct muscle. If this is unsuccessful, surgical ligation (1–5 years) is required or possibly an umbrella occlusion device. Cyanosis contraindicates surgery.

Ventricular septal defect

- *Small defect*: is also called *maladie de Roger*. There is a loud murmur with a normal-sized heart, chest X-ray and ECG.
- *Large defect*: the clinical importance of this depends on the pulmonary vascular resistance, which determines how much shunting is present and its direction of flow.

Symptoms

There are none unless the VSD is large, when there may be dyspnoea.

Signs

There may be a small-volume pulse and LVH may be present (and right ventricular hypertrophy too, if there is pulmonary hypertension). A pansystolic murmur (and thrill) is present in the fourth left intercostal space. A mitral diastolic flow murmur implies a large shunt.

Assessment

- *ECG* shows LVH.
- *Chest X-ray*: enlargement of the left atrium and ventricle may be present. The pulmonary arteries are enlarged if there is pulmonary hypertension.

Complications

- endocarditis can occur, with emboli into the pulmonary circulation
- Eisenmenger syndrome page 119, Chapter 10

Management

- A small VSD may close spontaneously. Surgery is not indicated for the endocarditis risk alone.
- A large VSD needs closure in most cases to prevent the development of irreversible pulmonary vascular damage.

Fallot's tetralogy

The four features (tetralogy) are:

1. VSD in which the shunt is from right to left because of;
2. pulmonary stenosis, infundibular or valvular;
3. right ventricular hypertrophy caused by the consequent load on the right ventricle;
4. associated dextroposition of the aorta so that it sits over the defect in the septum.

Symptoms

- syncope
- squatting (this may help decrease the right-to-left shunt by increasing systemic resistance and reducing venous return)
- dyspnoea
- retardation of growth

Signs

- Cyanosis and finger clubbing.
- The typical murmur is of pulmonary stenosis with a quiet or inaudible pulmonary second sound.

Assessment

- The *ECG* usually shows moderate right atrial and ventricular hypertrophy.
- *Chest X-ray* shows a normal-sized but boot-shaped heart and a large aorta with a small pulmonary artery and pulmonary oligaemia. It is boot-shaped because of the small left pulmonary artery.
- Polycythaemia is common.

Complications

- cyanotic and syncopal attacks (sometimes fatal)
- cerebral abscesses
- endocarditis
- paradoxical emboli
- strokes (thrombotic–polycythaemia)
- epilepsy is more common than in the general population

Management

Surgical correction.

Coarctation of the aorta

It is associated with Marfan and Turner syndromes. Ninety-eight percent are distal to the origin of the left subclavian artery.

Signs

- Classically, there is radial–femoral arterial pulse delay, with a smaller volume femoral pulse than radial. The blood pressure may be raised in the arms (especially on exercise), different between the two sides and low in the legs. Asymmetry of radial pulses may be present.
- Visible and/or palpable scapular collateral arteries.
- Left ventricular hypertrophy.
- The murmurs are:
  - a systolic murmur at front and back of the left upper thorax
  - collateral murmurs over the scapulae
  - an aortic systolic murmur (of an associated bicuspid valve in some cases) that is usually obscured by the coarctation murmur.

Assessment

- *ECG* for LVH.
- *Chest X-ray:* a double aortic knuckle results from stenosis and post-stenotic dilatation. There is rib notching (and notching at the scapular margin) and normal or large cardiac shadow.

Associations

Bicuspid aortic valve, cerebral aneurysms and patent ductus arteriosus.

Management

Percutaneous intervention (angioplasty with or without stenting or surgical correction).

Eisenmenger syndrome

There is a reversal of a left-to-right shunt (e.g. VSD, ASD, PDA) because of pulmonary hypertension. With left-to-right shunts there is pulmonary circulatory overload, and an increase in pulmonary vascular resistance follows with the development of pulmonary hypertension. When the pressure on the right side of the shunt exceeds that on the left side, the shunt flow reverses. The patient becomes cyanosed and develops symptoms of dyspnoea, syncope and angina. The lesion must be surgically corrected before this stage is reached. If not, heart–lung transplantation should be considered.

Infective endocarditis

Acute

Heart valves are infected as part of an acute septicaemia. Healthy valves are often affected. It follows infection with staphylococcus, often in association with in-dwelling intravenous catheters or primary infection of the lungs or skin. *Streptococcus pneumoniae, Haemophilus influenzae,* gonococcus and meningococcus may also be responsible.

Subacute

This is usually bacterial – subacute bacterial endocarditis (SBE).

Predisposing abnormalities

- *Congenital*: VSD, PDA, coarctation of the aorta and bicuspid aortic valves.
- *Acquired*: rheumatic valve disease now accounts for less than one-quarter of all UK cases. Mitral valve prolapse, calcified aortic stenosis and syphilitic aortitis (rare) predispose to endocarditis. It occurs on prosthetic valves. The normal tricuspid valve is at special risk in drug addicts.

Organisms

The origin of infection varies with the infecting organism and includes teeth and tonsils (*Streptococcus viridans*), urinary tract and bowel (*S. faecalis*), central venous catheterisation (*Staphylococcus*) and the skin (*Staphylococcus*). Rarer causes include *Coxiella burnetii* (Q fever) and fungi.

Diagnosis

The diagnosis of infective endocarditis should be considered in any patient with a predisposing cardiac lesion who develops any illness. The most efficient way to establish the diagnosis is by:

- repeated examination, particularly for changing murmurs
- blood cultures (at least three sets)
- urinalysis for microscopic haematuria
- echocardiography for vegetations, including transoesophageal echocardiography (TOE) if not detected by transthoracic echocardiogram.

Clinical features

The symptoms and signs may be considered in three groups.

1. *Signs of general infection*: lethargy, malaise, anaemia and low-grade fever are frequent but not invariable. Clubbing of the fingers and splenomegaly are fairly late signs (6–8 weeks). There may be transient myalgia or arthralgia. The white cell count may be low, normal or high.
2. *Signs of underlying cardiac lesions* must be sought. New lesions and changing murmurs are highly suggestive and the patient must be examined for these daily.
3. *Embolic phenomena*: large emboli may travel to the brain and viscera or cause occlusion of peripheral arteries. Emboli from left-to-right shunts (VSD and PDA) and on right-sided heart valves go to the lungs, giving pleurisy and lung abscesses.

Vasculitic phenomena cause splinter haemorrhages in the nail bed and microscopic haematuria. Osler's nodes in the finger pulp are pathognomonic but rare. Roth spots in the eye also occur rarely.

The renal lesions are of two kinds:

- a diffuse, proliferative glomerulonephritis
- focal emboli.

Immune complexes are present in serum and complement levels reduced.

Management

Prophylaxis

Patients with acquired valvular heart disease, valve replacement, structural congenital heart disease, hypertrophic cardiomyopathy and previous infective endocarditis are at increased risk of endocarditis. NICE has reviewed the need for antibiotic prophylaxis in these patients and recommends that antibiotic prophylaxis against infective endocarditis should not be offered to people undergoing dental procedures or procedures involving the upper and lower gastrointestinal tract, genitourinary tract or upper and lower respiratory tract. Episodes of infection in people at risk of infective endocarditis should be investigated and treated promptly.

Chemotherapy

It is essential to obtain blood culture before starting chemotherapy. Antibiotic therapy is guided by identification of the causative organism, but it should not be delayed in the presence of good clinical evidence even if cultures are negative. Eighty percent of cases are due to streptococcal and staphylococcal organisms. *Staphylococcus aureus* is the most frequent organism when the source of infection has been an intravenous catheter and in intravenous drug abusers who commonly infect tricuspid valves. It also frequently causes endocarditis in patients with insulin-dependent diabetes mellitus. A wide spectrum of organisms can infect prosthetic valves. Gram-positive and Gram-negative bacilli are relatively uncommon causative organisms. Fungal endocarditis, particularly *Candida,* usually occurs in patients with prosthetic valves, compromised immune systems and intravenous drug abuse.

Therapy should be continued for at least 4 weeks (intravenously for at least the first 2 weeks), if effective blood concentrations can be achieved. The patient should be carefully followed for recurrence. Emboli may occur for up to 1–2 months after cure.

Indications for surgery

Surgery must be considered early for valve rupture, intractable heart failure, resistant infection particularly of a valve prosthesis, and if the organisms are drug-resistant.

Culture-negative endocarditis

This diagnosis is considered after six successive negative cultures when culture technique is known to be good. The following should be considered:

- unsuspected organisms, e.g. *Coxiella burnetii* (Q fever), especially if the aortic valve is diseased. The diagnosis depends on finding a rise in antibody titre. *Bacteroides:* anaerobic culture is required (and kept for up to 3 weeks). Fungi: *Candida, Aspergillus, Histoplasma*
- partly treated bacterial causes
- right-sided endocarditis
- systemic vasculitis, systemic lupus erythematosus (SLE), atrial myxoma or the antiphospholipid syndrome (page 318, Chapter 18)
- non-bacterial thrombotic endocarditis associated with carcinoma.

Constrictive pericarditis

Aetiology

This is now rare. It may be caused by tuberculosis following spread from the pleura or mediastinal lymph glands. It may follow acute viral or pyogenic pericarditis, but the cause is often unclear. Haemo-pericardium, irradiation and carcinoma account for a few cases. It may be simulated by restrictive cardiomyopathy (page 123, Chapter 10).

Clinical features

Symptoms result from cardiac constriction with decreased filling and low cardiac output. Right heart failure predominates over left. Fatigue and ascites with little or no ankle swelling are characteristic, but dyspnoea and ankle swelling may occur later. Pulmonary oedema and paroxysmal nocturnal dyspnoea are rare.

Examination

The pulse is rapid and volume small and there may be arterial paradox (pulsus paradoxus), as with acute pericarditis. Atrial fibrillation may be present. Ascites may be the presenting feature and the elevated JVP may be missed because it is so high. The classical JVP signs of diastolic collapse (steep 'y' descent) and a further rise on inspiration (Kussmaul's sign) are often not observed. The liver, and sometimes the spleen, is enlarged. Ventricular contraction may cause localised indrawing of the chest wall at the apex. The heart sounds may be normal, although quiet. A third sound, brought about by an abrupt end to ventricular filling, may be present.

Investigation

- *ECG:* there may be widespread ST changes with low voltage complexes, and atrial fibrillation.
- *Chest X-ray:* there may be calcification of the pericardium. Cardiomegaly may be present.
- *Echocardiography* shows the rigid, thickened pericardium, particularly if calcified, large atria with normal (or small) ventricles, and ventricular filling predominantly in early diastole.

Management

No action is needed if the patient is symptom-free and the assessment confirms mild disease. Close follow-up is essential. Pericardiectomy is performed if severe constriction is present.

Acute pericarditis

Aetiology

Pericarditis is common within the first week of acute myocardial infarction. Dressler syndrome is uncommon and occurs between 2 weeks and 2 months after myocardial infarction or cardiac surgery. It is characterised by fever, pleurisy and pericarditis.

Infective pericarditis is usually a complication of chest infection. Acute benign pericarditis often follows a respiratory infection and is probably viral. A rising antibody titre to Coxsackie B virus is sometimes found. Suppurative pericarditis is rare. It results from infection with staphylococcus or, occasionally, haemolytic streptococcus. Tuberculous pericarditis is very rare and non-suppurative.

Pericarditis occurs as part of systemic syndromes, including rheumatic fever, SLE, severe uraemia, local extension of carcinoma of the bronchus and following trauma.

Clinical features

There is central, poorly localised tightness in the chest that varies with movement, posture and respiration. There may be pain referred to the left shoulder if the diaphragm is affected. The pericardial rub varies with time, position and respiration.

The signs of pericardial effusion without tamponade are an absent apex beat, a silent heart and disappearance of the rub. Tamponade, which is rare, produces the following:

- Pulsus paradoxus: the pulse volume decreases in the normal person on inspiration. This is more marked with tamponade and is then known as pulsus paradoxus. The paradox that Kussmaul noted was that the heart continued to beat strongly while the peripheral arterial pulse virtually disappeared during inspiration.
- A rise in the JVP on inspiration (Kussmaul's sign).

Both pulsus paradoxus and Kussmaul's sign result from decreased cardiac filling on inspiration because of the descending diaphragm stretching the pericardium and increasing the intrapericardial pressure.

Assessment

- *ECG*: there is raised concave elevation of the ST segment in most leads (especially II and V3–4) and T-wave inversion. The voltage is low in the presence of effusion.
- *Chest X-ray*: it is unchanged in the absence of effusion. Effusion classically produces an enlarged pear-shaped cardiac shadow with loss of normal contours.
- *Echocardiography* is the most sensitive way of detecting pericardial fluid with free space between the heart and pericardium.

Management

Aspiration for tamponade (if the systolic arterial blood pressure falls below 90–100 mmHg). Treat the underlying condition. Recurrent effusion with tamponade is treated by insertion of a drain or creation of a pericardial window.

Syphilitic aortitis and carditis

Late syphilis is rare in the UK. Acquired syphilis affects the aorta, the aortic ring to produce dilatation or aneurysm, and aortic regurgitation and the coronary artery orifices to cause angina.

Cardiomyopathy

This word means disorder of the heart muscle. It is classified into three major groups depending upon the effect on the left ventricle, which may be: hypertrophied, dilated or restricted.

Hypertrophic cardiomyopathy

Also known as HCM, it is usually familial. It results in asymmetrical LVH associated with:

- loss of left ventricular distensibility, which leads to symptoms of dyspnoea, pulmonary oedema and syncope – some patients develop angina

- hypertrophy, particularly of the left ventricle and septum with mitral regurgitation – in some patients this disappears with progression of the disease as the heart muscle fails.

Signs

There is a steep-rising, jerky pulse (unlike the slow-rising, plateau pulse of aortic valve stenosis), cardiac hypertrophy, a palpable atrial beat followed by a late systolic aortic ejection murmur, usually heard best in the left third and fourth intercostal spaces. There may be associated signs of mitral regurgitation. Complications include arrhythmias, systemic embolism, congestive heart failure and sudden death.

Investigation

Echocardiography shows asymmetrical septal hypertrophy, systolic anterior movement of the mitral valve and a narrow left ventricular cavity with hypertrophied trabeculae and papillary muscles. A 24-h ECG record may identify those most at risk from sudden death from dysrhythmias.

Management

Beta-blockade is given to increase left ventricular compliance and reduce the incidence of dysrhythmias and angina. Other anti-arrhythmic therapies or implantable cardioverter-defibrillator should be considered. Patients who develop atrial fibrillation should be anticoagulated and digoxin can be added. Patients are at risk from endocarditis. Treat for cardiac failure and if medical therapy fails, consider transplantation. Patients should receive genetic counselling and screening of their families should be offered.

Dilated (congestive) cardiomyopathy

This is very rarely familial. The label 'congestive cardiomyopathy' covers a large group of aetiologically unrelated disorders that tend to present as low-output congestive heart failure. By convention, the more common and more easily diagnosed myocardial disorders are excluded, i.e. ischaemic, hypertensive and rheumatic heart diseases. Angina, systemic and pulmonary infarcts, conduction defects and arrhythmias occur.

Aetiology

- Alcoholism and thiamine deficiency.
- Infections: viruses, e.g. influenza A_2, Coxsackie B, *Toxoplasma,* diphtheria.
- Infiltrations: sarcoidosis, amyloidosis (primary and secondary to myeloma), haemochromatosis.
- Auto-immune disease: SLE, polyartertis nodosa, diffuse systemic sclerosis.
- Muscular dystrophies and Friedreich's ataxia (page 232, Chapter 15).
- Endocrine: hyper- and hypothyroidism.
- Postpartum.

Management

Treat heart failure, page 103, Chapter 10. Anticoagulants are given because of the risks of embolism. Treat any underlying pathology (e.g. thyroid disease, auto-immune disease).

Restrictive cardiomyopathy

The efficiency of the ventricles as pumps is restricted by endocardial fibrosis or by granulation tissue – respectively, endomyocardial fibrosis (EMF) of equatorial Africa or Löffler eosinophilic endomyocardial disease. In the UK, amyloidosis is the most common cause of this rare condition.

Peripheral arterial disease

There are four common clinical syndromes: intermittent claudication, acute obstruction, ischaemic foot and Raynaud's phenomenon.

Intermittent claudication

Most cases are found in males >50 years of age. The disorder is associated with smoking, diabetes mellitus and hyperlipidaemia, and occasionally precipitated by anaemia. Obstruction is most commonly femoro-popliteal, and less often aorto-iliac or distal.

Diagnosis

The history is of pain in the calf on effort with rapid relief by rest. The Leriche syndrome is buttock claudication with impotence. The major peripheral arterial pulses are reduced or absent. There may be arterial bruits over the aorta, iliac or femoral arteries. The tissues of the leg atrophy with reduced muscle bulk and hair loss is common. There may be cyanosis, pallor or redness, oedema, ulcers or gangrene.

Doppler ultrasound is useful. Arteriography is required if surgery is contemplated.

Prognosis

Claudication usually indicates generalised vascular disease and most patients die from cardiovascular or cerebrovascular disease. Diabetes mellitus and persistent smoking are associated with a worse prognosis.

Management

- Stop smoking.
- Manage hyperlipidaemia and take aspirin.
- Exercise within the effort tolerance to help develop collateral vessels. Treat obesity and hypertension.
- Check for and treat diabetes, polycythaemia and anaemia.
- Attend carefully to foot hygiene.
- Dilatation of narrowed arteries using balloon catheter angioplasty and stenting may be successful.

Endarterectomy is indicated if there is a high block with good distal blood flow on angiography. Bypass (prosthetic or vein graft) surgery may be indicated if angiography shows the vessels to be satisfactory distal to the block.

Acute obstruction

This may be caused by thrombosis or due to embolism (usually blood clot in atrial fibrillation). Most cases are in the legs.

Diagnosis

Pain is associated with numbness, paraesthesiae and paresis. There is pallor and coldness of the limb below the obstruction followed by cyanosis. The limb becomes anaesthetic and the arterial pulses weak or absent.

Management

Treatment should involve vascular surgeons and radiologists, and approaches include anticoagulation and antiplatelet agents, thrombolytic agents and embolectomy, angioplasty and arterial bypass surgery.

Ischaemic foot

This is usually caused by chronic arterial obstruction distal to the knees. It is most commonly seen in diabetes and is associated with neuropathy and local infection.

Symptoms

- Areas of necrosis and ulceration.
- Pain in the foot (often not present in diabetics because of associated peripheral neuropathy).
- Intermittent claudication.

Signs

If the large arteries are narrowed there is pallor and/or cyanosis, empty veins in the feet with trophic changes in nails and absence of hair. The feet are cold and pulses diminished or are absent.

In diabetes, it is often chiefly the small vessels that are affected. The foot pulses can be present despite ischaemia of the toes.

Management

Foot hygiene is important, especially in diabetes. Pain may be severe and require morphine. Angioplasty, stenting or vascular bypass surgery are often not technically feasible. If amputation is required it is frequently above the knee.

Raynaud's phenomenon

Definition

Intermittent, cold-precipitated, symmetrical attacks of pallor and/or cyanosis of the digits without evidence of arterial obstructive disease. The digits become white (arterial spasm), then blue (cyanosis) and finally red (reactive arterial dilatation).

Aetiology

- Idiopathic and familial, usually in young women (Raynaud's disease).
- Auto-immune disease, especially SLE and scleroderma.
- Arterial obstruction, e.g. cervical rib.
- Trauma, usually in occupations involving vibrating tools (vibration white finger).
- Drugs, including β-blockers, the contraceptive pill and ergot derivatives.

Management

Treatment is disappointing. The hands and feet should be kept warm and free from infection. The patient is reassured about the long-term prognosis (usually good) and advised to stop smoking. Electrically heated gloves can be very helpful. Calcium antagonists (e.g. nifedipine) or patches of glyceryl trinitrate can be tried. Sympathectomy is sometimes successful as a last resort, particularly in the presence of recurring skin sepsis. Intravenous prostacyclin (epoprostenol) has been used in severe cases.

 REFERENCE

Thygesen, K., Alpert, J.S., White, H.D. (2007) Joint ESC/ACCF/AHA/WHF Task Force for the Redefinition of Myocardial Infarction. Universal definition of myocardial infarction. Circulation 116: 2634–2653.

11

Respiratory disease

The most common respiratory diseases are infections of the upper respiratory tract, e.g. the common cold. The most common diseases of the lower respiratory tract are pneumonia, asthma and carcinoma of the bronchus.

Chronic obstructive pulmonary disease (COPD)

Definitions

The WHO-sponsored 'Global initiative for chronic obstructive lung disease' (http://www.goldcopd.com) defines COPD as 'a common preventable and treatable disease, characterized by persistent airflow limitation that is usually progressive and associated with an enhanced chronic inflammatory response in the airways to noxious particles or gases. Exacerbations and comorbidities contribute to the overall severity in individual patients.'

COPD covers many previously used labels, including:

- *Emphysema* – enlargement of the air spaces distal to the terminal (smallest) bronchioles with destructive changes in the alveolar wall. In centrilobular emphysema, damage is limited to the central part of the lobule around the respiratory bronchiole, whereas in panacinar emphysema, there is destruction and distension of the whole lobule. If the air spaces are >1 cm in diameter they are called bullae.
- *Chronic obstructive airways disease.*
- *Chronic airflow limitation.*

Poorly reversible airflow limitation may also occur in bronchiectasis, cystic fibrosis, tuberculosis and some cases of chronic asthma.

- *Chronic bronchitis* is daily cough with sputum for at least 3 months a year for at least 2 consecutive years.

Pathogenesis

There is typically chronic inflammation throughout the airways and pulmonary vasculature. In the trachea, and bronchi and bronchioles that are >2–4 mm in internal diameter, inflammatory cells infiltrate the surface epithelium and there is hypersecretion from enlarged mucus-secreting glands and increased numbers of goblet cells. In small bronchi and bronchioles that have an internal diameter <2 mm, chronic inflammation is associated with remodelling of the airway wall, with fibrosis, narrowing the lumen and producing fixed airways obstruction.

Destruction of the lung parenchyma typically occurs as centrilobular emphysema. In mild cases lesions usually involve upper lung regions, but in advanced disease they may appear diffusely throughout the entire lung. Vascular changes occur early. Intimal thickening of the vessel wall is followed by smooth-muscle proliferation and an inflammatory cell infiltrate. These pathological changes lead to characteristic physiological changes. Mucus hypersecretion and ciliary dysfunction cause a chronic productive cough. Airflow limitation, hyperinflation and gas exchange abnormalities cause breathlessness. Pulmonary hypertension and cor pulmonale are late features.

Aetiology

- tobacco smoking
- atmospheric pollution

Clinical Medicine Lecture Notes, Eighth Edition. John R. Bradley, Mark Gurnell, and Diana F. Wood.
© 2019 John Wiley & Sons Ltd. Published 2019 by John Wiley & Sons Ltd.

- α_1-antitrypsin deficiency is a heritable disorder accounting for about 5% of patients with emphysema (and about 20% of neonatal cholestasis). Five percent of homozygotes tend to develop emphysema by the age of 40 years and heterozygotes are at risk. The emphysema is predominantly of the lower zones and is much worse in smokers.

Most patients with COPD die from one of three diseases: CHD; COPD; lung cancer (the risk of many cancers is increased by smoking).

Clinical presentation

Often the patient has a productive morning cough and an increased frequency of lower respiratory tract infections producing purulent sputum. The organisms responsible are usually *Haemophilus influenzae, Streptococcus pneumoniae* and the respiratory viruses. Over years there is slowly progressive dyspnoea with wheezing, exacerbated in the acute infective episodes. There is emphysema with hyperinflation of the lungs. Respiratory failure (page 28, Chapters 4 and 11) and chronic right heart failure (cor pulmonale) are long-term complications.

Investigation

Ventilatory function tests

The diagnosis of COPD is established by spirometry, which shows a post bronchodilator $FEV1 : FVC$ ratio <70%.

Chest X-ray

This may be normal. Abnormalities correlate with the presence of emphysema and are caused by:

- over-inflation with a low, flat diaphragm
- vascular changes with loss of peripheral vascular markings but enlarged hilar vessels – the heart is narrow until cor pulmonale develops
- bullae if present.

The chest X-ray is an important investigation to exclude other disease (carcinoma, tuberculosis, pneumonia, pneumothorax).

Arterial blood gas estimations

These may be normal. In later stages the PaO_2 falls and the $PaCO_2$ rises, particularly with exacerbations.

Electrocardiogram (ECG)

This records the presence and progression of cor pulmonale (right atrial and ventricular hypertrophy).

Sputum for bacterial culture and sensitivity

This is useful in acute infective episodes when infections other than *Haemophilus influenzae* or *Streptococcus pneumoniae* may be present.

Haemoglobin

This may show secondary polycythaemia.

Management (Box 11.1)

Management should include assessment and reduction of risk factors in addition to the management of stable COPD and exacerbations. There should be a stepwise increase in treatment according to disease severity.

Patients benefit from rehabilitation and exercise programmes. Education can help patients to cope and achieve goals, including stopping smoking.

Long-acting bronchodilators are used to prevent or reduce symptoms: the β_2-agonists, e.g. salbutamol (Ventolin®), terbutaline (Bricanyl®), the anticholinergic ipratropium (Atrovent®) or a combination of these drugs are given by metered aerosol or nebuliser on an as-required or regular basis. Theophylline is of limited value due to limited efficacy and side effects.

Regular treatment with inhaled steroids can benefit patients with a documented spirometric response to steroids, or who have repeated exacerbations requiring treatment with antibiotics or oral steroids. Chronic treatment with systemic steroids should be avoided. Long-term home oxygen (>15h/day) increases survival in patients with chronic respiratory failure.

The phosphodiesterase-4 inhibitor roflumilast may be of benefit if symptoms are not controlled by long-acting bronchodilators.

Patients should receive annual influenza vaccination.

Exacerbations are treated with inhaled bronchodilators; systemic steroids can be effective. Although a

---

 Box 11.1 Management of COPD

A systematic review to evaluate the effectiveness of COPD management strategies concluded that long-acting inhaled therapies, supplemental oxygen and pulmonary rehabilitation are beneficial in adults who have bothersome respiratory symptoms, especially dyspnoea, and FEV1 less than 60% predicted. Source: *Annals of Internal Medicine* 2007; **147**(9): 639–653.

cause is often not identified, infection is a common trigger and patients with signs of infection are given antibiotics – amoxicillin or a macrolide (erythromycin or clarithromycin). Bacterial sensitivities are useful if clinical improvement has not occurred.

Non-invasive intermittent positive pressure ventilation (NIPPV) can decrease the need for intubation and mechanical ventilation.

Asthma

Asthma is thought to affect 10–20% of the population of Europe and North America. It is characterised by recurrent shortness of breath, wheeze or cough caused by reversible narrowing of airways. The principal cause is contraction of smooth muscle cells as a result of hypersensitivity to many different stimuli. Thickening of the airways by oedema and cellular infiltrates, as well as blockage of airways by mucus and secretions, also contribute. Wheeze is not an essential feature.

Clinical features

Acute attacks

These may be fairly abrupt in onset and brief in duration (hours), or longer (days or weeks). Longer severe attacks are called 'status asthmaticus'. In an attack the patient feels tightness and there may be a cough. Symptoms tend to be worse at night and in the early morning. The patient usually sits up with an overinflated chest, an audible expiratory wheeze, using the accessory muscles of respiration. The respiratory rate may be little altered but the pulse is invariably rapid. Acute attacks may be triggered by allergens (e.g. pollens or house dust mite), exertion, cold air, a respiratory infection, aspirin and β-blockers. The patient or family members may have a history of atopy.

Recurrent asthma

Mild asthmatics usually have normal respiratory function between attacks, but those with long-standing severe asthma tend to develop some degree of dyspnoea and persistent airways obstruction between acute attacks.

Investigation

Investigation includes chest X-ray (for regional collapse, pneumonia, pneumothorax) and measurement of ventilatory function (*FEV1* or PEFR, preferably at several times a day on several days at home) and the response to bronchodilators. Variability through the day, especially with a 'morning dip' in PEFR, is characteristic. Skin hypersensitivity tests performed by pricking standard allergens into the skin can help the patient avoid environmental precipitants.

Management of chronic asthma

Self-management education, which includes written personalized asthma plans, improves outcome. The patient should be asked about precipitating factors, including upper respiratory tract infection, season (grass pollen and fungal spores), cold, exercise, food, house dust (contains the mite *Dermatophagoides*), smoke, emotion and drugs (e.g. aspirin, NSAIDs, β-blockers). Patients should be trained to use a peak flow meter reliably and to document values at home. Increasing morning dips provide an early warning of deterioration.

Most patients respond to simple therapy and may be controlled by:

- avoiding known allergens
- inhaled short-acting β_2-agonists, e.g. salbutamol, as required – the response is a guide to severity
- inhaled corticosteroids in a regular regimen
- inhaled sodium cromoglicate
- inhaled antimuscarinic preparations, e.g. ipratropium (Atrovent™)
- theophylline preparations, given as a slow-release preparation at night to control overnight symptoms
- leukotriene receptor antagonists, e.g. montelukast, are used as add-on therapies in the prophylaxis of moderate asthma not controlled by the above therapies
- oral steroids may be required for exacerbations
- hyposensitisation is of value in only a small number of patients who demonstrate specific allergies.

Pharmacological treatment involves use of inhaled short-acting β_2-agonist as needed, with additional agents as required to maintain control, increasing or decreasing treatment as necessary. The British Thoracic Society/Scottish Intercollegiate Guidelines Network (https://www.brit-thoracic.org.uk/) guidelines recommend incremental addition of inhaled corticosteroids, followed by long-acting β_2-agonists. Depending on the response, a fourth drug (e.g. leukotriene receptor antagonist, slow-release theophylline, long-acting muscarinic receptor antagonist, β_2-agonist tablet) can be added, before addition of steroid tablets.

NB: When metered aerosols are used, always check inhaler technique. A number of simple inhalers are available: spacers, discs, rotahalers, breath-activated aerosols.

Acute severe asthma

Acute severe asthma is a life-threatening condition. It typically occurs in poorly controlled individuals whose condition has been deteriorating over days or weeks, but death can be sudden and sometimes unexpected, as the patient may not appear severely ill. It is this lack of recognition of severity plus inadequate early treatment that is so dangerous. Most patients have some degree of respiratory failure at presentation. The term status asthmaticus is sometimes used to describe severe asthma attacks that have not responded to conventional therapy.

Features of life-threatening asthma are as follows.

Clinical

- severe breathlessness (unable to complete sentence in one breath)
- tachypnea, tachycardia, silent chest, cyanosis, collapse
- PEF < 33% of best or predicted
- $SpO_2 < 92\%$

Laboratory

- $PaO_2 < 8$ kPa

Chest X-ray

- to exclude suspected pneumothorax, pneumomediastinum or consolidation

Management

- *Oxygen* to maintain SpO_2 of 94–98%.
- *Bronchodilators*: β_2-agonists (e.g. salbutamol, terbutaline) and ipratropium by oxygen-driven nebuliser or intravenous infusion if inhaled therapy cannot be used reliably.
- *Corticosteroids*: oral prednisolone, or intravenous hydrocortisone if unable to swallow. Continue oral prednisolone 40–50 mg daily for at least 5 days or until recovery.
- *Intravenous fluids* are required for as long as oral fluids are not taken. Monitor urine output.
- *Bacterial infection* is a rare trigger but *antibiotics* are given if it is present or strongly suspected. The usual organisms are *Strepcococcus pneumoniae* or *Haemophilus influenzae*.
- *Mechanical ventilation* may be necessary. Persistent or increasing elevation of arterial $PaCO_2$, worsening hypoxia, or acidosis, especially with accompanying exhaustion, feeble respiration or drowsiness, indicates the need for referral for artificial ventilation.

Discharge from hospital after PEFR returns to >75% of best, with day variability <25%, with early clinic follow-up.

Respiratory failure

Respiratory failure can be defined as a reduction in arterial PaO_2 below 8 kPa with a normal arterial $PaCO_2$ (hypoxaemic respiratory failure), or with an increase in arterial $PaCO_2$ above 6.6 kPa (hypercapnic respiratory failure).

NB: The normal range for PaO_2 is about 10–13 kPa. Values of PaO_2 are lower in the elderly.

The PaO_2 may fall while the $PaCO_2$ remains normal. This may occur with alveolar parenchymal lung disease: infiltrations, fibrosing alveolitis and 'pure' emphysema. Much more commonly, both arterial gas levels are abnormal. This occurs with ventilatory failure.

Acute

- patients with normal lungs, with upper airways obstruction (e.g. croup and acute anaphylaxis) or mechanical failure (e.g. flail chest) or central nervous system depression of respiratory drive (e.g. sleep apnoea, drug overdosage, stroke)
- patients with abnormal lungs (e.g. asthma, chronic bronchitis)

Chronic

Usually in patients with abnormal lungs, especially COPD. These patients are particularly likely to develop acute failure if infection occurs.

In restrictive disorders, lung expansion is limited by:

- lung disease, such as fibrosis collapse, oedema, consolidation
- pleural disease, such as fibrosis, effusion or mesothelioma
- chest-wall disease, such as costospinal rigidity and deformity, or abdominal splinting by obesity, ascites or pregnancy
- neuromuscular disease, such as muscular dystrophy, myasthenia or phrenic nerve paralysis.

Acute on chronic respiratory failure

This usually occurs on a background of COPD.

TRIALS BOX 11.1 Home oxygen therapy in COPD

A systematic review of the effect of domiciliary oxygen therapy in patients with COPD found that long-term home oxygen therapy improved survival in a selected group of COPD patients with severe hypoxaemia (arterial PaO_2 less than 8.0 kPa). Home oxygen therapy did not appear to improve survival in patients with mild to moderate hypoxaemia or in those with only arterial desaturation at night. Source: *Cochrane Database Systematic Review* 2005; (4): CD001744.

Clinical presentation

- peripheral vasodilatation with headache, engorged veins in the fundi, warm hands and a bounding pulse, all caused by carbon dioxide retention
- varying degrees of agitated confusion, drowsiness and coma
- increasing cyanosis
- signs of right heart failure
- flapping tremor of the outstretched hands and papilloedema are late signs

NB: Physical signs are a poor guide to the presence and degree of respiratory failure; measure blood gases in all patients in whom the diagnosis is suspected.

Management

Consists of the measures used for COPD, with the addition of controlled oxygen therapy. The danger to life in this situation is hypoxia, but, paradoxically, relief of hypoxia may make the situation worse by causing hypercapnia. Give oxygen at 24 or 28% by face mask or nasal prongs if the arterial PaO_2 or oxygen saturation is low, targeting oxygen saturation at 94–98% unless the patient is at risk of hypercapnia, when the target should be lower at 88–92%. Oxygen is given continuously until the acute situation (including infection and heart failure) has recovered. $PaCO_2$ is monitored. For chronic respiratory failure controlled oxygen can be given continuously at home with improvement in symptoms and an increase in life expectancy (Trials Box 11.1).

Indications for respiratory support and mechanical ventilation

If the $PaCO_2$ falls, conservative therapy should be continued and reassessed periodically. If the $PaCO_2$ rises, this indicates that the patient's ventilation is inadequate and is the prime indication for non-invasive positive pressure ventilation using a full facial or nasal mask that delivers ventilatory support from a flow generator (Trials Box 11.2), or if this fails mechanical positive-pressure ventilation. Patients should be ventilated before they become exhausted. The final decision to ventilate a patient is determined mainly on the basis of respiratory function before the acute illness: if very poor, it may not be possible to wean the patient off the ventilator.

Acute anaphylaxis

This rare condition occurs following exposure to allergens such as certain foods, e.g. peanuts; drug therapy, e.g. penicillin; and insect stings. Clinical features

TRIALS BOX 11.2 Non-invasive positive pressure ventilation in acute respiratory failure

A systematic review of non-invasive positive pressure ventilation (NPPV) in patients admitted to hospital with acute respiratory failure secondary to an exacerbation of COPD showed the benefit of NPPV as first-line intervention as an adjunct therapy to usual medical care in all suitable patients. The review concluded that NPPV should be considered early in the course of respiratory failure and before severe acidosis ensues, as a means of reducing the likelihood of endotracheal intubation, treatment failure and mortality. Source: *Cochrane Database Systematic Review* 2004; (3): CD004104.

range from mild with flushing of the face, pruritus and blotchy wheals, to severe with asthma, respiratory obstruction from oedema of the larynx (angioedema) and circulatory collapse.

Immediate treatment is with adrenaline (epinephrine) 0.5 ml of 1 : 1000 (1 mg/ml) solution, i.e. 500 mg given intramuscularly and repeated after 5 min if no improvement is observed. Oxygen, if available, is important early on. An intravenous fluid challenge is given if there is hypotension. Hydrocortisone takes several hours to act. It is given (after the first injection of adrenaline (epinephrine)) in a dose of 200 mg slowly intravenously or intramuscularly, with chlorphenamine 10 mg slowly intravenously or intramuscularly.

In patients with a history of anaphylaxis allergens should be identified and avoided. Most patients will wish to carry self-administration preassembled pens containing adrenaline (epinephrine) for intramuscular injection.

Hereditary angioedema is a rare condition caused by C_1 esterase deficiency (autosomal dominant). It gives rise to erythema, patchy oedema and colicky abdominal pain. It responds to danazol prophylaxis and fresh frozen plasma (or if available plasma-derived C_1 inhibitor) to correct the deficiency during attacks.

Pneumonia

Community-acquired pneumonia affects approximately 5–10/1000 adults per year. One in 1000 requires hospitalisation, and mortality in these patients is around 10%.

Clinical presentation

Symptoms of cough, sputum, pleurisy and dyspnoea are less common in the elderly.

Clinical findings include fever, tachypnoea, crackles and signs of consolidation. The likely causative agent cannot be predicted from clinical findings.

The most common organism in UK studies of hospitalised patients is *Streptococcus pneumoniae* (approximately one-third of cases in which an organism is identified), followed by *Chlamydia pneumoniae* and *Mycoplasma pneumoniae*. *Haemophilus influenzae*, *Legionella* species, *Chlamydia psittaci* and *Staphylococcus aureus* account for most of the remainder. Gram-negative bacilli, *Coxiella burnetii* and anaerobes are rare. Viruses (including influenza) account for 10–15% of cases.

Investigations

Investigations are performed to establish the diagnosis and assess severity.

- *Chest X-ray* shows infiltrates. Computed tomographic (CT) scanning is more sensitive and may be useful in detecting interstitial disease, cavitation and empyema.
- *Blood gases* to assess severity and guide oxygen treatment.
- *Blood count* – white cell count $>15 \times 10^9$/l suggests bacterial infection; white cell count $>20 \times 10^9$/l or $<4 \times 10^9$/l indicates poor prognosis. Haemoglobin for haemolysis.
- *Creatinine and liver function tests* for underlying or associated renal or hepatic disease.
- *Gram staining and culture of sputum* – but cough is unproductive in one-third of patients, and negative results are common, particularly if antibiotics have been given.
- *Blood culture.*
- *Pleural fluid*, if present, should be aspirated for culture.

Management

- *Oxygen* – to maintain PaO_2 above 8 kPa and oxygen saturation >92%.
- *Antibiotics* – the organism is usually unknown initially. Treatment is started immediately and should cover *Streptococcus pneumoniae*. In uncomplicated pneumonia, treatment is usually started with oral amoxicillin or a macrolide (erythromycin or clarithromycin). In severe pneumonia intravenous therapy is given. The choice of antibiotics should take account of local guidelines, which will take account of other factors, including the incidence of *Clostridium difficile* enteritis.
- *Intravenous fluids* may be required.
- *Analgesia* for pleuritic pain.

Pneumococcal pneumonia is the most common bacterial pneumonia. *S. pneumoniae* is a Gram-positive diplococcus. It affects all ages, but is more common in the elderly, after splenectomy, in the immunosuppressed, alcoholics, patients with chronic heart failure and those with pre-existing lung disease. It typically presents acutely with fever, pleuritic pain and rust-coloured sputum. It causes both lobar and bronchopneumonia. Treatment is with penicillin, or erythromycin in the penicillin-sensitive. A polysaccharide pneumococcal vaccine is available for those at high risk. It should be given at least 2 weeks before splenectomy and before chemotherapy.

Staphylococcal pneumonia produces widespread infection with abscess formation. It may complicate influenzal pneumonia, and this makes it relatively common during epidemics of influenza. It also occurs in patients with underlying disease, which prevents a normal response to infection, e.g. chronic leukaemia, lymphoma, cystic fibrosis. Flucloxacillin is the drug of choice, although increasingly *Staphylococcus aureus* is methicillin-resistant (MRSA) and requires treatment with vancomycin. Lung abscess, empyema and subsequent bronchiectasis are relatively common complications.

Legionnaire's disease was first described in a group of American army veterans (legionnaires). The causative Gram-negative bacillus flourishes in the cooling waters of air conditioners and may colonise hot-water tanks kept at <60 °C. It begins as an influenza-like illness with fever, malaise and myalgia, and proceeds with cough (little sputum), dyspnoea and sometimes severe anorexia, marked confusion and coma. Diarrhoea and vomiting are common and renal failure may develop. Examination shows consolidation that usually affects both lung bases. X-ray changes may persist for more than 2 months after the acute illness. Erythromycin or ciprofloxacin are the antibiotics of choice, but the mortality remains high.

NB: Legionnaire's disease (and *Mycoplasma pneumoniae* or psittacosis) should be suspected in all patients who develop pneumonia that does not respond to standard antibiotics.

Mycoplasma pneumonia is caused by *M. pneumoniae,* the only mycoplasma definitely pathogenic to humans. The clinical picture resembles bacterial pneumonia, although cough and sputum are absent in one-third of cases.

Respiratory symptoms and signs and X-ray changes (patchy consolidation with small effusions) are usually preceded by several days of influenza-like symptoms. Polyarthritis occurs and may persist for months. Malaise and fatigue may persist long after the acute illness is over. The diagnosis is confirmed by a positive *Mycoplasma*-specific immunoglobulin M (IgM) titre. Erythromycin or tetracycline are the antibiotics of choice.

Psittacosis pneumonia is caused by *Chlamydia psittaci.* It is transmitted in the excrement of infected birds (the bird need not be ill). Headache, fever and dry cough may be accompanied by a rash and splenomegaly. Hepatitis, encephalitis, renal failure and haemolysis also occur. Treatment is with tetracycline or erythromycin.

Viral pneumonia in children is commonly due to the respiratory syncytial virus (RSV), so called as it is a respiratory virus that produces syncytium formation when grown in culture. Infection may be indistinguishable from acute bacterial bronchitis or bronchiolitis in children and infants. The presence of a skin rash supports the likelihood of RSV infection.

Acute viral pneumonia in adults is less common but occurs during epidemics of influenza. Fever, headache and myalgia are followed after a few days by dry cough and chest pain. Treatment is largely symptomatic (paracetamol, rest, fluids). Influenza vaccines are available for those at high risk. The most common cause of pneumonia during influenza epidemics results from secondary bacterial infection, the most serious being *Staphylococcal pneumonia.* The viruses of measles, chickenpox and herpes zoster may directly affect the lung. The diagnosis is confirmed by a rise in specific antibody titre.

Aspiration pneumonia. Aspiration of gastric contents may produce a severe chemical pneumonitis with considerable pulmonary oedema and bronchospasm (Mendelson syndrome). The acute respiratory distress and shock can be very rapidly fatal and very difficult to treat. It tends to occur in states of reduced consciousness such as general anaesthesia and drunkenness. Aspiration of bacteria from the oropharynx may follow dental anaesthesia. Recurrent episodes occur in dysphagia due to neurological or oesophageal disorders, including hiatus hernia, stricture, achalasia of the cardia, and in patients with diverticula or pharyngeal pouch. Treatment with augmentin or amoxicillin and metronidazole should provide cover for oropharyngeal bacteria, including *Bacteroides,* until any sensitivities of isolated organisms are known.

Recurrent bacterial pneumonia in the absence of chronic bronchitis arouses suspicion of:

- bronchial carcinoma preventing drainage of infected areas of lung
- bronchiectasis
- cystic fibrosis
- achalasia of the cardia, 25% of which present as chest disease, pharyngeal pouch and neuromuscular disease of the oesophagus, e.g. bulbar palsy, all producing aspiration
- hypogammaglobulinaemia and myeloma.

Opportunistic infection of the lungs occurs in patients immunosuppressed as a result of treatment, or HIV infection (page 399, Chapter 21).

Lung abscess

Aetiology

- aspiration (see earlier)
- bronchial obstruction, usually by carcinoma or a foreign body (especially peanuts and teeth)

- pneumonia partially resolved or treated, particularly when caused by the *Staphylococcus, Klebsiella* or *Pneumococcus* organisms

Clinical features

There is often a swinging fever with haemoptysis and foul, purulent sputum. Clubbing may develop.

Investigation

Sputum is sent for Gram stain and culture, and blood for culture. Chest X-ray shows round lesion(s) often with a fluid level, and serial X-rays monitor progress. It may be necessary to proceed to bronchoscopy to exclude obstruction and to obtain a biopsy.

Treatment

Antibiotic therapy is given according to sensitivities and continued until healing is complete. Repeated postural drainage is started. CT-guided aspiration or surgical excision may be required.

Bronchiectasis

Bronchiectasis means dilatation of the airways. It becomes of clinical significance when infection and/ or haemoptysis occurs. Severe forms are now rare, especially in the young.

Aetiology

- following acute childhood respiratory infection, particularly measles, whooping cough or pneumonia
- cystic fibrosis
- bronchial obstruction predisposes to bronchiectasis (e.g. peanuts)
- tuberculosis has become less common as a cause
- congenital (rare): primary ciliary dyskinesia, e.g. Kartagener syndrome (bronchiectasis, sinusitis, situs inversus)
- immunodeficiency

Clinical features

- chronic cough, often postural
- sputum, often copious, especially with acute infections
- halitosis
- febrile episodes
- haemoptysis: may be the only symptom ('dry bronchiectasis') and can be severe

- dyspnoea, coarse basal crepitations and wheeze
- cyanosis and clubbing
- loss of weight and cor pulmonale in advanced cases

Management

The object is to get rid of chronic sepsis. Postural drainage helps empty dilated airways and decreases the frequency of further infections. Bronchodilators will often help improve clearance of sputum. Antibiotics are given for acute infections and exacerbations, and long-term oral or nebulized antibiotics are sometimes used for recurrent infections. Surgery can be of benefit if disease is limited to isolated lung segments.

Pneumothorax

Aetiology

Spontaneous pneumothorax

Primary spontaneous pneumothorax in the absence of underlying lung disease is the most common type and usually occurs in normal, tall, thin, young, male smokers following rupture of a small subpleural bulla. There is history of sudden onset of one-sided pleuritic pain and/or dyspnoea. Dyspnoea rapidly increases in tension pneumothorax and the patient becomes cyanosed. The classical signs are diminished movement on the affected side with deviation of the trachea to the other side. There is hyperresonance to percussion and reduced pulmonary sounds (breath sounds, tactile fremitus and vocal resonance). Pneumothoraces are best diagnosed by seeing a lung edge on X-ray; it is clearest on an expiratory film (Fig. 11.1). It recurs in 25% of cases within 5 years, usually in the first year.

Secondary spontaneous pneumothorax occurs as a complication of underlying lung disease. Conditions predisposing to pneumothorax include:

- COPD
- cystic fibrosis
- infections, including pneumocystis (page 399, Chapter 21) and tuberculosis (see later and page 403, Chapter 21)
- interstitial lung disease
- asthma

Other rare causes include *Staphylococcal pneumonia,* carcinoma, occupational lung disease and connective tissue disorders, e.g. Marfan and Ehlers–Danlos syndromes. Familial spontaneous pneumothorax is associated with mutations in the folliculin gene.

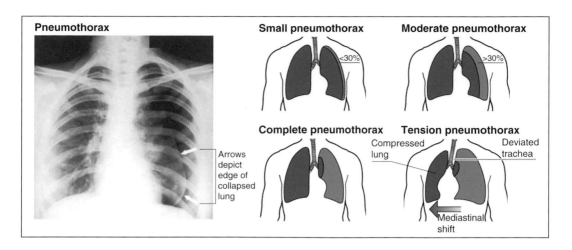

Figure 11.1 Pneumothorax. Source: Ward, J., Ward, J. and Leach, R. (2010) *The Respiratory System at a Glance*, 3rd edn. Oxford: Blackwell Publishing. Reproduced with permission.

Management of spontaneous pneumothorax

Often no therapy is required if the pneumothorax is small and symptoms minor. Spontaneous recovery occurs in 3–4 weeks. Indications for aspiration of air are:

- tension pneumothorax (an acute emergency)
- breathlessness
- moderate or complete collapse of the lung (>50% of the total lung field on chest X-ray).

Small pneumothoraces, with a visible rim of less than 2 cm between the lung margin and the chest wall at the level of the hilum, can be aspirated using a 16–18-gauge cannula if there is no clinical compromise.

If there is a small bore (<14 Fr) intercostal catheter is usually required.

Rarely, a continuing air leak persists from the lung into the pleural space (bronchopleural fistula), and surgical pleurectomy is required. Chemical pleurodesis with talc is an alternative.

Secondary spontaneous pneumothorax has a higher morbidity and mortality, and usually requires admission to hospital, supplemental oxygen and active intervention.

Cystic fibrosis

This is an autosomal recessive disorder affecting 1 in 3000 live births that occurs equally in males and

---

CASE STUDY Pleural disease

A 19-year-old male student presented to the Accident and Emergency Department with a sudden onset of left-sided chest and shoulder pain, worse on inspiration. There was no associated cough or breathlessness. He smoked 15 cigarettes per day and was on no regular medication. His height was 190 cm and weight 68 kg (BMI 18.8). There were no signs on examination of the chest.

The presentation with sudden onset of pleuritic chest pain in a young tall thin male smoker suggests a spontaneous pneumothorax, and chest X-ray confirmed the presence of a small apical left-sided

pneumothorax, with a visible rim of lung that was no more than 1.5 cm from the chest wall. The chest X-ray was otherwise normal.

The small primary spontaneous pneumothorax was managed conservatively. The patient was given guidance about stopping smoking to reduce the risk of recurrence, and discharged with advice to return to hospital if his symptoms worsened and not to fly until resolution had been confirmed. Chest X-ray at outpatient review 5 days later showed almost complete resolution, and chest X-ray after a further 2 weeks was normal.

females and usually presents in early childhood. It is caused by mutations of the cystic fibrosis transmembrane conductance regulator (*CFTR*) gene located on chromosome 7. *CFTR* functions as a cyclic adenosine monophosphate (cAMP)-regulated chloride channel on the apical surface of airway and other epithelial cells. Abnormally thick secretions are produced by glandular tissue. It predominantly affects the pancreas and respiratory tract, leading to pancreatic insufficiency and lung damage from recurrent chest infections. Secondary bronchiectasis or lung abscess may result. Recurrent small haemoptyses and finger clubbing are common, and pneumothorax occurs. Persistent productive cough is associated initially with *Staphylococcus aureus, Haemophilus influenzae* and Gram-negative bacilli. Later, *Pseudomonas aeruginosa* predominates and is associated with a poor prognosis.

Other manifestations are meconium ileus in newborns, diabetes mellitus, biliary obstruction and azoospermia (over 90% of males).

With improved survival cystic fibrosis is a disease of both adults and children. Most males are sterile and women subfertile. A high sodium concentration in the sweat (>70 mmol/l) is characteristic.

Management

- pancreatic enzymes and fat-soluble vitamins
- clearance of pulmonary secretions and treatment of infections
- chest physiotherapy with postural drainage
- bronchodilators
- inhaled recombinant human deoxyribonuclease 1 (rhDNase) reduces the viscoelasticity of sputum by digesting viscous extracellular DNA in mucus (it is expensive)
- antibiotics – exacerbations are usually treated with two parenteral antibiotics (to reduce antibiotic resistance). Choice is guided by sensitivity of isolated organisms but often includes an aminoglycoside with an anti-pseudomonal penicillin (e.g. ticarcillin), cephalosporin or quinolone. The benefits of maintenance antibiotic therapy have to be weighed against the risks of antibiotic resistance. Inhaled aminoglycosides may allow delivery of high concentrations to the lungs with less risk of toxicity. Although macrolide antibiotics are not directly active against *Pseudomonas aeruginosa,* several studies have shown a benefit from maintenance treatment with azithromycin (three times a week) with a small improvement in lung function, improved nutritional status and less frequent pulmonary infections.

- The protein modulator lumacaftor–ivacaftor (lumacaftor corrects and ivacaftor potentiates the CFTR) has a marketing authorisation in the UK for treating cystic fibrosis in people 12 years and older who are homozygous for the F508del mutation found in ~70% of patients with cystic fibrosis.

Lung transplantation should be considered for respiratory failure.

The social and emotional problems can be enormous and, for this reason, as well as the complexity of clinical management, the condition should be supervised from specialist centres.

Lung cancer

Incidence

This causes about 40 000 deaths per year in the UK, 55% in men and almost 90% in patients aged 60+. About 87% are non-small cell lung cancer and 12% small cell. One percent are carcinoid tumours. Most non-small cell cancers are squamous cell, but about 5% are undifferentiated large cell tumours and about 10% are adenocarcinoma. Alveolar cell carcinoma, an adenocarcinoma, is very rare.

Aetiology

Cigarette smoking. The risk of carcinoma of the bronchus (squamous and small cell) increases with both smoking duration and amount. Duration has the most effect. Most of the risk of lung cancer can be avoided by stopping smoking in middle age.

Other atmospheric pollution (coal smoke and diesel fumes) may prove to be aetiologically relevant, but quantitatively small compared with cigarettes. Exposure to chromium, arsenic, radioactive materials or asbestos (which in addition produces interstitial fibrosis and mesothelioma) is associated with a higher incidence of lung cancer.

Clinical presentation

The patient is usually a cigarette smoker, sometimes with tobacco-stained fingers. Cough or the accentuation of an existing cough is the commonest early symptom. Haemoptysis, dyspnoea, central chest ache and pleuritic pain, and slowly resolving chest infection are common early manifestations. Occasionally, patients are identified following a routine chest X-ray. The patient may also present with inoperable disease.

- Metastatic deposits involving brain, bone, liver, skin, kidney, adrenal glands or other site.
- Symptoms from local extension, e.g. superior vena cava obstruction (puffy, dusky head, neck and arms, a raised pulseless jugular venous pulse, headache, dilatated veins over the chest wall), cervical lymph glands, dysphagia from oesophageal involvement, cardiac arrhythmia and pleural effusion. The Pancoast syndrome consists of symptoms from local extension at the apex of the lung. There may be pain in the shoulder, upper back or arm, weakness and atrophy of the hand muscles from brachial plexus involvement, hoarseness from involvement of the recurrent superior laryngeal nerve, or a Horner syndrome (page 57, Chapter 6).

The presence of systemic and non-specific symptoms (anorexia, weight loss and fatigue) usually, but not always, implies late and possibly inoperable disease.

Blood and marrow

Anaemia (often normochromic or normocytic). Polycythaemia is uncommon. Marrow infiltration is common in small cell carcinoma.

Neuromuscular

Dementia or focal neurological deficit (caused by cerebral secondaries or rarely cortical atrophy), cerebellar syndrome, mixed sensorimotor peripheral neuropathy, proximal myopathy, polymyositis (page 323, Chapter 18) and the myasthenic (Eaton–Lambert) syndrome (223).

Skin, connective tissue, bone

Clubbing, hypertrophic pulmonary osteoarthropathy, dermatomyositis and acanthosis nigricans.

Endocrine

Syndromes caused by ectopic hormone production, the pituitary-like ones (adrenocorticotrophic hormone [ACTH], antidiuretic hormone [ADH], prolactin) usually from oat cell tumours, and parathyroid hormone from squamous cell tumours. Hypercalcaemia is usually caused by bone secondaries.

Cardiovascular

Atrial fibrillation (local extension) and migratory thrombophlebitis. Pericarditis.

Diagnosis

Chest X-ray may show:

- the tumour, often visible as a unilaterally enlarged hilum or peripheral circular opacity, occasionally cavitated
- collapse/consolidation caused by bronchial obstruction by the tumour
- effusion, raised hemidiaphragm of phrenic paralysis and bone erosion suggest local extension.

Magnetic resonance imaging (MRI) or CT scan show the tumour position better and demonstrate bronchial narrowing and mediastinal involvement. Positron emission tomography (PET) scan can be used for detecting metastatic spread. Exfoliative cytology may be diagnostic.

Fibre-optic bronchoscopy with biopsy is performed if possible to establish histological diagnosis and assess operability. The site of the tumour is a guide to operability (not less than 2 cm from the carina). CT-guided percutaneous needle biopsy is used for peripheral lesions.

Treatment

Patients are staged using a TNM (tumour, node, metastasis) classification. Overall survival rates are poor: in the UK around 20% survive 1 year and just over 5% survive 5 years. Surgery offers the only 'cure'. Surgery is contraindicated by metastasis (present in 60% of cases at the time of presentation – chiefly in bone and liver), local spread and inadequate respiratory function. Radical radiotherapy or continuous hyperfractionated accelerated radiotherapy (CHART) can be offered to patients who are inoperable, or in whom resection is incomplete. Chemotherapy with a third-generation drug (docetaxel, gemcitabine, paclitaxel or vinorelbine) plus a platinum drug (cisplatin or carboplatin if tolerated) can be offered to patients with more advanced disease.

Small cell carcinoma may be palliated with chemotherapy, using a platinum-based multidrug regime. Radiotherapy may have a role if the disease is limited or responds to chemotherapy.

Bronchial adenoma

This rare tumour is usually benign but locally invasive. Ninety percent of cases are histologically 'carcinoid' tumours, but only a few patients present with the carcinoid syndrome. They usually present with cough and haemoptysis. The tumour may occur either anywhere within the thoracic cavity and appear as a well-circumscribed peripheral mass on chest X-ray or, more often, in the major bronchi and appear as a pedunculated intrabronchial mass seen broncho-scopically. The tumours are removed surgically or endoscopically.

Sarcoidosis

Sarcoidosis is characterised by a systemic non-case-ating granulomatous infiltration that may involve any tissue. It most commonly affects the lungs, mediasti-nal lymph nodes and skin. The aetiology is not known.

Clinical presentation

See Fig. 11.2.

Pulmonary sarcoid

In the UK, the annual incidence of clinical disease is 3–4/100 000. It typically occurs in young people of 20–40 years and in females more commonly than males. It usually presents as a subacute syndrome with fever, malaise and lassitude, erythema nodosum, polyarthralgia and mediastinal hilar lymphadenopa-thy. Dyspnoea is not usually a feature of this acute form, which is self-limiting (2 months to 2 years).

Less commonly and more seriously, it presents as a chronic insidious disease with respiratory symp-toms of cough and progressive dyspnoea with malaise and fever leading to progressive pulmonary fibrosis.

Non-pulmonary sarcoid

Apart from erythema nodosum, this is relatively uncommon.

- skin – erythema nodosum (not sarcoid tissue) in the acute syndrome; infiltration of scars: lupus pernio
- hypercalcaemia occurs in about 10% of patients with sarcoidosis, and hypercalciuria is even more common. It may be the presenting abnormality

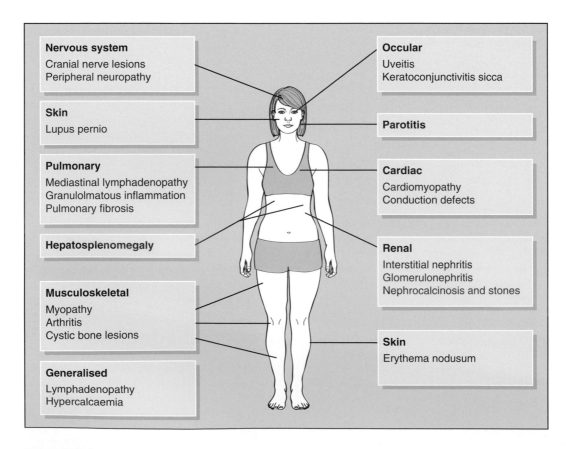

Figure 11.2 Common manifestations of sarcoidosis.

and responds to steroids. It is due to the uncontrolled synthesis of 1,25-dihydroxyvitamin D_3 by macrophages
- eyes – uveitis and keratoconjunctivitis sicca
- parotitis
- hepatosplenomegaly
- generalised lymphadenopathy
- bone and joints, producing cystic lesions most commonly in the phalanges
- nervous system, causing isolated cranial nerve lesions and peripheral neuropathy
- heart – conduction defects and arrhythmias
- endocrine, producing diabetes insipidus from pituitary involvement (very rare)
- renal damage from hypercalcaemia or an associated interstitial nephritis or glomerulonephritis

Investigation

In pulmonary sarcoid the chest X-ray shows symmetrical lobulated bilateral hilar and paratracheal gland enlargement (interbronchial rather than tracheobronchial) or, less commonly, parenchymal mottling or diffuse fibrosis. CT scan will help distinguish gland enlargement from prominent pulmonary artery shadows.

Angiotensin-converting enzyme (ACE) is produced by epithelioid cells of sarcoid granulomata. Elevated serum ACE can be useful in diagnosis and monitoring disease activity, although it can also be elevated in other granulomatous diseases.

'Blind' transbronchial lung biopsy at bronchoscopy often shows non-caseating epithelioid granulomas. Liver biopsy may reveal granulomas. The Mantoux test is usually negative; a positive test is not uncommon but a strongly positive test is very unusual. Polyclonal increase in γ-globulins is non-specific but common.

Management

The differential diagnosis of bilateral hilar lymph node enlargement is from Hodgkin's disease (and other lymphoproliferative disorders), and any deviation of the patient's syndrome from the usual pattern makes a definite diagnosis by biopsy imperative. Treatment, other than simple analgesics, is usually unnecessary.

Indications for corticosteroids in sarcoidosis (e.g. prednisolone 20 mg/day, reducing after 1 month to the minimum dosage necessary to suppress activity for 1 year) include the following:

- Progressive lung disease, to try to prevent fibrosis. The indication is progressive pulmonary shadowing or increasing breathlessness. The effect of therapy is monitored by symptoms, chest X-rays and lung function tests, including transfer factor of the lung for carbon monoxide, TLCO.
- Hypercalcaemia.
- When vital organs are threatened, e.g. eyes, nervous system, kidneys and heart.

Steroid-sparing drugs, including methotrexate and azathioprine, are often used when long-term treatment is needed. Tumour necrosis factor blockade has been effective in refractory cases.

Prognosis (of pulmonary sarcoid)

Complete clinical resolution in 3–4 months, and radiological resolution in 1–2 years, occurs in 70–80% of cases. The chest X-ray remains abnormal in about half of all cases (Table 11.1). Clinical disability brought about by the disease is much less common and is related to:

- age – the younger, the better
- presence of erythema nodosum, where over 95% recover by 1 year

---

Table 11.1 Prognosis of pulmonary sarcoid

Stage	X-ray appearance	Spontaneous remission (% of cases)
0	Normal	
I	Bilateral hilar lymphadenomegaly without pulmonary infiltrates	60–90
II	Bilateral hilar lymphadenomegaly plus pulmonary infiltrates	40–70
III	Parenchymal infiltrates without bilateral hilar lymphadenomegaly	10–20
IV	Extensive fibrosis with distortion or bullae	0

- extent of extrapulmonary involvement – bone or chronic skin lesions indicate chronicity, and the more widespread it is, the worse the prognosis
- extent of intrathoracic involvement.

Tuberculosis

Infection with the acid-alcohol-fast bacillus (AAFB) of *Mycobacterium tuberculosis* affects predominantly the lungs, lymph nodes and gut (Fig. 11.3). Some features of the disease vary with the patient's sensitivity to tuberculin. NICE has published guidelines on the diagnosis and treatment of tuberculosis (https://www.nice.org.uk/guidance/ng33).

Primary tuberculosis

This is the syndrome produced by infection with *M. tuberculosis* in non-sensitive patients, i.e. in those who have not previously been infected. There is a mild inflammatory response at the site of infection (subpleural in the mid-zones of the lungs, in the pharynx or in the terminal ileum), followed by spread to the regional lymph nodes (hilar, cervical and mesenteric, respectively). The combination of a focus with regional lymph node involvement is called the *primary complex*. One to two weeks following infection, with the onset of tuberculin sensitivity, the tissue reaction changes at both the focus and in the nodes, to the characteristic caseating granuloma. Patients are usually symptomless. The complex heals with fibrosis and, frequently, calcifies without therapy. The enlarged lymph node may be obvious in the neck or cause obstruction to a bronchus with consequent collapse. Blood dissemination of the organisms occurs rarely from the primary complex to cause widespread miliary disease, especially in infants.

Post-primary tuberculosis

This is the syndrome produced by infection with *M. tuberculosis* in the previously infected and therefore tuberculin-sensitive patient. Reactivation (or

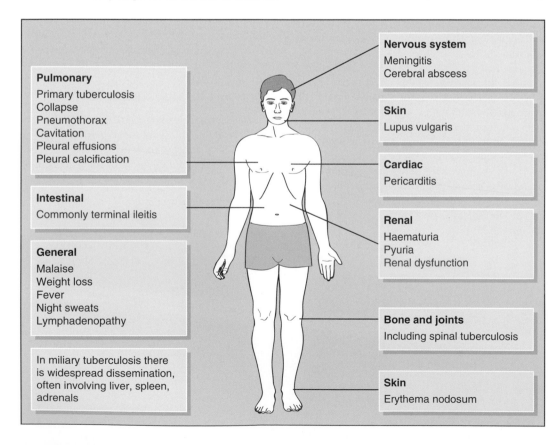

Pulmonary
Primary tuberculosis
Collapse
Pneumothorax
Cavitation
Pleural effusions
Pleural calcification

Intestinal
Commonly terminal ileitis

General
Malaise
Weight loss
Fever
Night sweats
Lymphadenopathy

In miliary tuberculosis there is widespread dissemination, often involving liver, spleen, adrenals

Nervous system
Meningitis
Cerebral abscess

Skin
Lupus vulgaris

Cardiac
Pericarditis

Renal
Haematuria
Pyuria
Renal dysfunction

Bone and joints
Including spinal tuberculosis

Skin
Erythema nodosum

Figure 11.3 Clinical features of tuberculosis.

reinfection) is followed by an immediate brisk granu-lomatous response that tends to localise the disease, and regional lymph node involvement is uncommon. As with primary tuberculosis, the lesion may:

- heal with fibrosis (and calcification)
- rupture into a bronchus, giving tuberculous bronchopneumonia
- spread via the blood to produce miliary tuberculosis of liver, spleen, lungs, choroid, bone and/or meninges.

Presenting features

Symptoms occur relatively late and therefore in established disease. The earliest are non-specific, such as malaise, fatigue, anorexia and weight loss. Of more specific symptoms, the most common is cough, often with mucoid sputum. Other symptoms include repeated small haemoptysis, pleural pain, slight fever or, occasionally, exertional dyspnoea. Frequently, the diagnosis is made presymptomatically on routine chest radiography. Signs also occur late in the disease and are not very specific, e.g. crepitations (usually apical) and, later, signs of consolidation, pleural effusion or cavitation.

Diagnosis

Clinical suspicion should be particularly high in high-risk groups:

- the homeless, and the alcoholic
- Pakistani and Indian immigrants (lymph node tuberculosis is common in Indian and Pakistani patients)
- diabetics
- patients with AIDS
- patients on immunosuppressive therapy (steroids or cytotoxic drugs).

Ideally, the diagnosis is made by repeated examination for AAFB in sputum and bronchial washing on direct smear or culture. At least three sputum samples, including one early morning sample, should be sent for culture and microscopy. Sometimes the diagnosis can only be made on imaging, where activity is suggested by:

- changing 'soft' shadows
- progression of apical lesions
- cavitation with a strongly positive Mantoux test.

It may be necessary to treat on clinical grounds alone and response to specific therapy is taken as proof of diagnosis.

Tuberculosis is notifiable in the UK.

NB: AAFB on microscopy may not be pathogenic mycobacteria, particularly in urine specimens.

Management

Admit patients who are sputum smear positive to a single room, with negative pressure and barrier nursing if multidrug-resistant tuberculosis is suspected. Risk factors for drug resistance include:

- prior treatment for tuberculosis or prior treatment failure
- contact with drug-resistant tuberculosis
- birth in a foreign country
- HIV infection
- age between 25 and 44
- male gender.

Close contacts should be screened with chest X-ray, Mantoux test and/or interferon-gamma assay depending on their age and bacille Calmette–Guérin (BCG) status (Box 11.2). People identified by screening as having latent tuberculosis are usually treated with 3 months of rifampicin or isoniazid, or 6 months of isoniazid.

For tuberculous meningitis see page 226, Chapter 15.

Common antituberculosis drug doses and complications

The first four drugs are considered 'first-line'.

 Box 11.2 Immune-based tests for tuberculosis

Tuberculin skin tests involve the detection of delayed-type hypersensitivity reaction to a purified protein derivative (PPD) containing a mixture of antigens shared by several mycobacteria. In the Mantoux test PPD is inoculated by intracutaneous injection and the size of any skin reaction is measured after 48–72 h.

In **interferon-gamma assays** blood from the person being tested is incubated with mycobacterial antigens, including early secretory antigen target 6 (ESAT-6) and culture filtrate protein 10 (CFP-10), which are specific for *Mycobacterium tuberculosis* and absent from the BCG vaccine strain. In people with latent or active *M. tuberculosis* infection, T lymphocytes within the blood sample produce interferon-gamma as a marker of infection or active tuberculosis.

- Rifampicin 450–600 mg/day: abnormal liver function tests. Colours the urine pink.
- Isoniazid (INAH) 300 mg/day (with pyridoxine 10 mg): peripheral neuropathy and encephalopathy – these are extremely rare, occur in slow acetylators and respond to pyridoxine, often given prophylactically.
- Pyrazinamide 1.5–2.0 g/day: hepatotoxic (rare but severe).
- Ethambutol 15 mg/kg/day: optic neuritis with colour vision and acuity reduced.
- Streptomycin 1 g/day by intramuscular injection: vertigo and nerve deafness. In the elderly and in the presence of raised blood urea, the dosage is reduced to 0.75 or 0.5 g/day to maintain blood levels of 1–2 mg/ml.

Treatment with four drugs for 2 months, is usually followed by treatment with isoniazid and rifampicin for a further 4 months. Fixed-dose combination tablets can be used to increase compliance. Drug-resistant tuberculosis should be suspected if there is a history of prior tuberculosis treatment or treatment failure, contact with drug-resistant tuberculosis, birth in a high incidence country, HIV infection, residence in London. It is commoner in males aged 25 to 44.

Occupational lung diseases

Occupational exposure may cause dust diseases, asthma and extrinsic allergic alveolitis.

Dust diseases

These include the pneumoconioses, asthma and allergic alveolitis. Pneumoconioses are caused by the inhalation and retention in the lung of dust, and include:

- coal pneumoconiosis
- silicosis in rock drilling and crushing – also occurs in coal miners
- asbestosis in insulation workers; this can produce fibrosis, carcinoma and pleural mesothelioma.

These are radiographic diagnoses made in the light of the patient's known occupational hazards; the shadows are caused by the metals themselves, e.g. siderosis (iron) and stannosis (tin). All are rare.

In the UK, workers who have developed pneumoconiosis or silicosis can receive compensation from the Industrial Injuries Scheme, administered by the Department for Work and Pensions.

Clinical features

In the early stages there are no symptoms but X-ray changes occur; later there is dyspnoea on exertion, cough, sputum and attacks of bronchitis. In coal miners, progressive massive fibrosis may occur and in Caplan syndrome pulmonary nodules occur in association with rheumatoid arthritis. The patients may eventually develop cor pulmonale.

Asthma

Occupational asthma can occur in response to precipitants of animal, vegetable, bacteriological or chemical origin. Some of the more common occupations are: animal laboratory workers (urinary proteins), grain and flour workers (mites and flour), sawmill operatives and carpenters (hardwoods), those who manufacture biological detergents (inhalation of *Bacillus subtilis* proteolytic enzymes), in the electronics industry (colophony in solder flux), paint sprayers and polyurethane workers (isocyanates), workers with epoxy resins or platinum salts, and those in the pharmaceutical industry. All these are recognised for compensation under industrial injuries legislation in the UK.

Extrinsic allergic alveolitis

Inhalation of organic dusts may give a diffuse allergic (type III precipitin-mediated) reaction in the alveoli and bronchioles.

Aetiology

Exposure to mouldy hay (*Micropolyspora faeni*) causes farmer's lung, to mouldy sugar cane causes bagassosis, to mushroom dust causes mushroom picker's lung, to bird droppings (containing avian serum proteins) causes bird fancier's lung, to contaminated malting barley (*Aspergillus clavatus*) causes malt worker's lung. Precipitating antibodies against the offending antigen can often be found in the patient's blood.

Clinical features

Acute (i.e. 4–6 h after exposure)

Dyspnoea, dry cough, malaise, fever and limb pains occur, and examination shows fine inspiratory crepitations with little wheeze. The symptoms subside in 2–3 days.

Chronic

After repeated acute attacks fibrosis occurs with persistent inspiratory crepitations, respiratory failure and cor pulmonale.

Investigation

Chest X-ray shows a diffuse haze initially and later micronodular shadowing, progressing to honeycombing. Ventilatory function tests initially show a reversible restrictive defect with low T_{LCO} during the acute attacks. This becomes permanent as the chronic disorder develops. There is little or no obstruction. The PaO_2 falls and $PaCO_2$ is normal or reduced by the hyperventilation.

Treatment

Separate the patient and the allergen. Ventilation and personal protective equipment may reduce dust exposure. Steroids can be tried in severe cases and should be continued only if there has been a measured response in lung function.

Obstructive sleep apnoea

The sleep apnoea syndrome has been defined as absence of airflow in periods of at least 10 s occurring at least five times per hour during sleep, with daytime drowsiness.

There are repeated episodes of upper airways obstruction during sleep with hypoxaemia and sudden arousal. This results in poor sleep, snoring, excessive daytime sleepiness and observed apnoeas in sleep. It is associated with male gender, obesity and evening alcohol consumption. It is a risk factor for the development of hypertension and has been associated with type 2 diabetes, ischaemic heart disease and stroke. Diagnosis requires overnight sleep studies where arterial oxygen saturation can be monitored. Management involves slimming and alcohol reduction, followed by continuous positive airways pressure (CPAP) if these fail. Surgery may be of value if there is evidence of anatomical obstruction.

Pulmonary embolism

Emboli usually arise in the veins of the pelvis or legs and, rarely, from the right atrium.

They occur more frequently:

- following surgery (classically, although not always, about 10 days)
- following myocardial infarction
- following a stroke
- in disseminated malignancy
- in prolonged bed rest associated with illness
- during air flights over 3 h or 3000 miles, not necessarily economy class
- following trauma, especially to the pelvis and legs (including caesarean section)
- in antiphospholipid syndrome (page 318, Chapter 18)
- in hypercoagulable states – antithrombin III, protein C and S deficiencies. In factor V Leiden a single point mutation in the factor V gene causes resistance to activated protein C.

The risk may increase if other factors are present:

- advancing age
- obesity
- pregnancy and postpartum
- treatment with oestrogens (oral contraceptive pill or hormone replacement therapy)
- previous venous thrombosis or family history of it.

Patients who die from pulmonary embolism have often had premonitory signs and symptoms of small emboli (unexplained breathless attacks) or venous thrombosis in the previous weeks. A deep vein thrombosis should be regarded as potential pulmonary embolus and must be suspected, diagnosed and treated as an emergency.

Clinical features

The clinical features of deep venous thrombosis include:

- erythema and warmth of the affected leg
- swelling and tenderness.

Thromboses that extend above the knee are more likely to produce clinically recognisable and life-threatening pulmonary emboli.

NB: Diagnosis is confirmed by ultrasound with vein compression or venography. Swelling of the calf also occurs in rupture of a Baker's cyst behind the knee. An effusion of the knee makes this more likely. The cyst can often be shown on ultrasound.

Clinical presentation (of pulmonary embolus)

This depends upon the size of the embolus. Multiple small acute emboli may remain undetected until up to 50% of the vascular bed is involved and present with effort dyspnoea.

- *Small.* Transient faints and dyspnoea, with slight pyrexia.
- *Medium.* Usually results in infarction and produces, in addition, haemoptysis, pleurisy and, occasionally, a pleural effusion.
- *Large.* Acute cor pulmonale with sudden dyspnoea and shock. There is a small-volume rapid pulse, with hypotension, cyanosis, peripheral vasoconstriction and a raised jugular venous pressure. There may be a gallop rhythm.

Investigation

Chest X-ray

This may demonstrate:

- pulmonary oligaemia of the affected segment (usually present but difficult to diagnose except in retrospect)
- the corresponding pulmonary artery is sometimes dilatated at the hilum
- small areas of horizontal linear collapse, usually at the bases, with a raised diaphragm
- a small pleural effusion.

With larger emboli, the heart enlarges acutely and the superior vena cava distends.

ECG

Electrocardiogram changes usually occur only with larger emboli but are then common. The characteristic changes are as follows (see also Fig. 10.4):

- tachycardia
- right ventricular 'strain' pattern (inverted T waves in leads V1–4)
- acute, often transient, right bundle branch block pattern
- S_1, Q_3, T_3 pattern
- transient arrhythmias, e.g. atrial fibrillation.

Arterial blood gases

With larger emboli, a fall in PaO_2 and $PaCO_2$ is common.

Lung perfusion scan

This may show underperfusion of one or more parts of the lung that are radiologically normal (and ventilated normally on ventilation scan).

Combined ventilation and perfusion scans

These may be helpful in pre-existent lung disease in which ventilation and perfusion defects are usually matched. A normal scan virtually excludes pulmonary embolism.

Pulmonary angiography

This is the most precise method of investigation for cases presenting difficulty in diagnosis. High-resolution CT pulmonary angiogram has a high accuracy rate for the evaluation of pulmonary embolism.

D-DIMER

D-DIMER is a fibrin degradation product formed by the enzymatic activity of plasmin on cross-linked fibrin polymers. Plasma levels can be measured and are raised in patients with pulmonary embolism or deep vein thrombosis. Negative test results rule out the likelihood of these diseases.

Treatment

Prophylaxis is given pre- and postoperatively, especially in lower abdomen and lower limb surgery, and in patients confined to bed or with predisposing disorders (e.g. cardiac failure). Aspirin with graduated-compression stockings are given to at-risk long-distance air travellers. Low-molecular-weight heparins are prepared by depolymerisation of standard (unfractionated) heparin. They have a longer duration of action than standard heparin and, given as a once daily subcutaneous dose, produce a more predictable anticoagulant response. They are safe and effective as low-dose prophylaxis, and can be used in weight-adjusted dosage for treatment of deep vein thrombosis without laboratory monitoring.

For established deep vein thrombosis or pulmonary embolism, oral factor Xa inhibitors provide an alternative to treatment with low-molecular-weight heparin, or fondaparinux (a synthetic pentasaccharide factor Xa inhibitor), followed by warfarin (Trials Box 11.3). Treatment is continued for a minimum of 3 months.

In massive pulmonary embolism, cardiac massage and correction of acidosis with urgent intravenous heparin may improve survival. With large emboli, oxygen in high concentration and thrombolytic therapy with urokinase or streptokinase may be valuable. The operative removal of large emboli with bypass surgery may be life-saving.

Placement of a vena caval filter should be considered when anticoagulation is hazardous or in patients who develop emboli despite adequate anticoagulation.

TRIALS BOX 11.3 Factor Xa inhibitors in venous thromboembolism

The EINSTEIN-PE investigators found that a fixed-dose regimen of rivaroxaban alone was non-inferior to standard therapy with enoxaparin followed by an adjusted-dose vitamin K antagonist for the initial and long-term treatment of pulmonary embolism. Rivaroxaban had a potentially improved benefit-risk profile. Source: *New England Journal of Medicine* 2012; **366**(14): 1287–1297.

The RE-COVER II trial investigators found dabigatran has similar effects on venous thromboembolism recurrence and a lower risk of bleeding compared with warfarin for the treatment of acute venous thromboembolism. Source: *Circulation* 2014; **129**(7): 764–772.

The Hokusai-VTE investigators found that edoxaban administered once daily after initial treatment with heparin was non-inferior to high-quality standard therapy and caused significantly less bleeding in patients with venous thromboembolism, including severe pulmonary embolism. Source: *New England Journal of Medicine* 2013; **369**(15): 1406–1415.

Hyperventilation syndrome

Breathlessness in the absence of abnormal clinical signs and increased by emotion (e.g. clinical examinations and ward rounds) should never be considered psychogenic until other diagnoses have been excluded.

Hyperventilation syndrome may be the presenting symptom of psychiatric illness and the patient should be asked about symptoms of anxiety and depression. The breathlessness is usually episodic and not directly related to exertion (often even occurring at rest). It may be described as an inability to take a deep breath or shortage of oxygen. There are associated symptoms of hypocapnia (tingling in the fingers, dizziness, headache, heaviness in the chest, cramp). Tetany may occur with carpopedal spasm. Spirometry may give a disorganised trace, but the *FEV1* and *FVC* are normal when obtained.

Idiopathic pulmonary fibrosis

Clinical features

The disease begins in middle age and presents with progressive dyspnoea and dry cough, usually without wheeze or sputum. The typical signs are clubbing, cyanosis and crepitations in the mid and lower lung fields.

Investigation

The arterial PaO_2 is reduced and hyperventilation may cause a reduction in $PaCO_2$. Spirometry (Fig. 4.6, Chapter 4) may be normal or demonstrate a restrictive pattern, sometimes with an obstructive pattern.

Chest X-ray shows diffuse bilateral basal nodular–reticular shadowing that extends upwards as the disease progresses. The differential diagnosis of the chest X-ray includes other causes of diffuse pulmonary fibrosis and infiltration: occupational dust lung diseases, sarcoidosis, scleroderma, lymphangitis carcinomatosa, collagen diseases, miliary tuberculosis, radiation pneumonitis, drugs (busulphan and other cytotoxic drugs, nitrofurantoin, paraquat), histoplasmosis, coccidioidomycosis and histiocytosis X. Clinically, the problem is less difficult. Lung biopsy, if performed, shows alveolitis with lymphocytic and plasma cell infiltration and diffuse pulmonary fibrosis.

Management

Pulmonary rehabilitation and ambulatory oxygen therapy can help, but the disease is progressive. Pirfenidone, an immunosuppressant with anti-inflammatory and antifibrotic effects, can reduce progression in mild to moderate disease. Lung transplantation should be considered.

Adult respiratory distress syndrome

Adult respiratory distress syndrome (ARDS) refers to acute progressive respiratory failure starting hours to days after a number of pulmonary or systemic insults. These include sepsis, trauma (lung contusion or non-thoracic), aspiration (gastric contents, toxins, smoke), shock from any cause, disseminated intravascular coagulation, and air and fat emboli. It can occur in association with pneumonia, and may be drug-induced (heroin, barbiturates). The pulmonary oedema is caused by capillary leakage rather than the elevated left atrial pressure of heart failure.

It is characterised by:

- arterial hypoxia
- reduced thoracic compliance
- normal pulmonary capillary wedge pressure
- diffuse infiltrates on chest X-ray.

Treatment

This should be aimed at the underlying condition, although in many cases the lung injury has already occurred. Ventilation with positive end-expiratory pressure is usually necessary. Neither steroids nor surfactant have been shown to be of benefit in sepsis-associated ARDS. Mortality is high and associated with sepsis, organ failure and age.

12

Gastroenterology

Symptoms arising in the gastrointestinal tract are extremely common. Irritable bowel syndrome, peptic ulcer, hiatus hernia, appendicitis, diverticulitis, haemorrhoids, ulcerative colitis and carcinoma of the colon are common. Carcinoma of the stomach and carcinoma of the oesophagus are less common.

Gastric and duodenal ulceration

Aetiology

Infection with *Helicobacter pylori* and the use of anti-inflammatory drugs, both steroidal and non-steroidal (including aspirin), are the most common precipitating factors. Smoking increases the rate of ulcer recurrence and slows ulcer healing. Very rarely, ulceration is associated with Zollinger–Ellison syndrome (see later, page 151), multiple endocrine neoplasia (MEN) type 1 syndrome (page 254, Chapter 16), hyperparathyroidism (page 296, Chapter 17) and stress (e.g. extensive burns – Curling's ulcer).

Helicobacter pylori colonises the mucus layer overlying the gastric epithelium. The associated chronic superficial gastritis may be asymptomatic, but infection is associated with peptic ulceration and an increased incidence of gastric cancer. Production of urease and cytotoxins and disruption of the gastric mucosal barrier are thought to contribute to disease production.

There is an association between *H. pylori* infection and the development of B-cell gastric lymphomas of mucosa-associated lymphoid tissue (MALT). Early stage MALT lymphomas may respond to eradication of *H. pylori*.

Clinical presentation

It is impossible, on the basis of history and examination alone, to differentiate between non-ulcer dyspepsia, duodenal ulceration, benign ulceration of the stomach and carcinoma of the stomach, but carcinoma is much less common.

Pain may be retrosternal or epigastric or occur anywhere in the anterior upper abdomen, and be associated with anorexia, vomiting and weight loss.

Examination

There may be epigastric tenderness. The presence of an epigastric mass suggests carcinoma. A gastric splash (or succussion) indicates the rare pyloric obstruction caused by benign duodenal stricture or due to carcinoma of the pyloric antrum.

Complications

- bleeding
- perforation (usually duodenal ulceration)
- pyloric stenosis

Investigation

Endoscopy with gastric biopsy is important in establishing the diagnosis and allows identification of *H. pylori* infection (see Box 12.1).

Duodenal ulcers are virtually always benign. Gastric carcinomas are more common on the greater curve and in the antrum, but lesser curve ulcers may be malignant. The size of the ulcer is no guide to whether a carcinoma is present. Carcinomas may have a rolled edge. Biopsy can give histological confirmation. Repeat endoscopy after 4 weeks of treatment should show healing of a gastric ulcer. If this has not occurred the presence of a carcinoma becomes more likely.

Clinical Medicine Lecture Notes, Eighth Edition. John R. Bradley, Mark Gurnell, and Diana F. Wood.
© 2019 John Wiley & Sons Ltd. Published 2019 by John Wiley & Sons Ltd.

Box 12.1 Tests for *H. pylori*

H. pylori is rich in the enzyme urease which hydrolyses urea to NH_4 and CO_2. In the rapid urease test a gastric biopsy is placed in a solution containing urease and phenol red. Urease present in the biopsy hydrolyses urea to ammonia causing a rise in pH and a change in colour from yellow to red, confirming the presence of *H. pylori*.

The urea breath test measures the amount of $^{14}CO_2$ released after a dose of ^{14}C-labelled urea. Infection can also be detected by testing for antibodies in the serum by enzyme-linked immunosorbent assay (ELISA) and a stool antigen test.

Management

Antacids and diet often ameliorate symptoms but do not hasten healing. The patient should stop smoking.

Patients with proven *H. pylori* infection are given eradication therapy with a proton-pump inhibitor and antibiotics (Box 12.2).

H^+/K^+-ATPase (proton-pump) inhibitors (PPI) cause a profound reduction in gastric acidity.

H_2-receptor antagonists reduce gastric acid output, and may be used if there is an inadequate response to a PPI.

Box 12.2 *H. pylori* eradication

NICE guidance on *H. pylori* eradication recommends a 7-day course of a proton-pump inhibitor (PPI) with amoxicillin and either clarithromycin or metronidazole. People who are allergic to penicillin should be offered a PPI with clarithromycin and metronidazole unless there has been previous exposure to clarithromycin, when a PPI should be combined with bismuth, metronidazole and tetracycline. Patients who remain symptomatic after a 7-day course of treatment are offered a 7-day course of second-line treatment with a PPI and a combination of antibiotics, chosen taking account of previous exposure and allergies.

NICE guidance CG184. Dyspepsia and gastro-oesophageal reflux disease: Investigation and management of dyspepsia, symptoms suggestive of gastro-oesophageal reflux disease, or both. November 2014.

Misoprostol, a synthetic prostaglandin analogue, is effective in reducing gastrointestinal damage induced by non-steroidal anti-inflammatory drugs (NSAIDs).

Gastric carcinoma

Gastric carcinoma is a leading cause of cancer mortality worldwide. It is associated with *H. pylori* infection. It affects mainly the pylorus and antrum. It can present with dyspepsia, anorexia, weight loss or evidence of bleeding.

The prognosis is poor. Resection with removal of the primary tumour and regional lymph nodes is the most effective treatment, and survival may be improved by adjuvant chemotherapy and radiotherapy.

Hiatus hernia and gastro-oesophageal reflux

Aetiology

Weakness of the diaphragmatic sphincter allows the lower oesophagus and cardia of the stomach to rise into the thorax. Gastro-oesophageal reflux may occur in the presence or absence of a hiatus hernia and is aggravated by smoking and alcohol.

Symptoms

Retrosternal burning pain, usually episodic, with acid regurgitation that is worse on lying flat or bending and relieved by antacids. Bleeding may give positive occult blood tests and anaemia. Oesophagitis may lead to ulceration and/or stricture.

Investigations

If persistent and symptoms are severe or if associated with dysphagia (to exclude benign or malignant stricture) or weight loss (to exclude oesophageal or gastric carcinoma), endoscopy or barium swallow will reveal the hernia and the presence of gastric acid reflux.

Management

- Weight reduction and stop smoking. Avoid clothes that constrict and increase intra-abdominal pressure, and avoid foods that induce symptoms if recognised. Sleep propped up (raise head of the bed).
- Antacids for symptoms. Metoclopramide increases oesophageal sphincter contraction and increases gastric emptying. It is a dopamine antagonist and

may induce acute dystonic reactions, which respond to procyclidine. A course of an H_2-receptor antagonist or a proton-pump inhibitor usually relieves symptoms if severe.

- Surgery for hiatus hernia is very rarely indicated in the absence of stricture formation as it is a major procedure and the results are uncertain. In Barrett's oesophagus, reflux is associated with columnar metaplasia of the normal stratified squamous epithelium of the lower oesophagus. It can progress to low-grade dysplasia, high-grade dysplasia and carcinoma. Surveillance allows earlier treatment by endoscopic resection or ablation, or oesophagectomy.

Inflammatory bowel disease (ulcerative colitis and Crohn's disease)

Aetiology

In ulcerative colitis and Crohn's disease environmental factors are thought to trigger inflammation of the bowel in genetically prone individuals.

Ulcerative colitis

Ulcerative colitis is a distal non-transmural inflammatory disease of the rectum (proctitis) with a variable extension proximally up the large bowel. Although it is restricted to the large bowel, ileal inflammation (backwash ileitis) can occur.

Clinical features (Table 12.1)

Ulcerative colitis may occur at any age, but usually presents in the 20- to 40-year age group with bloody diarrhoea, passage of mucus or pus and abdominal pain. In severe colitis, fever, tachycardia, marked abdominal tenderness, anaemia and weight loss are usually present, and marked dilatation of the colon (toxic megacolon) may lead to perforation. The disease follows a chronic relapsing–remitting course, with variation in the activity and extent of the disease changing in individual patients over the years. At any one time about 50% of patients are in remission.

Diagnosis

This is suggested by the clinical picture and may be confirmed by sigmoidoscopy with biopsy. The extent

Table 12.1 Clinical features of ulcerative colitis and Crohn's disease

Clinical feature	Ulcerative colitis	Crohn's disease
Rectal bleeding	+	+/−
Passage of mucus or pus	+	+/−
Disease confined to large bowel	+	−
Bowel obstruction	+/−	+
Fistula formation	−	+
Extraintestinal manifestations	+	+
Transmural inflammation	−	+
Granulomas	−	+
Antineutrophil cytoplasm antibodies	+	+/−
Anti-*Saccharomyces cerevisiae* antibodies	+/−	+

+, yes; +/−, uncommon; −, no.

of disease is confirmed by colonoscopy or imaging studies. Infectious causes should be excluded.

Sigmoidoscopy

The rectal mucosa is always abnormal in ulcerative colitis. Abnormal appearances, in order of severity, are:

- granular mucosa with loss of normal vascular pattern
- presence of pus and blood
- visible ulceration with contact bleeding at the rim of the sigmoidoscope.

Histology

Histology shows superficial inflammation with chronic inflammatory cells infiltrating the lamina propria with crypt abscesses, with little involvement of the muscularis mucosa and with reduction of goblet cells.

Imaging

Imaging by barium enema, CT or MR shows loss of normal haustral pattern with shortening of the large intestine (Fig. 12.1). The bowel takes on the appearance of a smooth tube (hosepipe appearance).

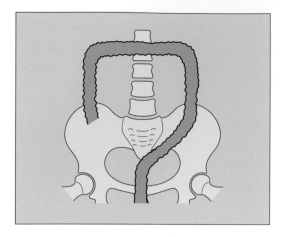

Figure 12.1 Long-standing ulcerative colitis. Widespread shallow ulceration leads to shortening and narrowing of the colon.

Undermined ulcers and pseudopolypi may be seen. Stricture formation or carcinoma produces fixed areas of narrowing.

Plain abdominal film will show acute dilatation when present, and bowel gas may outline mucosal ulceration. Barium enema examination in such circumstances may produce perforation.

Differential diagnosis

- Carcinoma of the colon, which may present with bloody diarrhoea.
- Infective enteritis. The acute case may resemble *Campylobacter* enteritis or bacillary dysentery, and the chronic case amoebic colitis (these should be excluded by stool examination).
- Antibiotic-associated pseudomembranous colitis is caused by toxins of *Clostridium difficile* when it colonises the colon, usually following antibiotic-induced suppression of the normal bacterial flora of the gut. On sigmoidoscopy, characteristically there are patchy yellowish areas of necrotic mucosa. Histology shows mucosal destruction with characteristic exudation of fibrin and inflammatory cells in the cross-sectional shape of a mushroom. *C. difficile*-derived glutamate dehydrogenase (detects all strains, including non-toxogenic *C. difficile*) and its toxin may be found in the stool. The condition responds to oral metronidazole or vancomycin.
- Very rarely, acute ischaemic colitis may occur and affect the rectosigmoid junction.
- Irritable bowel syndrome.

Treatment

Oral 5-aminosalicylic acid compounds are used to induce remission in mild to moderate colitis. Sulfasalazine is a combination of 5-aminosalicylic acid (5-ASA) and sulfapyridine, which acts as a carrier to deliver 5-ASA to its site of action in the colon. Mesalazine is 5-ASA by itself, and olsalazine is two linked molecules of 5-ASA that separate in the lower bowel. These newer aminosalicylates lack sulfonamide-related side effects, although their benefit over sulfasalazine in ulcerative colitis is unclear. 5-ASA compounds can be delivered by suppository in proctitis. In moderate colitis that does not respond to 5-ASA or severe colitis, oral steroids should be started, and azathioprine can be added for its steroid-sparing effect. Rectal steroids can be used in proctitis. In patients refractory to 5-ASA and steroids, the anti-TNF (tumour necrosis factor) agent infliximab can induce remission and reduce the need for colectomy in the short term.

Treatment can usually be tapered once remission is achieved, but all of the above agents have been used to maintain remission.

Patients with severe colitis should be admitted to hospital for intravenous steroids and fluids and managed jointly by the gastroenterologist and surgeon. Patients who do not respond to intravenous steroids may respond to ciclosporin, tacrolimus or infliximab, but the need for colectomy should be continuously reviewed.

Surgery

Surgery is indicated if there is:

- severe haemorrhage
- perforation
- acute toxaemia with dilatation of the colon which fails to respond to high-dose steroids.

Elective surgery is indicated if regular colonoscopy shows high-grade dysplasia or cancer, or in patients who are intolerant of or refractory to long-term medical treatments.

Crohn's disease

Crohn's disease is a relapsing inflammatory disease that can affect any site in the alimentary tract from mouth to anus.

Aetiology

Current evidence suggests that genetic and environmental factors contribute to an abnormal mucosal immune response that is facilitated by the gut microflora. Nucleotide binding oligomerisation domain 2/caspase recruitment domain-containing protein (NOD2/CARD15) was identified as the first susceptibility gene in Crohn's disease in 2001. NOD2 contains an intracellular receptor for components of microbial pathogens, and other genes encoding proteins that regulate microbial responses (autophagy, ER stress, phagocytosis), and innate and adaptive immunity have since been implicated in disease pathogenesis.

Clinical features (Table 12.1)

Peak incidence is between ages 10 and 40. The terminal ileum is most frequently diseased, followed by the colon and less commonly the upper gastrointestinal tract. It usually presents as intermittent abdominal pain with diarrhoea, sometimes with passage of blood or mucus. Less commonly it presents as an 'acute abdomen' with signs of acute appendicitis with or without a palpable mass or obstruction. A mass in the right iliac fossa from terminal ileitis must be differentiated from a caecal carcinoma and an appendix abscess. Amoebic abscess and ileocaecal tuberculosis are less common causes.

The granulomatous inflammatory process affects short lengths of the intestine, leaving normal bowel between skip lesions. The wall is thickened and the lumen narrowed. Mucosal ulceration and regional lymphadenopathy are present. The characteristic microscopic features are of submucosal inflammation, less marked than in ulcerative colitis. There are numerous fissures down to the submucosa with or without chronic granulation tissue.

Imaging (Fig. 12.2)

Barium enema

The terminal ileum is most commonly involved and may produce incompetence of the ileocaecal valve. Mucosal ulceration may be deep and 'spikes' of barium may enter deep into the bowel wall (rose thorn). Lesions may be multiple with normal bowel between (skip lesions, Fig. 12.2). Coarse cobblestone appearance of the mucosa appears early. Later in the disease, fibrosis produces narrowing of the intestine (string sign) with some proximal dilatation.

Small-bowel enema

There may be mucosal ulceration, luminal narrowing or pooling of barium in irregular clumps at the site of an inflammatory mass.

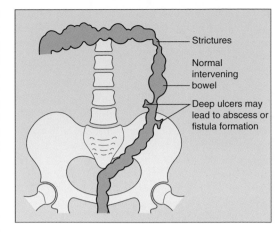

Figure 12.2 Crohn's disease. Patchy involvement of the bowel with: (1) deep ulcers which may lead to abscess or fistula formation; (2) strictures; (3) normal intervening bowel. Areas of disease with normal intervening bowel are known as skip lesions.

Cross-sectional imaging with multi-slice CT, MR with oral contrast and MR enteroclysis, in which contrast is inserted through a naso-duodenal tube, provide alternative approaches.

Indium-labelled white cell scanning is helpful in localising active inflammatory bowel disease.

Histology

In Crohn's disease the characteristic microscopic features are of submucosal inflammation, less marked than in ulcerative colitis. There are numerous fissures down to the submucosa with or without chronic granulation tissue consisting of non-caseating granulomas.

Complications

Fever, anaemia and weight loss. Hypoalbuminaemia results from loss of protein and in small-bowel disease malabsorption. Fistulae, peri-anal fissures, and sepsis may all complicate Crohn's disease.

Treatment

Aminosalicylates and corticosteroids have been used to induce remission. The newer aminosalicylates may be of more benefit in treating Crohn's disease. Mesalazine suppositories can be useful for localised rectal disease. Budesonide that is formulated to be released in the terminal ileum and colon can be effective with fewer side effects than conventional steroids. It is a steroid that is rapidly metabolised in the liver after absorption. Enteral nutrition has been used to induce remission but is less effective that steroids. Anti-TNF treatment with infliximab, adalimumab or certolizumab pegol are usually reserved for patients who do not enter remission with mesalazine or steroids. Methotrexate or ciclosporin may be of value in patients who are refractory to these treatments. Attention to nutritional deficiencies (page 284, Chapter 17) and electrolyte imbalance is essential.

Azathioprine, anti-TNF therapies and enteral nutrition have been shown to be effective in maintaining remission. Smoking cessation is important in maintenance of remission.

Antibiotics (ciprofloxacin and metronidazole) are widely used for the treatment of fistulas in Crohn's disease. Azathioprine may be effective, and anti-TNF treatments with infliximab and adalimumab are increasingly used to heal fistulas.

Surgery

In Crohn's disease surgery is used for relief of acute emergencies (obstruction), abscesses and fistulae. Resection of diseased intestine and bypass operations may become necessary for severe, chronic ill health, but unlike in ulcerative colitis these are not curative. Fistula formation may result and recurrence is the rule. Intestinal obstruction is best managed conservatively in the first instance with gastric aspiration and intravenous feeding to allow time for the acute inflammation to resolve.

The benefit of colonoscopy surveillance for colorectal carcinoma in ulcerative colitis and Crohn's disease remains unclear. The risk is greater if the entire colon is involved, if the history is prolonged (10% after 10 years), if the first attack was severe and if the first attack occurred at a young age. Medical treatment appears to lessen the risk of carcinoma.

Extraintestinal manifestations of inflammatory bowel disease

Extraintestinal complications usually respond to treatment of the inflammatory bowel disease. Clubbing, uveitis, arthritis and skin rashes (erythema nodosum and pyoderma gangrenosum) can occur.

Renal stones are more common, and primary sclerosing cholangitis is often associated with inflammatory bowel disease.

Intestinal cancer in inflammatory bowel disease

Patients with ulcerative colitis are at increased risk of colorectal cancer. In Crohn's disease there is an increased risk of both colorectal and small-bowel cancer. The risk of cancer depends on the duration and extent of the disease, and may be reduced by medical treatment to reduce disease activity and surveillance colonoscopy.

Endocrine tumours of the gut

All are very rare.

Apudomas

Amine precursor uptake and decarboxylation (APUD) cells are the hormone-secreting cells found chiefly along the length of the gastrointestinal tract. They have molecular and functional similarities with each other and may form various kinds of functioning tumour. They secrete a number of hormones including gastrin, cholecystokinin, secretin, glucagon and vasoactive intestinal peptide (VIP).

Carcinoid tumours

Carcinoid tumours originate in cells of the neuroendocrine system, usually in tissues derived from the embryonic gut. Twenty-five percent arise in the lung, thymus, stomach, or duodenum (foregut), 50% in the small intestine, appendix, or proximal colon (midgut), and 15% in the distal colon or rectum (hindgut). Secretory products depend on the site and include gastrin (gastric antrum and duodenum); histamine (gastric fundus and body); somatostatin, serotonin, motilin, and substance P (stomach, duodenum, jejunum, colon, rectum); cholecystokinin, gastric inhibitory polypeptide, motilin, secretin, pancreatic polypeptide (duodenum, jejunum); polypeptide Y (jejunum, ileum, colon, rectum); neurotensin (jejunum, ileum).

Carcinoid syndrome with flushing, abdominal pain, diarrhoea, bronchospasm, and carcinoid heart disease is rare in the absence of hepatic metastases because vasoactive amines are metabolised in the liver. In carcinoid heart disease valvular fibrosis is associated with tricuspid and pulmonary regurgitation, pulmonary stenosis, mitral and aortic regurgitation, and cardiac arrhythmias.

Treatments include surgical resection and somatostatin analogues. Lanreotide is a longer acting somatostatin analogue than octreotide that can be administered every 10 to 14 days with similar efficacy. Interferons can slow disease progression and provide symptom relief.

Zollinger–Ellison syndrome

This rare disorder is characterised by multiple recurrent duodenal and jejunal ulceration associated with a very high plasma gastrin level (>300 mg/l with the patient off H_2-receptor blockade), gross gastric acid hypersecretion and the presence of a gastrin-secreting adenoma (which may be malignant), usually in the pancreas but sometimes in the stomach wall.

Diarrhoea sometimes with steatorrhoea may be a feature (lipase is inactivated by the low pH). The volume of gastric secretion is enormous (7–10l/24h) and acid secretion persistently raised (and raised little further by pentagastrin). Normal fasting gastrin is <100 pg/ml. In Zollinger–Ellison syndrome there is a rise in serum gastrin level >200 pg/ml after infusion of secretin 2 units/kg.

The presence of an adenoma may be associated with adenomas of other endocrine glands, i.e. adrenals, parathyroids and anterior pituitary (page 250, Chapter 15).

Treatment is by removal of the tumour, which is usually benign. If it cannot be found, give either long-term proton-pump inhibitor or H_2-blockade.

Vipoma

Vipoma is a variant of the Zollinger–Ellison syndrome with severe watery diarrhoea, hypokalaemia with or without achlorhydria caused by a benign or malignant pancreatic tumour producing a VIP. Abdominal pain and flushing are typical features. Vipomectomy may be curative.

Endocrine tumours of the pancreas

These are very rare but are sometimes discussed in examinations.

Insulinoma

Insulinoma is a tumour of the pancreatic islet β-cells that produces episodic hypoglycaemic attacks which may present as epilepsy or abnormal behaviour. Fasting produces prolonged hypoglycaemia with high insulin levels in the serum. Rarely tumours are multiple or malignant.

Glucagonoma

Glucagonoma is a tumour of the α-cells that produces a syndrome of mild diabetes with diarrhoea, weight loss, anaemia, glossitis and a migratory necrolytic rash.

Gastrointestinal haemorrhage

Upper gut

Aetiology

Acute

Peptic ulcer accounts for most cases of non-variceal bleeding (see 168 for variceal bleeding). Other causes include gastric erosions, Mallory–Weiss (mucosal oesophageal tears caused by retching) and oesophagitis. Concurrent use of NSAIDs or aspirin with selective serotonin reuptake inhibitors (SSRIs) greatly increases the risk of upper gastrointestinal bleeding.

Oesophagitis, oesophageal ulcer, gastric ulcer and malignancy are more common in elderly people. Mallory–Weiss syndrome, gastritis and duodenal ulcer are more common in young people. Oesophageal varices, oesophageal ulcer and gastrointestinal malignancy are associated with increased risk of death. Poor prognostic factors include older age, comorbid illness, evidence of continued bleeding or rebleeding, low initial haemoglobin and elevated urea, creatinine or serum aminotransferase.

Clinical presentation

Haematemesis is a reliable indication of bleeding above the duodeno-jejunal flexure as is bright-red rectal bleeding of the lower colon or rectum. The colour of altered blood passed per rectum is related to transit time more than to the site of bleeding.

Faintness, weakness, sweating, palpitation and nausea often precede evidence of bleeding. The patient is pale and sweating and has tachycardia and hypotension.

Chronic

Bleeding from hiatus hernia and gastric is usually insidious (but not always).

Management

Admit to hospital (trivial bleeding can quickly progress to exsanguination), where management should follow local protocol.

Patients should be evaluated immediately and resuscitated if there is evidence of intravascular volume loss:

- Establish venous access. Take blood for group and cross-match, creatinine and electrolytes, liver function tests including the prothrombin time and full blood count with platelets.
- Treat shock if present with transfusion of blood (or colloid if blood is not yet available) and monitor pulse and blood pressure. Oxygen may be needed and the urine output should be monitored.

Variceal bleeding (page 168, Chapter 13)

Investigation (for site and cause of bleeding)

Within 24 h, as soon as the patient's condition allows, upper gastrointestinal endoscopy should be performed; this shows the site of bleeding in most cases. Local diathermy or injection of a sclerosant may arrest bleeding. Selective angiography may show the site of active bleeding if not previously determined, particularly when angiodysplasia is the cause.

If bleeding continues or recurs, surgery may be necessary (see later).

Proton-pump inhibitors (PPI) reduce mortality, rebleeding and the need for surgical intervention (see Trials Box 12.1). Intravenous bolus followed by continuous infusion of PPI should be considered in high-risk patients. Patients should be advised not to smoke.

Indications for surgery (in haemorrhage from peptic ulcer)

Surgery should be considered in patients who bleed after endoscopic treatment. However, such patients are often elderly and high risk.

Lower gut

Acute loss may occur from haemorrhoids, fissures, ulcerative colitis and Crohn's disease, ischaemic colitis, rectal, colonic and caecal carcinoma and diverticular disease. Patients with chronic and occult bleeding usually present with lethargy and iron-deficiency anaemia and diagnosis is confirmed by positive faecal occult blood tests. Any of the causes of upper or lower gut bleeding given earlier may be responsible. Other very rare causes include polyps and vascular abnormalities, such as arteriovenous malformations, angiodysplasia of the ascending colon, Peutz–Jeghers syndrome (small intestinal polyposis and blotchy pigmentation around the mouth) and Rendu–Osler–Weber (hereditary (autosomal dominant) haemorrhagic

---

 TRIALS BOX 12.1 Proton-pump inhibitors in gastrointestinal haemorrhage

A Health Technology Assessment systematic review concluded that proton-pump inhibitor (PPI) treatment compared with placebo or H_2-receptor antagonists reduces mortality following peptic ulcer bleeding among patients with high-risk endoscopic findings, and reduces rebleeding rates and surgical intervention. PPI treatment initiated prior to endoscopy in upper gastrointestinal bleeding significantly reduces the proportion of patients with stigmata of recent haemorrhage at index endoscopy but does not reduce mortality, rebleeding or the need for surgery. The strategy of giving oral PPI before and after endoscopy, with endoscopic haemostatic therapy for those with major stigmata of recent haemorrhage, is likely to be the most cost-effective.

Treatment of *H. pylori* infection was found to be more effective than antisecretory therapy in preventing recurrent bleeding from peptic ulcers. *H. pylori* eradication alone or eradication followed by misoprostol (with switch to PPI if misoprostol is not tolerated) are the two most cost-effective strategies for preventing bleeding ulcers among *H. pylori*-infected NSAID users, although the data cannot exclude PPIs also being cost-effective. Source: *Health Technology Assessment* 2007; **11**(51): iii–iv, 1–164.

telangiectasia in which thin-walled dilatated blood vessels rupture causing gastrointestinal bleeding, epistaxis, haemoptysis or haematuria) syndromes. Meckel's diverticulum, polyps and endometriosis may also present with bleeding.

Steatorrhoea and malabsorption

Malabsorption signifies impaired ability to absorb one or more of the normally absorbed dietary constituents, including protein, carbohydrates, fats, minerals and vitamins.

Steatorrhoea signifies malabsorption of fat, and is defined as a faecal fat excretion of more than 18 mmol/day (6 g/day) on a normal fat intake (50–100 g). Apart from the occasions when the cause of steatorrhoea is obvious (such as obstructive jaundice), the diagnostic problem revolves around the differentiation between enteropathy (commonly gluten-induced) and other causes of steatorrhoea.

Diarrhoea is not necessarily a presenting symptom and malabsorption may present with one or more of its complications (e.g. anaemia, weight loss, osteomalacia).

Gluten-sensitive enteropathy (coeliac disease)

Aetiology

There is mucosal sensitivity to wheat gluten (in particular gliadin, a polypeptide in gluten) and to barley and rye, and occasionally oats (although not rice or maize). There is an increased incidence in near-relatives, and both MHC (in particular HLA-DQ 2.5) and non-MHC gene loci are associated with disease risk. The prevalence of coeliac disease is around 1%.

NB: Virtually all patients with dermatitis herpetiformis have gluten-sensitive enteropathy.

Clinical presentation

There is usually a history of tiredness and intermittent or chronic increased bowel frequency. There may be a history of intermittent abdominal pain and distension, and flatulence. Depending on the severity and duration of the disease, there may weight loss. If the malabsorption started in childhood, the patient may be short compared with unaffected siblings or parents. Children may present with irritability, failure to gain weight or failure to thrive. Occasionally patients

Table 12.2 Vitamin and mineral deficiency following malabsorption

Vitamin/mineral	Deficiency
Vitamin B$_{12}$	Produces megaloblastic anaemia (Chapter 20)
Iron	Produces iron-deficiency anaemia (Chapter 20)
Vitamin D and calcium	Results in osteomalacia (rickets in children) (291)
Vitamin B group	Glossitis and angular stomatitis
Vitamin K	Deficient coagulation
Potassium	May produce muscle pain and weakness
	Abnormalities of cardiac rhythm

do not have gastrointestinal symptoms, but present with anaemia, osteoporosis, abnormal liver function tests or rarely neurological manifestations (ataxia or peripheral neuropathy).

The malabsorption involves not only fat and the fat-soluble vitamins but also minerals and water-soluble vitamins (Table 12.2).

Examination

In addition to the features mentioned earlier there may be evidence of anaemia, weight loss or clubbing. Signs of subacute combined degeneration of the cord are very rare.

Diagnosis (Box 12.3)

Anti-tissue transglutaminase and anti-endomysial antibodies are used in combination with duodenal biopsy, which shows villous atrophy, and repeat biopsy showing a return to normal after several months of a gluten-free diet.

NB: There may be a predisposition to malignancy – small intestinal lymphomas and oesophageal and small and large intestinal carcinoma – in gluten-induced enteropathy and there is some evidence that gluten-free diets reduce the incidence of these.

Treatment

Lifelong adherence to a gluten-free diet is essential. Treat vitamin and mineral deficiencies. Assess bone mineral density and initiate treatment to prevent osteoporosis if indicated (page 289, Chapter 17).

Box 12.3 Coeliac disease: diagnosis and guidelines

British Society of Gastroenterology guidelines on the diagnosis and management of adult coeliac disease recommends that diagnosis of coeliac disease requires duodenal biopsy when the patient is on a gluten-containing diet and for the vast majority of adult patients also positive serology. The guidelines recommend that biopsy remains essential for the diagnosis of adult coeliac disease and cannot be replaced by serology. Follow-up should aim at strict adherence to a gluten-free diet. Source: *Gut* 2014; **63**: 1210–1228.

Other causes of malabsorption

Bile salt deficiency

Patients present with obstructive jaundice usually secondary to carcinoma of the head of the pancreas or to gallstones or, more rarely, in primary biliary cirrhosis or bile duct stricture.

Pancreatic enzyme deficiency

This is usually caused by chronic pancreatitis or carcinoma affecting the pancreatic ducts (more rarely, cystic fibrosis, pancreatic calculi and benign pancreatic cystadenoma). It may be very difficult to differentiate between chronic pancreatitis and carcinoma at presentation.

Tests for malabsorption, glucose tolerance, serum bilirubin and barium meal are of little help.

Imaging

- Straight abdominal X-ray can demonstrate the presence of calcification of the pancreas or of gallstones, which favour chronic pancreatitis.
- Ultrasound, which can be difficult to interpret, can show changes in pancreatic size and shape, calcification and cysts. The biliary tract, neighbouring structures and fluid collections can be shown. Endoscopic ultrasound allows more detailed study.
- CT scan may show gallstones, dilated ducts, calcification and cysts.
- Magnetic resonance cholangiopancreatography (MRCP) or endoscopic retrograde cholangiopancreatography (ERCP) can give information about the biliary tract and help define tumours and cystic lesions.

Investigation

Tests of exocrine pancreatic function

These are rarely used clinically because they are difficult to perform.

Stimulation tests

The duodenum is intubated and duodenal contents aspirated before and after a stimulus (e.g. secretin, cholecystokinin). The fluid is analysed for pancreatic enzymes and bicarbonate.

Bentiromide test

Bentiromide is a synthetic peptide that releases para-aminobenzoic acid (PABA) when cleaved by pancreatic chymotrypsin. PABA is absorbed and excreted in urine. The patient is given bentiromide

---

CASE STUDY Malabsorption

A 34-year-old male teacher presents with excessive tiredness, weight loss and abdominal symptoms of diarrhoea, bloatedness and flatulence. His elder sister had been diagnosed with coeliac disease 3 years previously. BMI was 18, and abdominal examination was normal.

The family history prompted investigation for coeliac disease and the associated malabsorption. Investigations revealed normochromic normocytic anaemia with haemoglobin 115 g/l and a dimorphic picture on blood film (Chapter 20). Serum iron was low with a high transferrin and low transferrin saturation and

serum and red cell folate were low (Chapter 20). Bone profile was normal, but serum vitamin D levels were low. Serology revealed the presence of IgA anti-tissue transglutaminase and anti-endomysial antibodies. The stomach and duodenum appeared normal on endoscopy, but duodenal biopsy revealed villous atrophy, crypt hyperplasia, intraepithelial lymphocytosis and mucosal inflammation.

A diagnosis of coeliac disease was established, and the patient was advised about lifelong treatment adherence to a gluten-free diet. Iron and vitamin deficiencies were corrected with oral supplements.

and urinary PABA measured. A reduction in PABA excretion indicates pancreatic dysfunction.

Symptoms of pancreatic malabsorption can be improved by a low-fat diet, replacing minerals and vitamins, and giving pancreatic enzyme supplements. Avoid alcohol.

Other intestinal disease

Postsurgical

Malabsorption may follow gastrectomy, gastroenterostomy or small bowel resection.

Abnormal intestinal organisms

Bacterial overgrowth can occur with stasis from blind loops, diverticula and strictures. It may occur after gastrectomy as a result of reduced acid and pepsin, and in diabetic autonomic nephropathy.

Bacterial overgrowth can be distinguished from ileal disease using the early (40 min) peak in breath hydrogen after lactulose or glucose.

Bacteria in jejunal juice break down dietary tryptophan to produce indoxylsulphate (indican), which is excreted in the urine. Overgrowth can be detected by finding an increased urinary indican excretion.

In the radioactive bile acid breath test, ^{14}C glycine-labelled bile salt is given orally, and anaerobic bacteria in the intestine deconjugate the bile acid. The released ^{14}C amino acid is transported to the liver and metabolised to $^{14}CO_2$, which can be detected in the breath.

Crohn's disease

See above.

Rare causes

The following are very uncommon but well recognised.

- Zollinger–Ellison syndrome.
- Disaccharidase deficiency. Malabsorption of lactose, maltose and sucrose may occur in isolation caused by primary enzyme deficiency, or as part of a general malabsorption picture in any disease that damages the intestinal brush border. The most important is isolated lactase deficiency which presents, usually in children, with milk intolerance and malabsorption. Patients have abdominal pain, diarrhoea, flatulence and distension (i.e. symptoms of bacterial fermentation of unabsorbed sugars) after oral lactose. The diagnosis is confirmed by finding

symptoms of intolerance and increased levels of breath hydrogen (lactose hydrogen breath test) following lactose, taken orally after an overnight fast. Symptoms of intolerance are recorded. Management consists of withdrawal of milk and milk products from the diet.

- Other intrinsic disease of the intestinal wall caused by tuberculosis, Hodgkin's disease, lymphosarcoma, diffuse systemic sclerosis, amyloidosis and Whipple's disease (intestinal lipodystrophy), associated with the organism *Tropheryma whipplei*.
- Tropical sprue is a disorder that produces steatorrhoea and occurs almost exclusively in Europeans in or from the tropics, especially in India and the Far East. The aetiology is unknown. The most common associated deficiency is folic acid. The disease frequently remits spontaneously on return from the tropics. In some cases that do not remit, a course of parenteral folic acid, metronidazole or oral tetracycline may be curative.
- Very rarely, malabsorption is associated with diabetes, cardiac failure and giardiasis.

Investigation of malabsorption

Blood tests

- Anaemia is common and may be iron-deficient, megaloblastic or both (dimorphic).
- Serum and red cell folate, iron and transferrin may be low.
- Serum albumin may be reduced and the prothrombin time prolonged.
- Serum calcium, phosphate and magnesium may be low and the serum alkaline phosphatase increased.

Faecal fat excretion

The diagnosis of steatorrhoea can be made formally by measuring faecal fat excretion over 3–5 days on a normal diet. In the triolein breath test, ^{14}C-triolein, a triglyceride triolein that releases CO_2 upon metabolism, is given to the patient and the amount of exhaled $^{14}CO_2$ is measured.

Radiology

A small intestinal barium meal with a flocculable contrast medium may show flocculation and segmentation of barium as evidence of excess mucus secretion. Of more significance are widening of the small intestinal calibre and increased distance between adjacent loops of the bowel, indicating thickening of the intestinal wall. All these changes are non-specific and the main purpose of the barium meal is to detect diverticula, fistulae or Crohn's disease. Small bowel MR enteroclysis is an alternative to barium studies.

The bones may show evidence of osteomalacia and/or osteoporosis, and sometimes hyperparathyroidism if very severe and prolonged.

Diverticular disease

Diverticula occur anywhere in the alimentary tract but occur chiefly in the colon causing diverticulosis. They affect chiefly the descending and sigmoid colon. It is a disorder of middle and old age, more common in women than men, and is usually discovered incidentally.

Clinical features

Inflamed diverticula produce diverticulitis with:

- pain, discomfort and tenderness, typically in the left iliac fossa (there may be a mass from pericolic abscess)
- change in bowel habit with constipation and/or diarrhoea sometimes alternating (NB: exclude carcinoma)
- rectal bleeding, which may be acute and sometimes massive and the first symptom
- subacute obstruction
- frequency of micturition, cystitis, and pneumaturia (air in the urine) resulting from vesicocolic fistula
- perforation with peritonitis or fistulae.

Management

Acute diverticulitis may be extremely painful and require rest in bed, analgesia and antibiotics. Occasionally surgery is required, including resection with defunctioning colostomy for obstruction or perforation.

Dietary fibre

Diverticulosis is rare in communities that take a fibre-rich diet, where there is also far less carcinoma of the colon and appendicitis. A diet high in dietary fibre results in bulkier stools and rapid intestinal transit times.

Irritable bowel syndrome

Clinical presentation

Irritable bowel syndrome is one of the most common bowel disorders, affecting about 10% of adults, more often female than male. It is associated with abnormal gut motility. Patients present with different combinations of characteristic symptoms, e.g. colicky abdominal pain, eased by bowel movement, which is often loose, alternating constipation/diarrhoea, bloating and a sense of incomplete evacuation. Examination is usually normal, although there may be tenderness in the left iliac fossa.

The cause of the disturbed gastrointestinal function is unknown, but increased sensitivity to distension of the bowel and abnormalities of motility are found in some patients.

Investigation

Diagnosis is usually made from the pattern of symptoms and signs on history and examination, but investigation to exclude more serious disease is often necessary, particularly in older patients.

Treatment (Trials Box 12.2)

A number of therapies may be beneficial, although there is no uniformly successful treatment. Antispasmodics may be tried, e.g. hyoscine (Buscopan) 10–20 mg t.d.s. before meals. If a cause of anxiety (e.g. cancer) can be identified and

---

 TRIALS BOX 12.2 Treatment of irritable bowel syndrome

Systematic reviews and meta-analyses have shown that fibre, antispasmodics and peppermint oil were all more effective than placebo in the treatment of irritable bowel syndrome. Source: *BMJ* 2008; **337**: a2313. In addition, antidepressants are effective in treatment. There is less high-quality evidence for routine use of psychological therapies in irritable bowel syndrome, but available data suggest these may be of comparable efficacy. Source: *Gut* 2009; **58**(3): 367–378.

Tegaserod (a 5-HT$_4$ partial agonist) appears to improve the overall symptomatology of irritable bowel syndrome and frequency of bowel movements in those with chronic constipation. Source: *Cochrane Database of Systemic Reviews* 2007; (4):CD003960.

treated, symptoms may be markedly reduced and psychological therapy may help. 5-HT$_3$ antagonists (e.g. ondansetron) or antidepressants (tricyclics and SSRIs) can help with abdominal pain and discomfort, urgency and stool frequency in patients with diarrhoea-predominant symptoms (but not those with constipation/bloating). Occasionally, specific foods (cereal, dairy, fructose) may produce symptoms of irritable bowel syndrome, and these should be excluded from the diet. Fibre may help, but makes symptoms worse in some patients.

Ischaemic colitis

Clinical features

This is a disorder of middle and old age that often presents as an acute abdomen with the sudden onset of pain followed by bloody diarrhoea, sometimes copious.

Diagnosis

If subacute, it must be distinguished from the bleeding of diverticular disease and of ulcerative colitis. Any part of the colon can be affected, although, because it has the most precarious blood supply, the splenic flexure is usually involved. If the colon looks normal on sigmoidoscopy, ulcerative colitis is virtually excluded, although large-bowel Crohn's disease or diverticular disease is not. Imaging shows mucosal oedema with characteristic 'thumb-printing', as if a thumb had been pressed along the outside of the affected colon.

Prognosis

In mild cases there may be complete recovery but colonic strictures can develop later. In colonic gangrene, surgical resection is necessary. The differential diagnosis includes *Campylobacter* enteritis, and diverticular disease, in which bleeding can be considerable. Pseudomembranous colitis does not usually cause bloody diarrhoea.

Pancreas

Carcinoma

Most pancreatic cancers are adenocarcinoma. Less common are mucinous cystadenocarcinoma and endocrine, adenosquamous, anaplastic, intraductal papillary mucinous and acinar cell carcinoma.

Clinical presentation

Patients present with one or more of the following features:

- anorexia and weight loss
- indigestion or epigastric pain often indistinguishable from duodenal or gastric ulceration. Back pain suggests pancreatic disease (and posterior ulcers)
- obstructive jaundice. Intermittent jaundice suggests a gallstone in the bile duct (rarely carcinoma of the ampulla of Vater)
- patients can present with diabetes, usually of short duration.

Investigation

Ultrasound or CT scan may show the tumour.

ERCP may confirm the diagnosis and allows palliative stenting of the obstructed common bile duct to relieve pruritus and jaundice.

Management

Resection is the only curative treatment, but less than 10% of patients are suitable for surgery. Adjuvant chemotherapy may be of benefit. Five-year survival is 25% in patients undergoing pancreatectomy and less than 5% overall.

Islet cell tumours

See Zollinger–Ellison syndrome and insulinoma.

Acute pancreatitis

Aetiology

Most cases are associated with gall bladder disease (especially gallstones) or excess alcohol.

Clinical presentation

There may be a previous history of cholecystitis or biliary colic associated with gallstones. Pancreatitis occurs occasionally in association with mumps, drugs (e.g. thiazides) and severe hypertriglyceridaemia.

Abdominal pain, often very severe, occurs suddenly, usually in the epigastrium or across the upper abdomen with radiation to the back or shoulder. It spreads to involve the entire abdomen, which is tender with guarding and rebound tenderness. Hypotension with sweating and cyanosis occurs in severe attacks. There may be bruising around the umbilicus or in the flanks.

Differential diagnosis

It presents initially as an 'acute abdomen' and resembles:

- cholecystitis
- acute myocardial infarction
- dissecting aortic aneurysm
- mesenteric vascular occlusion
- intestinal perforation.

Investigation

The serum amylase is usually very high (>1000 units/ml) within 24 h of onset. The level can fall rapidly. Posterior duodenal ulcers can also cause very high amylase levels.

Straight abdominal X-ray may show gallstones, pancreatic calcification (indicating previous inflammation) and a distended loop of jejunum or transverse colon if they are close to the inflamed pancreas. Serum calcium may fall. There is usually a leucocytosis.

CT is useful in establishing the diagnosis and excluding other pathology.

Management

- If the diagnosis is definite, conservative management is preferred.
- Relieve pain.
- Give intravenous fluids to correct electrolyte imbalance and maintain the circulating volume, while monitoring the central venous pressure.
- Give nutritional support with enteral or parenteral nutrition (see Trials Box 12.3).
- Monitor the blood glucose.

TRIALS BOX 12.3 Nutrition in pancreatitis

A multivariate analysis of trials comparing the effect of enteral versus parenteral nutrition in patients with severe acute pancreatitis found that enteral nutrition resulted in clinically relevant and statistically significant risk reduction for infectious complications, pancreatic infections and mortality in patients with predicted severe acute pancreatitis. Source: *Archives of Surgery* 2008; **143**(11): 1111–1117.

- Renal support with haemodialysis or haemofiltration may be required.
- Monitor oxygen saturation and give oxygen.
- Patients with severe pancreatitis or organ dysfunction should be managed in a high-dependency or critical care unit.
- Patients with extensive (>30%) or infected necrosis of the pancreas require surgical or laparoscopic drainage.

Other measures are of less certain value:

- therapeutic ERCP with sphincterotomy in patients with gallstones
- prophylactic antibiotics.

Prognosis

Overall mortality is less than 10%. Gallstones should be removed early after recovery. Alcohol should be avoided if it is a possible cause. Pancreatic pseudocysts may resolve spontaneously but can require drainage if they cause symptoms or become infected.

Chronic pancreatitis

Aetiology

Alcoholism and gallstones are the commonest causes; also pancreatic malformations, hyperparathyroidism, cystic fibrosis and haemachromatosis. Mutations in the *PRSS1* gene, encoding cationic trypsinogen, have also been associated with chronic pancreatitis.

Clinical presentation

- recurrent, although mild, attacks that resemble acute pancreatitis
- malabsorption and steatorrhoea from pancreatic insufficiency
- anorexia and weight loss
- diabetes mellitus when the islet cells are involved
- obstructive jaundice, which may be intermittent
- in association with cystic fibrosis and haemochromatosis

Investigation

The serum amylase is unhelpful in chronic pancreatitis although it is sometimes raised. Imaging (CT or MR) can be helpful but may be normal in early disease and it can be difficult to distinguish between inflammatory and malignant mass at a later stage.

Investigate for malabsorption and exocrine pancreatic function (Chapter 17), diabetes mellitus (Chapter 17) and obstructive jaundice (Chapter 13), if relevant.

Treatment

- There is no specific therapy for chronic pancreatitis.
- Treat pancreatic malabsorption with a low-fat diet, fat-soluble vitamins, calcium and pancreatic enzymes (e.g. Pancrex V®, Creon®).
- Treat diabetes mellitus (Chapter 17).
- Remove gallstones if present.
- Consider sphincterotomy or pancreatectomy if recurrent attacks.
- Alcohol is forbidden.
- Chronic severe pain is common and may lead to opiate addiction.

Gall bladder

Acute cholecystitis

Clinical features

The history is of fever, occasionally with rigors, and abdominal pain, usually right subcostal with acute pain on palpation over the gall bladder region. The disease is more common in obese females over 40, but may occur in young adults. Gallstones are present in over 90% of cases. Occasionally, acute cholecystitis may be difficult to distinguish from a high appendicitis and right basal pneumonia, peptic ulcer, pancreatitis and myocardial infarction may need to be considered.

Management

The acute inflammation usually settles with bed rest, analgesia (pethidine) and antibiotics according to local protocol. The gall bladder is removed and early laporoscopic cholecystectomy is the preferred option in many units.

Rarely, an empyema develops or the gall bladder perforates.

Chronic cholecystitis

Clinical presentation

Recurrent episodes of cholecystitis are usually associated with gallstones. The attacks are often less severe than classical acute cholecystitis, and may resemble peptic ulceration or oesophagitis. Myocardial ischaemia may be confused if the site of the pain is high.

Gallstones

Cholelithiasis is twice as common in women as men. Classically gallstones occur in the fat, fertile female over 40 years. They are usually cholesterol or mixed. Rarely, they are pigment stones associated with haemolytic anaemia.

Clinical features

Most stones produce no symptoms, but they may cause:

- flatulence upwards
- biliary colic
- acute cholecystitis
- chronic cholecystitis
- obstructive jaundice, which may be intermittent, giving attacks of fever, jaundice and upper abdominal pain – Charcot's triad. Gall bladder empyema from bile duct obstruction is uncommon.

Gallstones are associated with acute and chronic pancreatitis and their presence indicates a higher risk of gall bladder carcinoma, although this is still extremely rare.

Investigation

Ultrasonography will reveal most stones. CT or MR provide alternative imaging modalities. Although surgeons may explore the bile duct at surgery, stones are sometimes missed and may later produce symptoms. Operative cholangiography and/or fibreoptic examination of the bile duct make this less likely.

Management

If causing symptoms, the gall bladder and stones should be removed. It is at this stage that pigment stones are detected and indicate investigation for haemolysis. In elderly patients or if surgery is contraindicated, sphincterotomy via ERCP may release the stones if they are in the common bile duct. Ursodeoxycholic acid may prevent formation of stones and dissolve radiolucent stones if the stones are <2 cm in diameter and if the gall bladder is functioning. The stones may recur after treatment. Asymptomatic stones found incidentally are sometimes removed to prevent complications, particularly in younger patients.

13

Liver disease

The most common liver diseases are acute viral hepatitis, drug jaundice, gallstones, biliary tract obstruction and carcinomatous secondary deposits.

Acute hepatitis

This refers to inflammation of the liver with little or no fibrosis and little or no nodular regeneration. There may be minor distortion of lobular architecture. If there is extensive fibrosis with nodular regeneration (and hence distortion of architecture) the condition is called cirrhosis. These diagnoses are made histologically and there may or may not be clinical evidence of previous hepatic disease.

Inflammation with necrosis of liver cells results from:

- *Infection,* most commonly acute infectious hepatitis A, but also with the viruses of hepatitis B, C and E, infectious mononucleosis, cytomegalovirus (CMV) and yellow fever, and associated with septicaemia and leptospirosis. Amoebic hepatitis is common on a worldwide basis and usually presents as a hepatic abscess or amoeboma.
- *Chemical poisons* and *drugs* are less frequent causes of acute hepatitis. Toxic chemicals include carbon tetrachloride, vinyl chloride, and ethylene glycol and similar solvents (glue sniffing). Toxic drugs include alcohol (ethanol and methanol), halothane (after repeated exposures), isoniazid and rifampicin, paracetamol, methotrexate, chlorpromazine.
- *Pregnancy* (rare).

If the patient recovers this is usually complete, but, rarely, progressive necrosis may affect almost the entire liver (fulminant hepatic failure or acute massive necrosis) progressing to hepatic coma and death.

Viral hepatitis

The clinical features of acute hepatitis A, B, C and E are similar, although they differ in severity, time course and progression to chronic liver disease.

Hepatitis A

Hepatitis A (infectious hepatitis) is a single-stranded RNA picornavirus of the enterovirus family which is excreted in the stool towards the end of the incubation period and disappears as the illness develops. Antihepatitis A virus immunoglobulin M (IgM) appears at the onset of the illness and indicates recent infection. The disease is endemic but small epidemics may occur in schools or institutions. Spread is usually via the faecal–oral route by food products such as shellfish.

Clinical presentation

After an incubation period of 2–6 weeks there is gradual onset of influenza-like illness with fever, malaise, anorexia, nausea, vomiting and upper abdominal discomfort associated with tender enlargement of the liver and, less commonly, the spleen. In smokers, there may be a distaste for cigarettes. After 3–4 days the urine becomes characteristically dark and the stools pale – evidence of cholestasis. Symptoms usually become less severe as jaundice appears, although pruritus may develop. Jaundice and symptoms tend to improve after 1–2 weeks and recovery is usually complete, although mild symptoms continue for 3–4 months in a few patients. Recurrent hepatitis A is extremely rare and immunity probably lifelong.

Clinical Medicine Lecture Notes, Eighth Edition. John R. Bradley, Mark Gurnell, and Diana F. Wood.
© 2019 John Wiley & Sons Ltd. Published 2019 by John Wiley & Sons Ltd.

Diagnosis

Diagnosis depends on detecting antihepatitis A virus IgM in serum.

Differential diagnosis

- Obstructive jaundice, either in the early cholestatic phase or in the rare case where cholestatic jaundice persists after other clinical and biochemical evidence of liver cell damage has settled. It is dangerous to diagnose infective hepatitis in patients over 40 years old – a safeguard against misdiagnosing major bile duct obstruction.
- Drug jaundice.
- Glandular fever.
- Yellow fever (travellers).
- Acute alcoholic hepatitis may present with enlargement and tenderness of the liver and, sometimes, obstructive jaundice. There are usually other signs of alcoholism.
- Wilson's disease should not be overlooked (page 231, Chapter 15).

Management

If hospitalised, the patient should be isolated. Virus is present in stools for 1–2 weeks before the onset of jaundice and for 1 week after. Symptomatic treatment only is required in the active disease state. No dietary restriction, other than alcohol, is necessary. Liver function tests usually return completely to normal in 1–3 months.

Recovery is the rule in virtually every case. Occasionally jaundice may be prolonged by intrahepatic cholestasis, and corticosteroids can be used to reduce the jaundice rapidly, particularly if associated with pruritus.

Fulminant hepatic failure is rare but has a high mortality, and management should be in a specialised centre where liver transplantation can be considered.

Prophylaxis

Active immunisation with inactivated virus is recommended for travellers to endemic areas.

Passive immunisation with pooled human immunoglobulin gives partial, short-lived immunity, but is effective immediately after the injection.

Hepatitis B (Fig. 13.1)

Hepatitis B is a double-stranded DNA hepadnavirus. It is spread by infected blood and serum and also occurs in saliva, semen and vaginal secretions. It is most frequently transmitted by sexual activity, shared needles used by drug addicts, and from mother to child. Health workers and other at-risk groups are now screened and offered vaccination.

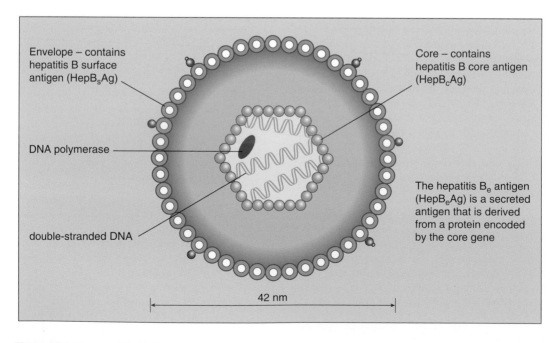

Envelope – contains hepatitis B surface antigen (HepB$_s$Ag)

DNA polymerase

double-stranded DNA

Core – contains hepatitis B core antigen (HepB$_c$Ag)

The hepatitis B$_e$ antigen (HepB$_e$Ag) is a secreted antigen that is derived from a protein encoded by the core gene

42 nm

Figure 13.1 The hepatitis B virion.

Hepatitis B virus causes acute liver disease that ranges from subclinical to fulminant hepatitis, and chronic diseases including chronic hepatitis, cirrhosis and hepatocellular carcinoma.

Clinical features

After a long incubation period of 6 weeks to 6 months, there is typically a gradual onset of lethargy, anorexia, abdominal discomfort, jaundice and hepatomegaly. It is often asymptomatic in infants. Occasionally immune-mediated extrahepatic manifestations occur with polyarthritis, skin rashes and glomerulonephritis. Cholestatic hepatitis is rare. Mutated viral strains may be associated with fulminant hepatic failure.

Diagnosis

Hepatitis B virus has three different antigens: a surface antigen ($HepB_sAg$), a core antigen ($HepB_cAg$) and an internal component ($HepB_eAg$). $HepB_sAg$ appears in the blood about 6 weeks after acute infection and has usually gone by 3 months. $HepB_eAg$ occurs at a similar time and denotes high infectivity. $HepB_cAg$ is usually found only in the liver. The development of antibodies to $HepB_sAg$ usually follows acute infection and indicates immunity. In about 5% of cases antibodies do not appear and $HepB_sAg$ persists in the blood (carrier state).

Hepatitis D virus (Delta virus) is an incomplete RNA virus that depends on the hepatitis B virus to replicate. It can cause an aggressive chronic hepatitis in $HepB_sAg$-positive patients. Chronic infection is usually associated with progressive liver disease.

Management

In the majority of cases spontaneous recovery occurs and treatment is supportive, as for hepatitis A. Of the estimated 50 million new cases of hepatitis B diagnosed worldwide 75% occur in Asia, and 5–10% of adults and up to 90% of children become chronically infected. Prevalence in the UK is <2%. The carrier state is usually asymptomatic but is associated with chronic hepatitis, which may progress to cirrhosis and hepatocellular carcinoma. Antiviral agents include interferon-α2b, pegylated interferon-α2a, the nucleoside analogue telbivudine, and the nucleotide analogue entecavir (Box 13.1).

Immunisation

Immunisation using recombinant $HepB_sAg$ is advised for occupational high-risk groups, including health workers, patients with chronic renal failure, intravenous drug abusers, individuals who change sexual partners frequently, patients who receive regular blood products, and family contacts of a case or carrier. Immunisation takes up to 6 months to confer immunity, and booster is recommended after 5 years.

Hepatitis C

Hepatitis C is a single-stranded RNA flavivirus. It predominantly affects intravenous drug abusers and patients who have received multiple blood transfusions. It accounts for 20% of acute hepatitis, 70% of chronic hepatitis, nearly half the cases of end-stage cirrhosis, 60% of primary liver cancer and 30% of liver transplants in the UK.

 Box 13.1 Hepatitis B (chronic): Diagnosis and management of chronic hepatitis B inchildren, young people and adults. NICE guidelines [CG165]. June 2013

NICE guidelines recommend offering antiviral treatment to adults aged 30 years and older who have HBV DNA>2000 IU/ml, and ALT≥30 IU/L in males and ≥19 IU/L in females, on two consecutive tests conducted 3 months apart. For adults younger than 30 years the criteria include evidence of necroinflammation or fibrosis on liver biopsy or a transient elastography score greater than 6 kPa.

Antiviral treatment should also be offered to adults with cirrhosis in the presence of detectable HBV DNA, or HBV DNA>20 000 IU/ml and ALT≥30 IU/L in males and ≥19 IU/L in females on two consecutive tests conducted 3 months apart regardless of age or the extent of liver disease.

Either peginterferon-α2a or entecavir or tenofovir disoproxil are recommended as options for the initial treatment of adults with chronic hepatitis B (HBeAg-positive or HBeAg-negative), within their licensed indications. Telbivudine is not recommended for the treatment of chronic hepatitis B.

Clinical features

Frequently asymptomatic – fewer than 10% of adults become jaundiced. Acute hepatitis following blood transfusion has been virtually eradicated by the introduction of testing of blood products for hepatitis B and C. The incubation period varies from 2 to 26 weeks. Sixty to eighty percent of those acutely infected develop chronic infection, which leads to cirrhosis in around 25% of patients over a 20- to 30-year period. Hepatocellular carcinoma has an annual incidence of around 3% in those with cirrhosis.

Diagnosis

Diagnosis is usually by antibody detection. First-generation enzyme-linked immunosorbent assay (ELISA) using recombinant antigen C100 is relatively non-specific. Newer assays using putative core antigens are more specific, although false positives still occur. The mean time from infection to antibody detection is 12 weeks. Hepatitis C virus RNA determination by PCR (polymerase chain reaction) is used to monitor hepatitis C infection. Hepatitis C is classified into six distinct genotypes, with subtypes in each genotype class.

Management

Progression to chronic active hepatitis and cirrhosis is much more common in hepatitis C than hepatitis B infection. Direct-acting antivirals (DAA) with activity against hepatitis C have been classified into three groups: NS3/4A serine protease inhibitors (include telaprevir, boceprevir, grazoprevir, paritaprevir, simeprevir); NS5A inhibitors (include daclatasvir, ledipasvir, ombitasvir, elbasvir, velpatasvir); and NS5B polymerase inhibitors (include sofosbuvir, beclabuvir). DAAs alone or combined, or in combination with pegylated interferon-α can achieve a sustained virological response, depending on the genotype. Pegylated interferon-α and ribavirin completely eradicates hepatitis C in up to 40–50% of patients with high viral loads of genotype 1b who have not previously received antiviral therapy.

Hepatitis E

Hepatitis E virus is an RNA hepevirus that is endemic in the developing world. Transmission is faecal–oral.

Clinical features

Infection is usually self-limiting, and it does not have a carrier state, but can cause fulminant hepatic failure in pregnant women, with mortality rates of around 20%.

Hepatitis G

Hepatitis G is a positive-stranded RNA flavivirus. There is no evidence at present that it causes acute or chronic liver disease.

CASE STUDY Hepatitis

A 42-year-old female clerical officer is found to have abnormal liver function tests at a routine insurance medical. She is asymptomatic and apart from two uneventful pregnancies 10 and 12 years previously has no significant medical history. She is a non-smoker, drinks less than 10 units of alcohol per week, and is on no regular medication. Her blood pressure is 124/76 and physical examination is unremarkable. Urinalysis is normal.

Investigations have shown raised serum alanine aminotransferase (ALT) at 120 (normal laboratory range less than 40 IU/L), aspartate aminotransferase (AST) at 145 (normal laboratory range less than 50 IU/L), and gamma glutamyl transferase at 168 IU/L (normal laboratory range less than 60 IU/L). Serum alkaline phosphatase, bilirubin and albumin are normal. Full blood count (haemoglobin 135 g/l, MCV 90 fl) and prothrombin time are normal.

The patient has elevated liver enzymes, with no evidence of biliary obstruction (normal serum bilirubin and alkaline phosphatase levels), and preserved synthetic liver function (normal serum albumin and prothrombin time).

The clinical picture is of a hepatitis. Further questioning confirms that alcohol use is not excessive (supported by the normal MCV), there has been no recent use of over-the-counter medicines, and no recent foreign travel. The patient admitted to a brief period of illicit intravenous drug use as a student 20 years previously.

A screen for viral hepatitis revealed the presence of IgG antibodies to hepatitis C, and the presence of hepatitis C viral RNA of genotype 1 was confirmed by PCR indicating persistent infection. Screening for hepatitis B was negative. Ultrasound of the liver was normal, but liver biopsy showed a chronic active hepatitis. Treatment with peginterferon-α and ribavirin was started.

Autoimmune hepatitis

Autoimmune hepatitis is characterised by hepatocellular inflammation and necrosis, which tends to progress to cirrhosis. It may be triggered by hepatic injury, including acute viral hepatitis, in predisposed individuals, and can coexist with chronic viral hepatitis. It is associated with MHC genes, particularly those encoding the HLA class II DRB1 alleles. It has been classified into two types based on the presence of autoantibodies:

Type I autoimmune hepatitis is the commonest type, with a female to male ratio of 8 : 1. It is characterised by the presence of antinuclear antibodies and/or anti-smooth muscle cell antibodies, and sometimes perinuclear antineutrophil cytoplasmic antibodies (p-ANCA). IgG concentrations and serum aminotransferases are elevated. Liver histology reveals plasma cell infiltrates, liver cell rosettes and piecemeal necrosis.

Type II autoimmune hepatitis typically affects girls aged 2–14 years, although 20–30% of cases occur in adults. Onset is often acute, with rapid progression to liver failure. It is characterised by the presence of anti-liver kidney microsome antibodies or anti-liver cytosol type 1 antibodies in the absence of antinuclear or anti-smooth muscle cell antibodies.

Management

Immunosuppressive therapy improves survival in the majority of cases. The majority of patients respond to steroids, alone or in combination with azathioprine.

In patients who fail to respond to immunosuppression, liver transplantation is the treatment of choice.

Alcoholic hepatitis

Moderate alcohol consumption is associated with a reduction in mortality compared with either abstinence or heavy drinking (Trials Box 13.1). Drinking in excess of 3 units of alcohol daily may increase mortality, but sensitivity to alcohol varies between individuals (8 g = 1 unit of ethanol = present in a single [25-ml] measure of spirits; a small [125-ml] glass of 12% wine contains 1.5 units). The clinical features of alcoholic liver disease vary from no clinical evidence at all, through nausea, episodes of right abdominal pain associated with tender hepatomegaly, fever and polymorphic leukocytosis, to cirrhosis with portal hypertension and fulminant hepatic failure. Jaundice is not always present.

The pathological spectrum includes fatty liver, alcoholic hepatitis, cirrhosis and hepatocellular carcinoma. Alcoholic hepatitis is characterised by liver cell damage, inflammatory cell infiltration and fibrosis. Injured hepatocytes are swollen, with pale granular cytoplasm ('ballooning degeneration'). In some cells Mallory bodies are seen by haematoxylin and eosin stain as purple-red aggregates of material, predominantly around the nucleus. The γ-glutamyltransferase, which reflects levels of microsomal enzyme induction, and the mean corpuscular volume may be the best indices of persistent ethanol ingestion.

 TRIALS BOX 13.1 Alcohol consumption and mortality

Doll et al. studied mortality prospectively in 12 321 male doctors. Moderate alcohol consumption (1 or 2 units/day) was associated with lower all-cause mortality than consumption of no or substantial amounts. Alcohol consumption reduced ischaemic heart disease, irrespective of amount. Source: *BMJ* 1994; **309**: 911–918.

Fuchs et al. followed 85 709 women aged 34–59 over a 12-year period. Light-to-moderate alcohol consumption (1.5–4.9 g/day) was associated with a reduced mortality rate, principally because of a decreased risk of death from cardiovascular disease. Heavier drinking was associated with increased risk of death from other causes, particularly breast cancer and cirrhosis.

Source: *New England Journal of Medicine* 1995; **332**: 1245–1250.

Grønbæk et al. studied different types of alcohol and death in 13 064 men and 11 459 women aged 20–98. J-shaped relations were found between total alcohol intake and mortality at various levels of wine intake. They found that wine intake may have a beneficial effect on all-cause mortality that is additive to that of alcohol. Source: *Annals of Internal Medicine* 2000; **133**: 411–419.

Woods et al. found that the minimum mortality risk in 599 912 current drinkers was around or below 100 g / week. Source: *Lancet* 2018; **391**: 1455–1548.

The only effective treatment is total abstinence from alcohol, if necessary with the help of support services. Nutritional deficiencies are common. Vitamin B preparations and dietary supplementation are usually given.

Chronic liver disease

Chronic hepatitis and cirrhosis are pathological diagnoses and therefore imply liver biopsy in suspected cases.

Non alcoholic fatty liver disease

Non alcoholic fatty liver disease (NAFLD) is emerging as one of the commonest causes of chronic liver disease. It is more common in obese patients with type 2 diabetes, hypertension and hyperlipidaemia, and can progress over years from (1) simple fatty liver (steatosis), to (2) non-alcoholic steatohepatitis (NASH) leading to (3) fibrosis and (4) cirrhosis. The liver is echogenic on ultrasound and there may be increased stiffness on elastography. Treatment is aimed at correcting underlying risk factors.

Cirrhosis

Cirrhosis is characterised by widespread fibrosis with nodular regeneration. Its presence implies previous or continuing hepatic cell damage. Liver function tests are normal in inactive disease. Cirrhosis can be classified as compensated or decompensated, depending on the absence or presence of ascites, variceal haemorrhage, encephalopathy or jaundice.

Classification of cirrhosis

Micronodular (portal cirrhosis) is characterised by regular thick fibrotic bands joining the portal tracts to hepatic veins and by small regenerative nodules. The liver is initially large with a smooth edge but subsequently shrinks with progressive fibrosis. It is often alcoholic in origin.

Macronodular (postnecrotic cirrhosis) is less common and characterised by coarse, irregular bands of fibrosis and loss of normal architecture and large regenerative nodules. It is believed usually to follow viral hepatitis with widespread necrosis. The liver is enlarged and very irregular as a result of large nodules.

Biliary cirrhosis is less common and is characterised by fibrosis around distended intrahepatic ducts. It may follow chronic cholangitis and biliary obstruction, or be idiopathic (primary).

Primary biliary cirrhosis

There is progressive damage to intrahepatic bile ducts. Antimitochondrial antibodies are present in 95% of patients and this helps with the differential diagnosis from drug cholestasis, sclerosing cholangitis, carcinoma of the bile duct and biliary cirrhosis from chronic obstruction. It chiefly affects women between 40 and 60 years of age and presents with features of cholestasis, namely pruritus, jaundice with pale stools, dark urine and steatorrhoea, pigmentation and xanthelasma.

Osteodystrophy results from a combination of osteomalacia secondary to impaired vitamin D absorption and osteoporosis. The liver and spleen are usually palpable.

Histology

Histology shows progression from granulomatous changes around the bile ducts through bile duct proliferation to fibrosis and finally cirrhosis.

Management

The anion exchange resin cholestyramine, which binds bile acids in the gut, relieves pruritus. Supplementary fat-soluble vitamins are given. Osteoporosis is common, and bisphosphonates prevent bone loss, although their effect on fracture rate is unclear. The bile acid ursodeoxycholic acid slows disease progression, leading to an improvement in both liver biochemistry and long-term survival. Immunosuppressive agents are of no proven benefit. Liver transplantation should be considered in patients with advanced disease.

Primary sclerosing cholangitis

There is progressive inflammation and fibrosis of intra- and extrahepatic ducts. The condition is diagnosed by endoscopic retrograde cholangiography or MRI. Inflammatory bowel disease coexists in 70% of cases. Cholangiocarcinoma is a recognised complication.

Management

Immunosuppression increases the risk of secondary bacterial cholangitis, although this may be required for coexistent inflammatory bowel disease.

Endoscopic stenting of strictures carries the same risk. Liver transplantation is the only therapeutic option for advanced disease.

Other causes of cirrhosis

Other rare causes of cirrhosis include autoimmune hepatitis, haemochromatosis and Wilson's disease. Cardiac cirrhosis may occur in chronic cardiac failure. Centrilobular congestion leads to necrosis and fibrosis, but nodular regeneration is not marked.

NB: Schistosomiasis causes periportal fibrosis and is not a form of cirrhosis. Liver involvement is more common in *Schistosoma mansoni* (bowel) infections than in *S. haematobium* (bladder) as a result of the portal rather than the systemic drainage of the primary infected area in the former. The schistosomes cause a granulomatous fibrosis in the portal tracts and enlargement of the liver. In severe cases the liver shrinks and extensive fibrosis develops, leading to portal hypertension. There is little or no hepatocellular failure because the disease is presinusoidal. Late spread may occur to the lungs (cor pulmonale) and to the spinal cord (paraplegia).

Clinical features

Clinical features of chronic liver disease relate mostly to the development of hepatocellular failure and complications of portal hypertension.

Hepatocellular failure

Marked jaundice is uncommon. The oestrogen effects of gynaecomastia, spider naevi, liver palms and testicular atrophy may be present. In alcoholics, other features of alcoholism may be present (wasting, polyneuropathy, Korsakoff's psychosis, dementia, delirium tremens and Wernicke's encephalopathy, page 284, Chapter 17). Pigmentation, fetor hepaticus, clubbing, white nails, cyanosis and peripheral oedema may occur.

Encephalopathy may be absent or may completely dominate the picture, with irritable confusion, drowsiness, flapping tremor, fetor and other signs of hepatocellular failure progressing to coma. Exaggerated reflexes and upgoing plantar responses may be present.

Constructional apraxia may be demonstrated in inability to draw or copy a star.

Acute liver failure

There are two main clinical situations in which hepatocellular failure may be precipitated and in which there are different management objectives:

1. A previously healthy person with a serious hepatic illness, such as paracetamol overdose or viral (C, B, A in that order) hepatitis. This can also occur with other drugs and with chemical poisoning. This is less common. The history is short and there is no evidence of chronic liver disease. The object is to support the patient to give time for the liver to recover.
2. A person with previously 'compensated' chronic liver disease, with an acute precipitating cause:
   - excess protein in the bowel, e.g. after gastrointestinal haemorrhage
   - acute alcoholic intoxication
   - intercurrent infection, particularly Gram-negative septicaemia
   - drugs, especially sedatives, and morphine or other alkaloids
   - trauma, including minor or major surgical procedures and paracentesis
   - electrolyte imbalance (potassium and/or sodium depletion), usually from the diuretics used to treat oedema and ascites.

The underlying damage to the liver is not treatable.

Fulminant hepatic failure refers to hepatic encephalopathy occurring within weeks of the onset of other symptoms of acute liver failure. Profound hypotension and multiple organ failure are common. Cerebral oedema and sepsis are the most common causes of death.

Management

Preferably, this should be in a specialist unit.

- *Assess the conscious level.* The conscious level is a guide to prognosis, and can progress from
   - drowsy, poor concentration
   - confused and disorientated
   - responding only to forceful, simple command, often aggressive and incoherent
   - unrousable, responding either only to painful stimuli or to none.

NB: In alcoholic liver disease, conscious level may also be affected by delirium tremens, thiamine (and other B vitamins) deficiency, epilepsy and acute alcohol intoxication.

- *Establish venous access* and consider nasogastric tube and central line.

- *Identify any site of bleeding* by fibroscopy and treat as appropriate: gastric or duodenal ulceration; variceal bleeding (see later).
- *Correct and maintain fluid and electrolyte balance.* Sodium restriction may be required despite hyponatraemia, which may be dilutional. Hypokalaemia is treated with standard oral potassium preparations. The blood glucose may be very low and require dextrose infusions.
- *Infection is common* so prophylactic broad-spectrum antibiotics and antifungal are often given. Take blood cultures and send ascitic fluid for bacteriological examination, including tuberculosis. Gram-negative and -positive (often staphylococcal) infections occur. Treat suspected infection immediately and then modify the antibiotic therapy as indicated by microbiological results, remembering that altered liver function may influence drug choice and dosage.
- *Minimise the protein load.* Identify any site of bleeding (see earlier). In those not bleeding, reduce the risk of gastrointestinal bleeding with H_2-blockers or proton-pump inhibitors. Lactulose 50 ml t.d.s. produces osmotic diarrhoea to remove protein and blood (if present) from the bowel and prevents proliferation of ammonia-producing organisms. Selective intestinal decontamination by the administration of non-absorbable antibiotics may eliminate ammonia-producing colonic bacteria. $MgSO_4$ enema may be added.
- *Correction of coagulation defects* is not usually needed in the absence of clinically significant bleeding. Use fresh frozen plasma or blood and platelet infusion if the platelet count is low. Add vitamin K, 10 mg intravenously, in case there is any cholestatic element.
- *Inotropic support* may be indicated.
- *Support respiration.* Early elective ventilation may be needed to maintain PaO_2.
- *Renal failure* may require dialysis or haemofiltration.
- *Give B vitamins* parenterally. Thiamine deficiency is common in alcoholics.
- *Assess for liver transplantation.*

NB: A reduced level of consciousness in hepatocellular failure may be caused by septicaemia, hypoglycaemia, raised intracranial pressure from cerebral oedema, subdural haematoma or epilepsy. Administration of *N*-acetylcysteine may be of benefit in acute liver failure caused by paracetamol overdose (Chapter 22) and other causes.

Portal hypertension

Portal hypertension is usually associated with cirrhosis. Other postsinusoidal causes (which have poor hepatic function) are exceedingly rare and result from cardiac failure, constrictive pericarditis and hepatic vein thrombosis (Budd–Chiari syndrome, see later). Presinusoidal obstruction causes portal hypertension with normal hepatic function in schistosomiasis (granulomatous portal tract fibrosis) and in obstruction to the portal vein by tumours or following venous thrombosis with umbilical sepsis.

Collateral circulation may be evident in the oesophagus (varices), anus (anorectal varices rather than haemorrhoids) and at the umbilicus where a venous hum may be heard. Tests of liver cell function are usually slightly abnormal, though not always so, and there may be hypersplenism.

Haematemesis is the commonest presenting symptom and may be precipitated by NSAIDs, including aspirin. Bleeding is often from peptic ulceration or erosions in the alcoholic, and H_2-blockade or proton-pump inhibitors are then useful.

Non-selective β-blockers are not effective in preventing the development of varices in patients with cirrhosis and portal hypertension and are associated with increased side effects.

Management of bleeding varices

The initial aim is to replace blood and correct coagulation defects. Short-term antibiotics to reduce bacterial infection reduces variceal rebleeding and death. Specific treatment with a combination of pharmacological and endoscopic therapy is better than either treatment alone.

- Endoscopic variceal ligation is safer and more effective than sclerotherapy.
- Vasopressin, octreotide, somatostatin and terlipressin reduce splanchnic blood flow and can be started prior to more definitive treatment.
- Non-selective β-blockers reduce portal pressure and are effective in preventing first bleed from varices, and as secondary prophylaxis after variceal bleeding.
- Surgical oesophageal transection or trans-jugular porto-systemic shunting can be considered in patients with recurrent or intractable variceal bleeding.

Management of ascites

Ascites can be due to a combination of factors, including portal hypertension, hypoalbuminaemia and secondary hyperaldosteronism. Management involves:

- sodium restriction
- diuretics – aldosterone antagonists (e.g. spirono-lactone), alone or in combination with loop diuretics in patients with marked sodium retention
- paracentesis is safe and effective, although expansion of plasma volume with albumin may be required if large quantities of ascitic fluid are removed
- peritoneo-venous shunting or ultrafiltration and reinfusion of ascitic fluid are rarely employed in the setting of refractory ascites.

Spontaneous infection of ascites is common in cirrhotic patients. Most episodes respond to intravenous cephalosporins or oral quinolones (e.g. ciprofloxacin), but the overall prognosis is poor.

Budd–Chiari syndrome

This results from obstruction of the hepatic veins. Causes are:

- hepatic venous thrombosis, usually in association with a hypercoagulable state such as the antiphospholipid syndrome
- occlusion of the hepatic veins by tumour, abscess or cyst
- webs of the suprahepatic segment of the inferior vena cava (IVC).

Patients present acutely with tender hepatomegaly (without hepatojugular reflux), resistant ascites and hepatic failure. Chronic onset is associated with weight loss, upper gut bleeding and spider naevi. All patients have abnormal liver function tests, but the pattern is variable and similar to other chronic liver diseases. Liver biopsy shows congestion around the hepatic venules. Laparotomy may produce abrupt deterioration. Treatment is surgical by side-to-side portocaval shunting or orthotopic liver transplantation. If there is a web, surgical correction may be attempted by transatrial membranectomy.

Rare cirrhoses

Idiopathic haemochromatosis (bronzed diabetes)

Idiopathic haemochromatosis is an autosomal recessive disorder of iron metabolism characterised by increased iron absorption and deposition, chiefly in the liver, pancreas, heart, synovial membranes and pituitary. The majority of patients are homozygous for the p.C282Y variant in the *HFE* gene. The HFE protein is a MHC class I-like protein that interacts with transferrin receptor 1 and modulates the uptake of transferrin-bound iron from plasma.

First-degree relatives should be screened with serum iron and transferrin saturation. Females may present postmenopausally because continuous menstruation until then reduces the iron load.

Clinical presentation

It usually occurs in men over the age of 30 years who present with:

- diabetes mellitus
- skin pigmentation (caused by melanin rather than iron)
- hepatomegaly (large, regular, firm); portal hypertension and hepatocellular failure are not common
- progressive pyrophosphate polyarthropathy and chondrocalcinosis
- arrhythmias and cardiac failure
- testicular atrophy, loss of body hair and loss of libido
- osteoarthritis of the first and second metacarpophalangeal joints.

Diagnosis

The serum iron is raised so that the serum iron-binding capacity is nearly saturated. The serum ferritin is also raised. The patient is not anaemic or polycythaemic. The glucose tolerance test is usually abnormal.

Biopsy of most tissues (skin, marrow, testes) shows excess iron deposits, but diagnosis is often made on liver biopsy, which shows iron staining of the liver with perilobular fibrosis.

Treatment

Deplete the body of the excess iron (up to 50 g) by weekly venesection of 500 ml (which contains 250 mg of iron). This is continued until a normal serum iron is established and/or the patient becomes anaemic (in about 2 years). Maintenance venesection will be required (about 500 ml every 3 months, depending on the serum iron).

Treat appropriately the diabetes, hypogonadism, heart failure and arrhythmias, hepatic cell failure and portal hypertension. High alcohol intake must be stopped. The arthropathy and testicular function do not improve but other features do.

NB: Primary hepatic carcinoma occurs in up to 20% of cases, whether treated or not. Alpha-fetoprotein is a suitable screen.

Overload of the tissues with iron can follow either repeated blood transfusions (about 100 units), as for instance in thalassaemia, or, rarely, after excessive iron ingestion. If the iron is in the reticuloendothelial cells only, the patients tend not to develop serious sequelae and the condition is called haemosiderosis.

Hepatolenticular degeneration (Wilson's disease)

Wilson's disease is an autosomal recessive disorder of copper transport, resulting in copper accumulation and toxicity to the liver and brain, caused by mutations in the copper-transporting gene *ATP7B*. Neurological manifestations (page 231, Chapter 15) and signs of cirrhosis appear during adolescence or early adult life. Low ceruloplasmin is found in the serum. The Kayser–Fleischer ring is a deep copper-coloured ring at the periphery of the cornea, which is thought to represent copper deposits. Hypercalciuria and nephrocalcinosis are not uncommon in patients with Wilson's disease.

Drug jaundice

Cholestasis

Clinically and biochemically this is an obstructive jaundice. Histologically, there are bile plugs in the canaliculi and there may be an inflammatory infiltrate of eosinophils in the portal tracts.

The classical example is chlorpromazine jaundice, which occurs 3–6 weeks after starting the drug. The prognosis is excellent if the drug is discontinued (and never given again).

Other drugs producing cholestasis are other phenothiazines, carbimazole, erythromycin estolate (but not the stearate), sulfonylureas, sulfonamides, rifampicin and nitrofurantoin. Occasionally there may be a more generalised reaction with fever, rash, lymphadenopathy and eosinophilia.

Acute hepatitis

Drugs occasionally cause acute necrosis. This is much less common but much more serious. It occurs 2–3 weeks after starting the drug and can be caused by halothane (after multiple exposure), monoamine oxidase inhibitors, methyldopa (which more commonly gives haemolytic jaundice) and the antituberculosis drugs ethionamide and pyrazinamide (403).

Direct hepatotoxicity

In some cases hepatotoxicity is dose-dependent, although individual susceptibility is extremely variable. The mechanisms are:

- cholestasis (without inflammatory infiltrate or necrosis). Chiefly as a result of C17-substituted testosterone derivatives, i.e. anabolic and androgenic steroids, including methyltestosterone and most contraceptive pills
- necrosis resulting from organic solvents, e.g. methotrexate, 6-mercaptopurine, azathioprine.

Haemolytic jaundice

This is a rare complication of therapy. It may occur with methyldopa (which more commonly gives a positive Coombs' reaction without jaundice) and the 8-aminoquinolines (e.g. primaquine) in patients with glucose-6-phosphate dehydrogenase deficiency.

14

Renal disease

Disease of the renal tract presents in only a few ways. Urinary tract infection is the most common, especially in females. In males it is prostatic hypertrophy and its consequences. Proteinuria, haematuria and disorders of excretory function often cause no symptoms if mild, being picked up during routine screening (e.g. insurance medical).

Urinary tract infection

There are two main clinical syndromes:

1. *Cystitis,* characterised by suprapubic tenderness, dysuria and frequency. NB: These symptoms can occur without urinary infection. Other causes include non-specific urethritis, gonococcus, interstitial cystitis, drug-induced cystitis (e.g. cyclophosphamide), bladder stones and tumours, and vaginitis (infections or senile).
2. *Acute pyelonephritis* presents with dysuria, frequency, loin tenderness and fever, often with rigors and vomiting. Fever may be the only feature in children, in whom recurrent infection may be associated with vesicoureteric reflux that tends to diminish with age.

Bacteriuria is confirmed by finding a urinary excretion of more than 100 000 organisms/ml urine (counts of <10 000/ml are usually caused by contamination). Infection may be symptom-free. *Escherichia coli* is the most frequent organism. Other organisms (*Proteus, Staphylococcus, Streptococcus, Klebsiella* and *Pseudomonas*) are usually associated with structural abnormality or catheterisation, and reinfection. Tuberculosis classically causes a sterile pyuria. White blood cells release leukocyte esterase into the urine, which can be detected on urinalysis, and many urinary pathogens,

including Enterobacteriaceae (*Escherichia coli* and *Proteus* sp.), convert nitrates to nitrite, yielding a positive nitrite test. Microscopic haematuria is common.

Management

Uncomplicated cases are treated with oral antibiotics such as trimethoprim and ampicillin (3-day course for cystitis, at least 7 days for pyelonephritis) after obtaining urine for culture and antibiotic sensitivity. Resistant organisms may be sensitive to co-amoxiclav (Augmentin®) or ciprofloxacin. Patients with acute pyelonephritis who are vomiting or have evidence of septicaemia require intravenous antibiotics.

There may be an obvious predisposing cause, e.g. pregnancy, urinary obstruction or catheterisation. Diabetes mellitus must be excluded. Acute pyelonephritis or more than two episodes of cystitis in a woman, or any infection in a man, suggest a structural abnormality. Ultrasound of the renal tract is performed to look for perinephric abscess, renal scarring, stone, tumours or obstruction. CT scanning and possibly cystoscopy may be necessary (frequent infections, persistent haematuria, dysuria or loin pain) to exclude small stones/tumours or bladder diverticula.

Women prone to recurrent infections should be given advice about complete emptying of the bladder (double micturition) and voiding soon after intercourse. Low-dose antibiotic prophylaxis (e.g. trimethoprim or cephalexin) reduces the incidence of infection and can be used for long periods.

Children require investigation as infection in the presence of vesicoureteric reflux can lead to permanent kidney damage.

Imaging the kidneys

A *plain abdominal film* usually shows the renal outlines and identifies any calcification in the renal tract.

Clinical Medicine Lecture Notes, Eighth Edition. John R. Bradley, Mark Gurnell, and Diana F. Wood.
© 2019 John Wiley & Sons Ltd. Published 2019 by John Wiley & Sons Ltd.

Renal ultrasound is useful in determining renal size and contour, and defining the size, location and consistency (solid or cystic) of any renal mass, and looking for pelvicalyceal dilatation of obstruction.

Intravenous urography (IVU) has largely been replaced by ultrasound, computed tomographic (CT) scanning and radionuclide scanning. *Ultrasound* and *CT* are particularly useful for anatomical studies, and radionuclide scanning for providing functional information.

Isotope scanning (most commonly ^{99m}Tc-diethylen-etriaminepentacetic acid (DTPA) or ^{99m}Tc-dimercap-tosuccinate (DMSA)) can be used to assess renal blood flow, renal function and transit time of filtrate across the parenchyma into the collecting system. It can be useful in the diagnosis of renal artery stenosis and obstruction. In addition, the renal parenchyma can be visualised for evidence of scarring.

Stones

Eighty percent of urinary tract stones contain calcium, usually as calcium oxalate. Less common constituents are uric acid (10%) or cystine. Staghorn calculi contain struvite, made up of calcium, ammonium and phosphate. Classical features are severe loin pain, with microscopic or macroscopic haematuria.

Clinical features

The most common presentation is with severe loin pain radiating to the groin (renal colic), with microscopic or macroscopic haematuria. About 1 in 1000 men and 1 in 3000 women present with their first kidney stone in a single year. Fifteen percent of patients develop recurrent stones within a year of first presentation, 30% by 5 years.

Recurrent stones should be investigated for a metabolic cause:

- hypercalciuria – 50% of stone-formers have increased urinary calcium excretion
- elevated serum calcium – usually caused by hyperparathyroidism in stone-formers
- hyperuricaemia
- cystinuria.

Management

The diagnosis is confirmed by imaging. Abdominal X-ray may detect calcium-containing stones. Ultrasound usually identifies stones and will detect dilatation of the renal pelvis or ureter, indicating obstruction.

IVU or CT scanning provide the most sensitive methods of detecting stones. Most small stones (<4 mm) will pass spontaneously, but those >6 mm are rarely passed. In such cases stones are cleared by extracorporeal shock wave lithotripsy, endoscopic removal, either percutaneously or through cystoscopy with retrograde urethroscopy, or open surgical procedure.

Measures to prevent stone formation

- Increased fluid intake – at least 2 l/day.
- Diet – increased risk of stone formation is associated with low rather than high calcium diet, and with diets high in sodium and protein.
- Thiazide diuretics reduce urinary calcium in hypercalciuria.
- Allopurinol reduces urinary uric acid excretion.
- Penicillamine and captopril form a complex with cystine, which renders it more soluble, and can be used to prevent or dissolve stones.
- Alkalinisation of urine increases solubility of uric acid and cystine and may be of value in preventing uric acid or cystine stone formation by increasing solubility of these compounds.

Chronic interstitial nephritis

The term *chronic pyelonephritis*, which implies infection, has been replaced by *chronic interstitial nephritis*, which is characterised by a chronic tubulointerstitial inflammatory infiltrate. Interstitial involvement is usually secondary to papillary or tubular damage by infection, ischaemia, radiation, toxins or metabolic disease. The most common cause is reflux nephropathy (see later). Other causes include obstructive uropathy, drugs (cyclosporin, lithium, chronic analgesic ingestion), renovascular disease, sickle-cell disease, long-standing hypokalaemia, hypercalcaemia or hyperuricaemia, tuberculosis, sarcoid, heavy metal poisoning (lead, cadmium), radiation nephritis, Sjögren's syndrome and hereditary nephritides (e.g. Alport's syndrome).

Clinical features

There is usually altered tubular function (glycosuria, aminoaciduria, renal tubular acidosis and tubular proteinuria) with a variable degree of renal failure. Ultrasound and radionuclide scans may show obstruction, and the kidneys are often small and scarred.

Management

Treat any underlying cause. Give antibiotics (prophylactic if necessary) for infection. Patients are commonly unable to concentrate their urine, and need a high fluid intake.

Reflux nephropathy

Reflux of urine through a congenitally abnormal vesicoureteric junction occurs in about 1% of infants. Reflux of sterile urine into the kidney may cause renal damage through hydrostatic injury, but there is clear evidence that reflux of infected urine leads to renal scarring. Reflux is present in 50% of infants who develop urinary infection during their first year, and one third of children who have infection before the age of 12 years. Reflux can also present with enuresis, hypertension and proteinuria. There is a familial incidence.

Management

Children with urinary infections (and possibly those with affected siblings or parents) should be screened with an ultrasound of the renal tract followed if necessary by a direct or indirect radionuclide micturating cystogram. Ureteric reimplantation and conservative treatment with antibiotics to prevent infection are equally effective in preventing scarring. Without surgery reflux generally resolves as the child grows older.

Proteinuria

Small amounts of low-molecular-weight proteins are normally filtered by the glomerulus, and reabsorbed or catabolised by proximal tubular cells. The kidneys normally excrete 50–80 mg protein daily, of which 30–50 mg is Tamm–Horsfall protein, a mucoprotein secreted by tubular cells. Proteinuria >150 mg/day is abnormal, but proteinuria is more commonly quantified as urinary albumin creatinine ratio (ACR) or protein creatinine ratio (PCR), which are more easily obtained on a spot urine sample and tend to be more reproducible than 24 h collections. ACR > 2.5 mg/mmol in men and 3.5 mg/mmol in women or PCR > 15 mg/mmol are abnormal. A PCR of 100 mg/mmol or ACR of 70 mg/mmol is approximately equal to 1 g of protein per 24 h. The conversion is non-linear for levels below this. Dipsticks primarily detect albumin and are relatively insensitive at detecting immunoglobulins or Bence Jones protein (immunoglobulin light chains). Microalbuminuria (urinary albumin excretion of 30–300 mg/day) is an early sign of diabetic nephropathy.

Causes

- glomerular disease: glomerulonephritis, glomerulosclerosis (diabetic and hypertensive), glomerular amyloid deposition
- tubular disease (because of impaired reabsorption of filtered proteins): chronic interstitial nephritis, polyuric phase of acute tubular necrosis, Fanconi syndrome, tubular toxins (aminoglycosides, lead, cadmium)
- non-renal disease: fever, heavy exercise, heart failure. Orthostatic proteinuria, a benign condition in which proteinuria is present when upright but not when recumbent
- urinary tract disease: infection, tumours, calculi
- increased production of filterable proteins: immunoglobulin light chains (Bence Jones protein) in myeloma, myoglobinuria, haemoglobinuria

Clinical presentation

Often asymptomatic (routine screening). Nephrotic syndrome if severe. There may be evidence of underlying cause (e.g. urinary infection, diabetes, hypertension).

Assessment

The history should include enquiries about recent infections, renal disease (including any family history), drugs and occupation. Examination may be normal, but there may be oedema, hypertension, heart failure or evidence of renal failure.

Investigation

- Serum creatinine and electrolytes and ACR or PCR.
- Serum for albumin and protein electrophoresis for monoclonal gammopathy. Blood glucose for diabetes. Urine for free light chains.
- Antinuclear antibodies (systemic lupus erythematosis, SLE), antineutrophil cytoplasmic antibodies (systemic vasculitis), cryoglobulin levels.
- Plain abdominal X-ray and ultrasound of renal tract for stones, structural abnormalities and renal size.

In the majority of cases these investigations fail to define the underlying cause, and renal biopsy may be necessary, particularly if nephrotic or there is impaired excretory function. This usually establishes the diagnosis and may identify a treatable cause (particularly some forms of glomerulonephritis).

In the absence of oedema, treatment should be directed towards any underlying cause or associated conditions (e.g. hypertension).

Nephrotic syndrome

The triad of:

- proteinuria
- hypoalbuminaemia
- oedema.

Aetiology

Any cause of severe proteinuria. Usually it is a consequence of glomerular disease – commonly glomerulonephritis, diabetic glomerulosclerosis or renal amyloid. More than 75% of childhood and × 20% of adult nephrotic syndrome is a result of minimal change disease. Tubular proteinuria is usually less than 2 g/day and does not cause nephrotic syndrome.

It is associated with thrombosis (loss of anticoagulant proteins such as antithrombin III, protein S, protein C), infection (loss of immunoglobulins) and hyperlipidaemia.

Management

Identify and treat any underlying cause. General management is aimed at the following:

- Reducing oedema with salt restriction and diuretics.
- Angiotensin-converting enzyme inhibitors reduce proteinuria, probably by lowering glomerular capillary pressure. NSAIDs also reduce proteinuria, but these agents reduce renal blood flow and glomerular filtration rate and cause salt retention.
- Treatment of hypertension: angiotensin-converting enzyme inhibitors and diuretics in the first instance, but additional agents may be required.
- Most physicians recommend a normal protein intake.
- Anticoagulate if immobile or thrombotic episode, or severe nephrotic syndrome. Look for and treat intercurrent infection.
- Hyperlipidaemia may be severe. Very-low-density lipoprotein cholesterol, low-density lipoprotein cholesterol and total plasma cholesterol are elevated, as are triglyceride levels. Although this pattern is associated with increased cardiovascular risk, the value of treatment with diet or lipid-lowering agents has not been fully assessed.

Haematuria

Isolated haematuria on dipstick testing of urine can occur in normal individuals. Microscopic haematuria is confirmed by finding more than three red cells per high-power-field of spun urine. Macroscopic haematuria is always abnormal.

Aetiology

Common

- urinary tract infection
- urinary tract stones (calcium oxalate 80%, triple phosphate 10%, urate 10%, cystine <1%)
- tumours of the bladder, kidneys and prostate
- glomerulonephritis
- schistosomiasis is common worldwide

Uncommon

- hypertension
- renal trauma
- papillary necrosis
- renal infarction
- drugs – cyclophosphamide (haemorrhagic cystitis), anticoagulants
- medullary sponge kidney (usually benign developmental abnormality with medullary cysts which may be complicated by infection or calculi)

Familial causes

- polycystic kidneys
- Alport syndrome
- thin basement membrane disease (a generally benign condition in which haematuria is usually the only clinical feature)
- medullary cystic disease (tubulointerstitial nephritis with medullary cysts which usually progresses to renal failure)

The causes vary with age. Glomerular causes predominate in children and young adults, whereas tumours and calculi are common in the elderly.

Investigation

The likely source may be suspected from the history and examination.

Microscopy of a fresh urine sample is performed in all patients to confirm the presence of red cells. The presence of red-cell casts or dysmorphic (abnormally shaped) red cells indicates glomerular bleeding (red cells are deformed by mechanical and osmotic stress as they pass through the tubules). Heavy proteinuria suggests a glomerular lesion, while white-cell casts indicate renal inflammation. Bacteria may be seen and culture should be performed. Urine should also be sent for cytology.

Plasma creatinine to assess renal function.

Plain abdominal film and *ultrasound of the renal tract* to look for structural lesions (calculi, tumours, cysts).

If glomerular bleeding is suspected (young age, hypertension, proteinuria, renal impairment, absence of structural lesion), consider *renal biopsy* to identify cause of proteinuria or renal dysfunction.

If a lesion of the renal tract is suspected (older age, no evidence of intrinsic renal disease) proceed to *cystoscopy* with *CT* if the upper renal tract has not been clearly identified by ultrasound.

NB: Normal urine (centrifuged deposit) contains:

- Red cells 1×10^6 cells/24 h (3 per high-power-field).
- White cells 2×10^6 cells/24 h (6 per high-power-field).
- Hyaline casts are composed of uromucoid (Tamm–Horsfall protein which is excreted by normal tubular cells).
- Epithelial cells may be found in normal urine as a result of contamination by cells from the vulva or prepuce.
- Cellular casts result from adherence of either red cells (implying glomerular bleeding) or white cells (implying tubular inflammation) to the surface of hyaline casts.

Acute kidney injury

Characterised by a rapid rise in serum creatinine, usually with a decrease in urine output. The causes can be divided into prerenal, renal and postrenal.

Prerenal

Aetiology

Acute kidney injury occurs most commonly in elderly patients in the context of an acute illness (Box 14.1). Common causes are

- hypovolaemia from any cause (e.g. diarrhoea or vomiting, diuretics, haemorrhage)
- sepsis, usually complicating surgery or pneumonia

NB: Angiotensin-converting enzyme inhibitors may reduce glomerular perfusion sufficiently to cause renal failure if given in the presence of bilateral renal artery stenosis (see later).

 Box 14.1 Acute kidney injury: Prevention, detection and management of acute kidney injury up to the point of renal replacement therapy

NICE guidelines [CG169]. August 2013

NICE recommends that adults with acute illness should be investigated for acute kidney injury if there is evidence or suspicion of chronic kidney disease, heart failure, liver disease, diabetes, history of acute kidney injury, oliguria (urine output less than 0.5 ml/kg/hour), neurological or cognitive impairment or disability, which may limit access to fluids, hypovolaemia, use of potentially nephrotoxic drugs (such as non-steroidal anti-inflammatory drugs [NSAIDs], aminoglycosides, angiotensin-converting enzyme inhibitors, angiotensin II receptor antagonists and diuretics or use of iodinated contrast agents within the previous week, especially if hypovolaemic, symptoms or history of urological obstruction, or conditions that may lead to obstruction, sepsis, deteriorating early warning scores, age 65 years or over.

In accelerated (malignant) hypertension, acute, severe hypertension is associated with marked renal abnormalities. The most striking of these is gross intimal hyperplasia, leading to occlusion of the lumen in small arteries and arterioles. Renal failure is a rapid consequence of this condition if the blood pressure is not controlled.

Renal failure commonly complicates advanced liver disease. Plasma urea and creatinine may be normal because of reduced hepatic urea synthesis, low dietary protein intake and loss of muscle mass. There is often a precipitating cause (e.g. hypovolaemia following diuretic therapy, paracentesis or gastrointestinal bleeding, sepsis). Unexplained renal failure complicating liver disease is the *hepatorenal syndrome*. The prognosis is poor. Reinfusion of ascites into the internal jugular vein via a peritoneo-venous shunt can expand plasma volume and improve renal function, but does not improve survival.

Pathophysiology

Despite high blood flow (20% of cardiac output) the kidneys are particularly susceptible to ischaemia or toxin-induced renal cell injury.

The medulla receives less than 10% of renal blood flow and is at greatest risk of injury. The common response to severe injury (regardless of cause) is *acute*

TRIALS BOX 14.1 Management of HUS and TTP

A systematic review of interventions for haemolytic uraemic syndrome (HUS) and thrombotic thrombocytopenic purpura (TTP) concluded that plasma exchange with fresh frozen plasma is the most effective treatment available for TTP. For patients with HUS, supportive therapy including dialysis appears to be the most effective treatment, but all studies in HUS have been conducted in the diarrhoeal form of the disease. Source: *Cochrane Database of Systematic Reviews* 2009; (1): CD003595.

tubular necrosis (ATN). The necrosis of tubular epithelial cells is most prominent in the proximal tubules and thick ascending limb of the loop of Henle. The tubular lumen may be obstructed by cell debris and casts. Regeneration of tubular cells leading to recovery can take weeks. Severe prolonged ischaemia can cause acute cortical necrosis from which there is little chance of recovery.

The distinction between prerenal failure (in which concentrating powers are retained) and ATN (in which concentrating powers are lost) can be made on urinalysis. In prerenal failure urine osmolality is high (>500 mOsmol/kg), urine sodium is low (<20 mmol/ l) and the urine to plasma urea ratio is >10 : 1. In ATN urine is isotonic with plasma (<400 mOsmol/kg), urine sodium is >40 mmol/l and the urine to plasma urea ratio is <10 : 1.

Renal

Causes

- glomerulonephritis
- nephrotoxic drugs (e.g. aminoglycosides, cyclosporin A, amphotericin B)
- poisoning (e.g. heavy metals)
- myoglobinuria – following rabdomyolysis myoglobin may cause tubular toxicity or form tubular casts. Creatine kinase is markedly elevated
- acute tubular (or cortical) necrosis complicating prerenal disease
- acute interstitial nephritis (usually a drug-induced hypersensitivity reaction which responds to withdrawal of the drug and a short course of corticosteroids. Eosinophils may be present within the predominantly mononuclear cell interstitial infiltrate)
- intrarenal obstruction (e.g. urate or oxalate crystals, calcium precipitation, tubular casts in myeloma)

NB: Hypercalcaemia causes renal failure through renal vasoconstriction, direct tubular cell toxicity and distal tubular calcium phosphate precipitation.

Haemolytic–uraemic syndrome (HUS) is characterised by thrombocytopenia (platelet consumption), microangiopathic haemolytic anaemia (red cell fragments on film) and acute renal failure. It commonly follows a diarrhoeal illness in infants infected with a verotoxin-producing strain of *Escherichia coli* (serotype O157). In adults it may follow an upper respiratory tract infection or be associated with calcineurin inhibitors (e.g. cyclosporin A), the oral contraceptive pill or cytotoxic agents. Renal biopsy shows occlusion of glomerular capillaries with fibrin and thrombi, without evidence of complement or immunoglobulin deposition. Recovery usually occurs over a few weeks in children, but the prognosis for adults is poor. *Thrombotic thrombocytopenic purpura* (TTP) is closely related to HUS but is most common in women, and central nervous system involvement and fever are typical additional features. See Trials Box 14.1.

Atypical haemolytic uraemic syndrome (aHUS) occurs in patients with a genetic or acquired abnormality of the complement system. The prognosis is poor with patients being at risk of sudden and progressive damage to vital organs. Familial forms can result from a mutation in complement factor H. Eculizumab is a humanized monoclonal antibody that binds to complement protein C5 and inhibits terminal complement-mediated haemolysis, and is licensed for treatment of aHUS (Box 14.2) and paroxysmal nocturnal haemoglobinuria (page 382, Chapter 20). In 2015 NICE estimated the cost of eculizumab per adult to be about £340 200 (initial and maintenance treatment) in the first year of treatment, and about £327 600 for 1 year of treatment on the recommended maintenance dose.

Postrenal

Acute urinary tract obstruction from:

- prostatic hypertrophy
- renal and ureteric stones
- tumour of the renal pelvis, ureters or bladder
- blood clot

Box 14.2 Eculizumab for treating atypical haemolytic uraemic syndrome

NICE highly specialised technologies [HST1]. January 2015

NICE recommends funding eculizumab for treating atypical haemolytic uraemic syndrome, only if its use is coordinated through an expert centre, AND monitoring systems to record the number of people with a diagnosis of atypical haemolytic uraemic syndrome and the number who have eculizumab, and the dose and duration of treatment are in place, AND there is a national protocol for starting and stopping eculizumab for clinical reasons, AND a research programme with robust methods to evaluate when stopping treatment or dose adjustment might occur.

- sloughed papillae
- external compression from retroperitoneal fibrosis or tumours
- surgical mishap (e.g. ureteric involvement in hysterectomy).

NB: Lesions above the bladder must involve both urinary tracts if there are two functioning kidneys.

Investigation

Where there is no obvious cause following careful history and examination, and preliminary biochemical and haematological assessment:

- Check that there is no obstruction. Rectal examination can exclude prostatic disease in men, or a pelvic mass. The bladder is enlarged in urethral obstruction. Ultrasound to look for urinary tract dilatation is the simplest method of excluding obstruction, although dilatation may be absent, particularly if obstruction is acute. This will also give information about renal size (small kidneys indicate chronic renal disease; scarring usually indicates chronic interstitial nephritis or ischaemia).
- Proceed to renal biopsy if renal size is normal and there are no clues on investigations, including urinalysis (exclude infection; heavy proteinuria, granular or red cell casts indicate intrinsic renal disease), calcium, uric acid, protein electrophoresis (myeloma), antineutrophil cytoplasm antibodies (vasculitis), antiglomerular basement membrane antibodies (Goodpasture's disease),

antinuclear antibodies (SLE), blood film, platelet, eosinophil count and coagulation (disseminated intravascular coagulation [DIC], TTP, HUS, drug-induced hypersensitivity).

Management

Identify and correct underlying causes – often multiple (e.g. hypotension, sepsis, DIC and aminoglycoside toxicity).

Rapid correction of prerenal causes (intravenous fluids or blood for hypovolaemia, antibiotics for sepsis, inotropes, avoidance of nephrotoxic drugs) may prevent ATN and restore renal function. Loop diuretics (e.g. furosemide) are often given and may prevent tubular cell ischaemia through inhibition of active sodium chloride reabsorption, thereby reducing oxygen requirements.

Relieve urinary tract obstruction from below (urethral catheterisation with or without ureteric stents) or above (nephrostomy). Prostatic obstruction in elderly men is the most common cause.

Initiate treatment for any intrinsic renal disease (e.g. immunosuppression for certain forms of glomerulonephritis, 183).

Continuing assessment of fluid status through input–output records, physical examination, daily weight, lying and standing blood pressure. Fluids should be restricted if there is oliguria or anuria, but patients are usually catabolic and nutrition should not be neglected. In severely ill patients enteral or parenteral nutrition may be necessary.

Careful monitoring of electrolytes, urea, creatinine and acid–base status.

If renal failure persists, renal replacement therapy with haemodialysis or haemofiltration will be required. Absolute indications include hyperkalaemia (potassium above 6–7 mmol/l), markedly elevated plasma creatinine (>1000 mmol/l, but absolute level must take clinical state into account), severe acidosis (bicarbonate below 10–15 mmol/l) and fluid overload with pulmonary oedema.

Acute kidney injury in adults should be detected in line with the RIFLE, AKIN or KDIGO definitions using any of the following criteria:

- a rise in serum creatinine ≥26 μmol/l within 48 hours
- a rise in serum creatinine of ≥50% within the previous week
- a fall in urine output to <0.5 ml/kg/h for more than 6 hours in adults and more than 8 hours in children and young people

Chronic kidney disease

Common causes

- Diabetic nephropathy (Chapter 17).
- Chronic glomerulonephritis.
- Chronic interstitial nephritis.
- Hypertension: estimates of the prevalence of chronic renal failure caused by hypertension vary widely, reflecting the fact that the diagnosis of renal disease caused by hypertension depends on the exclusion of other causes. Many cases may have undiagnosed renal disease. Renal failure because of hypertension is much more common in black people than white people, and within the black population there appears to be familial clustering of renal disease caused by hypertension, suggesting a genetic susceptibility to hypertensive renal damage.
- Renovascular disease.
- Hereditary renal disease.
- Polycystic kidney disease: an autosomal dominant condition in which there is progressive cystic degeneration of the kidneys. Patients present with hypertension, abdominal pain, haematuria or chronic kidney disease. The diagnosis is confirmed by ultrasound, and family members should be offered screening. Progression to renal failure with hypertension is usual, although the age at which renal replacement therapy becomes necessary varies. Approximately 85% of cases are caused by a defect in *PKD1*, which encodes a large transmembrane protein that can interact with the product of *PKD2* gene, which is an ion channel and responsible for most non-*PKD1* associated cases.

The disease should be considered a multisystem disease in which cysts occur in other organs (liver, pancreas, testes). There is an increased incidence of cardiac valve disease, cerebral aneurysms, hernias and diverticular disease.

- Alport syndrome: 85% of cases are due to mutations in the *COL4A5* gene on the X chromosome, which encodes the α_5 chain of type IV collagen. Progressive chronic kidney disease associated with sensorineural deafness and eye lesions occurs in affected males, whereas females typically only have abnormalities on urinalysis. Autosomal forms have variable presentations and are due to mutations in the *COL4A3* or *COL4A4* genes on chromosome 2, encoding the α_3 and α_4 chains of type IV collagen.

Alport syndrome is characterised by thinning and splitting of glomerular basement membrane (GBM). Thin basement membrane disease is a related condition in which thinning of the basement membrane is associated with microscopic haematuria, but renal function is usually preserved. Some patients with thin basement membrane disease have heterozygous mutations at the *COL4A3*/*COL4A4* locus.

- Long-standing urinary tract obstruction.

NB: About 20% of patients with established renal failure present with bilaterally small kidneys and no diagnosis is reached. Under these circumstances renal biopsy is hazardous and unlikely to show reversible changes.

The vasopressin V_2-receptor antagonist Tolvaptan can slow disease progression in polycystic kidney disease, but is associated with a high incidence of adverse effects (Box 14.3).

Clinical features

Screening for renal disease and the availability of dialysis mean that the classical manifestations of *uraemia*

 Box 14.3 Tolvaptan in polycystic kidney disease

The TEMPO 3:4 TRIAL trial investigators found that the vasopressin V_2-receptor antagonist tolvaptan slowed the increase in total kidney volume and the decline in kidney function over a 3-year period in patients with autosomal dominant kidney disease and eGFR 60 ml/min or more, but was associated with adverse events including thirst, polyuria, nocturia, and polydipsia and elevated liver enzymes. Source: *New England Journal of Medicine* 2012; **367**(25): 2407–2418. A post hoc analysis suggested clinically similar benefits across chronic kidney disease stages 1–3. Source: *Clinical Journal of the American Society of Nephrology* 2016; **11**(5): 803–811.

NICE recommends tolvaptan as an option for treating autosomal dominant polycystic kidney disease in adults to slow the progression of cyst development and renal insufficiency in patients who have chronic kidney disease stage 2 or 3 at the start of treatment, and evidence of rapidly progressing disease (tolvaptan for treating autosomal dominant polycystic kidney disease. Technology appraisal guidance [TA358]. October 2015. https://www.nice.org.uk/guidance/TA358).

(literally *urine in the blood*) are now seen infrequently. Chronic kidney disease is typically slow to progress and usually presents with lethargy, general malaise, anorexia and nausea. Generalised pruritus is common. Impotence, menstrual irregularities and loss of fertility are common complaints in younger patients. In severe uraemia there is a characteristic fishy fetor, hiccups, vomiting, severe pruritus with skin excoriations, skin pigmentation, peripheral neuropathy and central nervous system derangements leading to lethargy, stupor and coma with fitting. Pericarditis may be associated with effusion and tamponade.

Investigations

Biochemical

Plasma creatinine provides a guide to the severity of renal failure and can be used to estimate glomerular filtration rate (eGFR). *Creatinine* is derived from metabolism of creatine in muscle. The rate of production correlates with muscle mass, and depends little on protein intake. Fifty percent loss of renal function is often needed before the serum creatinine rises above the normal range; it is therefore not a sensitive indicator of mild to moderate renal injury.

Urea H_2N-CO-NH_2 (molecular mass 60 Da) is toxic and is the most abundant nitrogenous compound to accumulate in renal failure. It is the end-product of protein metabolism and is synthesised primarily in the liver. It is freely filtered by the glomerulus, but approximately 50% is reabsorbed so urea clearance is less than glomerular filtration rate (GFR). Urea production increases with cellular catabolism

(infection, trauma, steroid therapy) or following protein load (dietary or following gastrointestinal haemorrhage). It is reduced in liver failure.

Renal function is now most commonly reported as estimated GFR (eGFR), which is used to assess the severity of CKD (Table 14.1) and calculated as:

$$eGFR(ml/min/1.73m^2 =$$
$$175 \times [(plasma\ creatinine(\mu mol/l)/88:4)^{-1.154}]$$
$$\times age\,(years)^{-0.203} \times 0.742\,if\ female\ and$$
$$\times 1.21\,if\ African\ American$$

This is usually calculated by using a web-based calculator (for example, see http://www.renal.org/eGFRcalc/GFR.pl).

- *Cr ethylene diaminetetra-acetic acid (EDTA) clearance* more accurately reflects the GFR. It is calculated from the rate of disappearance of a bolus injection of ^{51}Cr EDTA from the blood. The normal GFR is $\times 100\,ml/min$ per $1.73\,m^2$.
- *Hyperkalaemia* is common.
- A number of abnormalities of *calcium* and *phosphate* homeostasis occur. *Phosphate* retention is associated with:

  o reciprocal depression of serum calcium level
  o rise in the calcium $\times$ phosphate product.

The diseased kidneys fail to hydroxylate *25-hydroxycholecalciferol* (25-HCC) to the more active form 1–25dihydroxycholecalciferol (1–25-DHCC). This results in:

- reduced calcium absorption from the gut
- osteomalacia.

Table 14.1 Classification of chronic kidney disease (CKD) by severity

Stages of CKD	GFR (glomerular filtration rate) (ml/min/1.73m²)	Description	Population prevalence (%)
1	>90	Kidney damage with normal or ↑ glomerular filtration rate	3.3
2	60–89	Kidney damage with mild ↓ glomerular filtration rate	3.0
3A	45–59	Moderate ↓ glomerular filtration rate	4.3
3B	30–44		
4	15–29	Severe ↓ glomerular filtration rate	0.2
5	<15 or dialysis	Kidney failure	0.1

The criteria for the definition of chronic kidney disease are either kidney damage or glomerular filtration rate <60ml/min for ≥3months. Kidney damage is defined as pathological abnormalities or markers of damage, including abnormalities in blood or urine tests or imaging studies.

Hypocalcaemia stimulates the parathyroid glands which are thus in a state of chronic hypersecretion, tending to return the serum calcium level to normal. Thus, dihydroxycholecalciferol is reduced (because of reduced 1α-hydroxylase activity in the kidney) with increased parathyroid hormone (PTH). The increased PTH may result from phosphate retention and a decrease in ionised calcium. The clinical consequences are:

- osteoporosis produced by hyperparathyroidism
- osteomalacia caused by lack of vitamin D
- ectopic calcification.

Hypocalcaemia rarely leads to tetany because acidosis and hypoproteinaemia reduce protein binding and increase ionised levels of calcium.
- Plasma *uric acid* is often raised (but clinical gout is rare).

Haematology

Haematological investigations usually reveal a *normochromic normocytic anaemia* which responds to parenteral erythropoietin. Gastrointestinal blood loss, iron, vitamin B$_{12}$ or folate deficiency, decreased red cell survival, hyperparathyroidism and aluminium toxicity may also contribute to anaemia and should be considered if there is a failed response to erythropoietin.

Urinalysis

Urinalysis should be performed to quantify proteinuria, look for non-visible haematuria, exclude urinary infection and look for cellular casts indicating active renal inflammation.

Ultrasound

Renal ultrasound identifies obstruction or renal scars and defines renal size (Table 14.2). *Plain abdominal*

Table 14.2 Causes of small and large kidneys

Causes of small kidney	
Unilateral	Hypoplasia, reflux nephropathy, obstructive atrophy, tuberculosis, renal artery stenosis
Bilateral	All of the above plus chronic glomerulonephritis, hypertension, diabetes, chronic interstitial nephritis
Causes of enlarged kidney	
Unilateral	Compensatory hypertrophy, bifid collecting system, renal mass, hydronephrosis, renal vein thrombosis
Bilateral	Polycystic kidneys, amyloid, acute glomerulonephritis

X-ray also defines the renal outline and excludes renal tract calcification. If renal size is normal and the cause of renal disease unknown, *renal biopsy* should be considered.

Management

There are two main aims:

1. to slow the decline in renal function;
2. to prevent or treat complications (bone disease, cardiovascular disease, endocrine effects, anaemia, socioeconomic).

Risk factors for progression of renal disease are:

- persistent activity of underlying disease
- uncontrolled hypertension
- proteinuria
- infection
- nephrotoxins (drugs).

Pathophysiology

Possible mechanisms of progression of renal failure include:

- increased glomerular pressure (as a result of increased systemic blood pressure, or efferent arteriolar constriction as a consequence of increased angiotensin II levels)
- glomerular protein leakage
- lipid abnormalities
- large and small vessel vascular disease

Hypertension in chronic kidney disease

Progression of chronic kidney disease is attenuated by treatment of hypertension. Thiazide diuretics, β-blockers, angiotensin-converting enzyme inhibitors and calcium antagonists are all effective in patients with early renal damage. Angiotensin-converting enzyme inhibitors, angiotensin II receptor antagonists, and calcium-channel blockers do not modify glucose or lipid metabolism, have a favourable effect on left ventricular hypertrophy and have a potentially nephro-protective effect by reducing increased renal vascular resistance. Angiotensin-converting enzyme inhibitors and angiotensin II receptor antagonists have the additional advantage of producing a fall in proteinuria in patients with both diabetic and non-diabetic renal disease. Renal function should be monitored as they can cause hyperkalaemia and reduce renal blood flow and precipitate acute renal failure, particularly in the presence of renal artery stenosis. Serum creatinine and potassium should be checked before starting therapy, after 1–2 weeks, and

---

CASE STUDY **Chronic kidney disease**

A 34-year-old male computer programmer was found to have a blood pressure of 156/98 at a routine check when registering with a new GP. Physical examination was otherwise normal, but urinalysis revealed blood ++ and was negative for protein. His father died at the age of 54 from a subarachnoid haemorrhage.

The patient is hypertensive (page 107, Chapter 10), and in view of his age and the presence of non-visible haematuria warrants further investigation. Serum creatinine was 112 mmol/l (calculated eGFR 69 ml/min/1.73 m²) with normal electrolytes and bone profile, and haemoglobin was 145 g/l. Ultrasound of his urinary tract showed multiple cysts in both kidneys, which measured 13.2 cm in length on the left and 13 cm in length on the right.

The presence of multiple cysts in kidneys that are slightly enlarged confirms a diagnosis of polycystic disease, and it is likely that he has inherited this from his father. The abnormalities on ultrasound confirm a diagnosis of chronic kidney disease (see above), but he does not yet meet the criteria on the basis of eGFR. He is started on ramipril and advised about the importance of blood pressure control, the long-term need for surveillance and likely progression of his chronic kidney disease, and the complications associated with polycystic kidney disease (see above). The possible use of Tolvaptan if there is evidence of rapid progression is discussed. He is referred for genetic counselling for advice about screening his own and his deceased father's siblings, and his children aged 6 and 8, which would normally be delayed until they reach adult life.

---

after subsequent dose increases. **If the creatinine rises >30% or eGFR falls >25%,** the tests should be repeated, angiotensin blockade stopped and investigation for renal artery stenosis considered.

Complications

Bone disease

Hypocalcaemia from decreased renal 1,25-$(OH)_2D_3$ synthesis (Fig. 14.1), hyperphosphataemia and resistance to peripheral actions of PTH all contribute to renal bone disease. Parathyroid hormone secretion increases as a result of phosphate retention and reduced 1α-hydroxylation of vitamin D and its consequences. Treatment is by dietary phosphate restriction with or without phosphate binders (calcium carbonate or acetate, or non-calcium containing binders such as sevelamer or lanthanum carbonate if there are concerns over calcium load), and early use of low-dose 1α-hydroxylated vitamin D derivatives. The calcimimetic cinacalcet or parathyroidectomy may be indicated if there is tertiary hyperparathyroidism (page 298, Chapter 17).

Cardiovascular disease

Cardiovascular disease is the most common cause of mortality in patients with chronic kidney disease. It is likely to reflect an increased incidence of hypertension, lipid abnormalities, glucose intolerance and haemodynamic abnormalities, including left ventricular hypertrophy, and possibly vascular calcification. Of these, hypertension is probably the most susceptible to treatment.

Anaemia

Circulating erythropoietin levels are inappropriately low. Parenteral recombinant erythropoietin increases haemoglobin, improves exercise tolerance and reduces the need for blood transfusion. In patients with pre-dialysis advanced renal failure, erythropoietin corrects anaemia and improves well-being, without affecting the rate of decline in renal function. Dose-dependent hypertension occurs in 35% of patients and can usually be controlled with hypotensive agents, although hypertensive encephalopathy can develop suddenly. Treating with erythropoietin to higher haemoglobin targets (within the normal range) is associated with increased cardiovascular risk (Trials Box 14.2).

Sexual dysfunction

Decreased libido and impotence are common. Hyperprolactinaemia is present in at least one-third of patients, resulting in an inhibitory effect on gonadotrophin secretion. Prolactin levels may be reduced by bromocriptine, although side effects are common (nausea, headache, drowsiness, postural hypotension).

Renal replacement therapy

Renal function can be replaced in end-stage renal disease by the following:

- *Haemodialysis.* Diffusion of solutes occurs between blood and dialysate which flow in opposite directions, separated by a semi-permeable membrane.

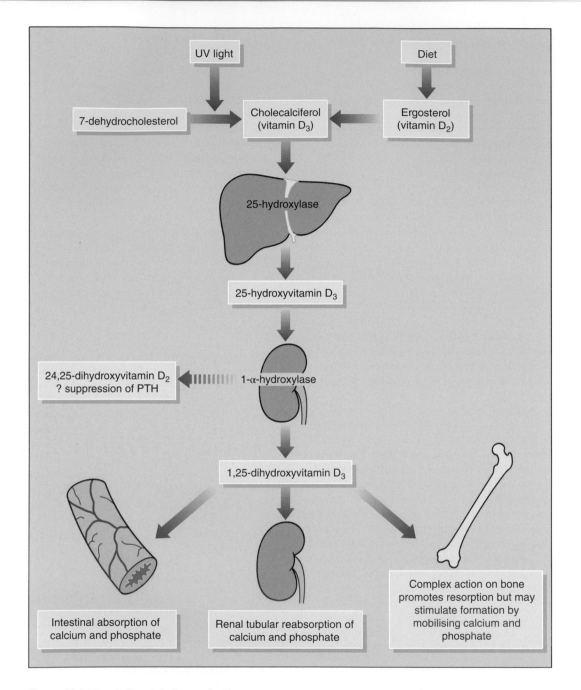

Figure 14.1 Vitamin D metabolism and actions.

The most common problems are cardiovascular instability during dialysis, and difficulty establishing vascular access. This is achieved by:
○ arteriovenous fistula;
○ double-lumen tunnelled line, usually jugular;

○ synthetic graft looping subcutaneously between an artery and vein in the forearm or leg.
● *Continuous ambulatory peritoneal dialysis.* Patients instil up to 21 of isotonic or hypertonic solutions into the peritoneal cavity via a permanent

TRIALS BOX 14.2 Target haemoglobin in chronic kidney disease

The CHOIR investigators studied 1432 patients with chronic kidney disease who were treated with erythropoietin. The use of a target haemoglobin level of 13.5 g/dl (as compared with 11.3 g/dl) was associated with increased risk and no incremental improvement in the quality of life. Source: *New England Journal of Medicine* 2006; **355**(20): 2085–2098.

The CREATE investigators randomly assigned patients with an eGFR of 15.0–35.0 ml/min/1.73 m² of body-surface area and haemoglobin 11.0–12.5 g/dl to a target haemoglobin value in the normal range (13.0–15.0 g/dl) or a subnormal range (10.5–11.5 g/dl). Early complete correction of anaemia did not reduce the risk of cardiovascular events.

Source: *New England Journal of Medicine* 2006; **355**(20): 2071–2084.

The TREAT investigators found that the use of erythropoietin in patients with diabetes, pre-dialysis chronic kidney disease, and moderate anaemia resulted in only a modest improvement in patient-reported fatigue, did not reduce the risk of either death or a cardiovascular event or death or a renal event, and was associated with an increased risk of stroke. Source: *New England Journal of Medicine*. 2009; **361**(21): 2019–2032.

NICE recommend an aspirational haemoglobin range between 100 and 120 g/litre for adults with chronic kidney disease (https://www.nice.org.uk/guidance/NG8).

indwelling catheter. The fluid equilibrates, across the 2 m² of peritoneal membrane, with blood in peritoneal capillaries. After several hours the fluid containing toxic waste products is drained out. This procedure is repeated three or four times daily. Excess fluid is removed by hypertonic solutions. The major complication is peritonitis, usually caused by *Staphylococcus epidermidis* or *S. aureus*. Automated peritoneal dialysis involves using a machine to cycle the fluid during the night.

- *Renal transplantation* is the treatment of choice in most patients, but is limited by supply of donor organs.

Assessment of dialysis adequacy

Plasma urea and creatinine are poor predictors of outcome in dialysis patients – low pre-dialysis urea, not high, has been found to be associated with increased mortality. This is because when protein intake is deficient or muscle mass is reduced, pre-dialysis urea and creatinine may remain low even in the presence of inadequate dialysis. Assessment of dialysis adequacy is achieved by the use of kinetic measurements – referred to as *urea kinetic modelling.* Two parameters, *urea clearance* corrected for volume of distribution (Kt/V urea, where Kt=urea clearance and V=volume of distribution) and *protein catabolic rate,* have been found in several studies to be useful predictors of outcome.

Glomerulonephritis

This describes a number of disorders that affect one or more of the glomerular components in both kidneys (Fig. 14.2). Patients present with one or more features of renal disease – hypertension, haematuria, proteinuria, nephrotic syndrome and reduced excretory renal function.

The classification of glomerulonephritis is based on histology and immunofluorescence of renal tissue. Contraindications to renal biopsy include:

- one functioning kidney
- small kidneys
- hypertension
- bleeding disorders.

Confusion arises because renal biopsy findings do not necessarily correlate with clinical features, although they are sometimes useful in guiding management and predicting outcome.

Histological changes are described as:

- *focal* – affecting <50% of glomeruli
- *diffuse* – affecting >50% of glomeruli
- *segmental* – affecting part of the glomerulus
- *global* – affecting all of the glomerular tuft
- *proliferative* – an increase in glomerular cells (mesangial, epithelial and endothelial) with leucocytic infiltration

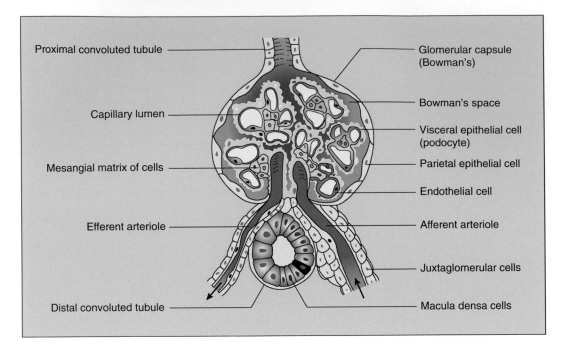

Proximal convoluted tubule

Capillary lumen

Mesangial matrix of cells

Efferent arteriole

Distal convoluted tubule

Glomerular capsule (Bowman's)

Bowman's space

Visceral epithelial cell (podocyte)

Parietal epithelial cell

Endothelial cell

Afferent arteriole

Juxtaglomerular cells

Macula densa cells

Figure 14.2 Glomerulus.

- *crescent* – a crescent-shaped proliferation of epithelial cells and mononuclear cells in Bowman's capsule. It occurs in any severe form of glomerular injury
- *membranous* – thickening of the glomerular capillary wall
- *sclerosis* – capillary collapse with loss of the lumen.

IgA-Nephropathy

Granular mesangial deposition of immunoglobulin A (IgA, and usually C3) with variable segmental mesangial proliferation (measurement of serum immunoglobulins is usually unhelpful: 20–50% have raised IgA).

Clinical features

Usually presents with haematuria (often provoked by infection).

Aetiology

Unknown. It is associated with liver disease (particularly alcoholic cirrhosis), coeliac disease, seronegative arthritis, neoplasia and infection.

Prognosis

It is probably the most common form of glomerulonephritis. Approximately 20% of cases progress to renal failure. Control of hypertension (ACE inhibitors are preferred) slows the decline of renal function. Steroids may be of benefit.

Henoch-Schönlein purpura

(See page 332, Chapter 18.)

Membranous nephropathy

Diffuse uniform thickening of glomerular capillary wall, usually without cellular proliferation.

Classification

- Stage I: small subepithelial electron-dense deposits (diffuse granular IgG staining).

- Stage II: outgrowth of basement membrane between subepithelial deposits (seen as 'spikes' on silver stain).
- Stage III: deposits incorporated into basement membrane, which becomes less electron-dense.
- Stage IV: thickened vacuolated membrane, sclerosis.

Clinical manifestations

Proteinuria (often nephrotic), hypertension, haematuria, deteriorating renal function.

Aetiology

Idiopathic – 70% of patients with 'idiopathic' membranous glomerulonephritis have antibodies against phospholipase A2 receptor 1.

Drugs (penicillamine, gold), neoplasia, SLE, infections (hepatitis B, malaria), diabetes.

Prognosis

The course of idiopathic membranous nephropathy is highly variable. Approximately 25% of cases undergo complete spontaneous remission, 25% have a partial remission with stable impaired renal function, 25% have persistent nephrotic syndrome with stable renal function and 25% progress to end-stage renal disease. Poor prognosis is suggested by heavy proteinuria, hypertension, elevated creatinine at presentation, and stage IV lesion. Deterioration in renal function can be halted or reversed by immunosuppression (Box 14.4).

Box 14.4 Treatment of membranous glomerulonephritis

A Cochrane review of immunosuppressive treatment for idiopathic membranous nephropathy in adults with nephrotic syndrome found that a combined alkylating agent and corticosteroid regimen had short- and long-term benefits, although adverse effects were common. Cyclophosphamide was safer than chlorambucil. Cyclosporine or tacrolimus have been recommended by the Kidney Disease Improving Global Outcomes (KDIGO) Clinical Practice Guideline 2012 as the alternative regimen for adult idiopathic membranous glomerulonephritis with nephrotic syndrome; there was no evidence that calcineurin inhibitors could alter the combined outcome of death or end-stage kidney disease.
Source: *Cochrane Database of Systematic Reviews* 2014; (10): CD004293. doi: 10.1002/14651858. CD004293.pub3.

Membranoproliferative (mesangiocapillary) glomerulonephritis

Mesangial expansion (caused by increased matrix and mesangial cells) and thickened capillary loops (caused by extension of matrix and mesangial cells between GBM and endothelium, giving the characteristic double contour).

Classification

- Type I: subendothelial immune deposits (stain for C3 and Ig – most common type).
- Type II: linear dense deposits along GBM (linear C3, occasional Ig).

Aetiology

Secondary causes include:

- infection, whether bacterial (infective endocarditis, 'shunt nephritis', leprosy), viral (hepatitis B) or protozoal (schistosomiasis)
- neoplasia
- SLE
- cryoglobulinaemia.

Nephritic factor occurs in >60% type I and 10–20% type II mesangiocapillary glomerulonephritis. It is an IgG autoantibody, which binds to and stabilises C3 convertase (C3bBb), permanently activating the alternative pathway and depleting C3. It is associated with partial lipodystrophy.

Clinical features

Proteinuria and haematuria, with variable degree of renal failure.

Prognosis

There is no evidence to support the use of immunosuppressive therapy. Half of cases progress to established renal failure in 10 years.

Minimal-change nephropathy

Normal light microscopy, with negative immunofluorescence. There is podocyte foot process fusion on electron microscopy (a relatively non-specific consequence of proteinuria).

Clinical features

It accounts for over 75% of childhood and × 20% of adult cases of nephrotic syndrome.

Aetiology

It is associated with allergy and malignancy (e.g. Hodgkin's disease).

Prognosis

The majority of cases respond to steroids. Cyclophosphamide is beneficial if relapsing. Cyclosporin may also be of benefit.

Focal glomerulosclerosis

Segmental sclerosis affecting some glomeruli (focal). Granular IgM and C3 may be present in areas of sclerosis.

Aetiology

Idiopathic – focal glomerulosclerosis accounts for 10–20% of adult and childhood nephrotic syndrome. About 20% of cases are secondary to systemic diseases, including hypertension, diabetes and obesity.

Clinical features

Proteinuria, often with hypertension and renal impairment.

Prognosis

There is a poor response to treatment – a trial of immunosuppression is often given if there is progressive renal dysfunction. Steroids or cyclosporin are most commonly used.

Systemic vasculitis

There is necrotising inflammation of blood-vessel walls. Any organ system can be involved.

Renal involvement is usually seen in Wegener's granulomatosis and microscopic polyangiitis. Typically, there is a focal proliferative glomerulonephritis, often with necrosis and crescent formation. Granulomatous inflammation of the upper and lower airway is usually present in Wegener's granulomatosis.

Vasculitis has been classified according to clinical features, size of vessel and the presence of antibodies against neutrophil cytoplasm antigens (ANCA most commonly directed against neutrophil proteases, including proteinase-3 and myeloperoxidase) (Table 14.3).

Renal lesion

Focal proliferation with necrosis and epithelial cell crescent formation. Immunofluorescence usually negative or sparse granular Ig and C3. Presents with rapidly progressive glomerulonephritis.

Prognosis

Remission occurs in over 90% of patients using oral cyclophosphamide and prednisolone. Maintenance immunosuppression, usually with steroids and azathioprine or mycophenolate, is required. Relapse occurs in one-third of patients during the first year. Intravenous immunoglobulin, monoclonal anti-CD52 antibody therapy or rituximab may be effective in patients with vasculitis refractory to further increases in immunosuppression.

Table 14.3 Classification of vasculitis			
	ANCA+	ANCA+/−	ANCA−
Small vessel	Wegener's granulomatosis Microscopic polyangiitis		Henoch–Schönlein purpura
Medium vessel	Churg–Strauss disease	Polyarteritis nodosa	
Large vessel			Takayasu's arteritis
			Giant-cell arteritis
ANCA, antibodies against neutrophil cytoplasm antigens. See also Fig. 18.4.			

Antiglomerular basement membrane disease (Goodpasture's disease)

Proliferative glomerulonephritis – usually severe glomerular inflammation with crescents and necrosis. Immunofluorescence reveals linear IgG along GBM (may also occur in SLE and diabetes).

Aetiology

Anti-GBM antibodies recognise a restricted epitope on type IV collagen. They bind with high affinity to basement membrane in glomeruli, alveoli, the eye and ear.

NB: Anti-GMB antibodies do not bind to Alport GBM in which type IV collagen is abnormal, but may develop following transplantation of a normal kidney into a patient with Alport syndrome.

Clinical features

There is an acute renal failure caused by a rapidly progressive glomerulonephritis. Pulmonary haemorrhage (in smokers) causes breathlessness and haemoptysis. Chest X-ray shows that pulmonary shadowing and transfer factor (T_{LCO}) is increased by the presence of haemoglobin in alveoli. The combination is known as Goodpasture syndrome, and anti-GBM disease (Goodpasture's disease) is a common cause. The other major cause is systemic vasculitis (see earlier).

Prognosis

The disease usually responds to plasma exchange (to remove the autoantibody) combined with steroids and cytotoxic therapy (usually cyclophosphamide). Recovery of renal function is rare once anuria or dialysis dependence has occurred.

Systemic lupus erythematosus

Renal involvement is common in SLE (page 315, Chapter 18) – over 90% of patients have abnormalities on renal biopsy. The World Health Organization (WHO) classification is shown in Table 14.4.

Table 14.4 World Health Organization classification of renal disease in systemic lupus erythematosus (SLE)

Class	Description
I	Normal (extremely rare)
II	Mesangial changes
IIa	Deposits by immunofluorescence and electron microscopy
IIb	Hypercellularity as well
III	Proliferative glomerulonephritis (<50%)
IV	Proliferative glomerulonephritis (>50%)
V	Membranous glomerulonephritis

Clinical features

There can be almost any manifestation of renal disease, including hypertension, haematuria, proteinuria, nephrotic syndrome, acute renal failure and end-stage renal disease.

Prognosis

The prognosis differs according to WHO classification. It is good in class II, but poor in classes III and IV. The significance of membranous change (class V) is unclear. Steroids in combination with azathioprine or cyclophosphamide can slow progressive renal damage. Plasma exchange may provide additional benefits.

Post-streptococcal glomerulonephritis

Diffuse proliferative glomerulonephritis with granular deposits of C3 and IgG.

Clinical features

Oliguria, oedema, hypertension, haematuria and renal impairment follow 2–3 weeks after infection with a nephritogenic strain of group A β-haemolytic streptococci.

Investigations

Throat or skin cultures may show group A streptococci if penicillin has not been given. Antibodies against streptococcal antigens provide evidence of recent infection, e.g. antistreptolysin (ASO). Hypocomplementaemia occurs with low C3 and CH_{50}.

Prognosis

Spontaneous recovery is usual. The disease is now very rare.

Fluid and electrolytes

Salt and water

Plasma sodium concentration and extracellular fluid volume vary independently of each other so alterations in plasma sodium reflect alterations in either sodium or water.

Serum sodium decreased (hyponatraemia)

This is when plasma sodium is <130 mmol/l.

Aetiology

Too little sodium or too much water, or both.

Clinical features

In salt depletion there is thirst, dry tongue, reduced tissue turgor and postural hypotension. In severe depletion, mental confusion, hypotension and shock occur. None of these features is present if water excess because of inappropriate antidiuretic hormone (ADH) or psychogenic polydypsia is the cause.

Investigation

Check serum osmolality and urine sodium. If:

- Serum osmolality is decreased and urine sodium is increased:
  - excess renal sodium loss (renal failure, Addison's disease, page 251, Chapter 16)
  - inappropriate ADH secretion. (NB: Some drugs such as chlorpropamide and carbamazepine can have an ADH-like action on the kidney.)
- Serum osmolality is decreased and urine sodium is decreased:
  - extrarenal loss of sodium (e.g. gastrointestinal tract, burns)
  - fluid retention associated with cardiac failure, hepatic failure or nephrotic syndrome
  - psychogenic polydipsia.

- Serum osmolality is normal:
  - usually spurious, e.g. in severe hyperlipidaemia when the amount of sodium in the aqueous phase of plasma is normal, but its concentration is expressed in terms of the volume of the aqueous and lipid phase.

Management

Salt depletion is corrected with NaCl, either orally (slow sodium tablets) or as intravenous normal saline (0.9%, 150 mmol/l each of Na^b and Cl^-). Water excess in inappropriate ADH secretion and psychogenic polydysia is treated by water restriction (<600 ml/24 h).

Serum sodium increased (hypernatraemia)

Aetiology

Too much sodium or too little water.

Investigation

Check urine sodium (normal 10–20 mmol/l) and whether urine osmolality is low (<300 mOsmol/l) or high (>800 mOsmol/l).
If:

- Urine osmolality decreased and urine sodium increased:
  - excess sodium load, either iatrogenic or endocrine (e.g. Conn syndrome, Cushing syndrome)
  - previous renal loss of water and sodium (e.g. osmotic diuresis resulting from glucose).
- Urine osmolality decreased and urine sodium decreased:
  - diabetes insipidus.
- Urine osmolality increased and urine sodium decreased:
  - previous and continuing extrarenal loss of sodium and water (e.g. from sweat, gastrointestinal tract).
- Urine osmolality increased and urine sodium increased or normal:
  - previous and continuing extrarenal loss of water but not sodium (e.g. from lungs during febrile illness).

Management

Patients with hypernatraemia need water, which can be given orally or as intravenous 5% dextrose. The underlying cause should be determined and treated.

Serum potassium

Around 98% of potassium is intracellular (in contrast to sodium which is predominantly extracellular). Normal potassium intake = 60–200 mmol/day.

Serum potassium decreased (hypokalaemia)
Aetiology

- Gastrointestinal losses: diarrhoea and/or vomiting (colonic tumours, particularly villous adenomas, may secrete large amounts of potassium), laxative abuse.
- Renal loss:
  - diuretic therapy (thiazides, loop diuretics)
  - mineralocorticoid excess. Renin secreted by the juxtaglomerular apparatus in the kidney converts angiotensinogen to angiotensin. Angiotensin stimulates aldosterone secretion from the adrenal cortex which causes urinary sodium retention and potassium loss. Causes include Conn syndrome, Cushing syndrome, corticosteroid therapy, ectopic adrenocorticotrophic hormone (ACTH, tumours) and Bartter syndrome (renal potassium loss associated with juxtaglomerular cell hyperplasia and hyperreninaemia)
  - osmotic diuresis (e.g. uncontrolled diabetes)
  - renal tubular acidosis (see below).
- Shift to intracellular compartment (e.g. insulin therapy, familial periodic paralysis).
- Poor intake (including eating disorders, which may be associated with laxative or diuretic abuse).

Clinical features

Weakness and lethargy. The electrocardiogram (ECG) shows flat T and prominent U waves.

Management

Treat the underlying cause.

- Give oral potassium as potassium chloride.
- Where oral administration is not possible (e.g. vomiting), potassium is given intravenously: 2 g/l (26 mmol/l) intravenous solution.

Serum potassium increased (hyperkalaemia)
Aetiology

- potassium retention:
  - decreased mineralocorticoids: Addison's disease, spironolactone (aldosterone antagonist), angiotensin-converting enzyme inhibitors
  - potassium-retaining diuretics (e.g. amiloride).
- increased supply of potassium – potassium is predominantly intracellular and released following cell destruction, e.g. haemolysis, trauma, cytotoxic therapy

Clinical features

Severe hyperkalaemia (>6–7 mmol/l) may be associated with life-threatening ECG abnormalities.

Management

Stop oral or intravenous intake.

Ion exchange resins, e.g. calcium resonium 15 g 6-hourly orally (or rectally).

In emergency states, intravenous calcium (10 ml 10% calcium gluconate) antagonises the cardiac effects of hyperkalaemia. Intravenous dextrose and insulin moves potassium into the intracellular compartment. Dialysis may be required.

Metabolic acidosis
Aetiology

- exogenous acids (e.g. poisoning by salicylate)
- accumulation of endogenous acids such as lactic acid (tissue hypoperfusion in cardiac arrest or shock) or acetoacetic acid in diabetic ketoacidosis
- loss of alkali (e.g. gastrointestinal loss in severe diarrhoea, biliary or enteric fistulae; or renal loss in proximal tubular acidosis)
- failure of renal elimination of acid (renal failure and distal tubular acidosis)

Management

Treat the underlying cause, e.g. diabetic ketoacidosis (page 268, Chapter 17), salicylate poisoning (Table 22.2).

In chronic kidney disease acidosis can be corrected with oral bicarbonate or dialysis against a bicarbonate-based dialysis fluid.

Bicarbonate deficit can be calculated as the measured serum bicarbonate below normal standard bicarbonate × 30% body weight in kilograms. In severe acidosis bicarbonate is sometimes replaced as 8.4% sodium bicarbonate solution (contains 1 mmol/ml). This should be rapid (give 50–100 ml) following sustained cardiac arrest as arrhythmias are difficult to revert in the presence of acidosis.

In *distal renal tubular acidosis (type 1)* there is a failure of hydrogen ion secretion in the distal tubule. Urine pH is inappropriately high despite hypokalaemic, hyperchloraemic acidosis. It may be inherited as an autosomal dominant trait or occur as a result of damage to the renal medulla from pyelonephritis, obstructive uropathy, medullary sponge kidney or ischaemia. Nephrocalcinosis and osteomalacia (or rickets in children) are common. Treatment is with oral bicarbonate, often with potassium supplements.

Proximal renal tubular acidosis (type 2) is less common. It is caused by a defect of proximal tubular bicarbonate reabsorption.

Metabolic alkalosis

Aetiology

- excess intake of alkali, e.g. milk-alkali syndrome, massive blood transfusion (citrate is metabolised to bicarbonate)
- loss of gastric acid, e.g. pyloric stenosis
- increased renal losses of acid with bicarbonate generation, as in hyperaldosteronism, elevated corticosteroids or severe hypokalaemia

Management

Identify and treat the underlying cause.

Hypercalcaemia

Aetiology

Hyperparathyroidism

- primary (parathyroid adenoma or hyperplasia)
- secondary: increased PTH secretion occurs in response to a fall in serum calcium (e.g. in renal failure, malabsorption) by definition the calcium is normal
- tertiary hyperparathyroidism: if secondary hyperparathyroidism gets 'out of control' autonomous parathyroid hormone secretion develops, causing elevation of both PTH and serum calcium

Malignancy

- bone metastases (commonly breast, lung, prostate, kidney, thyroid)
- multiple myeloma, leukaemia, Hodgkin's disease
- secretion of a PTH-like factor

Sarcoid

Increased sensitivity to vitamin D – hypercalcaemia often precipitated by exposure to sunlight.

Drugs

- excess vitamin D
- calcium-containing antacids (milk-alkali syndrome)
- rarely, thiazides

Endocrine (rare)

Thyrotoxicosis, adrenal insufficiency.

Hypocalcaemia

Aetiology

Hypoparathyroidism

- idiopathic
- post-thyroid or parathyroid surgery
- pseudohypoparathyroidism (reduced sensitivity to PTH)

Inadequate dietary intake of vitamin D or calcium (rarely, vitamin D resistance)

- malabsorption
- renal disease
- acute pancreatitis

Hypomagnesaemia

Magnesium is the second most abundant intracellular cation. Normal requirement is 150 mg/day. Normal intake is 300–400 mg/day.

Aetiology

Occurs in starvation, enteral nutrition with inadequate replacement, prolonged diarrhoea, enteric fistulae and drugs (diuretics, aminoglycosides, amphotericin, carbenicillin). Usually associated with hypocalcaemia.

Reduced calcium and magnesium are often found in the seriously ill where nutrition has been inaccurately estimated.

Clinical features

Paraesthesia, cramp, tetany, apathy.

Hyperphosphataemia

Aetiology

- reduced loss:
  - renal failure
  - hypoparathyroidism
- increased load:
  - excessive vitamin D intake

Hypophosphataemia

Aetiology

- increased loss:
  - diuretic therapy
  - hypoparathyroidism
  - renal tubular defects (e.g. Fanconi syndrome – glycosuria, aminoaciduria, phosphaturia, renal tubular acidosis)
- decreased absorption:
  - malabsorption
  - vitamin D deficiency or resistance
  - malnutrition

- intracellular shift:
  - diabetes mellitus
  - 'refeeding syndrome' (after starvation or severe illness)

Uric acid

Levels of uric acid are increased by stress and fasting.

Serum uric acid increased

Causes

- primary gout
- 25% of relatives with primary gout
- diuretics (particularly thiazides)
- doses of aspirin below 2 g/day
- renal failure
- increased destruction of nucleoproteins, usually in myeloproliferative disorders – particularly at the start of cytotoxic therapy or radiotherapy
- psoriasis (one-third of patients)

15

Neurology

Headache

Headache is the most frequently reported neurological symptom, accounting for considerable morbidity in the general population. The clinician's challenge is to exclude a treatable underlying intra- or extracranial secondary cause (Table 15.1) and to make a definitive diagnosis. The history provides important clues and should ascertain:

- date of onset, frequency and duration of episodes
- precipitating and relieving factors
- type and location of pain
- severity
- associated features
- family history.

Primary headache syndromes

Tension headache (chronic daily headache)

Characteristically a continuous severe pressure is felt bilaterally over the vertex, occiput or eyes. It may be 'band-like' or non-specific and of variable intensity. Aetiology remains unclear but may be musculoskeletal in origin. It may occur at any age and in either sex, especially in the context of stress or depression.

The headache often occurs daily and may persist for months or even years. Standard analgesics are reported to be ineffective and continuous analgesic use (simple analgesics for 15 or more days a month or more complex analgesia for 10 or more days a month) may exacerbate the situation, especially when the effects of medication wear off (so-called analgesic overuse headache or rebound headache). Aside from nausea, there are no other associated features and neurological examination is normal.

Treatment involves reassurance that there is no sinister underlying cause, as may teaching relaxation techniques and addressing underlying stressors. The patient should be advised to avoid analgesia use, but a small dose of amitriptyline taken at night may help.

Migraine

Migraine is usually episodic and affects approximately 10% of the population. It typically begins around puberty and continues intermittently to middle age. It is three times more common in women and there is often a family history. It may be associated with menstruation or triggered by contraceptive pill usage, physical exercise, alcohol, various specific foods (especially chocolate, cheese and red wine) or heightened emotions. There is a link with hypertension and prior head injury.

The pathophysiology remains poorly understood. Prodromal sensory phenomena ('aura') have been attributed to vasoconstriction within intracerebral vessels, although a wave of depolarisation spreading across the cerebral cortex may account for this early phase. Thereafter, vasodilatation of extracerebral vessels correlates with the onset of headache. A number of vasoactive peptides including calcitonin-gene related peptide (CGRP) and serotoninergic (5-HT) pathways have been implicated in the pathogenesis.

Clinical Medicine Lecture Notes, Eighth Edition. John R. Bradley, Mark Gurnell, and Diana F. Wood.
© 2019 John Wiley & Sons Ltd. Published 2019 by John Wiley & Sons Ltd.

Table 15.1 Causes of headache and facial pain

Type	Examples
Primary headache syndrome	Tension headache Migraine Cluster headache
Headache secondary to other disorders	Raised intracranial pressure Idiopathic ('benign') intracranial hypertension Meningeal irritation (e.g. meningitis, SAH) Post-traumatic (head injury) Hypertension Giant-cell arteritis Sinusitis Perioral disease (poor dentition, salivary gland disorders) Cervical spine disease Ocular, orbital and retro-orbital disease Ear disease Temporomandibular joint dysfunction Metabolic disturbance (e.g. hypoxia, hypercapnia, hypoglycaemia) Drugs (e.g. nitrates, vasoactive agents)
Facial pain	Trigeminal neuralgia Postherpetic neuralgia Atypical facial pain

SAH, subarachnoid haemorrhage.

Clinical presentation

Classical migraine with aura

Characteristically migraine starts with a sense of ill health (lasting up to several hours) followed by a visual aura (e.g. shimmering lights, fortification spectra, scotomata) usually in the field opposite to the side of the succeeding headache and lasting up to 1 h. In severe cases the patient may develop a homonymous hemianopia or even complete blindness. Sensory symptoms (e.g. unilateral numbness/paraesthesia) are less commonly seen. These 'spread' up a limb or limbs, making a distinction from a TIA straightforward in most cases. Speech disturbance or motor weakness are less common. Thereafter, a throbbing, usually unilateral, headache is associated with anorexia, nausea, vomiting, photophobia, phonophobia and a desire to be still, often in the dark and quiet. This distinguishes migraine from 'tension-type headache' where the patient can carry on with their usual activities, and cluster headache, where the patient wants to pace the room. The headache lasts from 3–72 h, and is aggravated by movement (e.g. coughing, sneezing, bending). Neurological examination is usually normal and between episodes the patient remains well.

Migraine without aura

Although the classical aura is absent, patients often feel non-specifically unwell prior to the onset of headache.

Hemiplegic migraine

Most hemiplegic migraines last <24 h, but rarely, focal neurological features may persist for several days. Other structural lesions (e.g. arteriovenous malformation, aneurysm) should be excluded.

Investigation

When the diagnosis is clear, investigation is generally not required; however, if there is any doubt, then brain imaging should be considered. If a patient presents with ongoing weakness associated with headache for the first time, imaging is considered mandatory.

Management

Acute attack

- Sleeping in a quiet, darkened room is effective in many patients.

- Simple analgesics (e.g. soluble aspirin, paracetamol) and an antiemetic agent (which can be administered by the buccal route if nausea/vomiting are present).
- 5-HT1B/D agonists (e.g. rizatriptan, sumatriptan, zolmitriptan) are effective when taken early and may abort an established attack. If one triptan fails, another may well work. They are contraindicated in patients with known/suspected coronary or cerebrovascular disease or uncontrolled hypertension and must be used cautiously in those with vascular risk factors.

Clinical trials with a novel class of agent, CGRP antagonists, are underway and may offer benefit for migraine sufferers who do not respond well to triptans.

Prophylaxis

Precipitating causes should be identified and avoided. Oestrogen-containing preparations must be used with caution. Preventative treatment for migraine should be considered for patients who suffer:

- >1 acute attack per month
- significant disability despite appropriate treatment for acute attacks.

Therapeutic options include:

- β-blockers – usually propranolol
- topiramate.

Cluster headache

These are relatively short-lived (30–120 min) episodes of severe pain, typically centered on one eye and affecting men more than women (~3 : 1), with an age of onset between 20 and 60 years. Attacks start without warning and are associated with red eye, eye and nose watering and vomiting. They may occur several times a day, often waking the patient from sleep. Usually cluster headaches are recurrent for several days, weeks or months before the disorder remits and the patient becomes pain-free for months or years. Alcohol is a recognised precipitant.

Sumatriptan (self-administered by subcutaneous injection) is the treatment of choice for cluster headaches – simple analgesics are not effective in this condition. High-flow oxygen, and corticosteroids are efficacious in many patients. The latter are given as a tapering dose and are particularly useful until prophylaxis (e.g. with verapamil or lithium) takes effect.

Secondary causes of headache

See Table 15.1.

Raised intracranial pressure

Usually secondary to an intracranial tumour, haematoma or abscess, the pain is worse on waking and associated with nausea and vomiting. It improves 1–2 h after rising and is exacerbated by coughing, sneezing, straining and bending down. Neurological symptoms and signs related to the primary lesion are usually evident.

Idiopathic ('benign') intracranial hypertension (IIH; pseudotumour cerebri)

IIH is commonest in young obese women. They present with symptoms and signs of raised intracranial pressure but no mass lesion on brain imaging. Altered cerebrospinal fluid (CSF) dynamics (with impaired absorption) have been suggested to underlie the disorder. The patient may report visual disturbance, including obscurations (abrupt onset transient visual loss secondary to changes in posture), and examination reveals bilateral papilloedema. Occasionally, bilateral sixth cranial nerve palsies are present and reflect raised intracranial pressure ('false-localising' sign). Pulsatile tinnitus is another recognised feature.

CT/MRI scanning of the brain is normal without hydrocephalus or mass lesion. CT or MRI venography is required to exclude a venous thrombosis. Lumbar puncture confirms raised CSF pressure with normal constituents. Intracranial venous sinus thrombosis, disorders of calcium metabolism, drugs (tetracyclines, isotretinoin, hormonal contraceptives, growth hormone and corticosteroids), systemic lupus erythematosus and hypervitaminosis A may all present with a syndrome similar to IIH, thus secondary causes should always be considered.

Weight loss often facilitates spontaneous remission. Serial therapeutic lumbar punctures can be used to lower CSF pressure. Medical therapy with acetazolamide or topiramate (or occasionally corticosteroids) is effective; surgical intervention (lumboperitoneal shunt or optic nerve sheath decompression) is occasionally required to relieve symptoms and/or protect vision – prolonged raised intracranial pressure predisposes to optic atrophy.

Meningeal irritation

Irritation of the meninges (meningism) occurring in meningitis or following subarachnoid haemorrhage characteristically produces a triad of symptoms:

- severe headache – global or occipital associated with nausea/vomiting
- photophobia
- neck stiffness.

In meningitis, the headache evolves over minutes to hours whereas in subarachnoid haemorrhage it is abrupt in onset and may be followed by loss of consciousness.

Post-concussion

Similar to tension headache but usually associated with dizziness (not vertigo) and impaired concentration, post-concussion headache may persist for months.

Giant-cell arteritis

This is a very important cause of headache in patients over 50 years of age (see rheumatology, Chapter 18).

Neuralgias

Neuralgias are intermittent, brief, severe, lancinating pains occurring along the distribution of a nerve.

Trigeminal neuralgia

Trigeminal neuralgia predominantly affects those over 50 years of age. It may reflect compression of the sensory root of the trigeminal nerve (e.g. by a tumour or aberrant vessel) or complicate multiple sclerosis. The agonising sharp pain is confined to the distribution of the trigeminal nerve on one side, commonly the maxillary or mandibular divisions. It lasts only seconds and is usually triggered from a place on the lips, side of the face or nose, by chewing, eating, speaking, or by a cold breeze. It tends to get worse with age, and eventually a continuous background pain may develop if left untreated. Physical examination is usually normal but may reveal neurological signs in the presence of an underlying mass lesion.

Simple analgesics are ineffective. Usually carbamazepine provides good symptom control, but gabapentin, sodium valproate, clonazepam and tricyclic antidepressants may be tried.

If medical options have failed, radiofrequency thermocoagulation or chemical (glycerol) ablation of the trigeminal ganglion produce benefits in some patients.

Glossopharyngeal neuralgia

A rare disorder precipitated by swallowing, which produces pain in the pharynx or deep inside the ear.

Postherpetic neuralgia

Patients have a history of herpes zoster infection (shingles) in the distribution of one of the branches of the trigeminal nerve (usually ophthalmic). Pain, itching and altered sensation develop along the course of the affected nerve and persist after the rash has healed. The pain may be difficult to treat, but sometimes responds to tricyclic antidepressants, carbamazepine or topically applied capsaicin.

Atypical facial pain

This describes episodic aching in the jaw and cheek (in a non-anatomical distribution), which lasts for several hours, and often coexisting with a history of anxiety or depression. It can be bilateral and may respond to antidepressants.

Epilepsy

Epilepsy results from intermittent paroxysmal electrical discharges of cerebral neurons causing stereotypical attacks of altered consciousness, motor or sensory function, behaviour or emotion. A single unprovoked episode (i.e. a seizure) is insufficient to make a diagnosis as the term 'epilepsy' is reserved for those with a recurring tendency to seizures. All patients with a first unexplained seizure should be assessed by a neurologist within 2 weeks.

Up to 1% of the general population suffers from epilepsy. Each year a small number of individuals with this condition (1–2 per 100 000) die prematurely as a consequence of status epilepticus (see later), accidental injury or sudden unexplained death – the latter is assumed to be related to seizure activity with associated cardiorespiratory dysfunction.

Classification

Partial seizures

These have a single focus of activity, which may be scar tissue related to previous trauma, to febrile convulsions (hippocampal sclerosis), a stroke or tumour. They are classified as:

- simple partial seizures: with no impairment of consciousness
- complex partial seizures: consciousness is impaired at some stage.

Partial seizures may progress to generalised seizures.

Generalised seizures

Generalised seizures are typified by widespread activity affecting both cerebral hemispheres and include:

- childhood absence seizures (petit mal) and atypical absence seizures
- myoclonic epilepsy
- tonic–clonic (grand mal) seizures
- tonic (spasm), clonic (jerking), atonic or akinetic seizures.

Aetiology

Most epilepsy is idiopathic. There may be a family history suggesting genetic susceptibility, particularly with absence seizures. Seizures may be secondary to cerebral disorders, metabolic dysfunction and drug ingestion (Table 15.2).

Provocation of seizures

A variety of factors can provoke seizures in patients not usually prone to epilepsy (e.g. drug overdose, hypoglycaemia). In those with known epilepsy, seizures may be provoked by sleep deprivation, stress, alcohol and, occasionally, stimuli such as television or strobe lighting. In some women, seizures may increase in frequency around the time of menstruation.

Differential diagnosis

- syncope: e.g. vasovagal faints, postmicturition and cough syncope
- cerebrovascular disease: e.g. transient ischaemic attacks, critical carotid artery stenosis
- vestibular disorders
- low cardiac output states
- metabolic: e.g. hypoglycaemia
- postural hypotension
- narcolepsy
- psychological: e.g. conversion disorders

Clinical features

Epilepsy in childhood

Absence seizures ('petit mal')
This usually presents between 4 and 10 years and is more common in girls. It is characterised by brief

Table 15.2 Causes of epilepsy	
Type	**Cause**
Idiopathic	Often unknown, but likely significant inherited component
Secondary to other disorders	
Neonatal	Birth trauma, including intracranial haemorrhage
	Hypoxia
Childhood	Congenital anomalies
	Tuberous sclerosis
	Metabolic storage disorders
Adulthood	Head injury
	Drug* and/or alcohol intoxication or withdrawal
Elderly	Cerebrovascular disease
	Degenerative disorders (e.g. Alzheimer's disease, Huntington's disease)
All/most ages	Metabolic disturbance (e.g. hypoglycaemia, hypocalcaemia, hyponatraemia)
	Cerebral infection (e.g. meningitis, encephalitis, abscess)
	Cerebral tumour or arteriovenous malformation
	Inflammation (e.g. vasculitis, SLE, demyelination [particularly in end- stage multiple sclerosis])

*A wide variety of drugs have been reported to provoke seizures – a list is available at www.epilepsy.com; SLE, systemic lupus erythematosus.

(10–15 s) moments of absence without warning (e.g. the child stops talking and stares blankly) followed by immediate recovery. It rarely continues beyond puberty, although 5–10% of children will develop adult seizures.

Febrile convulsions

These are seizures occurring in the context of fever, usually in young children under 5. The majority are 'one-off' events although up to 5% go on to develop epilepsy, generally as a consequence of scarring in the temporal lobe ('hippocampal sclerosis'). They are usually generalised and brief but occasionally longer lasting or focal in nature.

Infantile spasms

These are brief spasms (typically 'shock-like' with flexion of the arms, head and neck and drawing up of the knees) associated with progressive learning difficulties. Aetiology includes perinatal asphyxia, metabolic disorders, encephalitis and cerebral malformations.

Juvenile myoclonic epilepsy

This form of primary generalised epilepsy with typical onset in teenagers is characterised by relatively infrequent generalised seizures, daytime absences and myoclonus. Myoclonus typically occurs first thing from sleep and is frequently not volunteered unless directly asked about.

Epilepsy in adulthood

Primary generalised epilepsy (tonic–clonic seizures/grand mal)

Seizures may be preceded by a prodrome/aura in which the patient reports dizziness, irritability or other non-specific symptoms. This is followed by loss of consciousness and the tonic phase (characterised by generalised muscle spasms), which usually lasts up to 30 s. Cyanosis may occur. The clonic phase, characterised by sharp repetitive muscular jerks in all limbs, follows. Tongue biting, salivation and involuntary micturition may occur. Consciousness remains impaired typically for around 30 min, with drowsiness and confusion lasting several hours.

Temporal lobe epilepsy

Patients typically experience an aura which may include a sense of fear or déjà-vu, hallucinations (visual, olfactory or gustatory) or a rising sensation in the epigastrium. Confusion and anxiety may develop and some patients exhibit automatism (organised stereotyped movements, e.g. chewing, lipsmacking).

Jacksonian (focal) epilepsy

Epileptic activity originates in one part of the motor cortex. Each seizure begins in one body part and may proceed to involve that side of the body and then the whole body. Temporary paresis of the originally affected limb may persist after the attack (Todd's paralysis). Sensory epilepsy is a parallel condition originating in the sensory cortex.

Investigation

The object is to detect treatable underlying brain disease and identify provoking factors.

A full history and clinical examination should identify other causes of loss of consciousness. Biochemical evidence of excess alcohol, hypoglycaemia, hyponatraemia or hypocalcaemia should be sought.

An EEG may help to confirm the diagnosis, but both false positive (in 1% of the normal population) and, more commonly, false negative results occur. EEG diagnosis can be enhanced by prolonged recording or following sleep deprivation.

CT or MRI scanning is performed in all adult patients presenting with a seizure to identify structural lesions. Imaging is of particular value in late onset epilepsy, partial seizures and in patients with generalised epilepsy where the EEG discloses a focal abnormality.

Management

A single fit rarely requires treatment but an underlying cause should be sought. Most neurologists would begin treatment with prophylactic anticonvulsants after a second episode. However, it may be prudent to treat after a first seizure when neuroimaging reveals a structural lesion.

The choice of pharmacological therapy is determined by the type of epilepsy, for example:

- *Partial seizures (with or without secondary generalisation):* carbamazepine, lamotrigine, oxcarbazepine, levetiracetam and sodium valproate are the drugs of choice; second-line agents include clobazam, gabapentin, and topiramate.
- *Generalised tonic–clonic:* carbamazepine, lamotrigine, oxcarbazepine and sodium valproate are first-line agents; clobazam, levetiracetam, and topiramate are useful second-line options.
- *Absence:* ethosuximide, lamotrigine or sodium valproate are the drugs of choice for classical absence seizures.
- *Myoclonic:* sodium valproate, levetiracetam or topiramate are the drugs of choice for most cases.

In addition, age, sex, child-bearing potential, comorbidity and concomitant medication should be taken into account. Sodium valproate is particularly teratogenic and is no longer prescribed to any women of childbearing age. Seizure control with minimal adverse effects can be achieved using a single anticonvulsant in ~75% of patients. The addition of a second drug produces satisfactory control in a further subgroup.

Refractory epilepsy (inadequate control on multiple agents) may reflect:

- poor compliance
- non-epileptic attacks (either alone or in combination with genuine seizures)
- an underlying structural brain lesion
- excess alcohol or illicit drug usage.

Further information is available at https://www.nice.org.uk/guidance/cg137/chapter/appendix-e-pharmacological-treatment.

Status epilepticus

This is defined as recurring or continuous seizures, in which the patient does not regain consciousness between attacks. It is a medical emergency as hypoxia/anoxia can lead to permanent brain damage or even death. Key principles of management include:

- basic life support/resuscitation
- seizure control
- identification and correction of predisposing cause.

The choice of agent used to terminate seizure activity depends on the stage/duration, but may include:

- Intravenous lorazepam (4 mg) (clonazepam and diazepam are alternatives) – dose may be repeated after 10 min if seizures recur/continue.
- Intravenous phenytoin (15 mg/kg, maximum rate of 50 mg/min), fosphenytoin (prodrug of phenytoin), both of which require ECG monitoring, or phenobarbitone (10 mg/kg, maximum rate of 100 mg/min) should be used when there is established status.
- Intravenous thiopentone (bolus followed by infusion), combined with ventilation/neuromuscular blockade, is required when seizures continue beyond 30–60 min. Midazolam and propofol have also been used in this setting. EEG monitoring is required to confirm termination of seizure activity.

If the alcohol history and blood glucose level are not known (or the patient is hypoglycaemic), a bolus of 20% dextrose and intravenous thiamine must be given. Patients should be nursed in a high dependency/intensive care setting. Regular anticonvulsant therapy should be reinstituted as soon as possible in those with known epilepsy, if necessary intravenously or via the nasogastric route.

Surgical treatment of epilepsy

This should be considered in patients with intractable epilepsy if a focus for seizure onset can be identified using MRI and electrophysiology mapping.

Epilepsy and pregnancy

Uncontrolled seizures in pregnancy present a serious risk to both mother and fetus. Anticonvulsant drugs must be continued especially if there is a history of recent seizure activity. In women with no recent (2–3 years) history of seizures, a trial off therapy before pregnancy may be considered.

Women with epilepsy who wish to become pregnant should receive pre-pregnancy counselling about the risk of congenital abnormality and the individual pros and cons of continuing treatment. Wherever possible, the lowest dosage of a single agent should be used. Screening for neural tube defects is especially indicated in women taking sodium valproate (in practice all women taking valproate should be changed to an alternative agent prior to conception – see earlier) or carbamazepine, and folic acid supplementation is essential both pre-conception and throughout the pregnancy.

For mothers taking carbamazepine, phenobarbitone or phenytoin (enzyme-inducing agents), vitamin K should be prescribed before delivery and for the newborn.

NB: Carbamazepine, phenytoin and phenobarbitone all induce hepatic microsomal enzymes and increase metabolism of oestrogens and progestogens, making oral contraception unreliable.

Epilepsy and driving

In the UK, all patients with a history of seizures must report their condition to the Driver and Vehicle Licensing Agency (DVLA). Currently, for an isolated seizure, a 6-month 'off driving period' is stipulated providing the individual has undergone assessment by an appropriate specialist, no relevant abnormality has been identified on investigation, and the person is therefore not considered to be high risk for a further seizure. A 12-month 'off driving period' applies if there is deemed to be the potential for further seizures. Patients with a history of epilepsy must be seizure-free for 1 year before being allowed to drive. More stringent regulations apply to licences for heavy goods or passenger-carrying vehicles (https://www.gov.uk/epilepsy-and-driving). Patients with sleep-related epilepsy may be permitted to drive if they have an established pattern of seizures that have occurred only in relation to sleep.

Epilepsy and employment

There are certain statutory employment restrictions for individuals with epilepsy, including in relation to the emergency and armed services, pilots and train drivers.

Epilepsy and lifestyle

There are no 'absolute rules', but it is sensible to avoid heights/ladders, operating heavy machinery, working underground and activities such as unsupervised swimming until seizure control is established. Fires should be guarded and showers are recommended rather than baths.

Prognosis in epilepsy

The long-term prognosis of epilepsy is good, with most patients attaining a 5-year remission and many stopping treatment in due course. The decision to discontinue anticonvulsant therapy is determined by: type of epilepsy; duration of remission; potential deleterious effects of seizure recurrence (driving and employment) and side effects of treatment.

Stroke

Stroke is characterised by rapidly developing symptoms and/or signs of loss of central nervous system function. It is distinguishable from a transient ischaemic attack (see later) by virtue of symptoms persisting for more than 24 h (in reality, most TIA events are short-lived). Stroke has an annual incidence of 1–2 per 1000 population, is the third most common cause of death in industrialized countries and is a major cause of morbidity in those who survive.

Aetiology and pathophysiology

Approximately 85% of cases are ischaemic (thrombosis or embolism) in origin, 10% are caused by intracerebral haemorrhage and 5% by subarachnoid haemorrhage.

Thrombosis is due to one or more of the following:

- abnormal blood vessel wall, secondary to atherosclerosis
- polycythaemia
- altered blood flow.

Emboli may arise from vascular or cardiac sources, including:

- degenerative vascular disease
- atrial fibrillation
- cardiac valvular disease
- post-myocardial infarction.

Degenerative arterial disease is the most common cause of stroke. Risk factors include family history of premature vascular disease, smoking, hypertension, hyperlipidaemia, diabetes mellitus, excess alcohol ingestion and certain oral contraceptive preparations.

A small number of cases have a non-vascular lesion (tumour, subdural haematoma, migraine, intracranial infection, metabolic disturbance).

In the absence of a collateral blood supply, the brain territory supplied by an occluded artery undergoes infarction. Potentially salvageable surrounding areas of brain that lie within the so-called ischaemic penumbra remain viable for a period of time and may recover function if their blood supply is restored.

Both cytotoxic (accumulation of water in damaged neurones and glial cells) and vasogenic (extracellular fluid accumulation secondary to disruption of the blood–brain barrier) oedema may complicate infarction.

Clinical features

Symptoms and signs are dictated by the vascular territory that is rendered ischaemic. As a general rule, the carotids supply the anterior and middle cerebral arteries (anterior circulation), while the vertebrobasilar system feeds the posterior cerebral arteries which, together with branches supplying the cerebellum and the brainstem, constitute the posterior circulation.

Total anterior circulation infarct

- hemiplegia (corticospinal tract)
- homonymous hemianopia (optic tract/radiation)
- cortical deficits, e.g. dysphasia (dominant hemisphere), visuospatial loss (non-dominant hemisphere)

Partial anterior circulation infarct

- two of the above or cortical deficit alone

Lacunar infarct

- pure motor or sensory stroke or ataxic hemiparesis

Multiple/serial lacunar infarcts

These may produce cumulative neurological deficits including:

- cognitive impairment (multi-infarct dementia)
- gait disturbance/apraxia.

Posterior circulation infarct

- brainstem dysfunction, e.g. vertigo, diplopia, altered conscious level
- homonymous hemianopia

Spinal cord infarct

See later (spinal disorders).

Diagnosis and initial investigation

The introduction and promotion of 'diagnostic aids' such as 'FAST' (Box 15.1) and 'ROSIER' (Fig. 15.1) have facilitated earlier assessment and treatment, including thrombolysis or thrombectomy in selected cases.

Although the diagnosis of stroke is primarily clinical, CT scanning is required to distinguish cerebral infarction from haemorrhage. Early scanning is recommended in the majority of patients, (on CT a low-density area appears within a few hours of a cerebral infarct, whereas a high-density area appears immediately after a bleed; brainstem, cerebellar and small cortical infarcts may not be visible). MRI is more sensitive for detecting ischaemic stroke, but takes longer to perform and requires greater cooperation from the patient. Immediate CT/MRI scanning is especially important if any of the following are present:

- indication for thrombolysis, thrombectomy or early anticoagulation treatment
- on anticoagulant therapy or known bleeding diathesis
- reduced level of consciousness or unexplained progressive/fluctuating symptoms
- papilloedema, neck stiffness or fever
- headache at onset of symptoms.

Investigations to establish the aetiology

- full blood count (± ESR), coagulation (± thrombophilia) screen, urea and electrolytes, glucose/, fasting lipids
- ECG
- chest X-ray
- echocardiography
- duplex imaging of the extracranial carotid and vertebral arteries

Less common causes of stroke should be considered, particularly in young patients and those without risk factors (serum protein electrophoresis, autoantibody screen, protein C, S and antithrombin III levels, sickle test, blood cultures, urine for homocystinuria). An autoimmune profile, serum inflammatory markers and angiography may be helpful in detecting cerebral vasculitis.

Early management

Wherever possible, patients should be admitted as soon as possible to a specialist stroke unit, as research demonstrates significant improvements in outcome when patients are managed by a multidisciplinary specialist team. Thrombolysis with recombinant tissue plasminogen activator (alteplase) should be

---

 Box 15.1 The Face, Arm and Speech Test ('FAST')

Facial weakness	Ask the person to smile or show their teeth.
	Look for an unequal smile or grimace – has their mouth or eye drooped or is there obvious facial asymmetry?
Arm weakness	Lift the patient's arms together and ask them to hold the position for 5 s after you have let go.
	Does one arm drift down or fall rapidly?
Speech problems	Check for difficulties with speech.
	Can the person speak clearly and understand what you say? Is there any slurring of speech or difficulty finding words/naming common objects?

***T**ime to call emergency services*

Source: Adapted from Harbison et al., Stroke 2003; 34: 71–76. Reproduced with permission of Wolters Kluwer Health.

Assessment   Date [ ][ ][ ][ ][ ][ ]   Time [ ][ ][ ][ ]

Symptom onset   Date [ ][ ][ ][ ][ ][ ]   Time [ ][ ][ ][ ]

GCS   E=[ ]   M=[ ]   V=[ ]   **BP** [ ][ ]   ***BM** [ ]

*If BM <3.5 mmol/L treat urgently and reassess once blood glucose normal

Has there been loss of consciousness or syncope?   Y (−1) ☐   N (0) ☐

Has there been seizure activity?   Y (−1) ☐   N (0) ☐

Is there a <u>NEW ACUTE</u> onset (or on awakening from sleep)

I.   Asymmetric facial weakness   Y (+1) ☐   N (0) ☐

II.   Asymmetric arm weakness   Y (+1) ☐   N (0) ☐

III.   Asymmetric leg weakness   Y (+1) ☐   N (0) ☐

IV.   Speech disturbance   Y (+1) ☐   N (0) ☐

V.   Visual field defect   Y (+1) ☐   N (0) ☐

*Total Score_____(−2 to +5)

Provisional diagnosis

☐ Stroke   ☐ Non-stroke (specify) _____

*Stroke is unlikely but not completely excluded if total scores are ≤0.

Figure 15.1 The Recognition of Stroke In the Emergency Room scale ('*ROSIER*'). BM, blood glucose; BP, blood pressure (mmHg); GCS, Glasgow Coma Scale; E, eye; M, motor; V, verbal component. Source: Nor et al., *Lancet Neurology* 2005; **4**: 727–734. Reproduced with permission of Elsevier.

considered and commenced within 3 h of symptom onset for patients whose CT or MRI scan excludes cerebral haemorrhage. The efficacy of thrombolysis is highly time-dependent and the decision to thrombolyse should be taken by a specialist stroke physician/neurologist.

Thrombectomy involves removing the clot via an intra-arterial route in specialist neuroscience centres.

For patients with haemorrhagic stroke, any predisposing coagulopathy (including warfarin therapy) should be immediately corrected. Neurosurgical intervention is only rarely indicated in acute stroke, e.g. for symptomatic hydrocephalus or massive cerebral oedema; generally seen only after large MCA infarcts).

Once admitted to the stroke unit, further assessment/management includes:

- administration of aspirin 300 mg unless contraindicated; this is typically continued for 2 weeks after symptom onset, following which long-term antithrombotic therapy is instituted (see later)
- swallowing screen and institution of alternative feeding strategies if required
- malnutrition screen and nutritional support as required
- early mobilisation wherever possible
- specialist physiotherapy, occupational therapy and speech therapy input.

Prevention and treatment of complications

- Antithrombotic therapy: long-term aspirin (or clopidogrel) is indicated in most patients for secondary prevention. Anticoagulants should be considered for those with atrial fibrillation or other cardiac sources of emboli.
- Hypertension: in the longer term, good blood pressure control is crucial to reducing the risk of further cerebrovascular events. Unless there is evidence of hypertensive encephalopathy, hypertensive cardiac or renal failure, aortic dissection or pre-eclampsia/eclampsia, most physicians do not treat high blood pressure in the early stages following stroke, in recognition that lowering cerebral blood flow may exacerbate ischaemia.
- Chest infection: aspiration is common and treatment with antibiotics and physiotherapy should be started early.
- Deep venous thrombosis and pulmonary embolism: use graduated compression stockings and consider low molecular weight heparin prophylaxis.
- Pressure sores: avoidance requires careful positioning, regular turning and use of appropriate pressure-relieving mattresses.
- Urinary infections/septicaemia: especially in those requiring catheterization.
- Seizures: may require treatment with anticonvulsants.
- Hyponatraemia: may complicate intravenous fluid use or reflect syndrome of inappropriate antidiuretic hormone secretion.

Venous infarction

Thrombosis of the intracranial venous sinuses produces clinical syndromes which are generally distinct from those of arterial infarction. Superior sagittal sinus thrombosis may present with headache, papilloedema and features suggestive of raised intracranial pressure, together with seizures and bilateral neurological deficits. It may arise during extreme dehydration, in the puerperium and in those with a thrombotic tendency and those taking oral contraceptive preparations. It can also occur secondary to meningitis or middle ear infections.

Treatment is aimed at the underlying cause, with antibiotics for any predisposing infection. All patients with a cerebral venous thrombosis should be anticoagulated.

Transient ischaemic attack (TIA)

TIA describes sudden onset of focal neurological dysfunction of presumed vascular origin that, by definition, resolves within 24 h (usually much sooner). It is a predictor of progression to completed stroke. Non-focal features such as syncope, confusion or dizziness are not part of a TIA.

Aetiology

As for stroke, the most common cause is thromboembolism from atherosclerotic neck vessels. A cardiac source of emboli (e.g. atrial fibrillation) may be present or, rarely, cerebral vasculitis, hypercoagulable states or arterial dissection.

Non-vascular conditions that may mimic TIA include seizures, migraine, intracranial tumour and vascular malformation, subdural haematoma, multiple sclerosis, vestibular dysfunction, hypoglycaemia and psychogenic disorders.

Clinical features

Symptoms and signs again depend on the arterial territory involved:

- Carotid artery TIAs affect the cortex inducing ipsilateral monocular visual loss (amaurosis fugax) or contralateral weakness or sensory disturbance. Involvement of the dominant hemisphere may produce dysphasia.
- Vertebrobasilar TIAs affect the brainstem causing dizziness, ataxia, vertigo, dysarthria, diplopia with unilateral or bilateral weakness and numbness in the limbs. Bilateral sudden visual loss may occur.

At presentation, neurological signs have often fully resolved. Cholesterol emboli may be seen on fundoscopy in patients with amaurosis fugax. A detailed history, risk factor assessment and a full physical examination should be performed, checking for hypertension, cutaneous stigmata of hyperlipidaemia, atrial fibrillation, cardiac murmurs and carotid bruits.

Subclavian steal syndrome

Rarely, stenosis in the proximal subclavian artery is associated with retrograde flow down the vertebral artery when the arm is exercised. There may be an audible bruit in the root of the neck and reduced blood pressure in the affected arm.

Diagnosis and investigation

Recent recommendations, such as the UK National Clinical Guideline for Stroke, have emphasised the importance of early clinical assessment in patients suspected of suffering a TIA. As outlined earlier for stroke, effective early intervention in TIA is dependent on patients seeking medical help as soon as they develop symptoms/signs (https://www.nice.org.uk/guidance/cg68).

Assessment of those at highest risk of stroke following a TIA

Epidemiological studies have shown that the highest risk of progression to stroke is seen in older people (>60 years) and those with hypertension, diabetes mellitus, longer duration of symptoms, speech problems or motor weakness.

A scoring system such as 'ABCD²' may identify patients who need immediate specialist assessment (within 24 h) and those requiring assessment within 1 week (Table 15.3). A score of ≥4 is deemed 'high risk' (>4% risk of stroke over the next week) and requires immediate referral to a specialist unit. For patients with a score of <4, aspirin should be commenced immediately and the patient referred for specialist review as soon as possible.

NB: Scoring systems such as 'ABCD²' may fail to identify some 'high-risk' patients (e.g. those suffering recurrent events ['*crescendo TIA*' = ≥2 TIAs in a week] or receiving treatment with anticoagulation) who merit urgent evaluation. In addition, their relevance to patients who present late is unclear.

Management

Acute management

- Exclude hypoglycaemia: this is an important mimic of stroke/TIA – correct the blood glucose and reassess the patient.
- Confirm no ongoing/residual neurological deficit.
- Check full blood count (± ESR/CRP), electrolytes/renal function, glucose/HbA$_{1c}$, fasting lipids, ECG.
- Commence aspirin (300 mg/day, unless contraindicated).
- Establish 'high' or 'low risk' – i.e. do they need specialist review within 24 h or within 1 week?

Specialist management

- Confirmation of the diagnosis.
- Assessment/treatment of risk factors (e.g. hypertension, diabetes mellitus, dyslipidaemia, smoking, atrial fibrillation) and institution of secondary prevention measures/advice.
- Early pharmacological therapy.
- Timely referral for brain and carotid imaging.

Brain imaging is recommended when the diagnosis remains unclear, when the vascular territory affected is uncertain and the patient is a potential candidate for carotid endarterectomy, and to exclude intracerebral haemorrhage.

Table 15.3 The '*ABCD²*' score for assessment of risk of stroke following transient ischaemic attack (TIA)		
Age	≥60 years	=1 point
Blood pressure elevation	Systolic ≥140 mmHg or diastolic ≥90 mmHg	=1 point
Clinical features	Unilateral weakness	=2 points
	Speech impairment without weakness	=1 point
Duration of TIA	≥60 min	=2 points
	10–59 min	=1 point
Diabetes		=1 point

Source: Adapted from Johnston et al., Lancet 2007; 369: 283–292. Reproduced with permission of Elsevier.

Diffusion-weighted MRI is the imaging modality of choice for patients with suspected TIA. It should be performed within 24 h of onset of symptoms if the patient is deemed at 'high risk' ('ABCD^2' score $\geq$4) of subsequent stroke, and within 1 week in other cases. Patients with anterior circulation events who are deemed potential candidates for carotid endarterectomy should be referred for carotid imaging within 1 week.

Medical treatment

Aspirin reduces the risk of stroke, myocardial infarction and vascular death in patients with a history of TIA. Clopidogrel is an alternative in those who are aspirin intolerant. Anticoagulation is indicated for cardioembolic events, e.g. secondary to atrial fibrillation. However, in the absence of risk factors for cardioembolism, there are no conclusive data to support the routine use of oral anticoagulants. Antihypertensive and lipid-lowering therapies should also be instituted/optimized.

Surgical treatment

The decision to perform carotid endarterectomy depends on several factors, including the severity of the stenosis and the extent of comorbidities. In centres with low surgical morbidity/mortality, endarterectomy is of proven benefit in patients with a severe stenosis (70–99% according to the European Carotid Surgery Trial [ECST] criteria; 50–99% according to the North American Symptomatic Carotid Endarterectomy Trial [NASCET]) and should be undertaken within 2 weeks of symptom onset.

Extracerebral haemorrhage

Extradural haematoma

This results from traumatic damage to the middle meningeal artery as it passes upwards on the inside of the temporal bone. Momentary loss of consciousness is followed by apparent recovery, but if left untreated progressive neurological dysfunction with deteriorating consciousness and even death ensues. A high index of clinical suspicion and early imaging is required to facilitate early neurosurgical intervention.

Subdural haematoma

This occurs most frequently in the elderly, especially in those with a coagulopathy. It often follows trauma, which may seem relatively minor at the time. A small venous haemorrhage occurs and the clot slowly enlarges in size, absorbing fluid osmotically from the CSF.

Symptoms may develop over a period of weeks to months. Headache, confusion and progressive loss of conscious level occur with fluctuation of consciousness. Focal neurology and/or signs of raised intracranial pressure may be evident. If undiagnosed, patients with chronic subdural haematoma may present with features of dementia. Following radiological confirmation, evacuation of the haematoma may permit full recovery, irrespective of the patient's age. Subdural haematomas are often bilateral.

Subarachnoid haemorrhage

Subarachnoid haemorrhage presents with the abrupt onset of severe generalised headache, +/-loss of consciousness, vomiting or seizures. Meningeal irritation causes neck stiffness and photophobia. Neurological examination does not usually reveal focal signs.

It may result from:

- rupture of an aneurysm of the circle of Willis
- arteriovenous malformation
- trauma
- mycotic aneurysm
- pituitary apoplexy.

NB: In the case of an aneurysm, some patients give a history of previous similar but milder episodes, possibly caused by smaller leaks.

Unenhanced CT scanning shows subarachnoid blood in over 90% of cases and reveals haematoma, the site of a leaking aneurysm and associated hydrocephalus. If intracranial blood is not seen, but there is a reasonable clinical index of suspicion, then lumbar puncture should be performed to examine CSF for uniform bloodstaining (i.e. frank blood that fails to clear in subsequent bottles) and xanthochromia (the CSF supernatant becomes straw-coloured due to the presence of haemoglobin breakdown products). Lumbar puncture can be safely performed once imaging has excluded a mass lesion, providing there is no bleeding diathesis. It should be done from 12 hours post onset of headache and will be positive up to about a week.

Management

- resuscitation
- analgesia/bedrest
- nimodipine (to reduce vasospasm)

- cerebral angiography followed by surgical or neuroradiological intervention (e.g. clipping or coiling of the aneurysm)

The timing of investigation and surgery in patients with severe subarachnoid haemorrhage and impaired consciousness remains a matter of debate.

Aneurysmal subarachnoid haemorrhage carries a very high mortality (up to 30–40% of patients within the first few days). There is a significant risk of rebleeding, with the second bleed often more severe than the first. Hydrocephalus occurs in 20% of patients and may require ventricular drainage. Delayed ischaemic brain damage caused by cerebral vasospasm presents with deteriorating conscious level or focal neurological signs.

Dementia

Dementia is a major public health problem, with substantial social and financial implications in ageing populations. It is characterised by significant impairment in two or more domains of cognition, one of which must be memory (the others being abstract thought, language, praxis, personality, social behaviour or visuospatial skills). Typically, there is progressive, global impairment of intellectual function in the context of normal consciousness.

Dementia must be distinguished from *delerium* (i.e. an acute confusional state in which patients may exhibit lack of clarity of thought [and hence speech], memory impairment [especially with respect to new material/recent events], mood change, altered sleep [with disturbed sleep–wake cycle] and possible hallucinations), and psychiatric disorders (e.g. depression or schizophrenia) which may manifest some overlapping features ('*pseudodementia*').

Causes (Table 15.4)

Many diseases including infective, inflammatory, metabolic/endocrine and neurodegenerative disorders may predispose to cognitive impairment which may be reversible – hence the need to ascertain the underlying cause wherever possible.

Clinical assessment

The history should include both the patient's account of their problems and a 'collateral' account, generally from a relative or friend. A full physical examination and cognitive assessment should be performed. There are several cognitive assessments that can be done quickly. The TYM test is one example http://www.tymtest.com.

Table 15.4 Causes of dementia

Type	Examples
Inherited	Familial Alzheimer's disease Huntington's disease Some forms of spinocerebellar ataxia Wilson's disease
Infective	AIDS-related Herpes simplex encephalitis Progressive multifocal leucoencephalopathy Subacute sclerosing panencephalitis Syphilis
Inflammatory	Multiple sclerosis Sarcoidosis Systemic lupus erythematosus Vasculitis
Metabolic/ endocrine	Myxoedema Vitamin B_{12} deficiency Chronic renal (uraemic) or hepatic (encephalopathic) failure
Drug/toxin-induced	Alcohol Carbon monoxide, lead
Vascular Trauma	Multi-infarct Chronic subdural haematoma Severe/recurrent head injury (e.g. 'punch-drunk' syndrome)
Neoplasia	Frontal lobe tumours Multiple metastases Paraneoplastic Posterior fossa tumour with associated hydrocephalus
Degenerative	Alzheimer's disease Pick's disease Prion diseases Parkinson's disease and other akinetic-rigid syndromes
Other	Normal-pressure hydrocephalus, pseudodementia in depressive illness

AIDS, acquired immune deficiency syndrome.

Investigation

This is aimed at establishing the diagnosis and excluding treatable causes. The following should be considered:

- full blood count and ESR
- creatinine and electrolytes, glucose, liver, bone and thyroid function tests, CRP, HIV TPHA (*Treponema pallidum* hemagglutination assay for syphilis) and vitamin B_{12}

- chest X-ray (for bronchial carcinoma)
- CT/MRI scan of the head.

In other patients additional investigations may be required, including:

- functional imaging (e.g. with PET) may be useful in cases where diagnostic uncertainty persists
- EEG (useful if Creutzfeld–Jacob disease [CJD] or epileptic amnesia suspected)
- CSF analysis
- genetic testing (in patients with a relevant family history or appropriate clinical phenotype)
- brain biopsy (very rarely indicated).

Alzheimer's disease

Alzheimer's disease (AD) is the most common form of dementia in all age groups, with increasing prevalence with advancing age.

Aetiopathogenesis

AD is a neurodegenerative disorder. The so-called amyloid hypothesis proposes that altered metabolism of the transmembrane amyloid precursor protein (APP; genetic locus 21q21–22) results in the production of amyloid β-peptides (Aβ). Studies of patients with Down syndrome (trisomy 21) also support a pathogenic role for amyloid, where a 'gene dosage effect' has been implicated in early onset AD in this setting. Understanding of the pathogenesis of AD has been aided by the study of rare familial (autosomal dominant) cases, arising as a consequence of mutations in three different genes: APP, presenilin-1 and presenilin-2, all of which alter Aβ production. However, even when taken together, mutations in these genes account for <1% of all AD. Susceptibility to AD is also conferred by genetic variation at other loci, the most important to date being the ε4 allele of the lipid transport protein apolipoprotein E (ApoE). Genome-wide association studies have identified other potential susceptibility genes, several of which may influence Aβ metabolism.

Two characteristic pathological features are found in the brain of patients with Alzheimer's disease:

1. *Senile plaques,* consisting of extracellular aggregates of Aβ peptides (= oligomers).
2. *Neurofibrillary tangles,* which are dense bundles of abnormal fibres (paired helical filaments) in the cytoplasm of neurones, containing an altered form of the microtubule-associated protein, tau (τ).

NB: Neither senile plaques nor neurofibrillary tangles are specific to AD; they can occur in other chronic cerebral conditions and are found in elderly patients without dementia.

'Toxic' Aβ oligomers may exert effects on structural proteins of the neuronal cytoskeleton, while altered phosphorylation and aggregation of τ lead to reduced axonal transport, synaptic loss and ultimately neuronal death in specific areas of the cerebral cortex crucial to cognition. Cholinergic neurones appear to be particularly affected.

Clinical features

Loss of memory for recent events is the characteristic presenting feature. Patients have great difficulty learning and retaining new information. Although insight may be preserved in the early stages, some patients appear relatively unaware of their limitations. Later more marked memory disturbance results in disorientation with altered behaviour/personality. Ultimately there is global loss of cognitive function with complete dependence and death usually within 5–10 years.

Diagnostic criteria

Recent revisions to clinical diagnostic criteria incorporating new knowledge from neuroimaging findings, CSF biomarkers and genetic screening allow for earlier and more accurate diagnosis in more than three-quarters of all cases (Box 15.2). The revised *Diagnostic and Statistical Manual of Mental Disorders* (DSM) criteria for AD are also used (Box 15.3).

Management

The use of simple memory aids, avoidance of sedative drugs/alcohol and maintenance of general health can all contribute to preservation of function and independence in the early stages of the disease.

Cholinesterase inhibitors, e.g. donepezil, rivastigmine and galantamine, and memantine (an *N*-methyl-D-aspartate [NMDA] receptor antagonist) are the mainstays of pharmacological intervention. These agents are symptomatic, their effects are not long-lasting and they generally do not slow the progression to more advanced forms of the disease.

The development of potential disease-modifying agents is a focus of research in AD, with candidates

Box 15.2 Diagnostic criteria for Alzheimer's disease (AD)

Definite AD
- Clinical features + neuropathological confirmation *or*
- Clinical features + identification of a causative gene mutation

Probable AD

Core criterion:
- Early significant episodic memory impairment, including:
  - Gradual/progressive change in memory function over at least a 6-month period
  - Evidence of significantly impaired episodic memory on formal testing
  - Episodic memory impairment, isolated or associated with other cognitive changes at onset of AD

Together with one or more of the following 'supportive' features:
- Medial temporal lobe atrophy on MRI
- Abnormal CSF biomarker (e.g. ↑ total τ or phospho-τ; ↓ Aβ42)
- Specific pattern on functional neuroimaging with PET
- Proven autosomal dominant AD familial mutation

Aβ, amyloid β-peptides; CSF, cerebrospinal fluid; MRI, magnetic resonance imaging; PET, positron emission tomography; τ, tau protein. Source: Dubois et al., Lancet Neurology 2007; 6: 734–746.

 Box 15.3 DSM-5 criteria for major neurocognitive disorder due to Alzheimer disease

A. Evidence of significant cognitive decline from a previous level of performance in one or more cognitive domains*:
- Learning and memory.
- Language.
- Executive function.
- Complex attention.
- Perceptual-motor.
- Social cognition.
B. The cognitive deficits interfere with independence in everyday activities. At a minimum, assistance should be required with complex instrumental activities of daily living, such as paying bills or managing medications.
C. The cognitive deficits do not occur exclusively in the context of a delirium.
D. The cognitive deficits are not better explained by another mental disorder (eg, major depressive disorder, schizophrenia).
E. There is insidious onset and gradual progression of impairment in at least two cognitive domains.
F. Either of the following:
- Evidence of a causative Alzheimer disease genetic mutation from family history or genetic testing.
- All three of the following are present:
  i. Clear evidence of decline in memory and learning and at least one other cognitive domain.
  ii. Steadily progressive, gradual decline in cognition, without extended plateaus.
  iii. No evidence of mixed etiology (ie, absence of other neurodegenerative disorders or cerebrovascular disease, or another neurological, mental, or systemic disease or condition likely contributing to cognitive decline).

DSM, Diagnostic and Statistical Manual. * Evidence of decline is based on: Concern of the individual, a knowledgeable informant, or the clinician that there has been a significant decline in cognitive function; and a substantial impairment in cognitive performance, preferably documented by standardized neuropsychological testing or, in its absence, another quantified clinical assessment.
Source: American Psychiatric Association (2013) *Diagnostic and Statistical Manual of Mental Disorders, Fifth Edition* (DSM-5). Arlington, VA: American Psychiatric Association.

including immunotherapy (to target Aβ), *secretase inhibitors* (which prevent cleavage of APP to Aβ) and inhibitors of τ protein aggregation.

Adjunctive therapies, including behavioural approaches, and use of antidepressants, antipsychotics and anti-epilepsy drugs may be required. Later in the illness there is increasing dependence and requirement for fulltime care.

Multi-infarct dementia

Multi-infarct dementia is often of abrupt onset with a stepwise progression over time and focal neurological features may be evident. Predisposing factors (e.g. smoking, hypertension, hyperlipidaemia, diabetes mellitus) and more widespread vascular disease are often present. Postmortem studies have shown that pathological changes associated with vascular lesions and AD often coexist, in keeping with current beliefs that vascular dementia and AD are part of a continuum.

Fronto-temporal dementia (Pick's disease)

There is focal cortical atrophy with astrocytosis and intraneural inclusion bodies (Pick bodies) in surviving pyramidal cells. Patients present with frontal type dementia, i.e. altered personality, disinhibition (including violence), apathy, and poverty of speech with relatively preserved spatial skills and memory, which distinguish the disease clinically from AD. Pick's disease is also more common in a younger age group. Treatment is limited to supportive measures and symptomatic control of aberrant behaviours.

Dementia with Lewy Bodies (DLB)

Characterised by widespread distribution of Lewy bodies in the CNS, DLB is increasingly recognised as a relatively common cause of dementia. Clinical features include:

- fluctuating cognition (often with nocturnal confusion)
- visual hallucinations
- Parkinsonism
- worsening of features with neuroleptic and anti-parkinsonian drugs.

Treatment with cholinesterase inhibitors is often beneficial.

Parkinson's disease with dementia (PDD)

In PDD dementia arises several years after onset of the movement disorder. The clinical and neuropsychological phenotype of PDD overlaps with that of DLB. When the movement disorder and dementia present within a year of each other, the patient is deemed to have DLB.

Prion diseases including Creutzfeldt–Jakob disease (CJD)

This rare group of neurodegenerative disorders has attracted considerable media attention following linkage of a variant of CJD to human consumption of prion-contaminated beef (bovine spongiform encephalopathy, BSE).

Classical CJD presents in late middle age with dementia accompanied by cortical visual problems, myoclonus and muscle wasting/fasciculation, which progresses to death within months. The EEG may show a characteristic abnormality and spongiform changes are found in the brain at postmortem. CJD, together with the other spongiform encephalopathies scrapie and BSE, is both inheritable and transmissible, the phenomenon being due to prion proteins (PrP) that are highly resistant to inactivation by heat or chemicals. An isoform of PrP exists in normal cells and mutations in its gene may give rise to inheritable autosomal dominant forms of disease. 'Infectious' transmission between humans (e.g. accidental inoculation following corneal grafts or after the use of human pituitary extract-derived growth hormone) or species (e.g. variant CJD and BSE) may occur, although how the abnormal form of PrP leads to disease remains unclear. There appears to be a long latency between exposure to infected material and clinical presentation, meaning that the true extent of the BSE-related CJD 'outbreak' may still remain to be seen.

Variant CJD occurs in younger patients, and its onset may be heralded by the development of psychiatric features, ataxia and sensory disturbance before the appearance of dementia. MRI is characteristically abnormal in variant CJD: the pulvinar nucleus of the thalamus is often hyperintense (the 'pulvinar sign'). Diagnosis remains, however, largely clinical, and treatment is supportive.

Huntington's disease

Progressive dementia and involuntary chorea typically develop in middle age. Inheritance is autosomal dominant, although the disease may be late and variable in its presentation. Death usually occurs 10–15 years after the onset of symptoms.

The Huntington's gene (chromosome 4p16) contains an expanded CAG trinucleotide repeat which tends to increase as the gene passes from parent to offspring, providing an explanation for 'anticipation', the phenomenon by which the disease gets progressively more severe through successive generations.

Management

Tetrabenazine may help the chorea by depleting nerve endings of dopamine, but extrapyramidal dysfunction and depression are common side effects. Presymptomatic genetic screening of unaffected family members must be approached with great care because of the implications of a positive test for the patient and family whilst no disease modifying therapy is available. From a research perspective, fetal cell transplantation is attracting interest through direct targeting of striatal neuronal loss.

Alcohol-related dementia

This is distinct from Wernicke–Korsakoff syndrome (due to thiamine deficiency) and likely reflects synaptic and neuronal loss due to direct toxic effects of alcohol.

HIV-associated dementia

Although there has been a decline in the prevalence of frank HIV-associated dementia with the advent of highly active antiretroviral therapy (HAART), the prevalence of HIV-associated neurocognitive disorders is increasing with improved life expectancy.

Normal-pressure hydrocephalus

This condition presents with dementia, gait apraxia and urinary incontinence. Gross ventricular enlargement without cortical atrophy is evident on CT/MRI scanning. Isolated CSF pressure measurements are typically normal, but continuous monitoring may reveal intermittent periods of raised pressure. Some patients respond to ventriculoperitoneal shunting.

Multiple sclerosis

Multiple sclerosis (MS) is a demyelinating disease characterised by episodes of neurological deficit appearing irregularly throughout the CNS both in anatomical site and time. The UK prevalence is estimated at 1 : 1000 with a slight preponderance in women (male to female ratio ~1 : 1.5). First episodes usually occur in young adulthood, with a peak at around 30 years.

Aetiology

The aetiology of MS remains unknown. Currently, the favoured hypothesis is that an environmental trigger (e.g. a viral infection) precipitates the condition in a genetically susceptible individual.

The presence of chronic inflammatory cells in active plaques and linkage of the disease to certain major histocompatibility complex (MHC) genotypes suggests an immune basis for the disorder. MHC linkage, together with the observation that MS is more common in monozygotic than dizygotic twins, suggests a genetic component.

Pathophysiology

Patches of demyelination occur in discrete areas (plaques) in the white matter of the brain and spinal cord (with relative axonal sparing), especially in:

- optic nerves
- brainstem
- cerebellar peduncles
- dorsal and pyramidal (lateral) tracts.

Demyelination leads to a reduction in conduction velocity, with initial distortion and subsequent loss of impulse conduction. Oedema around acute lesions contributes to the neurological deficit. Function typically improves as oedema resolves. Later, scarring (gliosis) gives rise to the characteristic white plaque.

Clinical presentation

Symptoms include visual disturbance, clumsiness, weakness, numbness, tremor, cognitive impairment, bowel or bladder disturbance and sexual dysfunction reflecting the distribution of plaques.

- *Visual impairment:* optic (retrobulbar) neuritis is a common presenting feature. Symptoms include pain around one eye (exacerbated by movement), blurred vision and loss of colour vision. On examination, visual acuity/colour vision are reduced with a relative afferent pupillary defect, there may be a field defect (typically central scotoma) and the optic disc is pink and swollen. A single episode of optic neuritis does not necessarily herald the onset of MS and in isolation should not be used to make the diagnosis.
- *Diplopia with internuclear ophthalmoplegia.*

- *Upper motor neurone deficit*: paraparesis, hemiparesis or monoparesis.
- *Sensory deficit:* paraesthesia and proprioceptive loss in a limb or half of the body. Lesions in the posterior columns of the cervical cord may induce tingling sensations shooting down the arms or legs on neck flexion (L'Hermitte phenomenon).
- *Cerebellar signs:* intention tremor, nystagmus, vertigo and dysarthria.
- *Bladder dysfunction:* urgency and frequency, followed by incontinence.
- *Bowel disturbance:* constipation, urgency of defecation.
- *Erectile dysfunction and ejaculatory failure* are common.
- *Cognitive impairment:* IQ and language skills are preserved until late in the disease. Memory, learning and the ability to deal with abstract concepts may deteriorate in chronic forms.

Symptoms are commonly made worse by exertion and heat (Uhthoff's phenomenon).

Clinical features

Clinical features commonly evolve over days or weeks, reach a plateau and gradually resolve (partially or completely) over weeks or months. Recurrences are unpredictable and may affect the same or different parts of the CNS. There are no clearly identified precipitating factors, although relapses may be seen in the context of intercurrent illness and the postpartum period.

Several patterns of disease are recognised:

- Relapsing–remitting (~80% of cases): initial episodes may resolve completely or nearly so. Subsequent episodes usually result in some residual disability, with patients eventually progressing to the secondary progressive form.
- Secondary progressive: steady progression without remission.
- Primary progressive: no clear-cut relapses or remissions; more common in those presenting in middle age with a spastic paraparesis.

A rare fourth subtype (progressive–relapsing) was also previously recognised, but affected individuals would now be considered to have a form of primary progressive disease.

Diagnosis/investigation

Clinically the diagnosis is made on the basis of at least two characteristic episodes of neurological dysfunction, separated in time and space, with typical radiological findings on MRI (plaques of demyelination appear as bright lesions; clinically silent lesions are also frequently revealed), although these features are not specific to MS and false-negative scans may occur. Other investigations: visual evoked potentials (VEP) (demyelination causes an abnormality [usually delay] in occipital EEG tracings in response to a stimulus presented to the eyes – abnormalities are present in 95% of patients with MS, but are not specific; sensory and auditory evoked potentials may also show delay); and lumbar puncture, which typically reveals a lymphocytosis and raised CSF protein (up to 1 g/l) in the presence of active disease; CSF immunoelectrophoresis shows an increased proportion of immunoglobulin G (IgG) and oligoclonal bands.

Differential diagnosis

For relapsing–remitting disease:

- transient ischaemic attack
- systemic lupus erythematosus
- sarcoidosis.

For primary progressive disease:

- other causes of a spastic paraparesis
- motor neurone disease
- spinal/cerebellar degenerative disorders.

Management

Physiotherapy, rehabilitation, medical therapy, surgery and psychological support all have a role. Treatment is aimed at:

- management of an acute relapse
- modifying the course of the disease
- symptom control.

Acute relapse

High-dose corticosteroids (e.g. methylprednisolone orally or intravenously) may improve the speed of recovery during acute exacerbations. High-dose corticosteroids do not alter the final recovery, just the rate of recovery.

Disease-modifying agents

- *Interferon beta:* two forms are available – interferon β-1a (identical to its natural counterpart) and interferon β-1b (harbouring a single amino acid substitution); primarily for use in relapsing–remitting MS, but not all patients respond. The results of clinical trials have shown varying efficacy but, in general, treatment is associated with an approximately one-third reduction in relapse frequency and a small slowing of the rate of progression. Its role in secondary progressive disease remains unclear.

- *Glatiramer:* a mixture of random polymers of four amino acids, which is antigenically similar to myelin basic protein; may compete with myelin antigens for presentation to T-cells and induce expression of T-helper suppressor cells; reduces relapses and MRI abnormalities in patients with relapsing–remitting disease.
- Several other biological agents have also shown significant efficacy in MS.
  - *Alemtuzumab:* humanised monoclonal antibody targeting CD52 on the surface of mature lymphocytes (causing depletion of T-cells, B-cells, natural killer cells and monocytes), and used in relapsing–remitting disease; associated with a small increased risk of potentially serious infections and autoimmune disorders (e.g. immune thrombocytopaenia)
  - *Daclizumab:* humanised monoclonal antibody with specific binding to the alpha chain component of the high-affinity interleukin 2 receptor; effective for reducing relapse rates in relapsing–remitting MS
  - *Ocrelizumab:* recombinant human anti-CD20, which causes B-cell depletion; reduces relapses and may slow disability progression; contraindicated in those with active hepatitis B infection
  - *Natalizumab:* a monoclonal antibody that inhibits leucocyte migration into the CNS, is an option for the treatment of adults with highly active relapsing–remitting MS that has not responded to other disease-modifying agents. However, its more widespread use is limited due to an increased risk of opportunistic infections and the potentially fatal side effect of progressive multifocal leucoencephalopathy.
- Several oral therapies suitable for use in relapsing–remitting disease also exist and include: *dimethyl fumarate* (neuroprotective effects); *teriflunomide* (active metabolite of *leflunomide* (inhibits the interaction of T-cells with antigen-presenting cells) and *fingolimod* (sphingosine analogue, which alters lymphocyte migration, leading to their sequestration in lymph nodes).
- Other disease-modifying agents (e.g. *Mitoxantrone*) are generally reserved for those with rapidly advancing disease who have failed other therapies.

Symptom control in chronic disease

- Weakness: physiotherapy and rehabilitation are important.
- Spasticity/flexor spasms: may respond to stretching exercises, alone or in combination with antispasmodic agents such as benzodiazepines gabapentin or baclofen. Dantrolene acts directly on skeletal muscle to reduce spasm. Botulinum toxin injections may be tried. Intractable spasticity may require tendonotomy or neurectomy.
- Bladder dysfunction: antimuscarinic agents (e.g. oxybutynin, tolterodine) increase bladder capacity by diminishing unstable detrusor contractions and a-adrenoceptor blockers may be of benefit. Intermittent self-catheterisation enables some patients to remain free from a permanent indwelling catheter.
- Sexual dysfunction: oral phosphodiesterase type 5 inhibitors (e.g. sildenafil) or intracavernosal injection of papaverine may be of benefit for erectile dysfunction.
- Psychological support: patients may remain euphoric but often there is marked depression.

Prognosis

Traditionally, the average life expectancy from onset of symptoms has been 20–30 years. Overall, 80% of patients experience steadily progressive disability, 15% follow a relatively benign course and 5% die within 5 years. There may be a long latent period (15–30 years) after an episode of optic neuritis before further symptoms occur. Patients whose disease onset is sensory tend to have a better prognosis. Poor prognostic factors are older age at onset, early cerebellar involvement and cognitive problems. However, with the advent of many more disease-modifying therapies, improvements in prognosis might be anticipated for some subgroups.

Motor neurone disease

Motor neurone disease (MND) is an adult-onset neurodegenerative disorder characterised by progressive degeneration of:

- anterior horn cells in the spinal cord
- cells of the lower cranial motor nuclei
- neurones of the motor cortex with secondary degeneration of the pyramidal tracts.

MND causes progressive weakness of limb, bulbar and respiratory muscles, with death typically ensuing in 3–5 years, commonly due to respiratory failure.

It usually presents between the ages of 50 and 70 years, more frequently in men than women (1.5 : 1). The UK incidence is 1–3 per 100 000, with a prevalence of 5 per 100 000 of the population; 90–95% of MND occurs sporadically. Most familial MND is autosomal dominant and several loci have now been identified, including: repeat expansions of the *C9ORF72* gene (9p21), which are also linked with fronto-temporal dementia, and account for ~24–47% of familial amyotrophic lateral sclerosis (see later); mutations in the antioxidant enzyme copper-zinc superoxide dismutase (*SOD1*) gene in ~12–20% of cases; mutations in genes encoding RNA/DNA binding proteins (*TARDBP* and *FUS* genes), accounting for a further 10% of inherited cases.

Two main mechanisms are thought to contribute to motor neurone degeneration:

- excitotoxicity – overstimulation of glutamate receptors with consequent cellular calcium overload
- free radical damage.

Classification

- *amyotrophic lateral sclerosis* (ALS; most common): loss of upper and lower motor neurones (UMN and LMN) producing a mixed picture
- *progressive muscular atrophy* (PMA): predominantly LMN
- *primary lateral sclerosis* (PLS; rare): predominantly UMN

MND may be associated with extra-motor features, e.g. fronto-temporal dementia in ALS. Progressive bulbar palsy is considered a variant of ALS, affecting the bulbar region.

Clinical presentation

- LMN weakness, with wasting and fasciculation of the small muscles of the hand followed by wasting of upper and lower limb muscles
- LMN weakness, fasciculation and wasting of the tongue and pharynx producing dysarthria, dysphagia, choking and nasal regurgitation
- UMN spastic weakness starting in the legs and spreading to involve the arms

Fasciculation of some limb musculature is a hallmark of the disease. Lower limb lesions are often UMN type and upper limb lesions LMN type. The limbs may demonstrate marked muscular wasting, but still have exaggerated reflexes. Pseudobulbar palsy may occur. Although the sensory examination is usually normal, sensory symptoms may occur in 20–30% of patients (e.g. tingling paraesthesia). The bladder is not affected.

Diagnosis

Criteria for the diagnosis of ALS have been proposed and include:

- evidence (clinical, electrophysiological or neuropathological) of LMN degeneration
- evidence (clinical) of UMN degeneration
- progressive spread of symptoms or signs within a region or to other regions
- no radiological, electrophysiological or pathological evidence of other disease.

Investigation

There is currently no definitive test for MND. Investigations are geared towards excluding other (potentially treatable) conditions which can mimic the different subtypes of MND:

- ALS: multiple-level spinal cord/root compression, paraneoplastic syndromes, thyrotoxicosis, inclusion body myositis
- PLS: multiple sclerosis, spinal cord compression, hereditary spastic paraplegia
- PMA: multifocal motor neuropathy, Kennedy's disease, spinal muscular atrophy, porphyria, lead poisoning.

Investigations include:

- Electrophysiology: useful in identifying LMN features in both clinically affected and clinically silent regions; electromyographic features include evidence of active and chronic denervation.
- Imaging: not required in all cases but may be undertaken to exclude other pathology.
- Other tests: these are generally dictated by the clinical presentation, but may include full blood count, ESR, renal, liver, bone and thyroid function, glucose, creatine kinase, serum electrophoresis/urine Bence Jones protein, acetylcholine receptor antibody, CSF analysis, syphilis serology and genetic testing if familial disease is suspected.

Management

MND is optimally managed by a specialist multidisciplinary team, including:

- neurologist
- nurse specialist

- physiotherapist
- occupational therapist
- speech and language therapist
- dietician
- gastroenterology and respiratory teams for nutritional/feeding and ventilatory support
- psychologist
- social worker and local hospice support are also important.

In the UK, the MND Association provides useful advice and support for patients and their relatives.

Disease-modifying therapy

Riluzole (which reduces presynaptic glutamate release, non-competitively blocks N-methyl-D-aspartate [NMDA] receptor-mediated responses, and exerts direct actions on voltage-dependent sodium channels) has been shown in a small number of trials to extend the lifespan of patients with ALS by an average of 3–4 months. Its role in PMA and PLS remains unclear.

Edaravone (a free radical scavenger that is thought to reduce oxidative stress) has been found to slow functional deterioration in some patients with ALS and has recently been licensed in the USA.

Trials of immunomodulatory therapy (e.g. with interleukin-2) are currently underway to determine whether they might provide a novel approach to slowing disease progression.

Nutritional support

Good nutritional support from an early stage significantly contributes to quality of life and prognosis. Most MND patients eventually develop progressive bulbar problems, and advice regarding posture, airway protection and use of thickened fluids is important. Careful consideration is required regarding placement of a gastrostomy tube.

Respiratory support

Lung function tests should be performed at baseline and regularly thereafter – reduced forced vital capacity (FVC) in the supine versus upright position is an indicator of early respiratory failure. Aspiration pneumonia requires aggressive treatment.

Non-invasive positive pressure ventilation (NIPPV) confers a survival benefit and improves quality of life providing that bulbar dysfunction is not severe.

Other measures

- quinine for cramps
- baclofen and diazepam for spasticity
- carbocisteine (mucolytic), a 'cough assist' machine, suction and antimuscarinics for thick secretions
- laxatives for constipation
- tricyclic antidepressants or selective serotonin reuptake inhibitors for low mood/depression; these agents may also help with emotional lability due to pseudobulbar palsy

Prognosis

The median survival is 4 years, with a poorer prognosis in patients with bulbar onset.

Parkinson's disease and other extrapyramidal disorders

Parkinson's disease

Parkinson's disease (PD, originally described by James Parkinson in 1817 as 'Shaking Palsy') is a degenerative disorder predominantly affecting the extrapyramidal pathways (basal ganglia circuits – including the substantia nigra, striatum [caudate and putamen], globus pallidus, subthalamic nucleus, and thalamus). It is characterised by impaired dopaminergic neurotransmission, and is an akinetic-rigid syndrome (Table 15.5), estimated to affect ~1% of the population over the age of 60 years in the UK, with no significant gender bias.

Aetiology

In the majority of patients with PD the cause remains unknown. Most cases appear to be sporadic, but there is increasing evidence that genetic factors play a role in the pathogenesis (see later), especially in those with an age of onset <50 years. It has been speculated that an as yet unidentified environmental toxin may selectively damage dopaminergic neurones in the substantia nigra, possibly acting in a similar manner to MPTP (methyl-phenyltetrahydropyridine), a synthetic heroin by-product, which was responsible for causing parkinsonism in a group of illicit drug users in the USA in the 1980s (MPTP is converted by monoamine oxidase type B in glial cells to MPP$^+$, a free radical and mitochondrial toxin, which is taken up and concentrated in dopaminergic neurones). The dopaminergic neurones projecting from the substantia nigra in the midbrain to the striatum of the basal ganglia (in particular the caudate nucleus and

Table 15.5 Causes of an akinetic-rigid syndrome

Type	Examples
Inherited	Wilson's disease
Idiopathic	Parkinson's disease Multiple system atrophy Progressive supranuclear palsy Lewy body dementia
Inflammatory	Post-encephalitic (e.g. following the epidemic of *encephalitis lethargica* after World War I)
Drugs	Neuroleptics (e.g. chlorpromazine) Antiemetics (e.g. metoclopramide)
Toxins	MPTP (synthetic heroin by-product) Manganese Chronic carbon monoxide poisoning
Vascular	Multiple lacunar infarcts (although often associated with pyramidal and cognitive dysfunction)
Trauma	'Punch-drunk' syndrome in boxers (i.e. due to chronic head injury)
Neoplasia	Very rarely tumours arising in the region of the basal ganglia may cause contralateral hemi-parkinsonism

MPTP, methyl-phenyl-tetrahydropyridine.

putamen) are the primary site of neuronal loss in Parkinson's disease. An imbalance between dopaminergic and cholinergic signalling in the extrapyramidal pathways ensues (dopaminergic insufficiency or cholinergic excess results in an akinetic-rigid syndrome; dopaminergic excess or cholinergic insufficiency leads to involuntary movements, i.e. dyskinesia).

A number of established (*SNCA* (alpha-synuclein), *Parkin, PINK1, DJ-1, LRRK2, ATP13A2, PLA2G6*) and putative (*SNCAIP, NR4A2, FGF20*) genetic causes for PD have now been described.

Clinical presentation

Parkinson's disease is characterised by the triad of rigidity, tremor and bradykinesia plus postural abnormalities. The classical picture of parkinsonism is of immobile flexion at all joints (neck, trunk, shoulders, elbows, wrists and metacarpophalangeal joints) except the interphalangeal, producing a flexed or stooped posture. From the early stages, on walking the arms do not

swing fully and later in the disease the gait is stuttering and shuffling and the patient may show festination. He/she is slow and unstable on the turn and may 'freeze'. The face is expressionless ('mask-like facies'), eyes unblinking and speech quiet and monotonous.

As the disease progresses other symptoms include:

- difficulty in initiating movement
- poor balance with a tendency to fall because of slow correcting movements (± postural hypotension)
- small handwriting (micrographia)
- seborrhoea
- increased salivation (which, with dysphagia, may give rise to drooling)
- a soft unintelligible voice (dysarthria)
- constipation and urinary frequency, sometimes with incontinence
- oculogyric crises (forced upwards deviation of the eyes); this occurs characteristically in drug-induced and postencephalitic parkinsonism.

Parkinsonism is usually asymmetrical. The repetitive, rhythmic tremor (frequency: 4–6 Hz) is usually most obvious in the hands (where it is described as 'pill-rolling'). It is typically improved by voluntary movement and made worse by anxiety. Titubation refers to tremor involving the head. Repeated movements, such as tapping with the fingers, although regular in rate, are reduced in both amplitude and speed. The rigidity may be lead-pipe or, with the tremor superimposed, cogwheel. There may be a positive glabellar tap sign (blinking on repeated tapping of the forehead). With advanced disease, patients may suffer insomnia, depression and dementia.

Diagnosis

Diagnosis is based on the classical clinical triad. The history may help reveal an underlying cause for parkinsonism or other causes of an akinetic-rigid syndrome, thus helping to target treatment more effectively. Brain imaging is rarely helpful. An empirical trial of therapy may help confirm the diagnosis in less clear-cut cases.

Management

The object is to reduce each of the symptoms using a combination of pharmacological agents, physiotherapy, occupational and speech therapy. Coexistent depression should be treated. Postural hypotension may be exacerbated by certain drug treatments.

Two major classes of drugs are used: dopaminergic and anticholinergic agents, which help to address the imbalance between insufficient dopaminergic and relatively excessive cholinergic tone, respectively. The traditional approach has been to delay the onset of treatment until symptoms warrant it. However, there is now interest in the potential for earlier intervention with some agents to slow disease progression (i.e. to mediate neuroprotection).

Dopaminergic agents

Levodopa (L-DOPA) is a precursor of dopamine which crosses the blood–brain barrier following oral administration. It is given in combination with a peripherally acting DOPA decarboxylase inhibitor (e.g. benserazide [i.e. co-beneldopa] or carbidopa [i.e. co-careldopa]) to prevent its peripheral metabolism, which also helps to reduce side effects. It is effective in 75% of patients with idiopathic Parkinson's disease and excellent in 20%, particularly in those with bradykinesia.

After several years (typically 2–5) of treatment, the efficacy of L-DOPA therapy may be limited by the development of 'late' side effects including:

- Motor fluctuations: e.g. 'wearing-off' where the response to a given dose is shorter-lived than previously, and 'on–off' phenomenon where the patient may switch from being reasonably well controlled ('on') to an akinetic-rigid state ('off'), but without any obvious relationship to the timing of drug doses.
- Dyskinesias: related to high dopamine levels ('peak-dose dyskinesias'), or painful dystonia as dopamine levels fall ('wearing-off dystonias').

Helpful pharmacological manipulation includes increasing the dose frequency (but not the total daily dosage) of L-DOPA, using a slow-release preparation, or adding one of the following drugs:

- Selegiline and rasagiline: slow the enzymatic degradation of dopamine by monoamine oxidase type B (MAO-B).
- Entacapone: slows the enzymatic degradation of dopamine by catechol-O-methyl-transferase (COMT).
- Dopamine receptor agonists including ropinirole (a D2-agonist) and pramipexole (a D2- and D3-receptor agonist). These also may be used as monotherapy in early PD, potentially delaying the need for L-DOPA.
- Apomorphine: a potent D1- and D2-receptor stimulant.

NB: Ergot-derived dopamine receptor agonists (e.g. pergolide, cabergoline) have been linked with pulmonary, retroperitoneal and cardiac valvular/pericardial fibrotic disorders when used at the high dosages required for the treatment of PD, and are therefore no longer recommended. In addition, dopamine agonist therapy in general has been linked with an increased risk of impulse control disorders, including pathologic gambling, compulsive sexual behaviour or compulsive buying. All patients, and where possible their immediate relatives, should be advised of these potential adverse effects.

Domperidone (limited central antidopaminergic activity) for nausea, and atypical antipsychotic agents (e.g. olanzapine, quetiapine) or cholinesterase inhibitors (e.g. donepezil, rivastigmine) for hallucinations in those with cognitive impairment, may be used to alleviate the side effects of L-DOPA therapy.

Anticholinergic agents

Antimuscarinic drugs (e.g. trihexyphenidyl, benztropine, orphenadrine, procyclidine) can be tried as first-line therapy in mild disease, in patients poorly tolerant of dopaminergic therapy, and in drug-induced parkinsonism. Anticholinergic side effects limit their use especially in the elderly.

Amantadine

An antiviral agent with mild anti-parkinsonian activity. It appears to promote dopamine release and inhibit its reuptake, but is only mildly beneficial in early PD. It improves mild bradykinesia, tremor and rigidity. It may be useful for alleviating dyskinesias in more advanced disease.

Surgical treatment

Stereotactic thalamotomy is rarely used for intractable tremor in the non-dominant limbs on the contralateral side. Pallidotomy may alleviate drug-induced dyskinesias. However, deep brain stimulation (DBS) offers safer and entirely reversible physiological effects without destroying brain tissue, and is now preferred in those with advanced PD. Its use for patients with shorter duration PD is also being explored.

Cell transplantation (e.g. using fetal substantia nigra) remains primarily an experimental technique as therapeutic benefit remains to be established. Similarly, trials of gene therapy (e.g. to augment the reduced dopamine production) are ongoing.

Prognosis

Parkinson's disease is progressive in most cases, but with modern specialist treatment many patients die with, rather than from, PD.

Other idiopathic akinetic-rigid syndromes

Multiple system atrophy

Extrapyramidal features occur in combination with one or more of the following:

- autonomic failure (Shy–Drager syndrome)
- cerebellar dysfunction
- pyramidal features.

Supranuclear palsy (Steele–Richardson–Olszewski syndrome)

A very rare degenerative condition of the upper brainstem similar to Parkinson's disease. It is characterised by:

- expressionless facies
- axial rigidity
- limb extension rather than flexion
- lead-pipe rigidity and cogwheeling
- fixation of voluntary vertical, followed by lateral and convergence, eye movements
- pseudobulbar palsy
- falls
- later dementia.

Response to anti-Parkinson's therapy is poor.

Other movement disorders

Tremor

Causes include:

- physiological tremor, including exacerbation by anxiety, alcohol, drugs, thyrotoxicosis
- essential tremor
- postural tremor
- Parkinson's disease and other akinetic-rigid syndromes (associated with 'rest tremor')
- cerebellar disorders (associated with 'intention tremor').

Chorea

Irregular random and variable movements which may have a flowing/semi-purposeful quality. Any part of the body can be affected. Causes include:

- hereditary (e.g. Huntington's chorea)
- post-infectious (e.g. Sydenham's chorea in association with rheumatic fever)
- polycythaemia rubra vera
- thyrotoxicosis

- systemic lupus erythematosus
- pregnancy and oral contraceptive
- phenytoin, neuroleptics, alcohol.

Hemiballismus

Violent jerky movements, typically restricted to one side of the body and secondary to damage to the contralateral subthalamic nucleus.

Athetosis

Slow writhing movements most commonly seen with congenital brain damage in cerebral palsy.

Dystonia

Involuntary sustained muscle contractions resulting in abnormal postures which may be focal (e.g. blepharospasm, spasmodic torticollis, laryngospasm, trismus) or generalised (e.g. primary torsion dystonia).

Myoclonus

Rapid, abrupt, jerky movements of part or all of the body, which may occur in epilepsy or arise from elsewhere in the central nervous system causing myoclonic jerks.

Tics

Rapid, compulsive, repetitive stereotyped movements, also referred to as 'habit spasms'. In Gilles de la Tourette syndrome, complex tics are associated with involuntary utterances which may be repetitive ('echolalia') and obscene ('coprolalia').

Disorders of the spinal cord (Table 15.6)

Spinal cord compression

Aetiology

Disorders of vertebrae (extradural; ~45% of cases)

- cervical and lumbar spondylosis
- collapsed vertebral body (malignancy, osteoporosis)
- prolapsed intervertebral disc
- tuberculosis, abscesses, Paget's disease, reticuloses, angiomas

Table 15.6 Causes of spinal cord disease

Type	Examples
Inherited	Hereditary spastic paraplegia Spinocerebellar degenerative disorders
Congenital	Arnold–Chiari malformation with syringomyelia
Infective	Epidural abscess Tuberculosis (and Pott's disease of the spine) HIV Syphilis Tropical spastic paraparesis
Inflammatory	Multiple sclerosis Transverse myelitis (postviral) Sarcoidosis Vasculitis Spondylitis with cord compression
Metabolic	Subacute combined degeneration Paget's disease with cord compression
Vascular	Infarction of the spinal cord Arteriovenous malformation Epidural haematoma with cord compression
Trauma	Vertebral fractures or dislocations Disc prolapse Radiation damage
Neoplasia	Vertebral metastases Benign extrinsic tumours (e.g. meningioma) Intrinsic spinal cord tumours (e.g. glioma)
Degenerative	Motor neurone disease Spondylosis with cord compression

Meningeal disorders (intradural; ~45%)

- neurofibromas
- meningiomas

Disorders of the spinal cord (intramedullary; 5–10%)

- gliomas
- ependymomas

Clinical presentation

Patients present with a spastic paraparesis:

- upper motor neurone weakness in the legs
- loss of sphincter control

- loss of abdominal reflexes if the lesion is in or above the thoracic cord.

The level of the sensory loss ('sensory level') may, but does not necessarily, equate to the level of the lesion – it is vital not to unduly restrict imaging of the spine, otherwise a lesion at a higher level may be missed. Lesions in the high cervical cord cause a spastic tetraparesis. Patients typically complain of 'difficulty walking and numb clumsy hands'.

Bladder involvement is an early feature of spinal cord disease, presenting with urgency, frequency and urge incontinence; bowel involvement occurs later; men may report erectile dysfunction.

Cord compression is a neurosurgical emergency, particularly if of recent onset and rapid progression.

Investigations

- urgent MRI scan
- chest X-ray/CT chest/abdomen/pelvis to exclude malignancy
- serum electrophoresis/Bence Jones protein

Other investigations will be dictated by the clinical context.

Differential diagnosis

Other causes of spastic paraparesis include:

- multiple sclerosis
- subacute combined degeneration of the cord
- transverse myelitis
- anterior spinal artery thrombosis
- motor neurone disease
- parasagittal cranial meningioma

Cervical spondylosis

Over 70% of the adult population in the UK have X-ray changes of osteoarthritis of the joints of the cervical spine, usually osteophytes. These radiological changes are unrelated to the presence or severity of symptoms.

Clinical features

Most patients are symptom-free. Clinical features may include:

- neck pain associated with and precipitated by movements of the neck
- cervical nerve root pain, paraesthesiae, numbness and sometimes segmental weakness with muscle wasting

- brisk reflexes in the arms (although this varies with the level – e.g. absent biceps with brisk triceps with a C5/6 lesion), and upper motor neurone damage affecting the legs caused by narrowing of the cervical canal with compression of the spinal cord or occlusion of the spinal cord vessels (spinal stenosis).

Brown–Séquard syndrome

Damage to one side of the cord produces a very characteristic pattern of sensory and motor loss with:

- an upper motor neurone weakness on the same side as the lesion (the descending corticospinal tracts have already crossed in the medulla)
- ipsilateral loss of position and vibration sense (the ascending fibres in the dorsal columns do not cross until they reach the medulla)
- contralateral spinothalamic (pain and temperature) sensory loss (as these pathways cross at, or just above, their point of entry into the cord); however, a narrow band of ipsilateral spinothalamic sensory loss may be seen at/close to the level of the lesion, reflecting involvement of fibres which have not yet decussated.

In its most severe form (cord hemisection), this is known as the Brown–Séquard syndrome.

Syringomyelia

A rare condition characterised by development of a longitudinal CSF-filled cyst/cavity (syrinx) in the cervical cord and/or brainstem (syringobulbia) anterior to the central canal which spreads asymmetrically to each side. It may be caused by outflow obstruction of the fourth ventricle from a congenital anomaly such as the Arnold–Chiari malformation. It is usually slowly progressive over 20–30 years.

Damage to the cord occurs as follows:

- at the root level of the lesion in the decussating fibres of the lateral spinothalamic tracts (pain and temperature) and anterior horn cells where the lower motor neuron starts
- distant from the lesion in the upper motor neuron in the pyramidal tracts.

Syringomyelia presents with painless injury to the hands (sensory C6, 7, 8) and weakness and wasting in the small muscles of the hands (T1).

Examination may reveal more extensive asymmetrical dissociated sensory loss in the cervical segments, upper motor neuron signs in the legs and Charcot joints in the upper limbs. Surgical decompression of the foramen magnum and aspiration/drainage of cysts should be considered.

Syringobulbia

In syringobulbia the descending root of the trigeminal nerve (pain and temperature) may be involved with a Horner syndrome from involvement of the cervical sympathetic tract. The motor nuclei of the lower cranial nerves may cause rotatory nystagmus from involvement of vestibular and cerebellar connections.

Subacute combined degeneration of the cord

The neurological consequences of vitamin B_{12} deficiency include subacute combined degeneration of the cord, signs of peripheral neuropathy, dementia and optic atrophy.

Combined degeneration refers to the combined demyelination of both pyramidal (lateral columns) and posterior (dorsal) columns.

Clinical presentation

Sensory peripheral neuropathy with numbness and paraesthesia in the feet are the usual presenting symptoms. Less commonly, the disease presents as a spastic paraparesis. The signs are:

- posterior column loss (vibration and position senses, with positive Romberg's sign, page 55, Chapter 6)
- upper motor neurone lesion (weakness, hypertonia and hyperreflexia, with absent abdominal reflexes and upgoing toes)
- peripheral neuropathy (absence of all the jerks, reduced touch sense).

Investigation

- serum B_{12} and folate levels
- parietal cell and intrinsic factor antibodies

Management

Vitamin B_{12} (hydroxocobalamin).

Prognosis

Neurological symptoms and signs usually improve but may remain unchanged or, rarely, continue to progress. Sensory abnormalities resolve more completely than motor.

Spinal root disease (radiculopathy)

Spinal nerve roots may be compressed or damaged as they emerge from the intervertebral foramina on either side of the spinal column. Examples of radiculopathy include:

- Cervical radiculopathy: e.g. due to degenerative cervical intervertebral disc disease, spondylosis or tumour.
- Cauda equina: the spinal cord ends with the conus medullaris (usually at the lower border of the L1 vertebra), below which the lumbar and sacral nerve roots follow a long course in the spinal canal (comprising the cauda equina), before exiting through their respective foramina; compression of the cauda equina is typically associated with lower motor neurone signs and sensory features at several levels, and bladder involvement is common (retention with overflow); if there is also involvement of the lower end of the cord ('conus lesion'), then mixed upper and lower motor neurone signs may be present; disturbance of the blood supply to the cauda equina may result in transient/intermittent neurological symptoms and signs, which are exacerbated by exercise, and which can be confused with intermittent claudication due to vascular insufficiency – however, recovery from the latter is typically more rapid (1–2 min as opposed to 5–10 min at rest) and there are no sensorimotor features.
- Prolapsed lumbar intervertebral disc.
- Acute central disc prolapse: this is a neurosurgical emergency, typically presenting with severe back pain, bilateral lower limb weakness and urinary retention/bowel dysfunction. Urgent imaging and decompression are required.

Peripheral nerve disorders

Peripheral nerves may be affected:

- in isolation (e.g. by trauma) leading to a mononeuropathy
- as part of a systemic disorder that renders them susceptible to pressure (e.g. diabetes mellitus)
- by compromise of their vasculature, e.g. vasculitis in multifocal neuropathy (mononeuritis multiplex)
- as part of a polyneuropathy (classical peripheral neuropathy), commonly due to inflammatory, metabolic or toxic disorders.

Mononeuropathies

Carpal tunnel syndrome

Due to compression of the median nerve as it passes under the flexor retinaculum and through the carpal tunnel at the wrist; commonly bilateral. Predisposing conditions include:

- pregnancy
- local deformity (e.g. secondary to osteoarthritis, fracture)
- diabetes mellitus
- rheumatoid arthritis
- hypothyroidism
- acromegaly
- amyloidosis.

It is characterised by pain and tingling paraesthesia in the hand or arm, typically worse at night, with wasting of the muscles of the thenar eminence and sensory loss in the distribution of the median nerve (radial three-and-a-half digits).

Tinel's (tapping over the median nerve) and Phalen's (forced flexion of the wrist) tests may reproduce tingling paraesthesia.

Diagnosis can be confirmed with electromyography, and secondary causes should be sought. Treatment depends on severity, but may include splinting (especially at night), local injection of corticosteroids and surgical decompression.

Ulnar neuropathy

Typically due to compression of the ulnar nerve at the elbow. It is characterised by pain and/or paraesthesiae radiating along the ulnar border of the forearm, with wasting of the small muscles of the hand but sparing of the thenar eminence; there is also sensory loss in the hand in the distribution of the ulnar nerve.

Electromyography can be used to confirm the diagnosis; treatment may involve advice to avoid leaning/pressure on the elbow and/or surgical decompression/transposition of the ulnar nerve.

Radial neuropathy

Pressure on the radial nerve in the upper arm may lead to wrist drop – most commonly seen with prolonged abnormal posture of the upper arm (e.g. draped over the back of a chair).

Others

- Brachial plexus lesions – including: Erb's palsy (upper nerve roots) and Klumpke's palsy (lower nerve roots) typically due to traction injury (e.g. as a result of birth injury); cervical rib; Pancoast tumour (may be associated with Horner syndrome).

- Meralgia paraesthetica – numbness in the thigh due to compression of the lateral cutaneous nerve of the thigh as it passes under the inguinal ligament.
- Lateral popliteal palsy – the common peroneal nerve is susceptible to pressure damage as it travels around the neck of the fibula, resulting in foot drop (weakness of ankle dorsiflexion and eversion and extensor hallucis longus, with variable sensory disturbance); it is more common in diabetes mellitus.

Multifocal neuropathy/mononeuritis multiplex

An asymmetrical neuropathy affecting two or more peripheral nerves at one time, producing symptoms of numbness, paraesthesiae and sometimes pain in their sensory distribution with associated muscle weakness and wasting.

Causes are shown in Table 15.7.

Peripheral polyneuropathy

Diffuse disease of the peripheral nerves classified according to whether there is sensory or motor involvement or both, and whether the site of disease is the myelin sheath (demyelinating neuropathy) or the nerve fibre (axonal neuropathy). Long-standing disease may result in claw deformities of the foot

(pes cavus) and hand and sensory loss may lead to neuropathic ulceration and joint deformity (Charcot arthropathy). Coexistent autonomic symptoms may be present. Numerous causes are recognised (Table 15.8), but four disorders account for most cases:

- diabetes mellitus
- carcinomatous neuropathy
- vitamin B deficiency (including B_{12})
- drugs or toxins (especially alcohol).

In a significant number the aetiology remains unknown.

Diabetic neuropathy (see metabolic disorders, Chapter 17)

Diabetes mellitus causes a distal, predominantly sensory neuropathy commonly affecting the lower limbs in a stocking distribution. Symptoms of numbness, paraesthesiae and sometimes pain in the feet are

Table 15.7 Causes of multifocal neuropathy/mononeuritis multiplex

Type	Examples
Inherited	Hereditary neuropathy with predisposition to pressure palsies
Infective	Herpes zoster HIV Lyme disease Leprosy
Inflammatory	Rheumatoid arthritis Systemic lupus erythematosus Polyarteritis nodosa Wegener's granulomatosis Sarcoidosis
Metabolic	Diabetes mellitus
Neoplasia (malignant infiltration)	Carcinoma, lymphoma

Table 15.8 Causes of polyneuropathy (peripheral neuropathy)

Type	Examples
Inherited	Charcot–Marie–Tooth disease
Infective	HIV Lyme disease Leprosy Diphtheria
Inflammatory	Guillain–Barré syndrome Chronic inflammatory demyelinating neuropathy Sjögren syndrome Vasculitis Sarcoidosis
Metabolic	Diabetes mellitus Uraemia Myxoedema Amyloidosis
Nutritional	Vitamin deficiency (especially thiamine, niacin and B_{12})
Drugs	Isoniazid Vincristine Cisplatinum Amiodarone Phenytoin
Toxins	Alcohol Lead Arsenic Insecticides
Neoplasia	Paraneoplastic

associated with loss of vibration and position sense and loss of the ankle reflex. It may be associated with Charcot arthropathy.

Carcinomatous neuropathy

Cancer may be associated with either a sensory neuropathy in a 'glove-and-stocking' distribution or motor neuropathy in which there is muscle weakness and wasting, usually of the proximal limb muscles. The neuropathy may be mixed. It may also reflect the toxic effects of treatment.

Vitamin B Deficiency

Vitamin B_1 deficiency, usually seen in patients with alcoholism, presents with a sensory neuropathy characterised by numbness ('walking on cotton wool'), paraesthesiae, pain and soreness of the feet. In vitamin B_{12} deficiency the peripheral neuropathy may be associated with megaloblastic anaemia and subacute combined degeneration of the cord (see above).

Disorders of the neuromuscular junction

Myasthenia gravis

A rare disorder (estimated incidence <1/100 000, but prevalence ~1 : 10 000) in which muscle weakness results from failure of neuromuscular transmission. The number of functioning postsynaptic acetylcholine receptors (AChR) is reduced and a high titre of specific anti-AChR antibodies is found in ~85% of cases. Ten percent of patients have an associated thymoma. Excessive muscular fatigability may also occur in polymyositis and SLE and there is an increased incidence of myasthenia gravis in thyrotoxicosis. The Eaton–Lambert myasthenic syndrome is associated with malignant disease.

Clinical presentation

Painless muscular weakness is produced by repetitive or sustained contraction (fatigability typically worse at the end of the day or after exercise). This is most marked in the face and eyes, producing a symmetrical ptosis and diplopia. Dysarthria and dysphagia with nasal regurgitation of liquids may occur. Proximal muscles are more often affected than the distal, and the upper limb more than the lower. There is no

wasting and tendon reflexes are preserved. Involvement of respiratory muscles may require emergency treatment.

Diagnosis

Diagnosis is based on the clinical assessment, supported by targeted investigations:

- serum anti-AChR antibody titre (present in approximately 85% of patients with generalised disease and in virtually all patients with a thymoma); antibodies to a muscle specific receptor tyrosine kinase (MuSK) are detectable in up to 50% of those with generalised myasthenia gravis who are anti-AChR negative (possibly indicating a discrete underlying pathological mechanism); anti-striated muscle antibodies are found in approximately one-third of all case of myasthenia, but in 80% of those with thymoma.
- edrophonium ('Tensilon') test: intravenous injection of edrophonium (short-acting anticholinesterase producing a temporary increase in synaptic acetylcholine levels) produces rapid, albeit transient, improvement in clinical features. Cardiac monitoring/resuscitation should be available (risk of bradycardia/asystole). This test is now rarely used in clinical practice.
- electrophysiological studies, e.g. repetitive nerve stimulation and single-fibre electromyography
- thyroid function tests
- CT or MR scan of thorax for thymoma (especially in those with relevant positive immunological markers – see earlier).

Treatment

- Long-acting anticholinesterases orally often provide good symptomatic relief, e.g. neostigmine or pyridostigmine, preferably titrated by increasing the dosage slowly until measured muscular strength is optimised.
- Corticosteroids: (between 10 and 80 mg of prednisolone) – should be started under close supervision at a low dosage as there is a risk of increasing weakness in the early stages of therapy.
- A number of other steroid-sparing immunomodulatory agents have been used including azathioprine, methotrexate, cyclosporine and mycophenalate. In cases of refractory myasthenia, agents such as rituximab, pulsed cyclophosphamide and tacrolimus may be tried.
- Plasmapheresis or intravenous immunoglobulin may be valuable in intractable cases, but the effect

is short-lasting and best reserved for those preparing for thymectomy.

- Thymectomy at any age increases the chance of remission and is mandatory when the presence of thymoma is suspected.

NB: Certain antibiotics (e.g. aminoglycosides) may exacerbate neuromuscular blockade and should be avoided in patients with myasthenia gravis.

Differential diagnosis

- other causes of ptosis
- muscular dystrophies involving the face
- familial hypokalaemic paralysis

Prognosis

Myasthenia gravis may never progress beyond ophthalmoplegia and spontaneous periods of remission of up to 3 years occur. The outlook is poorer if the respiratory muscles are involved. Thymectomy usually improves the outlook unless a thymoma is present.

Eaton–Lambert myasthenic syndrome

A disorder of acetylcholine release in which myasthenia is usually associated with small cell carcinoma of the bronchus. It differs from classical myasthenia gravis in that the eyes are less frequently affected, proximal limb muscle weakness is common and their strength is initially increased by repeated movement. There is no response to edrophonium, but oral 3,4 diaminopyridine may help.

Disorders of muscles

Myotonia

Myotonia describes the inability of muscles to relax normally after contraction, producing a 'reluctant release' of handshake and percussion contraction ('percussion myotonia'), due to a slow relaxation phase.

Myotonic dystrophy (dystrophia myotonica)

This is a rare autosomal dominant disorder producing progressively more severe symptoms and signs with succeeding generations, i.e. 'anticipation'. Classical myotonic dystrophy type 1 (DM1) results from expansion of a CTG repeat in the 3′ untranslated region of the dystrophia myotonica protein kinase gene (*DMPK*, genetic locus 19q13). Myotonic dystrophy type 2 (DM2) is caused by an expanded CCTG tetranucleotide repeat expansion in intron 1 of the *ZNF9* (also known as the *CNBP*) gene on chromosome 3q21. In both DM1 and DM2 the repeat expansion is transcribed into RNA, but remains untranslated – thus providing an example of a novel mechanism of disease, RNA toxicity. Both males and females are affected with usual onset at 15–40 years. UK incidence is estimated at 1 in 20 000, but is higher in certain regions (e.g. Quebec in Canada and the Basque region of Spain).

Clinical features

- typical facies include frontal balding, ptosis, a smooth expressionless forehead, cataracts and a 'lateral smile'
- skeletal muscle weakness and wasting, typically affects the facial muscles (levator palpebrae superioris, temporalis), sternomastoids, distal muscles of the forearm, intrinsic muscles of the hand; less commonly weakness occurs in the quadriceps, respiratory muscles, palatal and pharyngeal muscles, tongue and extraocular muscles
- loss of limb reflexes with no fasciculation
- myotonia which increases with cold, fatigue and excitement and may reduce with repeated activity
- muscle pain
- primary hypogonadism with testicular atrophy
- insulin resistance and diabetes mellitus
- cognitive impairment (including mental retardation in congenital/childhood forms)
- cardiac abnormalities (e.g. conduction disorders, cardiomyopathy)
- sleep disturbance
- gastrointestinal disturbance (e.g. colicky pain, constipation or diarrhoea)
- cataracts
- some cohort studies have also suggested that patients with myotonic dystrophy are at increased risk of cancer

Diagnosis

Clinical and confirmed with genetic testing.

Treatment

Currently, there is no disease-modifying treatment for myotonic dystrophy. Phenytoin or mexiletine may reduce myotonia. Other complications (e.g. cardiac) are treated along conventional lines. A multidisciplinary approach is generally required.

Muscular dystrophies

Pseudohypertrophic (Duchenne; Becker)

An X-linked recessive disorder due to mutations in the gene encoding the muscle cytoskeletal protein dystrophin – hence the term dystrophinopathies. Prevalence is 3 in 100 000 and incidence 25 in 100 000 male births.

The severe childhood form (Duchenne muscular dystrophy [DMD]) presents from an early age with difficulty in walking, climbing stairs and rising from the floor (children use their hands to 'climb' up their legs). On examination lordotic posture and waddling gait are seen because of weakness of the muscles of the pelvic girdle and proximal lower limb. The calves are hypertrophied but weak and the creatine kinase level is raised. Diagnosis is confirmed by EMG and muscle biopsy. Subsequent leg muscle contracture may produce talipes equinovarus and muscle weakness may spread to the upper limbs. Glucocorticosteroids are the mainstay of treatment for DMD, and are typically commenced in early childhood when motor skills have plateaued or are declining. Measures to prevent bone loss should be considered in those on long-term glucocorticosteroid therapy. Respiratory interventions (e.g. assisted cough techniques) and assisted ventilation are important aspects of management. Historically, individuals with DMD usually died in their teens and 20s from associated complications including chest infections and cardiomyopathy. However, survival has improved in recent years, likely reflecting the increased use of glucocorticoid therapy and better supportive measures, although most patients will not live beyond their mid-30s.

Less severe mutations may present in adolescence or adulthood (Becker muscular dystrophy [BMD]) but are still usually associated with progressive disability. BMD has a better prognosis, with a mean age of death in the mid-40s.

Facio-scapulo-humeral (Landouzy–Déjérine)

A rare autosomal dominant trait which affects both sexes equally. The onset is at puberty with progressive wasting in the upper limb-girdle and face, with characteristic 'winging' of both scapulae. It may cease spontaneously or progress to the muscles of the trunk and lower limbs.

Limb-girdle (Erb)

A rare autosomal recessive trait which affects both sexes equally. It presents at 20–40 years and progressively involves the muscles of the shoulders and pelvic girdles.

Acquired muscular disorders

Inflammatory myopathies

Polymyositis may occur in isolation or in association with autoimmune connective tissue disorders (see rheumatology, Chapter 18). Dermatomyositis is characterised by an inflammatory myopathy in association with a characteristic 'heliotrope' facial rash and may indicate underlying malignancy in the elderly.

Neurological infections

Bacterial meningitis

Bacterial meningitis is usually caused by infection with one of three organisms: *Neisseria meningitidis, Haemophilus influenzae* type b and *Streptococcus pneumoniae*. The annual incidence of bacterial meningitis is 5–10 per 100 000 in developed countries.

Meningococcal meningitis

N. meningitidis (meningococcus) is carried in the nasopharynx and produces epidemics of infection chiefly in children and young adults. These occur in conditions of overcrowding and in closed communities.

Clinical presentation

After an incubation period of 1–3 days, the disease begins abruptly with fever, headache, photophobia, nausea, vomiting and neck stiffness. Mental confusion, seizures and coma may follow. Physical examination reveals signs of infection (fever, tachycardia, hypotension) and there may be a characteristic purpuric/petechial rash. Neurological signs include 'meningism' (neck stiffness, positive Kernig's sign), altered conscious level, features of raised intracranial pressure, cranial nerve palsies and other focal neurology.

Acute complications of meningitis include abscess formation, hydrocephalus, septic shock with cardiorespiratory collapse, disseminated intravascular coagulation and adrenal haemorrhage (Waterhouse–Friderichsen syndrome).

Investigations

CT head scan is now performed routinely before lumbar puncture to exclude raised intracranial pressure.

CSF analysis typically reveals:

- purulent/turbid fluid
- raised opening pressure
- marked polymorph leucocytosis
- raised protein
- low glucose (<50% of paired blood glucose level)
- Gram-negative diplococci may be identified on Gram stain, CSF culture or by molecular techniques.

Other investigations should include:

- full blood count (neutrophilia)
- coagulation profile (disseminated intravascular coagulation)
- renal function (hyponatraemia, renal failure)
- blood cultures (may be positive even with negative CSF findings).

Treatment must not be delayed while investigations are being performed – bacterial meningitis may be fatal within hours, and early diagnosis and treatment with high-dose antibiotics are essential. Urgent blood cultures should be taken and antibiotics started immediately.

Treatment

In suspected meningococcal meningitis, general practitioners should give a single dose of intravenous or intramuscular benzylpenicillin while arranging urgent transfer to hospital.

Acute bacterial meningitis of unknown cause

In clinical practice this is the most common scenario, especially when no organisms are seen with Gram staining of CSF. There is no time to wait for the results of culture, and antibiotics must be started immediately. In this setting, a third-generation cephalosporin (e.g. ceftriaxone or cefotaxime) is the drug of choice (chloramphenicol is an alternative for those with a history of hypersensitivity to cephalosporins). In recognition of the worldwide increase in the prevalence of penicillin-resistant pneumococci, vancomycin is often added to ceftriaxone or cefotaxime as empiric treatment until culture and sensitivity results are available.

Neisseria meningitis

Local guidelines should dictate which antibiotic is preferred based on pathogen isolation and susceptibility testing. Traditionally, high-dose benzylpenicillin (2.4 g, 4-hourly) has been the drug of choice for meningococcal infection. However, third-generation cephalosporins are often continued, and meropenem and chloramphenicol are alternative options.

Supportive therapy with analgesics, intravenous fluids, anticonvulsants, inotropes and clotting factors may be needed.

Prevention

Chemoprophylaxis

Rifampicin or ciprofloxacin should be considered to eliminate nasopharyngeal carriage and for household or close contacts in consultation with the infectious diseases or communicable disease control team.

NB: Meningitis is a notifiable disease in the UK.

Vaccination

Vaccines are now available against *Neiseria meningitidis* serogroups A, B, C, W and Y; most cases in the UK are caused by serogroups B and C. Childhood vaccination programmes are combined with targeted vaccination for non-immunised individuals considered to be at particular risk (e.g. students attending university, those with asplenia/splenic dysfunction and travellers to high-risk areas). The choice of vaccine depends on individual circumstances (for further information see the British National Formulary).

Pneumococcal meningitis

Infection may be secondary to pneumococcal pneumonia, or may spread from infected sinuses or ears or through skull base fractures. It is more common in children and the elderly and in patients with asplenia.

Benzylpenicillin is the drug of choice in penicillin-sensitive cases, but the emergence of resistant pneumococcal strains means that cefotaxime or ceftriaxone are preferred as first-line therapy, often with the addition of vancomycin. Meropenem is an alternative.

Pneumococcal vaccination is advisable in patients with asplenism, chronic cardiac, renal or liver disease (especially if >65 years), immunosuppression and conditions predisposing to CSF leakage. In addition, long-term phenoxymethylpenicillin (500 mg b.d.) is recommended for patients with asplenia.

Haemophilus influenzae meningitis

Usually occurring in the under-5s, the introduction of a vaccination programme has dramatically reduced the number of cases of meningitis due to *H. influenzae*. It often follows an influenzal type of illness, has a longer, insidious onset and presents with fever, nausea and vomiting.

Cefotaxime or ceftriaxone are the drugs of choice (chloramphenicol is an alternative). Adjunctive dexamethasone therapy should be considered – see later.

Chemoprophylaxis with rifampicin is advised to prevent secondary infection. Immunisation using *H. influenzae* type b vaccine is routinely recommended for children at the ages of 2, 3 and 4 months.

Adjunctive dexamethasone

Permanent neurological sequelae (e.g. hearing loss, focal neurologic deficits) are not uncommon in survivors of bacterial meningitis. Based on clinical trial data, the main current indication for dexamethasone therapy in adults is known or suspected pneumococcal meningitis, and in children known or suspected *H. influenzae* meningitis. However, since the aetiology is frequently unknown at the time of initiating treatment, dexamethasone is administered to the majority of patients. Rifampicin is sometimes added in those patients also receiving vancomycin whose entry into the CSF may be diminished due to the anti-inflammatory effects of dexamethasone.

Prognosis

The mortality from acute bacterial meningitis remains high (~10% overall) and is greatest in pneumococcal disease, which is also more likely to leave patients with long-term sequelae, e.g. hydrocephalus, cranial nerve palsies, epilepsy.

Tuberculous meningitis (see also tuberculosis, Chapter 11)

This may present as acute meningitis but usually as an insidious illness with fever, weight loss and progressive signs of confusion and cerebral irritation (seizures and focal neurological signs) leading to mental deterioration and finally coma. Immunocompromised individuals and those from certain ethnic groups are at greatest risk.

At lumbar puncture the opening pressure is raised, polymorphs and lymphocytes are typically present, with raised protein and very low glucose. Auramine or Ziehl–Neelsen staining may reveal organisms, but prolonged culture is often required. Polymerase chain reaction (PCR) for bacterial nucleic acids offers a faster diagnostic route.

Treatment is with rifampicin, isoniazid (with pyridoxine cover), pyrazinamide and either ethambutol or streptomycin (the fourth agent can often be stopped after 3 months). A prolonged course (12 months or more) is usually required under close supervision. Corticosteroids are used during the early phase of treatment to suppress the host's inflammatory response and risk of developing cerebral oedema.

Intracranial abscess

Brain abscess is rare. It may complicate otitis media or paranasal sinus infections or occur secondary to haematogenous spread from bacterial endocarditis or pulmonary infection. There may be a history of head injury or neurosurgery. The clinical features are typically those of an expanding mass lesion with fever and possible systemic illness. CT/MRI is required in any suspected case and lumbar puncture must **not** be performed where there is a risk of raised intracranial pressure.

Treatment involves surgical drainage, broad-spectrum antibiotics until an organism/sensitivities are available and high-dose corticosteroids once antibiotics have commenced. It is essential to identify and treat the source of primary infection.

The mortality rate is high in cerebral abscess, and of those who survive up to one-third develop epilepsy.

Parameningeal infections

Occasionally pus collects in the epidural space, especially in the spine. *Staphylococcus aureus* is the most common organism, usually from skin infections. Vertebral osteomyelitis and accompanying discitis may complicate the picture. Fever and systemic upset are accompanied by severe back pain and paraparesis.

MRI scanning of the spine is the investigation of choice. Treatment is with anti-staphylococcal antimicrobial therapy and surgical drainage if there is neural compression.

Lyme disease

The spirochaete *Borrelia burgdorferi*, transmitted by tick bite, may produce neurological manifestations including fever, meningism and arthralgia in the acute phase. In chronic disease, meningitis, encephalitis, cranial nerve palsies, and spinal root and peripheral nerve lesions can occur.

Serological diagnosis is available in specialist laboratories. Treatment is with cefotaxime or ceftriaxone.

Leprosy

Mycobacterium leprae directly invades peripheral nerves leading to a patchy sensory (poly)neuropathy with associated thickening of peripheral nerves, which become palpable. Skin in affected areas may be depigmented and anaesthetic.

Bacterial toxins

Botulism

Clostridium botulinum causes acute gastrointestinal upset followed by a 'descending paralysis' (ptosis, diplopia, difficulty with accommodation, then bulbar and limb involvement); assisted ventilation may be required.

Diphtheria

Corynebacterium diphtheriae may cause a polyneuropathy.

Tetanus

Clostridium tetani causes tonic spasms of the jaw ('lockjaw'; trismus) and trunk (opisthotonos) and whole body fever. Treatment is supportive with muscle relaxants and ventilation together with penicillin, human antitetanus immunoglobulin and wound cleansing.

Viral meningitis

Many viruses have been implicated including:

- enteroviruses (coxsackie A and B, echoviruses, polioviruses)
- herpes simplex viruses HSV-1, HSV-2
- Epstein–Barr virus
- varicella zoster virus
- mumps
- measles
- adenoviruses.

Symptoms of headache and meningism are self-limiting and complications rare. At lumbar puncture the opening pressure may be raised but the CSF is clear with normal or modestly raised protein content and normal glucose. Mononuclear cells (lymphocytes) may be seen but no organisms. PCR may identify the causative virus.

Viral encephalitis

Viral infection of the brain parenchyma resulting in a lymphocytic inflammatory reaction with necrosis. The most common cause is herpes simplex (HSV), but other pathogens include herpes zoster, cytomegalovirus, Epstein–Barr virus, adenovirus and mumps.

HSV encephalitis

Most episodes are thought to result from reactivation of latent virus and it is most common in immunocompromised subjects. A brief prodrome of headache, fever and malaise is followed by severe CNS dysfunction, with focal signs, seizures and reduced consciousness/coma.

CT/MRI may show low-density lesions with ring enhancement typically in the temporal lobes, although these can take several days to appear. EEG is abnormal with evidence of diffuse brain dysfunction and CSF findings are similar to those in viral meningitis. Identification of HSV viral DNA in CSF by polymerase chain reaction or detection of viral antigen by immunoassay, rising antibody titres to HSV and/or brain biopsy may all aid diagnosis. Treatment with intravenous aciclovir should be started as soon as the diagnosis is suspected.

Retroviral infections (Chapter 21)

HIV-AIDS may affect neurological function including:

- direct involvement of the nervous system causing a meningitic-like illness around the time of seroconversion and later a slowly progressive dementia with involvement of the spinal cord and peripheral nerves
- opportunistic infections such as cerebral toxoplasmosis, cryptococcal meningitis, cytomegalovirus, herpes simplex, herpes zoster
- progressive multifocal leucoencephalopathy (PML)
- cerebral lymphoma.

These events are rare in patients treated with HAART.

The human T-cell lymphotrophic virus type 1 (HTLV-1), prevalent in certain equatorial areas, including the Caribbean, is neurotropic and causes tropical spastic paraparesis (HTLV-1-associated myelopathy, HAM).

Protozoal infections

- malaria – *Plasmodium falciparum* can cause haemorrhagic encephalitis
- toxoplasmosis

- trypanosomiasis – may present with low-grade encephalitis, hypersomnolence and seizures ('sleeping sickness')

Metazoal infections

- hydatid disease – intracranial cysts present as mass lesions or rupture to produce meningitis
- cysticercosis – multiple cyst formation results in raised intracranial pressure, focal neurology and seizures

Rabies

Although eradicated from the UK and other countries, rabies remains endemic in certain parts of the world. Following a bite by an infected animal the virus migrates slowly to the CNS where it promotes an inflammatory reaction. Brainstem involvement induces fever, psychiatric disturbance and hydrophobia, whereas spinal cord involvement causes a flaccid paralysis. Prophylactic immunisation is advised when travelling to endemic regions and active and passive immunisation should be commenced after a 'suspect' animal bite, together with thorough wound cleansing.

Poliomyelitis

Polio remains endemic in the tropics despite its near eradication from the developed world following introduction of immunisation with the oral Sabin vaccine (live attenuated poliovirus).

Clinical features

Ninety to ninety-five percent of infected patients have mild upper respiratory or gastrointestinal symptoms that settle completely. The rest have a more severe early infection with fever, sore throat, diarrhoea or constipation and muscle pains. The **minor illness** usually settles, but 1–2% of patients go on to develop a **major illness** 5–10 days later with features of acute viral meningitis. A small number of patients with poliovirus meningitis develop flaccid lower motor neurone muscle paralysis with loss of reflexes following anterior horn cell damage. The legs are most commonly affected but paralysis may spread to the arms; involvement of the medulla oblongata and lower pons causes bulbar palsy.

Respiratory failure is a result of paralysis of the respiratory muscles and may be complicated by aspiration pneumonia secondary to dysphagia and an inability to cough caused by bulbar palsy.

There are no sensory neurological changes.

Diagnosis

CSF analysis reveals raised protein, increased polymorphs and lymphocytes and normal glucose. The virus can be grown from throat, stool and CSF and paired sera show a rising titre.

Management

There is no specific treatment but patients should be isolated and contacts immunised.

Management is supportive:

- artificial ventilation for respiratory failure
- careful nursing to prevent sores
- monitoring of fluid and electrolyte balance
- nutritional support
- physiotherapy and progressive rehabilitation are started after the fever has settled.

Prognosis

Patients with isolated bulbar palsy usually recover completely. In limb paralysis full muscle recovery is rare and paralysis of the respiratory muscles often requires continued artificial ventilation.

Syphilis of the nervous system

Neurosyphilis is now rare and can be avoided by early treatment. There are several distinct clinical entities:

- *Mild (self-limiting) meningitis.*
- *Meningovascular disease:* occurs 3–4 years after primary infection involving fibrosis and thickening of the meninges with nipping and paralysis of cranial nerves, endarteritis causing cerebral ischaemic necrosis or spinal transverse myelitis and paraplegia, spinal meningeal thickening involving posterior spinal roots to produce pain and anterior roots to cause muscle wasting.
- *Tabes dorsalis:* occurs 10–35 years after primary infection. Degeneration of the dorsal columns and nerve roots causes severe paroxysmal stabbing pains that occur in the limbs, chest or abdomen. Paraesthesiae may occur with ataxia and a wide-based gait due to numbness and loss of joint position and vibration sensation. There are absent reflexes, positive Rombergism and a typical facies with Argyll Robertson pupils.
- *Generalised paralysis of the insane:* occurs 10–35 years after primary infection and is characterised by the physical signs of tabes dorsalis, plus evidence of cerebral cortical degeneration, and loss of

memory and concentration with associated anxiety and/or depression. Later, insight is lost and the patient may become euphoric with delusions of grandeur and loss of emotional responses. Epilepsy is common.

Investigation

Serological tests for syphilis may be performed on blood and CSF. CSF analysis may also reveal lymphocytosis, raised protein and oligoclonal bands.

Management

- Penicillin by injection is the drug of choice for active syphilitic infection. Improvement, stabilisation or deterioration may occur in any one case despite adequate penicillin therapy.
- The Jarisch–Herxheimer reaction is an acute hypersensitivity reaction and results from toxins produced by spirochaetes killed on the first contact with penicillin. Death has been reported in some cases, and hence corticosteroids are often given during the first few days of penicillin therapy to mitigate this risk.

Miscellaneous neurological disorders

Cerebral tumours

Intracranial neoplasms can be classified as:

- Benign – generally arising from meninges, cranial nerves or other structures and leading to extrinsic compression of the brain. They may be life-threatening due to local mass effect.
- Malignant – predominantly arising from the brain parenchyma. They may be primary (~20%, most commonly gliomas) or secondary (~80%, usually from bronchus, breast, kidney, colon, ovary, prostate or thyroid cancer).

Symptoms and signs

Caused by raised intracranial pressure

- headache
- confusion, change in personality, apathy, drowsiness
- sixth-nerve palsy results from pressure on the nerve as it crosses the petrous temporal bone ('false localising sign')

Epilepsy

Progressive focal neurological signs

These depend upon the site of the tumour:

- *Prefrontal:* progressive dementia with loss of affect and social responsibility, anosmia and positive grasp reflex in the contralateral hand.
- *Precentral:* contralateral hemiplegia (± Jacksonian epilepsy).
- *Parietal:* falling away of the contralateral outstretched arm, astereognosis, tactile inattention, apraxia and spatial disorientation. Low-sited tumours may produce lower quadrantic homonymous hemianopia rather than complete homonymous hemianopia. Dysphasia occurs with lesions in the dominant temporoparietal region.
- *Temporal lobe:* temporal lobe epilepsy, aphasia (if on the dominant side) and an upper quadrantic homonymous hemianopia.
- *Occipital lobe:* homonymous hemianopia with macular sparing.

Investigation

- CT or MR scanning will identify the tumour.
- Screening for primary tumours at the sites that most frequently metastasise to the brain should be undertaken if secondaries are suspected and may involve CT and FDG-PET.

Management

Management depends upon the type of tumour and combines surgery, radiotherapy and chemotherapy. Some benign tumours may be amenable to complete excision. For malignant primary or secondary tumours, cure is generally not possible. Surgery may be indicated to establish a histological diagnosis and to relieve symptoms through debulking of the tumour. Pathological analysis confirms the nature of the lesion, excludes other treatable conditions (e.g. CNS lymphoma, cerebral abscess) and allows grading of the tumour which has prognostic value. Radiotherapy may treat both primary and secondary malignant CNS tumours and is also indicated in some benign lesions (e.g. recurrent pituitary adenoma, meningioma).

Chemotherapy may be used as an adjunct to surgery and/or radiotherapy. The oral alkylating agent temozolomide improves survival in gliomas when given in combination with radiotherapy.

Corticosteroids (e.g. dexamethasone) are used in patients with focal neurological features and/or raised intracranial pressure to reduce cerebral oedema. Anticonvulsants are used to control/reduce associated seizure activity.

Specific intracranial tumours

Acoustic neuroma (Schwannoma)

Arises from the nerve sheath cells of the acoustic (eighth) nerve in the region of the internal auditory meatus. It is more common in neurofibromatosis. Symptoms include progressive unilateral sensorineural deafness, diminished reaction on caloric testing, tinnitus and vertigo. Pressure on other ipsilateral cranial nerves at the cerebellopontine angle may produce:

- facial nerve palsy
- trigeminal nerve involvement.

Tumour growth produces ipsilateral ataxia (brainstem-cerebellar compression) and bulbar cranial nerve involvement.

Meningioma

Generally benign (although sometimes locally invasive or aggressive) tumours that arise from the meninges. In addition to clinical features common to all intracranial tumours, meningiomas in certain locations may manifest specific presenting symptoms/signs:

- olfactory groove: anosmia, papilloedema, frontal lobe dysfunction
- sphenoid wing: optic nerve compression with unilateral visual loss and optic atrophy
- parasagittal: spastic paraparesis
- cavernous sinus/parasellar region: cavernous sinus syndrome and/or hypothalamic-pituitary dysfunction.

Surgical excision or debulking is undertaken wherever possible, with radiotherapy reserved for surgically inaccessible, incompletely resected, or recurrent tumours.

Pituitary adenomas

These account for ~10% of all diagnosed intracranial neoplasms. Presentation is typically with one or more of the following:

- endocrine hyperfunction (e.g. hyperprolactinaemia, Cushing syndrome, acromegaly)
- endocrine hypofunction (i.e. varying degrees of hypopituitarism)
- local mass effects (e.g. optic chiasmal compression, cavernous sinus syndrome).

High resolution CT/MR scanning reveals pituitary 'incidentalomas' in 10–15% of the population, although most of these are non-functioning lesions that do not require treatment.

See pituitary disorders in Chapter 16.

Guillain–Barré syndrome (GBS)

GBS is characterised by ascending paralysis with subacute weakness and reduced tendon reflexes. Patients may manifest paraesthesias in the hands and feet, although sensory abnormalities on examination are often mild. There is an inflammatory demyelinating polyradiculoneuropathy affecting predominantly motor nerves. It has an annual incidence of 1–2 per 100 000 and is the most common cause of neuromuscular paralysis in the Western world.

Aetiology

GBS is due to an autoimmune peripheral neuropathy, usually in healthy individuals with no antecedent history of autoimmune disease. Around 75% of patients give a history of an infectious illness preceding the onset of weakness by 1–2 weeks. Some antecedent infections share structural similarities (so-called molecular mimicry) with peripheral nerve components, e.g. *Campylobacter jejuni* contains β-N-acetylglucosamine residues homologous to the terminal carbohydrate residue of ganglioside GM1 and antibodies to one or more gangliosides are found in up to one-quarter of patients. Antibodies to ganglioside GQ1b are found in patients with the Miller–Fisher syndrome/variant. Other infections that have been linked with GBS include CMV, EBV, HIV and Zika virus.

Clinical features

Paraesthesia in the toes is followed within hours by flaccid paralysis of the lower limbs ascending to involve the arms and sometimes facial muscles, the muscles of the palate and pharynx and the external ocular muscles. Less commonly, the disease affects the upper limbs or the cranial nerves alone, or proximal more than distal muscles. Sensory symptoms are minimal or absent. GBS can be difficult to diagnose in the early stages as it may manifest with vague symptoms of weakness, neck or back pain and paraesthesia.

Paralysis is of lower motor neurone type and maximal disability occurs at 2–4 weeks (plateauing by day 28).

The major complications are:

- respiratory failure from weakness of respiratory muscles
- bulbar failure
- autonomic involvement causing lability of blood pressure and arrhythmias
- venous thrombosis with pulmonary embolism.

The Miller–Fisher variant is characterised by brainstem features of ataxia, ophthalmoplegia and areflexia.

Differential diagnosis

- brainstem infarct
- acute spinal cord lesion
- infection (e.g. Lyme disease, poliomyelitis)
- inflammation (e.g. neurosarcoidosis)
- paraneoplastic syndrome
- malignant infiltration of nerve roots
- vasculitis
- porphyria
- metabolic dysfunction (e.g. vitamin B_1 deficiency)
- hysteria

Investigation

GBS is predominantly a clinical diagnosis, supported by excluding other diagnoses and demonstrating characteristic findings in tests including:

- Electrophysiology: may show dispersed motor potentials and prolonged distal motor latencies; also helps to subclassify as predominantly demyelinating or axonal.
- Lumbar puncture: characteristically reveals a high CSF protein (>1 g/l) with no, or very few, white cells – a raised white cell count should prompt consideration of other diagnoses, e.g. human immunodeficiency virus (HIV), Lyme disease, leptomeningeal malignancy.
- Antiganglioside antibodies: see earlier.

Management

The most important aspect of treatment is the prevention of complications. Complete recovery occurs over several months in 80–90% of patients. Clinical management involves:

- Careful nursing with physiotherapy usually in a high-dependency/intensive care setting. Attention to preventing pressure sores, chest infection and contractures.

- Anticoagulants, passive movements of the legs and graduated compression stockings help reduce the risk of deep venous thrombosis and pulmonary embolism.
- Careful fluid balance and nutritional support.
- Vital capacity (VC) monitoring regularly with oxygen saturations (not peak flow).
- Intubation with ventilation may be necessary.
- Cardiac monitoring; temporary cardiac pacing may be required for persistent bradycardia.

Randomised controlled trials suggest that the recovery of non-ambulant patients treated early (within 2 weeks of symptom onset) is hastened by intravenous immunoglobulin for 5 days or by four to six plasma exchanges (over 8–10 days). Plasma exchange may also help ambulant patients and those with more long-standing symptoms. Corticosteroids are of no benefit in GBS.

Rehabilitation is an important part of the recovery process.

Prognosis

GBS has a high mortality rate (up to 10%) in the acute phase even with supportive care and immunoglobulin therapy. Causes of death include cardiac dysrhythmias, pulmonary embolism and sepsis. Residual disability and chronic fatigue affect a significant proportion of sufferers. Poor prognostic indicators include older age, rapid onset of weakness, requirement for ventilation, evidence of axonal degeneration on EEG and detectable antiganglioside antibodies.

Hereditary disorders

Hepatolenticular degeneration (Wilson's disease)

An autosomal recessive disorder (due to mutation of the *ATP7B* gene) where the primary defect is a failure to excrete copper into bile. Accumulation of hepatic copper inhibits the formation of serum caeruloplasmin. When hepatocytic storage capacity is exceeded, copper is released into the blood and deposited in the:

- liver – producing cirrhosis, hepatosplenomegaly and jaundice
- basal ganglia – producing choreoathetosis
- cerebrum – producing dementia and emotional lability
- eyes – producing Kayser–Fleischer rings (a green-gold 'fuzz') around the cornea (detectable on slit lamp examination) and cataract

- renal tubules (rarely) – producing the effects of heavy metal poisoning and renal tubular acidosis
- bones – producing osteoporosis and osteoarthritis
- red cells – producing haemolytic anaemia.

The cerebral type is more common than the hepatic type.

Management

- low dietary copper intake
- d-penicillamine (a chelating agent to increase 24-h urinary copper excretion)

Prognosis with treatment is very good. Siblings should be examined and screened for serum copper and caeruloplasmin levels plus 24-h urinary copper output.

Huntington's chorea

Autosomal dominant CAG triplet repeats in the huntingtin gene, with symptom onset usually between 30 and 45 years. The chorea is distal initially and involves the legs (with ataxia), arms (with clumsiness) and face. Rapid and jerky movements occur together with epilepsy. Chorea may respond to tetrabenazine, which depletes nerve endings of dopamine. Cognitive changes develop gradually with progression to dementia and death in about 10–15 years.

Hereditary ataxias

These are rare familial disorders, usually transmitted as autosomal dominant traits. Pathological changes of degeneration are present in one or more of the optic nerves, cerebellum, olives and long ascending tracts of the spinal cord. Each family presents its own particular variants.

Friedreich's ataxia

A rare autosomal recessive disorder (due to triplet repeat expansion in the *FXN* gene) characterised by degeneration in the dorsal and lateral (pyramidal) columns of the cord and the spinocerebellar tracts.

Clinical presentation

Cerebellar ataxia is noted at 5–15 years of age, affecting first the lower and then upper limbs. Pes cavus and spinal scoliosis may be present. Pyramidal tract involvement produces upper motor neurone lesions of the legs, and dorsal column involvement, sensory

changes and absent ankle jerks. Cardiomyopathy causes arrhythmias and heart failure and there may be optic atrophy. Mild dementia occurs late in the disease and patients usually die from cardiac disease in their 40s.

Cerebellar degeneration

This rare group of hereditary ataxias affects primarily the cerebellum and the cerebellar connections of the brainstem. They present in late middle age and must be distinguished from:

- posterior fossa tumours;
- paraneoplastic syndromes;
- vascular, metabolic, toxic infective or inflammatory disorders.

Hereditary spastic paraplegia

The pyramidal tracts are affected and patients develop progressive spasticity. The onset occurs from childhood to middle age. The disorder, when first seen, must be distinguished from cord compression and multiple sclerosis.

Leber's optic neuropathy (atrophy)

Typically presents in adolescence or young adulthood with subacute unilateral, then bilateral, visual failure. Males are more commonly affected than females, although inheritance is mitochondrial.

Hereditary motor and sensory neuropathy (Charcot–Marie–Tooth disease; peroneal muscular atrophy)

This condition is often confused with the muscle dystrophies. It is rare and genetic counselling is advisable. It is usually transmitted as an autosomal dominant trait, but in some families, is recessive or sex-linked (i.e. multiple gene defects have been implicated). It may be classified into two groups of hereditary motor and sensory neuropathy affecting the peripheral nerves:

- type I with thickened peripheral nerves as a result of repeated demyelination and remyelination (ulnar at elbow, and common peroneal at the neck of the fibula)
- type II as a result of axonal degeneration, without thickening.

Clinical presentation

It presents about the age of 20 years with wasting and weakness of all the distal lower limb muscles and pes cavus. Later, the upper limbs may be affected. The wasting stops at mid-thigh, producing an inverted champagne-bottle appearance, and at the elbows. Fasciculation and sensory loss are sometimes present and reflexes depressed. The disease usually arrests spontaneously and life expectancy is normal. Contractions may produce talipes equinovarus.

Narcolepsy

This rare condition usually starts in late puberty. The onset is sudden, with episodes of irresistible and inappropriate sleep typically lasting 10–20 min and from which the patient awakes refreshed. It is associated with cataplexy (attacks of sudden, brief muscle atonia often causing falls but without loss of consciousness, precipitated by strong emotions such as stress or laughter). The aetiology of narcolepsy remains poorly understood although there is an association with human leucocyte antigen (HLA) DR2 (DQB1). Loss of signalling by the neuropeptides orexin-A and orexin-B (also known as hypocretin-1 and hypocretin-2) appears to be an important factor. Modafinil, a central nervous system stimulant, is the preferred first-line treatment, although the long-term risk of dependency remains unclear. Cataplexy may respond to clomipramine.

Head injury and the Glasgow Coma Scale

Brain injury following head trauma reflects:

- primary damage at impact – including contusion and laceration of the cerebral cortex (both at the site of impact and 'contre-coup'), and diffuse white matter injury (due to axonal shearing)
- secondary complications – including haematoma, oedema, ischaemia, coning and infection.

The latter are potentially treatable, and early intervention can reduce the extent of residual neurological deficit in those who survive the initial insult.

Clinical presentation

Important clinical features in the history (possibly obtained from a third party) include:

- circumstances of injury
- duration of loss of consciousness and post-traumatic amnesia
- occurrence of a 'lucid interval', suggesting development of a secondary complication (haematoma, oedema)
- persistent headache and vomiting (raised intracranial pressure).

Examination

Check carefully for

- external evidence of trauma
- features suggestive of skull base fracture (e.g. bilateral periorbital haematoma and/or haematoma over the mastoid ['Battle's sign']; bleeding from the ear; subconjunctival haemorrhage; CSF leakage).
- other neurological signs.

Conscious level should be charted using the Glasgow Coma Scale (GCS) score (Table 15.9).

Investigations

All centres now routinely perform cranial CT in any patient in whom there is concern (e.g. transient/persistent impairment of consciousness, focal neurological signs, features to suggest skull base fracture) following head injury.

Table 15.9 Glasgow Coma Scale

Category	Response	Score
Eye-opening	Spontaneously	4
	To speech	3
	To pain	2
	None	1
Best verbal response	Orientated	5
	Confused	4
	Inappropriate words	3
	Incomprehensible sounds	2
	None	1
Best motor response	Obeys commands	6
	Localises to pain	5
	Withdraws from pain (normal flexion)	4
	Flexes abnormally to pain (spastic flexion)	3
	Extends to pain	2
	None	1
TOTAL		15

Table 15.10 Criteria for brainstem death	
Preconditions	Ensure CNS depressant drugs are not contributing to clinical state
	Confirm requirement for ventilatory support due to inadequate spontaneous respiration (effects of neuromuscular blockade must be excluded)
	Exclude hypothermia (core temperature <35 °C)
	Exclude severe metabolic/endocrine disorders (e.g. myxoedema)
	Ensure cause of patient's condition is known and that it is compatible with irreversible brain damage (radiological findings should support the diagnosis)
Tests	Absent oculocephalic ('doll's head') reflex[a]
	No pupillary response to light
	Absent corneal reflexes
	No gag reflex and no response to tracheal suction
	No motor response in cranial nerve territory to painful stimulus (e.g. supraorbital pressure or pinching of the nose)
	No spontaneous respiratory effort when patient is disconnected from ventilator[b]

[a]When the head is gently, but fully, rotated to either side there is absence of the normal transient eye movement in the opposite direction.
[b]PaO_2 is maintained throughout by preoxygenation of the patient prior to disconnection of the ventilator, and continued supply of high flow oxygen (6 l/min) via endotracheal tube thereafter, but $PaCO_2$ is allowed to rise to >6.65 kPa.

Management

Minor head injuries may be managed locally with wound cleansing/suturing and neurological observation, but patients with more severe injuries should be transferred to a specialist neurosurgical unit once stabilised. Surgical intervention may be required in cases of intracranial haematoma and for depressed skull fractures.

Medical therapy may include:

- intravenous mannitol and/or artificial hyperventilation for raised intracranial pressure
- anticonvulsants
- prophylactic antibiotics for suspected/confirmed skull base fracture(s).

Prognosis

Survivors of serious head injury may be left with numerous sequelae including:

- residual neurological deficit/cognitive impairment including persistent vegetative state

- post-traumatic epilepsy
- post-concussion syndrome
- hypopituitarism
- late complications including meningitis in cases of undetected CSF leakage and chronic subdural haematoma.

Criteria for diagnosis of brainstem death

In certain circumstances, irreversible brain damage occurs with permanent loss of brainstem function, but with preservation of cardiovascular function. The decision to remove cardiorespiratory support in such cases is dependent on a number of factors, including formal demonstration that the patient meets the criteria for brainstem death (Table 15.10). The assessment must be carried out by two doctors with appropriate expertise, at least one of whom should be a consultant. All 'preconditions' must be met before the tests are performed, which should be repeated at an interval, with death being certified at the time of the second set of tests providing the criteria are met.

16

Endocrine disorders

Diabetes mellitus (Chapter 17) and disorders of the thyroid gland are the most commonly encountered endocrine conditions in clinical practice.

Thyroid

The term 'goitre' simply denotes enlargement of the thyroid gland. It may be diffuse or nodular, simple or toxic, benign or malignant, and physiological or pathological. Minor enlargement of the thyroid is common, especially in women. Both hypothyroidism and hyperthyroidism are also common. In contrast, thyroid cancer is relatively rare.

Non-toxic goitre

Aetiology

A variety of factors may predispose to thyroid enlargement:

- *Simple goitre:* iodine deficiency, especially in areas of endemic goitre. Sporadic goitre may reflect relative iodine deficiency for that patient. Iodine requirement is increased at puberty in girls and during pregnancy.
- *Goitrogens:* e.g. iodide in large doses, antithyroid drugs, lithium.
- *Inborn errors of thyroid hormone biosynthesis (dyshormonogenesis):* the production of thyroid hormones is mediated by iodide uptake and oxidation, organification of thyroglobulin to generate iodotyrosines followed by their coupling to yield thyroxine (T4) and triiodothyronine (T3). Several genetic disorders involving proteins in this biosynthetic pathway have been described. For example, Pendred syndrome, which is characterised by sensorineural deafness and goitre, is caused by defects in pendrin, which transports iodine into the colloid.

Clinical presentation

The patient (or a relative) usually notices a painless swelling of the thyroid. With time it may develop into a large nodular goitre and cause pressure on the trachea, oesophagus or veins, especially if there is significant retrosternal extension.

Differential diagnosis

The differential diagnosis of thyroid enlargement is shown in Table 16.1.

Investigation

- Thyroid function tests: serum-free thyroxine (FT4) and thyrotropin (thyroid-stimulating hormone, TSH); if TSH is suppressed, but with normal FT4, check serum-free triiodothyronine (FT3) for possible T3-toxicosis.
- Thyroid autoantibodies (e.g. antithyroid peroxidase) for Hashimoto's disease.
- CT scan of neck and thorax if pressure symptoms are present; respiratory flow-volume loops may also help to confirm/refute significant airway obstruction.
- Ultrasound can help distinguish solid or cystic masses and whether the patient has a single or multiple nodules; in addition, the likelihood of benign versus malignant disease in a nodule may be predicted based on specific features (e.g. microcalcification, vascularity, etc.). However, ultrasound is not required in all cases.
- Fine-needle aspiration biopsy (FNAB) with cytology is performed for solitary or dominant nodules or if there is clinical concern regarding possible malignancy; it is commonly performed under ultrasound guidance.

NB: Thyroid radioisotope scans are not generally performed unless the patient is thyrotoxic (see later).

Clinical Medicine Lecture Notes, Eighth Edition. John R. Bradley, Mark Gurnell, and Diana F. Wood.
© 2019 John Wiley & Sons Ltd. Published 2019 by John Wiley & Sons Ltd.

Table 16.1 Causes of thyroid enlargement (goitre and/or nodules)

	Type	Examples
Diffuse goitre	Physiological	Puberty, pregnancy
	Autoimmune	Graves' disease, Hashimoto's disease
	Thyroiditis	Subacute (De Quervain's), Riedel's
	Endemic	Iodine deficiency
	Goitrogens	Antithyroid drugs, lithium, iodine excess
	Dyshormonogenesis	Pendred syndrome (hearing loss and goitre)
Nodular goitre	Multinodular	Toxic, non-toxic
	Solitary nodule	Follicular adenoma, benign nodule or cyst, thyroid malignancy, lymphoma, metastasis
	Infiltration (rare)	Tuberculosis, sarcoidosis

Table 16.2 Causes of thyrotoxicosis

Type	Frequency	Condition(s)
Primary	Common	Graves' disease
		Toxic multinodular goitre
	Less common	Solitary toxic adenoma
		Thyroiditis (e.g. post-partum; subacute)
		Drug-induced (e.g. amiodarone; over-treatment with/inappropriate administration of L-T4 and/or L-T3 therapy)
		Excess iodine intake (e.g. health food supplements such as kelp, or drugs, e.g. amiodarone)
		'Hashitoxicosis' (hyperthyroid phase of Hashimoto's thyroiditis)
	Rare	Metastatic follicular thyroid carcinoma
		Struma ovarii (ovarian tumour containing thyroid tissue)
Secondary	Rare	TSH-secreting pituitary adenoma
		Resistance to thyroid hormone
		Trophoblastic tumour secreting hCG (shared/common α subunit with TSH)

TSH, thyrotropin (= thyroid-stimulating hormone); hCG, human chorionic gonadotrophin.

Treatment

If the patient is euthyroid and there are no concerns regarding possible malignancy, treatment is not required unless the swelling is unsightly or causing pressure symptoms, when surgery (or occasionally radioiodine therapy) may be indicated. If TSH is raised (subclinical hypothyroidism), thyroxine can be given to suppress TSH hypersecretion (TSH is trophic for thyroid growth).

Thyrotoxicosis (hyperthyroidism)

Thyrotoxicosis is the clinical disorder resulting from exposure to raised circulating levels of thyroid hormone (T4 and/or T3). It is most commonly due to thyroid gland dysfunction (hyperthyroidism), but can occur when exogenous T4 and/or T3 is taken in excess. The prevalence of hyperthyroidism in the UK has been estimated at 1–2%, with a female predominance female to male ~5–10 : 1.

Aetiology

The causes of thyrotoxicosis are shown in Table 16.2. Graves' disease is an autoimmune disorder in which autoantibodies against the TSH receptor (TRAb) provide continual (unregulated) stimulation of thyroid follicular cells leading to thyroid enlargement (diffuse smooth goitre) and thyrotoxicosis. Involvement of the retro-orbital tissues and skin may also result in Graves' ophthalmopathy and dermopathy (pretibial myxoedema), respectively. Environmental 'triggers' (e.g. stress, pregnancy, drugs) combined with genetic susceptibility (e.g. HLA-DR3, cytotoxic T-lymphocyte antigen 4 (CTLA4) variants) are implicated in many cases.

Clinical presentation

The symptoms and signs of thyrotoxicosis are shown in Fig. 16.1. Several of these are reminiscent of a 'hyperadrenergic state'. However, other features are specific for the underlying disorder (see Box 16.1).

Other presentations

- hyperactivity, increased linear growth and weight gain in children
- apathy and depression, atrial fibrillation and cardiac failure in the elderly
- thyroid crisis – mainly seen in patients with unrecognised or poorly controlled disease; intercurrent illness, surgery or radioiodine therapy may serve as precipitants; typical features include hyperpyrexia, profuse sweating, restlessness, confusion/psychosis, dysrhythmias and cardiac failure. If untreated coma and death may ensue.

Differential diagnosis

Thyrotoxicosis may be difficult to differentiate from an anxiety state (with hyperadrenergic features),

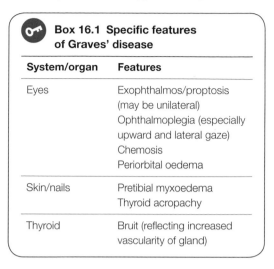

Box 16.1 Specific features of Graves' disease

System/organ	Features
Eyes	Exophthalmos/proptosis (may be unilateral) Ophthalmoplegia (especially upward and lateral gaze) Chemosis Periorbital oedema
Skin/nails	Pretibial myxoedema Thyroid acropachy
Thyroid	Bruit (reflecting increased vascularity of gland)

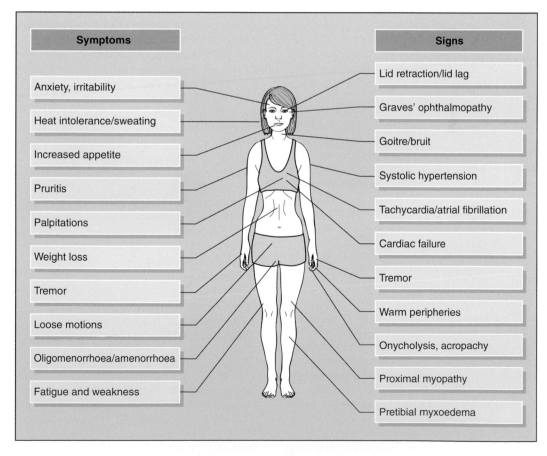

Symptoms	Signs
Anxiety, irritability	Lid retraction/lid lag
Heat intolerance/sweating	Graves' ophthalmopathy
Increased appetite	Goitre/bruit
Pruritis	Systolic hypertension
Palpitations	Tachycardia/atrial fibrillation
Weight loss	Cardiac failure
Tremor	Tremor
Loose motions	Warm peripheries
Oligomenorrhoea/amenorrhoea	Onycholysis, acropachy
Fatigue and weakness	Proximal myopathy
	Pretibial myxoedema

Figure 16.1 Schematic representation of the symptoms and signs associated with thyrotoxicosis.

particularly when this is coincidentally associated with a simple goitre.

Investigation

- TSH – fully suppressed (i.e. <0.1 mU/l. NB: Modern TSH assays may report even lower limits of detection, e.g. <0.03 mU/l).
- FT4 and FT3 – typically both are elevated, although FT4 may fall within the reference range, but with raised FT3 in cases of 'T3-toxicosis'.
- TSH receptor antibody (TRAb) – many laboratories now routinely offer TRAb measurement, which is both sensitive and specific for Graves' disease.

NB: Thyroid peroxidase (TPO) titres are not elevated in all patients with Graves' disease and are not therefore routinely measured.

- A radioiodine or (more commonly) technetium uptake scan can help distinguish Graves' disease, toxic nodular goitre, toxic adenoma or thyroiditis in cases where there are no specific clinical features of Graves' disease (Box 16.1) and TRAb is not raised.
- CT/MRI of the orbits may be required to assess the extent of eye disease in Graves' ophthalmopathy.

Treatment

Beta-blockers

- Preferably non-selective, e.g. propranolol 20–40 mg t.d.s. for rapid relief of symptoms.

Antithyroid drug (ATD) therapy

- Carbimazole (CBZ) or propylthiouracil (PTU): result in long-term remission in ~40–50% of cases of Graves' disease; regimens include (1) 'titration', i.e. beginning with a higher dose (e.g. CBZ 40–60 mg/day), then titrating to a lower maintenance level (e.g. CBZ 5–15 mg/day) and continuing for 12–18 months; (2) 'block and replace', in which the ATD dose is maintained at a higher level (e.g. CBZ 40 mg/day), with thyroxine added back (once FT4/FT3 levels are controlled), and typically continued for 6–12 months.
- ATDs control, but do not cure, thyrotoxicosis in toxic multinodular goitre/toxic solitary adenoma; ATDs are ineffective in cases of inflammatory/destructive thyroiditis where stored hormone is released – β-blockers are preferred to block peripheral actions of excess hormone.
- It is important to avoid inducing hypothyroidism, especially in patients with coexistent Graves' ophthalmopathy, which can be exacerbated.
- Side effects of ATDs include skin rashes (often minor and respond to antihistamines or changing agent) and the more serious agranulocytosis and/or thrombocytopenia. All patients on ATDs must therefore be warned of this possibility and given instructions (including in written format) advising them to immediately stop treatment and attend their GP or local hospital for a full blood count if they develop a sore throat, mouth ulceration or fever. If confirmed, the patient should **not** be restarted on/switched to an alternative ATD, as the risk of recurrence is high. Hepatic dysfunction (PTU) and cholestatic jaundice (CBZ) are also important recognised side effects.
- Traditionally treatment with PTU in a titration regimen was preferred in pregnancy because of the risk, albeit rare, of fetal malformation (in particular aplasia cutis) with CBZ therapy; however, concerns regarding potential PTU-induced hepatic dysfunction has led clinicians to favour a mixed regimen whereby PTU is used during the first trimester, but if ongoing treatment is required thereafter, the woman is switched to CBZ.

Radioactive iodine therapy (RAI; ^{131}I)

- May be used as first-line therapy (especially for toxic nodular goitre/nodule) or following ATD failure.
- Typically given in doses ranging from 300–800 MBq; using higher doses reduces rates of relapse but increases rates of hypothyroidism.
- ATDs must be discontinued prior to RAI (~1 week before for CBZ, but longer for PTU) to ensure adequate thyroidal uptake, but can be restarted 5–7 days later and continued for 2–3 months, at which point residual thyroid status should be assessed.
- Patients with a single toxic adenoma or a toxic multinodular goitre can receive a large dose of RAI with relatively little chance of subsequent hypothyroidism, because the unaffected parts of the thyroid lie dormant following suppression of TSH by excessive thyroid hormone secretion and therefore do not take up the RAI.
- RAI is contraindicated in pregnancy (which should be avoided for 6 months after treatment) and in breast-feeding mothers; men are advised not to attempt to father a child for 4 months after RAI.
- Most centres avoid RAI in patients with severe Graves' ophthalmopathy, but permit treatment in mild to moderate cases under steroid cover (e.g. prednisolone 30–40 mg/day).

Surgery

- Total or subtotal thyroidectomy may be performed.
- Normally reserved for those with relapsing thyrotoxicosis who decline or who are not suitable for RAI, or if there are significant compressive symptoms.
- Potential complications include haemorrhage, vocal cord paresis, hypoparathyroidism and hypothyroidism.

Treatment of complications

Eyes

- Control of the underlying thyrotoxicosis is essential in all patients; lid retraction usually resolves with restoration of euthyroidism.
- Simple lubricants and taping the eyelids closed at night may help in milder cases.
- In severe cases of Graves' ophthalmopathy, and in those failing to improve with correction of the thyroid disturbance, treatment with high-dose corticosteroids, other immunosuppressive agents, orbital decompression or radiotherapy may be required.
- Smoking exacerbates ophthalmopathy.

Atrial fibrillation

- Atrial fibrillation responds poorly to digoxin and larger doses are often needed until the patient is rendered euthyroid. Propranolol or other β-blockers may provide better rate control.
- Anticoagulation is also required as the risk of embolisation is relatively high.

Thyrotoxic crisis/thyroid storm

This is a rare but potentially life-threatening disorder, which requires urgent treatment targeted at various steps in the thyroid hormone synthesis/action pathway:

- Stop further hormone synthesis: CBZ (20 mg orally or via nasogastric tube 4–6-hourly) or PTU (200 mg orally or via nasogastric tube 4–6-hourly).
- Impair release of stored hormone: sodium iodide (0.5–1 g IV 12-hourly) or saturated solution of potassium iodide (6–8 drops orally every 6 h); the radiographic contrast agents ipodate and iopanoic acid may also be used and have the added benefit of markedly impairing T4 to T3 conversion.

- Block peripheral manifestations of excess thyroid hormones: propranolol (initially 0.5–2 mg IV slowly, followed by 40–80 mg orally 6–8-hourly). Verapamil can be used in those with a history of asthma.
- High-dose glucocorticoids: dexamethasone (2 mg orally or IV 6–8-hourly) reduces peripheral conversion of T4 to T3.
- Supportive measures: O_2 therapy, intravenous fluids, active cooling, diuretics, chlorpromazine as indicated.

Hypothyroidism

Hypothyroidism is the clinical condition resulting from low levels of circulating thyroid hormones. The term 'myxoedema' refers to the deposition of mucopolysaccharide beneath the skin, producing a non-pitting swelling of the subcutaneous tissues.

Hypothyroidism is common, with a prevalence of 1–2% in the general population. Females are much more commonly affected (female to male ratio ~10 : 1), reflecting the high proportion of cases due to autoimmune disease (see later).

Congenital hypothyroidism occurs in 1 in 3000 to 1 in 4000 live births in the UK.

Aetiology

The causes of hypothyroidism are shown in Table 16.3.

Clinical presentation

The symptoms and signs of hypothyroidism are shown in Fig. 16.2.

Other presentations

- Subclinical hypothyroidism – characterised biochemically by normal FT4 and FT3 levels in the

Table 16.3 Causes of hypothyroidism

Type	Frequency	Condition(s)
Primary	Common	Autoimmune (e.g. Hashimoto's thyroiditis – typically associated with a goitre: atrophic thyroiditis when the gland atrophies without producing a goitre) Previous treatment for thyrotoxicosis (e.g. surgery, RAI)
	Less common	Defects of hormone synthesis (e.g. iodine deficiency or excess, ATD therapy, lithium, amiodarone or, rarely, dyshormonogenesis) Thyroiditis (often transient)
	Rare	Infiltration Thyroid gland hypoplasia or agenesis
Secondary	Less common	Hypothalamic or pituitary disorders

RAI, radioactive iodine therapy; ATD, antithyroid drug therapy.

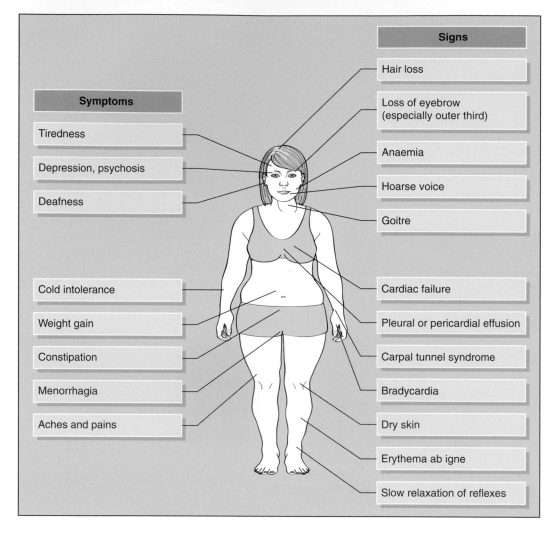

Figure 16.2 Schematic representation of the symptoms and signs associated with hypothyroidism.

presence of a mildly elevated TSH. The patient may be asymptomatic or manifest mild hypothyroid features or hypercholesterolaemia.

- Pregnancy – untreated maternal hypothyroidism is associated with higher rates of miscarriage, stillbirth and congenital abnormalities. Even mild maternal hypothyroidism may be associated with a reduction in IQ of the offspring. Thyroxine requirements can increase by 50–100% during pregnancy and thyroid function tests should ideally be checked prior to conception and at regular intervals during pregnancy.
- Myxoedema coma – a rare but life-threatening medical emergency.

Investigation

- Serum FT4 is reduced and this stimulates pituitary secretion of TSH (raised in primary hypothyroidism). FT3 is also low, although routine measurement is not required in most instances.
- Elevated antithyroid peroxidase (TPO) antibodies.
- Serum cholesterol is often raised and creatine kinase (CK) may also be elevated, reflecting hepatic and muscle hypothyroidism, respectively.
- Anaemia (microcytic if menorrhagia, macrocytic if coexistent pernicious anaemia, or normocytic).
- ECG shows slow rate and low voltage with flattened or inverted T waves.

NB: Check for use of drugs, e.g. lithium, amiodarone. Amiodarone is rich in iodine and also inhibits peripheral conversion of T4 to T3, making thyroid investigations more difficult to interpret. Ideally, before starting treatment with amiodarone, basal FT3, FT4 and TSH levels should be checked to identify any underlying thyroid disease.

- The finding of low FT4 and FT3 levels with an inappropriately low or normal TSH is strongly suggestive of a central (hypothalamic/pituitary) disorder.
- Low TSH with low FT3 and low/low-normal FT4 may also be seen in non-thyroidal illness (so-called sick-euthyroid syndrome).

Treatment

- Standard treatment is with levo-thyroxine (L-T4), typically beginning with a dose of 50 mcg/day.
- A full replacement dose (e.g. in an adult patient post-total thyroidectomy) is ~1.6–2.0 mcg/kg/day.
- Lower starting doses should be used in the elderly or in those with known or suspected ischaemic heart disease.
- Reassess clinically and check FT4 and TSH at 4- to 6-weekly intervals until stabilised on treatment.
- In primary hypothyroidism, titrate L-T4 to achieve TSH level in the lower half of the reference range (i.e. 0.4–2.0 mU/l); in central hypothyroidism TSH is unreliable and treatment should be titrated to alleviate symptoms and achieve an FT4 level in the normal (typically upper half of the) reference range.

NB: In subjects with suspected coexistent hypoadrenalism do not start L-T4 until the diagnosis has been excluded or confirmed and glucocorticosteroid replacement commenced.

- Myxoedema coma: treatment includes ventilatory and circulatory support, correction of hypothermia and hypoglycaemia, glucocorticosteroid replacement until normal adrenal reserve is demonstrated, treatment of precipitating event and thyroid hormone replacement (L-T4 or L-T3 – dose and regimen should be decided in conjunction with an endocrinologist).

Thyroiditis

Acute thyroiditis

- Although relatively uncommon, acute thyroiditis may follow an upper respiratory tract or other infection.

- There is fever and malaise, usually with some local swelling and tenderness of the gland and sometimes dysphagia.
- Initially the patient may experience thyrotoxic features as stored hormone is released from the gland, prior to developing hypothyroidism, which may be transient or occasionally permanent.
- Classical appearance on radioiodine/technetium scan with very low or absent uptake.
- Treatment with simple analgesia (e.g. NSAID) may suffice.
- Occasionally prednisolone 30 mg/day is necessary, but this can usually be tailed off rapidly.
- ATDs are ineffective in the treatment of the thyrotoxic phase; β-blockers control symptoms.

Post-partum thyroiditis

- typically occurs within the first 6 months post-delivery
- usually painless
- thyrotoxic phase must be distinguished from Graves' disease developing/relapsing in the post-partum period. TRAb antibodies are typically raised in the latter.

Thyroid cancer (Table 16.4)

- commonest endocrine cancer, although still relatively rare
- Table 16.4 summarises important features of each of the subtypes

Pituitary

Pituitary anatomy and physiology

The hypothalamus and pituitary lie in close proximity to each other and are connected by the pituitary stalk. Both are surrounded by a number of important structures and the pituitary gland sits within a bony seat, the sella turcica (Fig. 16.3). The optic chiasm lies just above the pituitary fossa, and on either side are the cavernous sinuses ('venous lakes') through which the intracavernous carotid artery passes. The third, fourth, upper division of the fifth and sixth cranial nerves lie within the lateral and inferior aspects of the cavernous sinuses, rendering them susceptible to compression by tumours with parasellar extension. The sphenoid sinus, which is below the pituitary fossa, is the route through which the pituitary gland is approached during trans-sphenoidal surgery (Fig. 16.3).

Table 16.4 Thyroid malignancy

Type	Epidemiology/aetio-pathogenesis	Clinical features/spread/metastases	Treatment/prognosis
Papillary thyroid cancer	• ~70–80% of all cases • ♂ : ♀ ~1 : 3 • Peak incidence during fourth and fifth decades of life, but also smaller peak in second and third decades • External irradiation or exposure to radioactive iodine isotopes (e.g. following the Chernobyl nuclear incident) at an age <20 years is associated with ↑ risk • Translocations in genes encoding effectors of the MAP-kinase (MAPK) pathway, e.g. RET-PTC proto-oncogene rearrangements, are often found, especially after irradiation • Activating mutations of RAS or BRAF are important drivers in some patients	• Slow growing • Local spread to cervical lymph nodes is common at presentation, but distant metastases are rare	• Total thyroidectomy for all but the smallest of tumours • Modified radical neck dissection for cervical node involvement • Ablative radioiodine therapy is also required in many cases • Life-long thyroxine therapy to suppress TSH used to be considered a mandatory requirement, although this is no longer universally the case (e.g. in completely excised small tumours with no evidence of spread/recurrence during follow-up) • For refractory/relapsing disease kinase inhibitors may be beneficial in some patients • Thyroglobulin levels serve as a useful tumour marker following total thyroidectomy • Cancer-related deaths occur in <5% of cases during 10 years' follow-up
Follicular thyroid cancer	• ~10–15% of all cases • ♂ : ♀ ~1 : 2–3 • Peak incidence during fifth decade of life	• More aggressive than papillary carcinoma • Local spread to cervical lymph nodes may occur • Haematogenous spread (e.g. to lung and bone) is more common than with papillary carcinoma	• Treatment as per papillary carcinoma • Cancer-related deaths in 5–10% of cases during 10 years' follow-up

| Medullary thyroid cancer | • ~5% of all cases
• ♂ : ♀ ~1 : 1
• Peak incidence during fourth and fifth decade of life for sporadic MTC, but much earlier (including in childhood) for hereditary cases
• Both sporadic and hereditary MTC are associated with mutations in the *RET* proto-oncogene
• A component of the MEN-2A and MEN-2B syndromes | • More aggressive than papillary or follicular carcinoma
• Locally invasive
• Distant spread by lymphatics and blood | • Possible phaeochromocytoma (as part of the MEN-2 syndrome) must be excluded before surgical intervention
• Total thyroidectomy may be curative in the early stages – hence the rationale for genetic screening of relatives
• Central compartment/lymph node dissection is required in most cases
• Radioiodine and TSH suppression are not indicated in MTC
• Systemic chemotherapy and external beam irradiation are of limited value
• For refractory/relapsing disease kinase inhibition (e.g. with vandetanib which targets RET) may be beneficial in some patients
• Plasma calcitonin levels serve as a useful tumour marker |
| Anaplastic thyroid cancer | • <5% of all cases
• ♂ : ♀ ~1–2 : 1
• Peak incidence during seventh and eighth decades of life | • Aggressive
• Typically presents with painful, rapidly expanding thyroid mass, which infiltrates local tissues and hence does not move on swallowing | • Although surgery, external irradiation and chemotherapy may be tried, few patients survive for more than 6–12 months |

MTC, medullary thyroid carcinoma; MEN, multiple endocrine neoplasia.

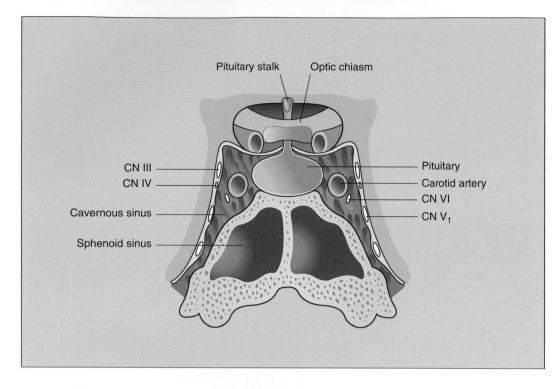

Figure 16.3 Pituitary anatomy: line drawing demonstrating the relationship of the pituitary gland to adjacent vascular and neurological structures. CN, cranial nerve.

The hypothalamus and pituitary work in concert to regulate a number of different endocrine systems involved in processes as diverse as growth, metabolism and reproduction. Hypothalamic releasing factors (e.g. growth hormone releasing hormone (GHRH), gonadotrophin releasing hormone (GnRH), corticotropin releasing hormone (CRH) and thyrotropin releasing hormone (TRH)) travel down the pituitary stalk to regulate release of growth hormone (GH), the gonadotrophins (luteinising hormone [LH] and follicle stimulating hormone [FSH]), adrenocorticotrophic hormone (ACTH) and thyrotropin (TSH) from anterior pituitary somatotrophs, gonadotrophs, corticotrophs and thyrotrophs, respectively. In addition, the inhibitory hormones somatostatin and dopamine are also released by the hypothalamus to regulate pituitary hormone synthesis and secretion. For example, somatostatin negatively regulates GH, TSH and to a lesser extent ACTH release, while pituitary lactotrophs are under tonic inhibitory control by dopamine (Fig. 16.4).

In contrast to the anterior pituitary, hormonal synthesis does not occur within the posterior pituitary, but instead hormones (antidiuretic hormone [ADH = vasopressin] and oxytocin) synthesised by hypothalamic neurones travel down the pituitary stalk in axonal projections that finish in the posterior pituitary where the mature hormones are stored in vesicles for release.

Knowledge of the anatomy and physiology of the hypothalamus and pituitary helps to understand the different presentations of patients with sellar and parasellar lesions. In essence, pituitary disorders typically present with one or more of the following:

- Hormone hypersecretion – e.g. excess production of growth hormone in acromegaly and ACTH in Cushing's disease.
- Hormone hyposecretion – e.g. partial or complete hypopituitarism as a consequence of damage to/suppression of the remaining normal pituitary tissue.
- Local mass effects – due to compression/infiltration of adjacent structures, e.g. bi-temporal field defects (due to optic chiasmal compression), third, fourth or sixth cranial nerve palsies (if there is involvement of the cavernous sinuses, especially if this occurs acutely, e.g. pituitary apoplexy) or headache (due to invasion of the bony wall of the sphenoid sinus).

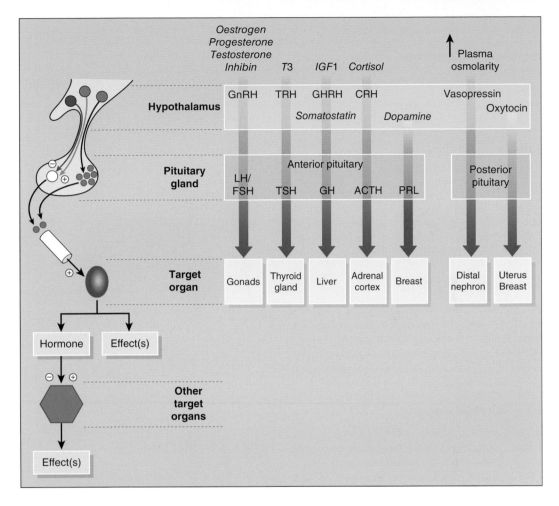

Figure 16.4 Hypothalamic-pituitary-target organ axes. Specific hypothalamic releasing (GnRH, TRH, GHRH, CRH) and inhibiting (somatostatin, dopamine) factors regulate synthesis/secretion of anterior pituitary hormones, which in turn control target organ function. In contrast, vasopressin and oxytocin are transported along axonal projections from the hypothalamus to the posterior pituitary and stored in vesicles prior to release. Negative feedback at the level of the pituitary and hypothalamus is mediated via hormones secreted by target organs (shown in italics).

Pituitary adenomas and hypopituitarism

The term hypopituitarism denotes an insufficiency of one or more of the anterior or posterior pituitary hormones. With pituitary tumours, the usual sequence in which pituitary hormone function is lost is GH, followed by LH/FSH, followed by ACTH and finally TSH. Interestingly, prolactin insufficiency is rare in this setting and indeed the lactotrophs are remarkably resistant to pressure effects, such that prolactin levels often rise as the tonic inhibitory control of dopamine is lost due to stalk compression. ADH insufficiency is also unusual in this setting. In contrast, inflammatory or infiltrative disorders of the pituitary may be associated with ADH deficiency and different patterns of anterior hypopituitarism.

Aetiology

Destruction/compression of the normal pituitary tissue or reduction in the blood supply (including the hypothalamic–pituitary portal circulation) accounts for the majority of cases of hypopituitarism (Table 16.5). Aside from a small number of familial cases (e.g. due to mutations in *MENIN, AIP*), the factors underlying pituitary adenoma formation remain poorly understood. Recently, however, somatic mutations in the *USP8* deubiquitinase

Table 16.5 Causes of hypopituitarism	
Frequency	**Condition(s)**
Common	Pituitary/peripituitary tumours (or as a complication of treatment, including surgery and radiotherapy)
Rare	Vascular (e.g. pituitary apoplexy, Sheehan syndrome) Pituitary infiltration (e.g. metastasis, sarcoidosis, histiocytosis) Infection (e.g. tuberculosis, pituitary abscess) Autoimmune (lymphocytic hypophysitis) Traumatic (e.g. post head injury) Congenital Idiopathic

gene (which putatively increases signalling via the EGF receptor) have been identified in a proportion of corticotroph tumours causing Cushing's disease.

Clinical presentation

This is variable and depends on not only the aetiology but also the extent of endocrine dysfunction and the rapidity of onset. In the majority of cases patients present with features of one or more of hormone hypersecretion, hormone hyposecretion or local mass effects, as outlined earlier.

Hormone hypersecretion

Prolactinomas are the most commonly encountered functioning pituitary adenoma, and tumours secreting growth hormone, ACTH and TSH are seen less frequently.

Hyperprolactinaemia per se is associated with reduced libido in both sexes and galactorrhoea in females. In addition, however, even in the presence of a small prolactinoma, which is insufficient to cause compression of the adjacent normal pituitary tissue, hypogonadotrophic hypogonadism is frequently seen as a consequence of the suppressive effect of high prolactin levels on the hypothalamic GnRH pulse generator. Accordingly, oligomenorrhoea/amenorrhoea in females and erectile dysfunction in males are commonly encountered. It is important to note, however, that hyperprolactinaemia is not always caused by a prolactinoma. Physiological stimuli such as stress, use of certain drugs (e.g. antidopaminergic agents), inhibition of dopaminergic tone through pituitary stalk compression (e.g. by a non-functioning pituitary adenoma), renal failure and several other disorders can all lead to elevated serum prolactin levels.

Clinical features of Cushing syndrome (due to hypercortisolism) and acromegaly (due to GH/insulin-like growth factor-1 [IGF-1] excess) are shown in Figs. 16.5 and 16.6, respectively.

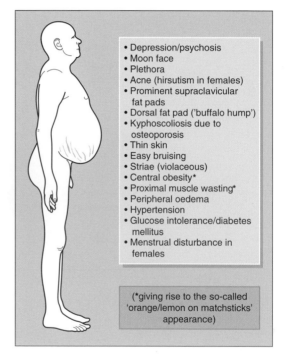

- Depression/psychosis
- Moon face
- Plethora
- Acne (hirsutism in females)
- Prominent supraclavicular fat pads
- Dorsal fat pad ('buffalo hump')
- Kyphoscoliosis due to osteoporosis
- Thin skin
- Easy bruising
- Striae (violaceous)
- Central obesity*
- Proximal muscle wasting*
- Peripheral oedema
- Hypertension
- Glucose intolerance/diabetes mellitus
- Menstrual disturbance in females

(*giving rise to the so-called 'orange/lemon on matchsticks' appearance)

Figure 16.5 Schematic representation showing the key clinical features associated with Cushing syndrome.

Hormone hyposecretion

In addition to features of hypogonadism, patients may manifest with features of GH deficiency (e.g. tiredness, reduced stamina, impaired cognition), ACTH deficiency (pallor, postural hypotension, reduced axillary/pubic hair, tiredness/lethargy) and TSH deficiency (tiredness/lethargy, cold intolerance, constipation, etc.).

Posterior pituitary dysfunction, and in particular diabetes insipidus (DI) due to ADH deficiency, is very rarely a presenting manifestation of a pituitary adenoma, and is more commonly encountered following

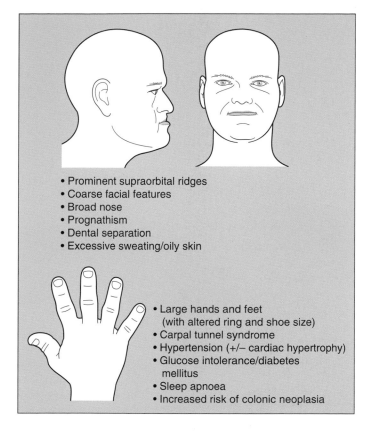

- Prominent supraorbital ridges
- Coarse facial features
- Broad nose
- Prognathism
- Dental separation
- Excessive sweating/oily skin

- Large hands and feet
  (with altered ring and shoe size)
- Carpal tunnel syndrome
- Hypertension (+/− cardiac hypertrophy)
- Glucose intolerance/diabetes
  mellitus
- Sleep apnoea
- Increased risk of colonic neoplasia

Figure 16.6 Schematic representation showing the key clinical features associated with acromegaly.

pituitary surgery (when it is often transient), but can also be seen with infiltrative disorders (e.g. sarcoidosis). When present, cranial (hypothalamic) DI must be distinguished from nephrogenic DI (in which there is renal resistance to the action of ADH) and also from habitual/compulsive water drinking (dipsogenic DI). Lack of ADH action results in polyuria (greater than 3 litres of urine output per 24 h), which in turn stimulates thirst and leads to polydipsia.

Local mass effect(s)

In addition to compression of the normal pituitary gland, sellar/parasellar lesions may cause compression of the optic chiasm, resulting initially in a superior quadrantic bi-temporal field defect (signifying pressure on the underside of the chiasm), which ultimately progresses to a complete bi-temporal hemianopia (Fig. 16.7). In contrast, lesions originating in the suprasellar region (e.g. craniopharyngioma) may initially give rise to inferior quadrantic field defects, reflecting chiasmal compression from above. Third, fourth and sixth cranial nerve palsies are relatively rare even with lateral tumour extension, but may be seen with infiltrative lesions or if there is rapid

expansion of a tumour, for example following haemorrhage, as occurs in pituitary apoplexy.

Investigation

Again, for ease of memory, the investigation of pituitary disorders can be considered under the headings of hormone hypersecretion, hormone hyposecretion and local mass effects.

Hormone hypersecretion

Hyperprolactinaemia

Wherever possible the confounding effects of medications and other disorders (e.g. renal failure, macroprolactinaema [a condition in which prolactin is bound by immunoglobulin thus rendering it biologically inactive but with preserved immunoreactivity in laboratory assays]) should be excluded; thereafter, genuine hyperprolactinaemia should be confirmed on at least two separate samples.

Cushing syndrome

(NB: Pituitary-dependent Cushing syndrome = Cushing's disease)

Superior quadrantic bitemporal field defect

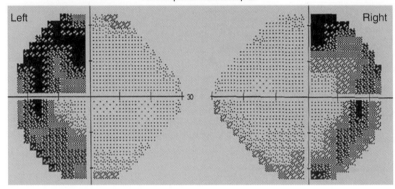

Bitemporal hemianopia

Figure 16.7 Visual field assessments in patients with pituitary adenomas causing compression of the optic chiasm.

Investigation of pathological hypercortisolaemia is approached in two stages:

1. Confirm diagnosis

   Most centres use one or more of the following for screening purposes, with confirmation/further investigation of positive results:

   - 24-h urinary free cortisol excretion (at least three separate collections)
   - loss of diurnal cortisol variation (measured either on serum or on salivary samples)
   - overnight dexamethasone suppression test (1 mg at 23:00 h with serum cortisol measured at 09:00 h the following morning)
   - low-dose dexamethasone suppression test (0.5 mg every 6 h for a total of 8 doses with serum cortisol measured at 09:00 h following the final dose).

   Normal subjects suppress serum cortisol to <50 nmol/l in both dexamethasone tests.

2. Define aetiology

   Once the diagnosis has been confirmed tests are undertaken to establish the cause. Measurement of plasma ACTH distinguishes between ACTH-dependent (pituitary adenoma [i.e. Cushing's disease] and ectopic ACTH secretion [e.g. due to small cell bronchial carcinoma or thymic carcinoid tumour]) and ACTH-independent (adrenal adenoma, adrenal carcinoma, adrenal nodular disease) causes.

   NB: It is important to exclude exogenous glucocorticoid administration (which is the commonest cause of Cushing syndrome in clinical practice) before embarking on extensive investigations.

   If an ACTH-dependent cause is suspected, then imaging (MRI of the pituitary, CT of the thorax and abdomen) and further biochemical tests (e.g. inferior petrosal sinus sampling for ACTH pre- and post-CRH injection, high-dose dexamethasone suppression test and peripheral CRH test) may be required to differentiate pituitary disease from an ectopic source of ACTH. ACTH-independent disease is investigated with adrenal CT/MRI in the first instance.

Acromegaly

The diagnosis of acromegaly is confirmed by the finding of:

- failure of GH suppression (to <0.4 mg/l) during an oral glucose tolerance test
- an elevated IGF-1 level.

NB: Complications of hormone hypersecretory states (e.g. hypertension, diabetes mellitus, osteoporosis in Cushing syndrome; hypertension, diabetes mellitus, osteoporosis, cardiac hypertrophy, sleep apnoea, colonic neoplasia in acromegaly) should also be screened for.

Hormone hyposecretion

Screening for hypopituitarism includes measurement of:

- free T4 and TSH (remember TSH alone is unreliable in hypothalamic/pituitary disease)
- LH, FSH and testosterone or oestradiol
- prolactin (rarely low; typically raised – see earlier)
- 09:00 h cortisol
- creatinine and electrolytes with paired serum and urine osmolalities if diabetes insipidus (DI) is suspected.

In addition, dynamic testing for growth hormone deficiency (e.g. with a glucagon stimulation test or insulin tolerance test [ITT]) may be required. The ITT is also the preferred means of excluding significant ACTH/cortisol deficiency but is contra-indicated in patients with a history of epilepsy, dysrhythmias or suspected/known ischaemic coronary disease. The short Synacthen® test is a reasonable alternative in this setting, but must be interpreted with caution (see below).

NB: Hypertension, dyslipidaemia and other features of the metabolic syndrome should also be screened for in patients with hypopituitarism.

Local mass effect(s)

- MRI/high-resolution CT of the pituitary fossa
- formal visual perimetry (Fig. 16.7)

Treatment

Hormone hypersecretion

Prolactinomas (both micro- and macro-adenomas) are usually treated with medical therapy with a dopamine agonist (e.g. bromocriptine, cabergoline or quinagolide), which achieves control of hyperprolactinaemia, tumour shrinkage and resolution of symptoms in the majority of patients. Although generally well-tolerated, common side effects include initial nausea, postural hypotension and drowsiness, which tend to settle with continued usage. Less common, but more concerning longer-term side effects include compulsive gambling/shopping and hypersexuality (it is important to warn patients and, when possible, their immediate relatives of this potential adverse effect). In addition, concerns regarding ergot-derived dopamine agonists (e.g. bromocriptine, cabergoline) and the development of cardiac valvular fibrosis in patients with Parkinson's disease (where the drugs are typically used at much higher dosages, e.g. 3 mg/day) have led to regulatory recommendations for routine surveillance echocardiography, although subsequent cohort studies in pituitary patients (where much lower doses, e.g. < 2 mg/week, are used) have so far proved reassuring.

Somatostatin analogues (e.g. octreotide, lanreotide) may be used as primary therapy to control symptoms in acromegaly and to promote tumour shrinkage. However, trans-sphenoidal surgery remains the mainstay of treatment for pituitary adenomas (micro or macro) causing Cushing's disease, acromegaly and also for non-functioning pituitary adenomas, which typically present with local mass effects. In cases where there is incomplete tumour resection, adjunctive radiotherapy may be considered, depending on the extent of residual tumour, threat to neurological structures (e.g. the optic chiasm), degree of pituitary dysfunction and patient preference.

For residual/recurrent secretory tumours medical therapy may be recommended either as a long-term option, or while the beneficial effects of radiotherapy are awaited (e.g. octreotide/lanreotide and/or the growth hormone receptor antagonist pegvisomant for acromegaly). Cortisol hypersecretion can be controlled with metyrapone or ketoconazole (which block adrenal steroid biosynthesis). Mifepristone, which antagonizes cortisol signalling via the glucocorticoid receptor, may also be used. Cabergoline and second-generation somatostatin receptor ligands (e.g. pasireotide) directly suppress ACTH secretion in a subgroup of corticotroph tumours. Bilateral adrenalectomy may be required in patients with severe hypercortisolism refractory to medical therapy; however, if radiotherapy is not given in this setting, then the patient is at risk of developing Nelson syndrome (progressive pituitary enlargement and pigmentation due to rising ACTH levels).

Non-pituitary causes of Cushing syndrome are usually treated surgically (e.g. unilateral or bilateral adrenalectomy [usually laparoscopic] for primary adrenal disease). Pre-operative control of hypercortisolism is important to reduce operative risk and post-operative complications, e.g. poor wound healing.

Correction of hormone hyposecretion

- GH insufficiency may be corrected with a daily SC injection of growth hormone titrated against IGF-1 levels and symptom control.
- Cyclical oestrogen/progesterone therapy in pre-menopausal females and testosterone replacement in males corrects hypogonadism, although combination hCG (substituting for LH) and recombinant FSH may be required for infertility.
- ACTH/cortisol deficiency is corrected with hydrocortisone typically given in a b.d./t.d.s. regimen.

NB: Fludrocortisone replacement is not required in cases of secondary hypoadrenalism, as aldosterone production is preserved (under renin control).

- Thyroxine replacement is used to correct hypothyroidism.
- Desmopressin is effective in treating cranial DI.

Local mass effect

Although bromocriptine/cabergoline may induce rapid tumour shrinkage in cases of prolactinoma, surgical decompression (trans-sphenoidal or tran-scranial) is required in the majority of patients with compression of the optic chiasm in order to avoid permanent loss of vision. This should not be delayed.

Prognosis and treatment

Untreated Cushing syndrome is often fatal, predominantly as a consequence of cardiovascular complications and increased susceptibility to infection. Control of hypercortisolism is therefore mandatory and may require combination therapy to achieve this. Similarly, uncontrolled acromegaly is associated with excess morbidity and mortality secondary to cardiovascular and respiratory disease. In addition there appears to be an increased incidence of colonic polyps/carcinoma in subjects with acromegaly. Control of growth hormone hypersecretion restores morbidity/mortality levels to that of the general population.

Hypopituitarism per se is associated with an increased mortality rate of approximately twice that of the general population.

Adrenal

The adrenal glands comprise two major 'functional units' – the cortex and the medulla. The cortex consists of three zones: an 'inner' zona reticularis (secreting androgens, e.g. dehydroepiandrosterone sulphate [DHEAS]), a 'middle' zona fasciculata (secreting glucocorticoids, e.g. cortisol) and an 'outer' zona glomerulosa (secreting mineralocorticoids, e.g. aldosterone). Glucocorticoid and androgen secretion is directly under the control of pituitary ACTH, which in turn is regulated by hypothalamic CRH. Aldosterone production is independent of the hypothalamus and pituitary and controlled by the renin-angiotensin system.

Cortisol has many vital metabolic and immunomodulatory effects and is important in the maintenance of normal circulatory function. Aldosterone promotes renal sodium retention and potassium excretion.

Cushing syndrome

See earlier section on pituitary disorders.

Primary hyperaldosteronism

Primary hyperaldosteronism is an important treatable cause of hypertension, accounting for 5–10% of all cases and 20–25% of refractory hypertension.

Aetiology

Approximately 40–50% of cases are caused by unilateral benign aldosterone producing adenomas (so-called Conn's adenomas), while bilateral adrenal hyperplasia/nodular disease accounts for the majority of the remainder. Rarely, adrenal carcinoma and familial hyperaldosteronism are seen. In recent years a number of somatic gene mutations have been identified in Conn's adenomas, including several ion channels and pumps (KCNJ5, ATP1A1, ATP2B3 and CACNA1D), which predispose to increased aldosterone secretion and possibly cell survival.

Clinical presentation

Most cases come to light during investigation of hypertension or unexplained hypokalaemia. Non-specific symptoms including weakness, lassitude and polyuria (hypokalaemia may be associated with nephrogenic DI) are reported by some patients. Evidence of end organ damage (e.g. hypertensive retinopathy and nephropathy) may be seen in long-standing, inadequately treated cases.

Investigation

Prior to investigation it is important to ensure satisfactory dietary sodium intake, which may otherwise mask the condition. Hypokalaemia should also be corrected as it suppresses aldosterone production.

Screening tests are traditionally performed having withdrawn agents (e.g. β-blockers [suppress plasma renin]; diuretics, ACE inhibitors [raise plasma renin]; mineralocorticoid receptor antagonists [raise plasma renin and aldosterone]) that interfere with the renin-angiotensin-aldosterone system, substituting other antihypertensives (e.g. doxazosin or verapamil) where necessary.

- Creatinine and electrolytes – the classical picture is one of hypokalaemic alkalosis: the accompanying serum sodium level is typically normal to high. However, many patients with primary hyperaldosteronism are normokalaemic at presentation.
- Urinary potassium and sodium – hypokalaemia is associated with an inappropriate kaliuresis. Urinary sodium estimation can be used to ensure adequate dietary sodium intake.
- Plasma renin and aldosterone – the hallmark of primary hyperaldosteronism is excessive autonomous production of aldosterone, occurring in the face of renin suppression, and resulting in a raised aldosterone to renin ratio (ARR).
- Salt loading – it may be necessary to 'salt-load' the patient to confirm ongoing inappropriate aldosterone production. However, this should only be undertaken under specialist supervision and not in patients prone to fluid overload (e.g. those with cardiac failure, renal impairment).

Once a diagnosis of primary hyperaldosteronism has been established, CT/MRI of the adrenals may help to distinguish unilateral adenoma from bilateral hyperplasia (especially in younger patients <35 years of age). However, the majority of patients require a lateralising procedure to help confirm the site of excess aldosterone production. This is most commonly selective adrenal vein sampling (AVS), although functional imaging (traditionally conventional radionuclide scintigraphy, or more recently PET-CT, e.g. with the radiotracer ^{11}C-metomidate) offer a non-invasive alternative.

Management

Spironolactone is the medical treatment of choice by virtue of its ability to block the action of aldosterone at the mineralocorticoid receptor. Treatment is titrated to normalise blood pressure and restore normokalaemia. Eplerenone (an aldosterone antagonist without the anti-androgenic side effect profile of spironolactone) and amiloride (which inhibits renal reabsorption of sodium via the epithelial sodium channel) are alternatives if spironolactone is poorly tolerated.

Thereafter specific therapy is directed at the underlying cause:

- adrenal adenoma – unilateral adrenalectomy (typically laparoscopic)
- idiopathic hyperaldosteronism/bilateral hyperplasia – long-term medical therapy.

Primary adrenal insufficiency

NB: Adrenocortical insufficiency may be:

- primary – arising as a consequence of destruction or dysfunction of the adrenal cortex (as described by Thomas Addison)
- secondary – consequent on ACTH insufficiency due to hypothalamic/pituitary dysfunction (see earlier).

Aetiology

Although tuberculosis probably remains the commonest cause of primary adrenal insufficiency worldwide, in the UK the majority of cases are due to immune-mediated destruction of the adrenal glands and may be associated with other autoimmune glandular hypofunction (see autoimmune polyglandular syndromes, Table 16.7). Rarer causes of primary adrenal failure include infection (e.g. histoplasmosis, AIDS) and infiltration, although it is important to note that despite adrenal metastases being a relatively common finding on imaging, clinically evident adrenal insufficiency is rare in this setting. Adrenal haemorrhage, severe sepsis (e.g. meningococcaemia), congenital adrenal hyperplasia (CAH) and adrenoleukodystrophy (rare X-linked disorder) may also present with primary adrenal failure.

Clinical presentation

The clinical picture varies widely from the acutely ill patient in Addisonian crisis (Box 16.2) to the relatively asymptomatic patient with increased pigmentation. When present, symptoms may be non-specific, leading to a delay in diagnosis. Tiredness, weakness, dizziness, anorexia, weight loss and gastrointestinal disturbance are frequently reported. Female patients may present with menstrual disturbance (oligo/amenorrhoea). Salt 'craving' is common.

Increased pigmentation in the palmar creases, buccal mucosa and scars may be noted on examination. Postural hypotension is also common and females may exhibit loss of axillary and pubic hair (due to lack of adrenal sex steroids e.g. DHEAS).

Box 16.2 Addisonian crisis

Features

- Fever
- Nausea and vomiting
- Weakness and impaired cognition
- Hypotension/shock
- Hypoglycaemia
- Hyponatraemia
- Hyperkalaemia

Investigation

NB: In the acutely ill patient in whom you suspect adrenal insufficiency treatment must not be delayed. Venous access should be established (taking blood for creatinine and electrolytes, glucose and cortisol) and intravenous hydrocortisone (100 mg) must be given immediately. A 0.9% saline drip should also be set up and blood glucose checked using both a finger-prick and laboratory sample.

In non-emergency cases consider the following:

- Creatinine, electrolytes and glucose. NB: The classic pattern of low sodium, high potassium, high urea and low glucose is not seen in all cases.
- Full blood count – normochromic normocytic anaemia, neutropenia and eosinophilia are all recognised associations.
- Short Synacthen test – serum cortisol measured pre- and 30 (±60) min post-250 mcg of Synacthen IM/IV. Normal subjects exhibit a peak response >450 nmol/l at 30 min (precise thresholds depend on individual laboratory reference ranges). Occasionally the longer 'depot' Synacthen test is used to distinguish primary and secondary adrenal dysfunction.
- Adrenal autoantibodies.
- Exclusion of other associated conditions (see autoimmune polyglandular syndromes, Table 16.7).

Management

Hypoadrenal crisis should be treated as above, with the patient then established on regular parenteral hydrocortisone (e.g. 50–100 mg t.d.s./q.d.s. IV or IM, or an IV infusion of 4–8 mg/h following the initial IV bolus of 100 mg)) until the acute phase has resolved. Underlying precipitants/causes should be sought and treated appropriately.

Routine replacement with hydrocortisone is typically given using a twice or thrice daily regimen (e.g. 10 mg on waking, 5 mg at lunch-time and 2.5–5 mg in the late afternoon). Adequacy of replacement is assessed clinically, with some centres also advocating cortisol day profiles. Larger patients and those on enzyme-inducing agents (e.g. phenytoin, carbamazepine, rifampicin) typically require higher doses of corticosteroid replacement therapy. Patients must be advised about the steroid 'sick day rules', should carry a card/emergency bracelet and be provided with an emergency pack (containing injectable hydrocortisone).

Fludrocortisone replacement is also required in primary (but not in secondary) adrenal insufficiency. The usual maintenance dose is 50–200 mcg/day.

NB: In patients with concomitant hypothyroidism, thyroxine replacement should not be commenced until glucocorticoid replacement has been established, due to the risk of precipitating an Addisonian crisis.

Congenital adrenal hyperplasia

Congenital adrenal hyperplasia (CAH) is not a single disease entity but encompasses several autosomal recessive disorders (due to inborn errors in adrenocortical enzyme function) that result in differing degrees of impairment in the synthesis of cortisol and aldosterone. Deficiency of 21-hydroxylase is the most common enzyme defect (approximately 90–95% of all cases) and classical 21-hydroxylase deficiency affects approximately 1/14 000 live births in Caucasians.

Reduced cortisol synthesis results in elevated circulating ACTH, thereby further stimulating steroidogenesis. However, precursors that cannot be metabolized by the deficient enzyme are then shunted down adjacent (e.g. androgenic) pathways, with the resulting clinical phenotype reflecting both hormone deficiency (e.g. cortisol and aldosterone) and excess (e.g. androgen) states.

Clinical presentation

Both 'classical' and 'non-classical' variants of CAH are recognised. The former denotes a more severe form, predominantly seen in the neonate/young child, and is characterised by hypoadrenalism with salt wasting (especially in males) or ambiguous genitalia and virilisation (in females). Non-classical CAH is typically 'milder' and may only come to light in adulthood (e.g. with hirsutism, menstrual irregularities and/or infertility).

Investigation

Depending on the enzyme defect, different steroid precursors/androgens accumulate and can be measured in plasma. In practice, most laboratories restrict screening to the following:

- 17-hydroxyprogesterone – this precursor accumulates in 21-hydroxylase deficiency
- testosterone ± DHEAS and androstenedione
- plasma ACTH – elevated (although serum cortisol may be low or normal)
- plasma renin activity/mass – usually elevated in proportion to mineralocorticoid deficiency.

Genetic screening to identify mutations/deletions within the genes encoding the different enzymes involved in adrenal steroidogenesis is increasingly undertaken and has particular application in prenatal diagnosis.

Management

Episodes of acute adrenal insufficiency should be managed along conventional lines (see earlier). Routine replacement in 'classical' forms typically requires glucocorticoids (titrated against symptoms/signs, plasma ACTH, 17-hydroxyprogesterone and testosterone levels) and mineralocorticoid replacement (titrated against symptoms/signs, electrolytes, postural blood pressure and plasma renin).

'Non-classical' cases presenting with hirsutism may be managed with prednisolone (sometimes given in a 'reverse circadian rhythm', i.e. with a higher dose at night time to suppress the nocturnal ACTH drive) together with cosmetic measures.

Interest is currently focused on the potential use of novel long-acting slow-release hydrocortisone preparations to control excess ACTH secretion.

Psychological support is often an important component of the long-term management. Patients with CAH wishing to fall pregnant require shared care between the endocrine and genetic teams to ensure optimisation of CAH therapy and appropriate counselling regarding risks to the offspring.

Phaeochromocytoma

Phaeochromocytoma is a rare but potentially life-threatening disorder. The majority of tumours arise within the adrenal medulla, but a smaller number are derived from sympathetic/parasympathetic ganglia (so-called paragangliomas). Tumours of adrenal origin commonly secrete noradrenaline (norepinephrine) and adrenaline (epinephrine), whereas paragangliomas as a rule do not secrete the latter (as they are unable to convert noradrenaline to adrenaline). In some (especially malignant) tumours significant amounts of dopamine may be released, while others appear to be non-secretory.

Although phaeochromocytomas were originally known as the '10% tumour' (10% extra adrenal, 10% bilateral/multiple, 10% malignant, 10% familial) this is now considered to be outdated. For example, increasing numbers of cases are recognised to be familial, and the prevalence of bilateral tumours is much greater than 10% in certain familial syndromes.

So far, germline mutations in a large number of genes have been found in association with familial phaeochromocytoma. These include the *RET* proto-oncogene (MEN-2A and MEN-2B), the *VHL* tumour suppressor gene (von Hippel-Lindau syndrome: comprising renal cysts/carcinoma, pancreatic tumours and cysts, retinal and craniospinal (e.g. cerebellar) haemangioblastomas, phaeochromocytomas, endolymphatic sac tumours), *NF1* (neurofibromatosis type 1), mitochondrial succinate dehydrogenase complex subunits (e.g. *SDHA, SDHB, SDHC, SDHD, SDHAF2* – giving rise to hereditary paragangliomas syndromes), *TMEM127, MAX, EPAS,* and the gene encoding fumarate hydratase.

Clinical presentation

Increasing numbers of phaeochromocytomas are identified incidentally on cross-sectional imaging undertaken for other purposes. These tumours may be asymptomatic. Other cases come to light during the investigation of poorly controlled hypertension, when closer questioning reveals an array of other manifestations of catecholamine excess including episodic or paroxysmal 'attacks/spells' in which the patient develops pallor/sweating, palpitations and headaches. Indeed, this triad of symptoms is considered to be highly suggestive of a diagnosis of phaeochromocytoma. Occasional cases may present with myocardial infarction, cerebrovascular accident, dilated catecholamine cardiomyopathy or pregnancy-associated hypertension.

Investigations

This typically involves two stages:

- confirm the presence of phaeochromocytoma/paraganglioma
- localise the tumour(s).

1. Confirmation of diagnosis
   - Urinary catecholamines and their metabolites – $2 \times 24\,h$ urine collections for estimation of urinary free catecholamines (adrenaline, noradrenaline and dopamine) were traditionally used for screening in many centres. However, these have been largely replaced with measurement of urinary fractionated metanephrines (normetanephrine and metanephrine) which offer increased sensitivity and specificity when compared with catecholamine measurements.
   - Plasma free metanephrines (normetanephrine and metanephrine) are currently the most sensitive test for detecting phaeochromocytoma.
   NB: False positive results may occur in some assays either as a consequence of the patient having true catecholamine excess, but for a non-tumoral reason (e.g. use of tricyclic antidepressant agents, obstructive sleep apnoea) or as a consequence of interference with the analytical method.

2. Localisation of tumour
   Various imaging strategies may be employed, including:
   - CT/MRI
   - radioiodine-labelled metaiodobenzylguanidine (^{123}I -MIBG) scintigraphy
   - ^{18}F-FDG or ^{18}F-DOPA PET(-CT).

Genetic testing is particularly indicated in younger patients, those with paraganglioma syndromes or if there is a family history of phaeochromocytoma or other associated conditions.

Management

Prior to surgical removal, medical treatment must be instituted with the aims of:

- ameliorating symptoms
- normalising blood pressure
- correcting intravascular depletion.

The non-competitive α-adrenoceptor antagonist phenoxybenzamine is the treatment of choice. The competitive antagonist doxazosin may be considered in those intolerant of phenoxybenzamine. Occasionally intravenous phentolamine is also required (e.g. in the setting of a phaeochromocytoma crisis).

Although β-blockade may be required for symptom control and relief of tachycardia/dysrhythmias (especially in those with elevated adrenaline levels), it is important to note that β-blockers must **not** be commenced in a patient with suspected or proven phaeochromocytoma until adequate α-blockade has been established, since there is a significant risk of precipitating a life-threatening hypertensive crisis due to unopposed α-adrenoceptor activity.

Once the patient is adequately 'blocked' surgical excision can be undertaken (either traditional or laparoscopic approach). Therapeutic ^{131}I-MIBG therapy may be used in patients with recurrent/metastatic disease, and several studies suggest a possible role for tyrosine kinase inhibitors in this setting.

Multiple endocrine neoplasia (MEN)

Three main multiple endocrine neoplasia syndromes are recognised: MEN-1, MEN-2A and MEN-2B. Each is characterised by autosomal dominant inheritance. Table 16.6 outlines the key features of each syndrome.

Investigation and management

Although the individual components of the MEN syndromes are generally managed along standard lines, there are some important differences:

- four gland parathyroid hyperplasia is more common than a single adenoma
- pancreatic tumours are often multiple
- phaeochromocytoma must be excluded in patients with suspected/confirmed MEN-2 before they undergo surgery for (MTC) or hyperparathyroidism.

In general, genetic testing has now effectively replaced biochemical screening in the identification of affected members in the majority of MEN kindreds. Because MTC is aggressive and the only effective cure is thyroidectomy, genetic screening is now increasingly offered to young children in affected kindreds, raising important ethical issues.

Autoimmune polyglandular endocrinopathies

Autoimmune-mediated dysfunction in two or more endocrine glands is recognised in the context of the autoimmune polyglandular endocrine syndromes (APS). Table 16.7 shows the key features of the two major syndromes.

Polycystic ovarian syndrome

Polycystic ovarian syndrome (PCOS) is the commonest cause of hirsutism and menstrual disturbance in females. It has been estimated to affect ~5% of all women of reproductive age. Increasing evidence suggests a complex interplay between genetic susceptibility and

Table 16.6 Key features of the multiple endocrine neoplasia syndromes

Type	MEN-1	MEN-2A	MEN-2B
Components	• Parathyroid hyperplasia • Pancreatic tumours • Pituitary tumours	• MTC • Phaeochromocytoma • Parathyroid hyperplasia	• MTC • Marfanoid habitus • Phaeochromocytoma • Mucosal neuromas • Intestinal ganglioneuromatosis
Genetic loci	• Chromosome 11: loss-of-function mutations in the *MENIN* tumour suppressor gene	• Both MEN-2 syndromes are associated with gain-of-function mutations in the *RET* proto-oncogene on chromosome 10	
Clinical features	• Hyperparathyroidism is the most common presenting feature • Of the functioning pancreatic tumours, gastrinomas and insulinomas constitute the majority • Prolactinomas and acromegaly are the most common pituitary disorders	• Phaeochromocytoma may be bilateral • Familial MTC without the other features of MEN-2 also occurs in certain kindreds harbouring mutations in *RET*	• Mucosal neuromas most commonly affect the oral cavity and gastrointestinal tract • MTC in the setting of MEN-2B is particularly aggressive • Phaeochromocytoma may be bilateral

MEN, multiple endocrine neoplasia; MTC, medullary thyroid carcinoma.

Table 16.7 Autoimmune polyglandular syndromes (APS)

Type	Type 1*	Type 2
Epidemiology	• Rare, autosomal recessive • Childhood onset	• Autosomal dominant, recessive or polygenic • Young adults • Females > males
HLA associations		• DR3, DR4
Genetic loci	Chromosome 21q: mutations in the *AIRE* gene	
Common endocrinopathies	• Hypoparathyroidism • Primary adrenal insufficiency	• Primary adrenal insufficiency • Primary hypo- (or hyper-) thyroidism • Type 1 diabetes mellitus
Less common endocrinopathies	• Primary gonadal failure • Primary hypo- (or hyper-) thyroidism • Type 1 diabetes mellitus	• Primary gonadal failure
Non-endocrine associations	• Mucocutaneous candidiasis • Chronic active hepatitis • Pernicious anaemia • Vitiligo • Alopecia	• Myasthenia gravis • Pernicious anaemia • Vitiligo • Alopecia

*Also known as autoimmune polyendocrinopathy, candidiasis-ectodermal dystrophy (APECED) syndrome; *AIRE*, autoimmune regulator gene.

environmental factors in the aetiopathogenesis of this disorder. Reduced insulin sensitivity, with consequent hyperinsulinaemia, are key features of the metabolic derangements that are typically seen in PCOS (including impaired glucose tolerance/type 2 diabetes mellitus and other features of the metabolic syndrome).

Clinical presentation

The symptoms of PCOS usually date from menarche and develop gradually. These include features of hyperandrogenism (e.g. hirsutism, acne) and menstrual irregularity (oligomenorrhoea or occasionally amenorrhoea). Weight gain and obesity tend to exacerbate the disorder. Clinical and/or biochemical evidence of hyperandrogenism, together with a history of anovulatory cycles (typified by oligomenorrhoea), are sufficient to make a diagnosis of PCOS. In addition, ultrasound of the ovaries may reveal the typical appearance of multiple peripherally sited follicles ('string of pearls') with increased ovarian stroma.

However, the presence of polycystic ovaries on ultrasound does not in itself indicate that the woman has PCOS (approximately 15–20% of all women have polycystic changes on ultrasound, although only one-third of these have PCOS).

Testosterone levels may be increased, but this is not an absolute requirement for diagnosis of the disorder – clinical evidence of hyperandrogenism suffices.

Fasting glucose/oral glucose tolerance test and lipid profiles should be checked for evidence of features of the metabolic syndrome.

Measurement of 17-hydroxyprogesterone (to exclude CAH) and adrenal androgens (e.g. DHEAS to exclude adrenal tumours) can help to distinguish from other causes of hirsutism/hyperandrogenism.

Weight loss often improves many of the features of PCOS. Other therapies are targeted to the principle complaint: for example, treatment of hirsutism with cosmetic measures or anti-androgens; infertility with clomifene. Cardiovascular risk factors should also be addressed.

17

Metabolic disorders

Diabetes mellitus

Diabetes mellitus (DM) is the term used to describe a group of metabolic disorders characterised by hyperglycaemia and due to:

- deficiency in pancreatic beta (β)-cell insulin production; and/or
- impaired insulin action (typically due to insulin resistance).

Diagnostic criteria

The World Health Organization (WHO) Expert Committee on the Diagnosis and Classification of Diabetes Mellitus recommends that DM should be diagnosed in the following circumstances:

- symptoms of diabetes and random venous plasma glucose ≥ 11.1 mmol/l;
- fasting venous plasma glucose (FPG) ≥ 7.0 mmol/l (confirmed on a second occasion in asymptomatic individuals).
- haemoglobin A_{1c} (HbA$_{1c}$) ≥ 48 mmol/mol (6.5%)

The term impaired fasting glycaemia (IFG) is used for those with fasting venous plasma glucose levels in the range 6.1–6.9 mmol/l. The WHO recommends that patients in the latter category should proceed to an oral glucose tolerance test (OGTT):

- Venous plasma glucose ≥ 11.1 mmol/l (2 h after 75 g of oral anhydrous glucose) confirms a diagnosis of DM; those with 2-h venous plasma glucose levels in the range 7.8–11.0 mmol/l are deemed to have impaired glucose tolerance (IGT).

Classification

Diabetes mellitus can be broadly classified into type 1 and type 2, although not all patients are easily assigned to one or other category. In addition, there are other specific types of diabetes (e.g. gestational DM and diabetes due to specific genetic defects), which are best considered independently (Table 17.1).

Type 1 diabetes mellitus

This was previously referred to as insulin-dependent diabetes mellitus (IDDM).

- An autoimmune disorder in which the insulin producing β-cells of the pancreas are destroyed; hence there is ultimately an *absolute* insulin deficiency.
- Although type 1 DM develops mostly during childhood and adolescence, it may also present in later life.
- Patients typically experience an acute onset of the disease (weeks rather than months) and often give a history of significant weight loss. They are dependent upon insulin therapy and are prone to ketoacidosis (see later).

Type 2 diabetes mellitus

This was previously referred to as non-insulin-dependent diabetes mellitus (NIDDM).

- The predominant form worldwide, accounting for ~90% of patients with DM.
- Tissue insensitivity to insulin action (i.e. insulin resistance), and an inability of the pancreatic β-cells to compensate adequately for this, leads to overproduction of glucose by the liver and under-utilisation by other tissues, with an inevitable rise in blood glucose levels – i.e. there is *relative* insulin deficiency.

Clinical Medicine Lecture Notes, Eighth Edition. John R. Bradley, Mark Gurnell, and Diana F. Wood.
© 2019 John Wiley & Sons Ltd. Published 2019 by John Wiley & Sons Ltd.

Table 17.1 Classification of diabetes mellitus

Classification	Examples (list is not exhaustive)
Type 1 DM	
Type 2 DM	
Gestational DM	
Other specific types	
Monogenetic disorders	MODY
	MELAS
	Lipodystrophy[a]
	Leprechaunism[b]
Diseases of exocrine pancreas	Pancreatitis
	Haemochromatosis
	Cystic fibrosis
	Neoplasia
	Trauma/surgery
Endocrine disorders	Acromegaly
	Cushing syndrome
	Phaeochromocytoma
	Glucagonoma
Drug induced	Corticosteroids
	Thiazide diuretics
	Olanzapine
	Alpha interferon Statins
Conditions associated with DM	Down syndrome
	Klinefelter syndrome
	Turner syndrome
	Laurence–Moon–Biedl syndrome
	Prader–Willi syndrome

DM, diabetes mellitus; MELAS, mitochondrial encephalomyopathy, lactic acidosis and stroke-like episodes; MODY, maturity-onset diabetes of the young.
[a] Lipodystrophy may be caused by mutations in several different genes.
[b] Leprechaunism is linked to defects in insulin receptor signalling.

- Traditionally this form of DM was considered predominantly a disease of obese, older adults, although now it is being increasingly diagnosed in adolescents and younger adults (and even in some children) due to the increasing prevalence of obesity in these age groups.

- Symptoms are often mild in the early stages, which can lead to a delay in the patient seeking medical attention; hence, diagnosis may occur later in the disease process, with some cases presenting with established complications (e.g. retinopathy, neuropathy or cardiovascular disorders).
- There may be a history of recurrent infections and injuries that are slow to heal.
- Ketosis is uncommon, except in situations of extreme stress, as patients usually have sufficient insulin to prevent lipolysis.
- Although initially controlled with diet and/or oral hypoglycaemic agents, many patients eventually need supplemental insulin.
- Type 2 DM is recognised as part of the so-called *metabolic syndrome,* where it is associated with central obesity, hypertension, dyslipidaemia (low HDL cholesterol [HDL-C] and hypertriglyceridaemia – see later) and premature cardiovascular disease.

Gestational diabetes mellitus (GDM)

Most women who develop DM during pregnancy have normal glucose homeostasis during the first half of gestation, but develop a relative insulin deficiency during the second half, leading to hyperglycaemia. The guidelines published in March 2010 by the International Association of Diabetes and Pregnancy Study Groups (IADPSG) recommend universal screening, and that all women without a prior diagnosis of DM be considered for a 75 g anhydrous glucose OGTT at 24–28 weeks' gestation. If one of the following criteria are met, then the woman is deemed to have a diagnosis of GDM:

- fasting venous plasma glucose ≥ 5.1 mmol/l
- 1-h venous plasma glucose level ≥ 10.0 mmol/l
- 2-h venous plasma glucose level ≥ 8.5 mmol/l.

The UK National Institute for Health and Clinical Excellence (NICE) guidance (2015), however, only advises screening the following 'at risk' groups:

- $BMI \geq 30 \, kg/m^2$
- previous macrosomic baby (weighing ≥ 4.5 kg)
- previous GDM
- first-degree relative with DM
- ethnic origin with a high prevalence of DM (South Asian, black Caribbean and Middle Eastern).

If screen positive (i.e. one positive risk factor), offer 75 g OGTT at 24–28 weeks. If previous GDM, offer early self-monitoring of blood glucose or early OGTT at 16 weeks, repeating at 24 weeks if initially negative.

Currently, NICE recommends GDM be diagnosed if fasting venous plasma glucose ≥ 5.6 mmol/l or if 2-h venous plasma glucose in an OGTT is ≥ 7.8 mmol/l.

Some women with undiagnosed type 2 diabetes may present for the first time in pregnancy, and so technically are classified as gestational diabetes, until confirmed otherwise post-delivery.

Other specific types of diabetes mellitus

This category includes a diverse spectrum of conditions, ranging from rarer genetic disorders to primary pancreatic pathology, endocrine diseases and drug induced DM (Table 17.1).

Epidemiology

According to the WHO, the number of adults with diabetes mellitus worldwide was estimated to be 108 million in 1980 and had risen to 422 million by 2014 (thus the global prevalence amongst adults over 18 years of age had increased from 4.7% in 1980 to 8.5% in 2014. Almost 3.6 million people in the UK had been diagnosed with diabetes by late 2016, with an estimated additional 1 million people remaining undiagnosed (with type 2 diabetes).

Aetiology

Genetics

Type 1 DM

The identical twin of a person with type 1 DM has a 30–50% chance of developing the disease, implicating both genetic and environmental factors in its aetiology. A number of genetic susceptibility loci have been identified and include:

- *IDDM1* in the major histocompatibility complex (MHC)/human leucocyte antigen (HLA) region on chromosome 6p21.3.
- *IDDM2* near the insulin gene locus on chromosome 11p15.
- *CTLA4 on chromosome 2q33.*

Overall, the risk of a sibling or offspring of an individual with type 1 DM developing the same condition is relatively low but increased compared to the background population. The risk is higher if the father has the condition (6–8% versus 2–4% if the mother is affected).

Type 2 DM

Typically, there is a positive family history. In most affected individuals, the inherited component is likely to be polygenic, involving interaction between multiple genes involved in both insulin secretion and insulin action. Overall, the risk of a sibling or offspring of a person with type 2 DM developing the condition is high (as much as 33%; identical twins are affected in 60–100% of cases). Lifestyle changes can modify this risk (see later).

MODY

MODY is an autosomal dominant condition. Individual subtypes are associated with mutations in a variety of different genes that encode factors involved in insulin production/release by pancreatic β-cells. For example, MODY type 2 is caused by mutations in the gene coding for glucokinase, a rate-limiting enzyme in the glycolytic pathway, which acts as a pancreatic 'glucose sensor', regulating insulin release in response to a rise in blood glucose levels. Mutations in glucokinase are associated with an altered 'set-point' for glucose sensing, i.e. insulin release is triggered at higher ambient blood glucose levels compared with the general population. Accordingly, hyperglycaemia tends to be mild and relatively stable over time, and is often detected incidentally or as part of family screening; severe hyperglycaemia and complications are rare. In contrast, in MODY type 3, mutations in a transcription factor, hepatocyte nuclear factor 1α (HNF1α), which regulates β-cell mass/insulin production, result in DM that typically presents in adolescence or young adulthood, with progressive hyperglycaemia over time such that treatment with oral hypoglycaemic agents and/or insulin is usually required. Patients with MODY 3 are particularly sensitive to the blood glucose lowering effects of sulfonylureas (see later), and patients started on insulin therapy prior to the diagnosis being made may be able to transition back to a sulfonylurea with maintenance of excellent glycaemic control; however, many patients ultimately require insulin therapy. Currently, HNF1α mutations account for ~70% of all MODY cases.

MELAS

MELAS is a rare disorder characterised by mitochondrial encephalomyopathy, lactic acidosis and stroke-like episodes. It is due to mutations in genes encoded by mitochondrial DNA (e.g. *MT-TL1* and *MT-ND1*) and maternally inherited.

Environmental/other factors

Type 1 DM

In genetically susceptible individuals, one or more environmental factors may 'trigger' immune-mediated destruction of islet β-cells ('*insulinitis*'). A variety of agents have been implicated including viruses (e.g.

coxsackie, rubella, mumps, cytomegalovirus), dietary constituents (e.g. bovine serum albumin in cow's milk, especially if fed to infants) and stress.

Type 2 DM

This is strongly linked to obesity, which predisposes to insulin resistance. Fetal malnutrition *in utero* may also be associated with an increased risk (so-called *fetal programming*). Statins are now associated with an increased risk of diabetes.

Clinical presentation

The classic triad of diabetic symptoms include:

- polyuria
- increased thirst (polydipsia)
- weight loss.

These features typically manifest in an acute or subacute fashion in those with type 1 DM, but may be of gradual onset in the setting of type 2 DM. Other presenting features include:

- tiredness/fatigue
- blurred vision
- opportunistic infections (e.g. balanitis, thrush, pruritus vulvae).

Individuals with type 1 DM are traditionally thought of as being 'lean' as opposed to their type 2 DM counterparts, who are often overweight/obese. However, with the rising 'obesity epidemic' the margins have begun to 'blur' as more obese type 1 cases are identified. Similarly, not all patients with type 2 DM are necessarily obese.

Occasionally, diabetes may present as part of another disorder (e.g. Cushing syndrome, acromegaly, haemochromatosis) where features of the primary condition dominate the clinical picture, or may be detected incidentally or during screening (e.g. on urinalysis or a fasting/random blood sample).

Once the clinical diagnosis of DM is suspected, it is usually relatively easily confirmed (see diagnostic criteria earlier). In cases where there is difficulty in distinguishing between type 1 and type 2 DM, measurement of plasma C-peptide (low/absent in type 1 DM; present/elevated in type 2 DM) and screening for islet cell, islet cell antigen 2 (IA2) and anti-GAD (glutamic acid decarboxylase) antibodies may be of help.

Research into first-degree relatives of those with type 1 diabetes, has led to staging of type 1 diabetes by the ADA (American Diabetes Association) 2017 – where stage 3 is the classical presentation, stage 1 is autoimmunity with normal glycaemia, and stage 2,

autoimmunity and impaired asymptomatic glycaemia. The ultimate goal is to prevent progression of positive autoimmunity to clinical presentation.

There is also a body of work looking at pre-diabetes in the context of type 2 diabetes, with one aim being the screening of high-risk individuals and concentrating resources on lifestyle interventions to reduce progression to type 2 diabetes.

Management

General principles

The major aim of management is to achieve near-normal glucose homeostasis (for which patient education/activation is a key component), initially to provide symptom relief and in the longer term to prevent/minimise complications – surveillance for, and treatment of, the latter is also a priority. Management should be coordinated by a specialist multidisciplinary diabetes team, based in either primary or secondary care, and individuals with DM should be reviewed at least once, and ideally twice, a year by this team. Table 17.2 shows aspects of the patient's care that should be assessed during each 'annual review' process.

In addition to the diabetologist/GP with a specialist interest, diabetes specialist nurse/practice nurse and dietician, patients with diabetes may also require input from the following disciplines: chiropody, psychology, orthopaedics, vascular surgery, ophthalmology and urology.

A plethora of clinical trials have confirmed the benefits of achieving/maintaining good glycaemic control in DM, but two landmark studies merit particular mention: the Diabetes Control and Complications Trial (DCCT – type 1 DM) and the United Kingdom Prospective Diabetes Study (UKPDS – type 2 DM) – see Box 17.1.

Glycaemic control

Monitoring

This is typically assessed using a combination of the patient's home blood glucose monitoring (HBGM) records and glycosylated haemoglobin A_{1c} (HbA_{1c}) measurement. The latter provides an estimate of overall glycaemic control during the past 6–8 weeks, and can be assayed either using a near-patient testing kit or in the clinical biochemistry laboratory. Due to potentially significant variations in analytical methods and quality control, all assays have traditionally been aligned to that used in the DCCT and previously

Table 17.2 Key elements of the diabetic 'annual review' process

Element	Comment(s)
Diet and eating habits	Promote healthy diet/eating habits with specific advice pertaining to DM
Weight	Encourage maintenance of optimal weight
Physical activity	Explain that exercise improves glycaemic control, blood pressure and lipid profile
Glycaemic control	Assess by reviewing home blood glucose diary/meter in conjunction with HbA$_{1c}$
Hypoglycaemia	Check: frequency; awareness; ability to recognise and treat appropriately
Complications:	
retinopathy	Confirm enrolment into retinal photography screening programme; ask about visual change/symptoms
nephropathy	Check serum creatinine and urine ACR
neuropathy	Enquire about symptoms and examine for evidence of impaired sensation
foot problems	As for neuropathy, but also check: peripheral pulses; for callus, ulceration and Charcot arthropathy
cardiovascular disease	Ask about/examine for features of IHD; stroke/TIA; peripheral vascular disease
Associated risk factors	Advise avoidance of/cessation from smoking; ensure within targets for blood pressure and lipids (see text)
Medications	Check: DM treatment regimen, antihypertensive/renal protection therapy, lipid-lowering agents and, where appropriate, antiplatelet therapy
Injection sites	Look for evidence of lipohypertrophy (or rarely lipoatrophy) and advise rotation of injection sites
Driving	Ensure awareness of DVLA regulations/advice (e.g. test blood glucose before driving – should be >5 mmol/l)
Alcohol	Advise variable impact on blood glucose – mainly risk of late hypoglycaemia and possible requirement for adjustment to insulin regimen
Sexual function	Ask about erectile dysfunction in men; advise on contraception and preconception glycaemic control in women
Psychological factors	Check for concerns, e.g. regarding coping with a chronic illness
Blood tests	Electrolytes, renal function, liver function, glucose, HbA$_{1c}$, fasting lipid profile, full blood count

ACR, albumin : creatinine ratio; DM, diabetes mellitus; DVLA, Driver Vehicle and Licensing Authority; HbA$_{1c}$, haemoglobin A$_{1c}$; IHD, ischaemic heart disease; TIA, transient ischaemic attack.

expressed as a percentage. However, since 2011, a new standard introduced by the International Federation of Clinical Chemistry and Laboratory Medicine (IFCC), which expresses HbA$_{1c}$ values in mmol/mol of unglycosylated haemoglobin. Table 17.3 shows DCCT and IFCC equivalents.

The frequency/necessity of HBGM continues to be widely debated. Its routine use in those with type 2 diabetes on diet and/or oral hypoglycaemic agents has not been shown to be beneficial, and so it is not routinely recommended (or funded). However, at a minimum, testing should be undertaken during periods of change or intercurrent illness, and in all patients on insulin therapy, with recommendations determined on an individual patient basis. Continuous glucose monitoring systems (CGMS) are available, but are expensive and generally reserved for 'difficult cases' and/or highly engaged individuals. Routine use is not funded by the NHS, but on an individual basis.

Box 17.1 Glycaemic control in diabetes: landmark trials

The **Diabetes Control and Complications Trial (DCCT)** compared intensive and standard treatment in 1441 patients with type 1 DM (mean age 27 years) over a 6.5-year period; 726 patients had no retinopathy (primary prevention cohort), whereas 715 had mild retinopathy (secondary prevention cohort). Intensive treatment involved insulin given by a pump, or by three or more daily subcutaneous injections, with dosages adjusted according to blood glucose measured at least four times daily. Standard treatment involved insulin given once or twice daily, with once-daily monitoring of blood or urinary glucose. The study showed that:

- Intensive treatment reduced the risk of developing retinopathy by 76% in the primary prevention group, and of worsening retinopathy by 54% (and of developing proliferative or severe non-proliferative retinopathy by 47%) in the secondary prevention group.
- In the two groups combined, intensive therapy reduced the risk of developing microalbuminuria by 39%, albuminuria by 54% and neuropathy by 60%.
- The major adverse event in the intensively treated group was a two- to threefold increase in severe hypoglycaemic episodes.

Source: *New England Journal of Medicine* 1993; **329**: 977–986.

The **United Kingdom Prospective Diabetes Study (UKPDS)** was a multicentre trial involving 5102 patients with newly diagnosed type 2 DM. It ran for 20 years (1977–1997) in 23 UK clinical centres and demonstrated conclusively that the complications of type 2 DM could be reduced by improving glycaemic and/or blood pressure control. UKPDS randomised newly diagnosed patients with type 2 DM into conventional (target FPG < 15 mmol/l) and intensive (FPG < 6 mmol/l) glucose control treatment arms. The study showed that:

- Retinopathy, nephropathy and possibly neuropathy are benefited by lowering blood glucose levels in type 2 DM with intensive therapy, which achieved a median HbA_{1c} of 7.0% (equivalent to 53 mmol/mol) compared with conventional therapy with a median HbA_{1c} of 7.9% (equivalent to 63 mmol/mol) compared.
- The overall microvascular complication rate was decreased by 25%, and for every percentage point decrease in HbA_{1c} there was a 35% reduction in the risk of complications; there was no evidence of any glycaemic threshold for any of the microvascular complications above normal glucose levels.
- A 16% reduction (which was not statistically significant, $p = 0.052$) in the risk of combined fatal or non-fatal myocardial infarction and sudden death was observed.
- For every percentage point decrease in HbA_{1c}, there was a 25% reduction in diabetes-related deaths, a 7% reduction in all-cause mortality, and an 18% reduction in combined fatal and non-fatal myocardial infarction. Again no glycaemic threshold for these macrovascular complications was observed.
- Lowering blood pressure to a mean of 144/82 mmHg significantly reduced strokes, diabetes-related deaths, heart failure, microvascular complications and visual loss.
- A log-linear relationship between the incidence of complications and increasing HbA_{1c} or systolic blood pressure indicated that any improvement in glycaemic or blood pressure control would be advantageous.
- Metformin appeared to confer particular benefits in obese subjects with T2DM, and was associated with less weight gain and fewer hypoglycaemic episodes.

Source: *Lancet* 1998; **352**: 837–853, 854–865; *BMJ* 1998; **317**: 703–713, 713–720. http://www.dtu.ox.ac.uk/ukpds. DM, diabetes mellitus; FPG, fasting plasma glucose; HbA_{1c}, haemoglobin A_{1c}.

Technology is advancing, self-funded 'flash glucose monitoring' systems are now commercially available for patients to purchase. They do not measure capillary blood glucose, but interstitial fluid glucose. They are currently not classified as a valid blood glucose measurement for the purpose of driving in the UK.

Similarly, 'ideal' blood glucose targets are often debated and 'one size does not fit all'; in general, HBGM levels of 4–8 mmol/l are likely to correlate with a satisfactory HbA_{1c} (53 mmol/mol; <7.0%). NICE guidelines on type 1 diabetes (NG17) state that care providers should 'Support adults with type 1

Table 17.3 Diabetes Control and Complications Trial (DCCT) and International Federation of Clinical Chemistry (IFCC) equivalent HbA$_{1c}$ values

DCCT-aligned HbA$_{1c}$ (%)	IFCC-standardised HbA$_{1c}$ (mmol/mol)
4.0	20
5.0	31
6.0	42
6.5	48
7.0	53
7.5	59
8.0	64
8.5	69
9.0	75
9.5	80
10.0	86

diabetes to aim for a target HbA$_{1c}$ level of 48 mmol/mol (6.5%) or lower, to minimise the risk of long-term vascular complications'. However, individualised targets should be agreed between the patient and his/her clinician, bearing in mind the large volume of trial data showing that good glycaemic control reduces the risk of microvascular and macrovascular complications, and that in some settings (e.g. pregnancy – see later) tight glycaemic control is particularly important (to reduce the risk of fetal malformations and macrosomia), but that for others (e.g. the frail/elderly living alone) the need to avoid hypoglycaemia may necessitate running the HbA$_{1c}$ at less than optimal levels.

Treatment of hyperglycaemia

Type 1 DM

Patients with type 1 DM require insulin to control their blood glucose levels. Education about the effects of diet, physical activity and illness upon glycaemic control, and hence insulin requirements, is critical. It is recommended that all those newly diagnosed with type 1 diabetes should be offered a validated, structured education course within a year of diagnosis. The most well-known is the DAFNE (Dose Adjustment for Normal Eating) course.

Insulin preparations

Based on source, insulins are classified as animal (porcine, bovine), human or analogue. The use of animal insulins has fallen significantly in recent years, but there are still a small number of patients who derive particular benefits from these preparations, although it is unclear how long they will continue to be available. Based on the duration of action, insulin can be classified as rapid-, short-, intermediate- or long-acting. In addition, various mixed preparations exist, containing different proportions of faster- and slower-acting insulins; for example, Novomix-30 is a pre-mixed insulin analogue that contains 30% *soluble* insulin aspart (rapid-acting form) and 70% insulin aspart *protamine* (intermediate-acting form) (Tables 17.4 and 17.5).

Insulin was previously standardized to 100 units per ml, and always prescribed as units. However, with the increasing problem of insulin resistance, increasingly large doses of insulin need to be injected. Insulins are now licensed in U500, 500 units per ml, and U200, 200 units per ml. Extreme care should be taken when prescribing these concentrated preparations.

Insulin administration

Options include:

- syringe and needle
- 'pen devices'
- insulin pump/continuous subcutaneous insulin infusion (CSII) therapy.

Insulin regimens

A variety of different insulin regimens exist (Table 17.6).

Other therapeutic options

A small number of patients may ultimately be considered for whole organ (pancreas – often combined with kidney) or islet cell transplantation, but currently these options are limited and only available in a small number of centres.

Type 2 DM

Patient education

Type 2 DM may be prevented, or at least its onset delayed, by making significant lifestyle changes in those at high risk of the condition. The US and UK are both running National Diabetes Prevention Programmes. Dietary modification and physical activity are critically important for achieving good glycaemic control. A comparable programme to *DAFNE* for type 2 DM – *DESMOND* (*D*iabetes *E*ducation and *S*elf-*M*anagement for *ON*going and *D*iagnosed) is recommended by NICE, again within a year of diagnosis.

Table 17.4 Classification of insulin preparations

Type of insulin (with examples)	Source	Characteristics
Super fast-acting Fiasp®	Analogue	Onset of action: within 5 min Peak action: 0.5–1 h Duration of action: 4 h
Rapid-acting Insulin aspart, insulin glulisine, insulin lispro	Analogue	Onset of action: within 15 min Peak action: 1 h Duration of action: 4 h
Short-acting/neutral Actrapid®, Humulin S®, Insuman® rapid	Human	Onset of action: 30 min Peak action: 1–2 h Duration of action: 5–6 h
Hypurin® bovine neutral, Hypurin® porcine neutral	Animal	Onset of action: 30 min Peak action: 2–4 h Duration of action: 5–6 h
Intermediate/long-acting Humulin I®, Insulatard®, Insuman® basal	Human	Onset of action: 30–60 min Peak action: 4–8 h Duration of action: 16–20 h
Hypurin® bovine isophane, Hypurin® bovine lente, Hypurin® porcine isophane	Animal	Onset of action: 60–120 min Peak action: 6–12 h Duration of action: 16–20 h
Long-acting Insulin detemir, insulin glargine	Analogue	Onset of action: 60–70 min Peak action: no peak, flat profile Duration of action: 20–24 h
Hypurin bovine protamine zinc insulin (PZI)	Animal	Onset of action: 240–600 min Peak action: 10–20 h Duration of action: 20–30 h
Ultra long-acting Insulin Degludec	Analogue	Onset of action: 30–90 min Peak action: no peak, flat profile Duration of action: 42 h

If these measures alone fail to control blood glucose levels, then oral hypoglycaemic agents are typically commenced. The majority of oral hypoglycaemic agents reduce HbA_{1c} by 5–10 mmol/l in clinical trials. Ultimately, many patients require combination therapy with oral hypoglycaemic agents and/or injectable therapies (e.g. incretin mimetics or insulin – see later).

Table 17.7 shows the oral hypoglycaemic agents currently available in the UK.

Biguanides
Metformin, the only biguanide licensed in the UK, reduces hepatic glucose production, mainly by inhibiting gluconeogenesis. It also increases peripheral

Table 17.5 Types of mixed/biphasic insulins

Examples	Source	Characteristics
Humulin M3®, Insuman® Comb 15, Insuman® Comb 25, Insuman® Comb 50	Human	Onset of action: 30 min Peak action: 1–8 h Duration of action: up to 20 h
Hypurin porcine 30/70 mix	Animal	Onset of action: 30 min Peak action: 4–12 h Duration of action: up to 22 h
Humalog® Mix25, Humalog® Mix50, NovoMix® 30	Human	Onset of action: within 15 min Peak action: 30–240 min Duration of action: up to 20 h

Table 17.6 Insulin regimens

Regimen	Example	Indication(s)
Once-a-day	Insulin detemir, insulin glargine, Insulin degludec, Insulatard	Type 2 DM together with oral hypoglycaemic agents
Twice-a-day	Mixed/biphasic insulins	Type 2 (or type 1) DM
Thrice-a-day	Mixed insulin (morning), rapid-acting (evening), long-acting (night) or mixed biphasic insulin thrice daily	Used mostly in children to avoid the need to inject while at school; rarely used in adults (e.g. if high total daily insulin requirement)
Four times a day ('basal-bolus')	Long-acting insulin once/twice daily and rapid-acting insulin with each meal	Preferred regimen in type 1 DM; also used for young type 2 DM failing oral hypoglycaemic agents with once daily insulin

insulin sensitivity, albeit through a poorly understood mechanism. Beneficial effects include promotion of weight loss, reductions in total and low-density lipoprotein (LDL) cholesterol and triglycerides.

Gastrointestinal side effects are common, especially during the early stages of treatment, but usually subside (hence the mantra 'low [dosage] and slow [dosage increments]'). It should be avoided in patients with renal impairment (serum creatinine > 150 mmol/l or GFR < 30 ml/min) to reduce the risk of lactic acidosis. In addition, its use should be suspended in those undergoing radiological contrast studies or general anaesthesia and not restarted until renal function has returned to baseline.

Vitamin B_{12} deficiency may develop as a result of decreased absorption – annual full blood count is therefore suggested.

Sulfonylureas

Sulfonylureas augment residual pancreatic β-cell function, hence the term 'insulin secretagogues' (Table 17.7). They are licensed for monotherapy (mainly used in patients who are intolerant of metformin or in whom there is a specific indication for sulfonylurea therapy, e.g. MODY 3 [see earlier]), or in combination with other oral hypoglycaemic agents or insulin. Sulfonylureas are generally not recommended for use during pregnancy, although glibenclamide (US approved name glyburide) can be used safely after the first trimester.

Their major side effects are hypoglycaemia (especially in the elderly) and weight gain.

Prandial glucose regulators ('meglitinides')

Repaglinide and nateglinide are rapid-acting insulin secretagogues with a fast onset and short duration of action. They should be taken 15–30 min before each

Table 17.7 Oral hypoglycaemic agents and non-insulin-based injection therapy for type 2 diabetes mellitus

Class	Comment(s)
Biguanides	Suppress basal hepatic gluconeogenesis (major contributor to fasting hyperglycaemia in type 2 DM); also reduce peripheral insulin resistance, thereby increasing glucose utilisation.
e.g. metformin	• preferred first-line agent in type 2 DM, especially in overweight/obese subjects • does not cause hypoglycaemia.
Sulfonylureas	Insulin secretagogues, which act on ATP-sensitive potassium channels in pancreatic β-cells to promote insulin secretion.
1st generation, e.g. chlorpropamide, tolbutamide	• rarely used due to less favourable side effect profile, e.g. long duration of action of chlorpropamide, which predisposes to hypoglycaemia
2nd and 3rd generation, e.g. gliclazide, glimepiride, glipizide	• more potent, but generally better tolerated than first-generation agents • predispose to hypoglycaemia, especially in the elderly and those with renal/hepatic impairment.
Meglitinides	Insulin secretagogues, which bind to ATP-sensitive potassium channels on pancreatic β-cells in a similar manner to sulfonylureas, but at a discrete binding site.
e.g. nateglinide, repaglinide	• rapid onset and very short duration of action; controls prandial hyperglycaemia • reduced risk of postabsorptive hypoglycaemia.
Thiazolidinediones (TZDs)	Selective agonists of the nuclear receptor PPARγ, which improve peripheral insulin sensitivity and promote more favourable adipose tissue distribution/function, but at a cost of overall weight gain.
e.g. pioglitazone	• hypoglycaemia is relatively uncommon with monotherapy, but risk may be increased by concomitant use of certain other oral hypoglycaemic agents (especially sulfonylureas) or insulin.
Alpha-glucosidase inhibitors	Impair the enzymatic degradation of complex carbohydrates (e.g. starch and sucrose) in the small intestine, thereby delaying their digestion and absorption.
e.g. acarbose	• modest effect on lowering blood glucose • not associated with hypoglycaemia when used alone.
DPP-4 inhibitors	Inhibit the function of DPP-4, thus impairing the degradation of the endogenous incretin GLP-1, which leads to an increase in GLP-1 levels, thereby promoting insulin release and suppressing glucagon secretion.
e.g. saxagliptin, sitagliptin, vildagliptin	• hypoglycaemia is relatively uncommon.
GLP-1 agonists/analogues e.g. exenatide, liraglutide	Incretin mimetics, which mimic endogenous GLP-1 action, thereby increasing insulin secretion, suppressing glucagon secretion and slowing gastric emptying. • hypoglycaemia is a recognised albeit uncommon side effect.
SGLT-2 inhibitors	Lowers the renal threshold for glucose, thereby increasing urinary glucose excretion
e.g. empagliflozin dapagliflozin	UTI and genitourinary infections can occur in 6–8%

ATP, adenosine triphosphate; DM, diabetes mellitus; DPP-4, dipeptidylpeptidase-4; GLP-1, glucagon-like peptide 1; PPARγ, peroxisome proliferator-activated receptor γ; SGLT, sodium-glucose linked transporter-2.

main meal. However, they are relatively expensive and although there are theoretical advantages to their use, in practice they offer few benefits over sulfonylureas.

Thiazolidinediones (TZDs; 'glitazones')

The TZDs are high-affinity ligands for the nuclear hormone receptor peroxisome proliferator-activated receptor γ (PPARγ), which is expressed ubiquitously, but at particularly high levels in adipose tissue.

Pioglitazone is the only remaining TZD in the UK. It is known to cause fluid retention and is contraindicated in those with/at risk of heart failure – this tendency is exacerbated when used in conjunction with insulin therapy. Other adverse effects of TZD therapy include weight gain, increased fracture rate at peripheral sites in women and, rarely, hepatic dysfunction; in addition, specific concerns have been raised regarding an increased risk of bladder cancer in those taking pioglitazone.

Alpha-glucosidase inhibitors

These agents inhibit the function of intestinal alpha-glucosidases, thereby delaying the digestion and absorption of complex carbohydrates (e.g. starch, sucrose). Currently, only one agent, acarbose, is licensed for use in the UK. It has a relatively small effect on lowering blood glucose levels and is associated with an unwelcome side effect – flatulence!

Dipeptidylpeptidase-4 inhibitors (DPP-4 inhibitors; 'gliptins')

Glucagon-like peptide 1 (GLP-1), an incretin that is secreted from the intestinal L-cells in response to nutrients, promotes glucose-dependent insulin secretion from pancreatic β-cells, while simultaneously suppressing glucagon release. In addition, GLP-1 slows gastric emptying and may confer additional 'protective effects' on the β-cells, through as yet unclear mechanisms. Endogenous GLP-1 has a very short half-life in the circulation and is rapidly degraded by the enzyme dipeptidylpeptidase-4 (DPP-4). Accordingly, inhibitors of DPP-4 (e.g. saxagliptin, sitagliptin and vildagliptin) enhance endogenous GLP-1 signalling and are of potential benefit in the treatment of type 2 DM. DPP-4 inhibitors are generally weight neutral. Hypoglycaemia is relatively uncommon.

Glucagon-like peptide 1 (GLP-1) agonists/analogues ('incretin mimetics')

Exenatide and liraglutide were the first agents to become available in this class, and mimic the effects of endogenous GLP-1. Both are given by subcutaneous injection. Unlike the DPP-4 inhibitors, they promote weight loss, which has been postulated to occur via a variety of mechanisms, including delayed gastric emptying, which results in early satiety, and central appetite suppressant effects. Weight loss may be profound with a resultant reduction in insulin resistance to such an extent that other oral hypoglycaemics can be reduced/withdrawn. The risk of hypoglycaemia is generally low, which is advantageous for those occupations where insulin use is prohibited. However, when used in combination with sulfonylureas (see later), there is a significant increase in the risk of hypoglycaemia, and patients should be advised of this.

Gastrointestinal side effects, particularly nausea, are common; severe (rarely fatal) pancreatitis has also been reported and patients should be carefully counselled and advised of symptoms to report.

Sodium-glucose linked transporter-2 (SGLT-2) inhibitors

SGLT2s are the newest oral hypoglycaemic agent, with a unique mechanism of action. SGLT-2 is a low-affinity, high-capacity glucose transporter located in the proximal renal tubule. SGLT-2 inhibitors prevent reabsorption of glucose and facilitate its excretion in urine. As glucose is excreted, its plasma levels fall leading to an improvement in all glycemic parameters. Mechanism of action is dependent on blood glucose levels, but independent of the actions of insulin, so hypoglycaemia is uncommon when used as monotherapy. Weight loss is common, due to calorie loss. Glycosuria, however, predisposes to genitourinary tract infection.

Post-marketing surveillance has led to an EMA warning regarding risk of toe amputation, while the FDA have issued a warning regarding the risk of ketoacidosis and severe urinary tract infection.

Insulin

The natural history of type 2 DM with insulin resistance is progressive pancreatic β-cell failure; so while good glycaemic control may initially be achievable through lifestyle measures alone, eventually most patients progress to require oral hypoglycaemic agents followed by incretin mimetics or insulin. Unfortunately, the use of insulin in type 2 DM is often complicated by weight gain. The different types of insulin regimen used in type 2 DM are shown in Table 17.6.

Diabetic emergencies

There are two common types of diabetic coma:

- hypoglycaemic (the most common)
- hyperglycaemic (diabetic ketoacidosis (DKA) or hyperosmolar hyperglycaemic state (HHS) (previously known as hyperosmolar non-ketosis [HONK]).

Hypoglycaemia ('hypo')

Hypoglycaemia in the context of DM occurs in patients who are treated with insulin and, less commonly, in those receiving certain oral hypoglycaemic agents (Table 17.7). It reflects an imbalance between insulin and carbohydrate, the most frequent precipitants being inappropriate medication use, excess physical activity, decreased food intake, excess alcohol ingestion or a combination of factors.

Hypoglycaemia is usually associated with the development of so-called warning symptoms – hypoglycaemic awareness involves:

- 'Autonomic' symptoms – a physiological response that is associated with the release of counter-regulatory hormones (adrenaline [epinephrine] and noradrenaline [norepinephrine]). Clinical signs include tremor, sweating, anxiety, palpitations and shivering.
- 'Neuroglycopenic' symptoms – manifest if hypoglycaemia is prolonged and more profound; as glucose is the only fuel source readily utilised by the brain, cognitive function is affected with symptoms of tiredness, dizziness, drowsiness, difficulty in speaking, inability to concentrate, confusion and aggression; as a general rule, neuroglycopenic symptoms develop when blood glucose is <2.6 mmol/l; if left untreated coma and death may ensue.

Although the blood glucose level at which people begin to experience hypoglycaemic symptoms varies, the consensus for defining hypoglycaemia in the context of DM is a blood glucose value of <4 mmol/l. *'Four is the Floor'* has proved to be a successful awareness campaign.

Management

The Joint British Diabetes Societies Inpatient Care Group (JBDS IP Group) has published recommendations for the treatment of hypoglycaemia, with the aim of standardising treatment within the UK National Health Service (NHS):

- If the patient is conscious, advise 15–20 g of rapidly acting carbohydrate (e.g. 3 dextrose tablets) *to correct* the hypoglycaemia, always followed with longer acting/complex carbohydrate *to maintain* glucose in the normal range (this may be the next meal if imminent; if not, offer toast or a sandwich).
- If the patient is semiconscious, then apply commercially available glucose gel to the buccal mucosa; this may allow sufficient improvement in conscious level to continue treatment as per a conscious individual.
- If the patient is unconscious, administer 50 ml of 20% dextrose IV (50% dextrose may cause significant phlebitis and is no longer recommended) via a large vein, followed by a generous flush; if intravenous access is not available, then 1 mg of glucagon can be given intramuscularly while awaiting further medical help.

Ascertaining the cause of recurrent hypoglycaemia is often neglected by the individual, or clinician. It should be sought and remedial action taken. Sometimes early morning headaches or a restless night may be the only indication of nocturnal hypoglycaemia.

NB: Recurrent and severe hypoglycaemia may cause a downregulation of the autonomic response to hypoglycaemia, resulting in reduced warning, so-called hypoglycaemic ('hypo') unawareness. Development of the latter has significant social/lifestyle implications, particularly with respect to driving.

Ninety to 120 ml of Lucozade™ used to be recommended but due to the UK 'sugar tax' (which is expected to be implemented in April 2018), whereby soft drinks with more than 5 g of sugar per 100 ml will have extra tax levied and even higher levies for drinks with more than 8 g per 100 ml, Lucozade has reduced its sugar content, so a larger volume is now required.

Hyperglycaemia

Diabetic ketoacidosis (DKA)

DKA most commonly occurs in the context of type 1 DM, but is also occasionally seen in type 2 DM under conditions of extreme stress. Glucose cannot be utilised as an energy substrate in the absence of insulin, and the body 'perceives' itself to be lacking in glucose, hence hepatic gluconeogenesis and glycogenolysis are enhanced, exacerbating the hyperglycaemia. An alternative energy substrate is sought, and lipolysis occurs with the mobilisation and increased production of fatty acids and amino acids; ketones are produced as a toxic metabolite of this process within the liver, resulting in the development of metabolic acidosis.

DKA is defined as a triad of:

- hyperglycaemia (plasma glucose > 11 mmol/l)
- acidosis (venous pH < 7.3)
- ketosis (either ketonaemia [>3 mmol/l] and/or ketonuria [>2+]).

The incidence, using all three criteria, is estimated at 4–8 episodes per 1000 diabetic individuals. It is a potentially life-threatening catabolic state, but fortunately mortality rates are now low in the developed world (<1%). Life-threatening complications include cerebral oedema (remains the commonest cause of mortality in the young), hypokalaemia and the development of adult respiratory distress syndrome.

The two major precipitating factors for DKA are inadequate insulin therapy, either deliberate or accidental, and intercurrent infection. All patients with type 1 DM should be educated regarding the nature, cause and prevention of DKA, often referred to as the 'sick day rules'.

Symptoms of DKA include thirst, dry mouth, polyuria, nausea, vomiting, weakness, myalgia, headache and abdominal pain. Drowsiness may progress to confusion and coma. It is rare for DKA to develop without a prodromal phase, and symptoms of hyperglycaemia have often been present for at least 24 h, but missed or ignored. Clinical signs include dehydration, tachycardia, hypotension, hyperventilation (Kussmaul breathing) and the characteristic smell of ketones. Hypovolaemic shock can ensue in more severe cases.

Management

The primary aim of treatment is to suppress ketogenesis, rather than normalise hyperglycaemia. The JBDS IP Group has released guidance on the management of DKA (March 2010, updated 2013). As with hypoglycaemia, the aims are to standardise care within the NHS, while at the same time incorporating recent advances in technology and recognising the changing presentation of DKA.

The major technological advance relates to near patient (i.e. bedside) routine testing of blood ketones (3-betahydroxybutyrate), and using the fall in ketonaemia as a guide to the response to treatment.

Recognition that 'euglycaemic acidosis' is now a more common presentation (with improved education, individuals often manage to partially treat their acidosis, often leading to lower blood glucose levels at presentation) is also emphasised in the guidance.

The management of DKA revolves around:

- fluid replacement
- insulin replacement
- metabolic treatment targets
- additional measures.

Fluid replacement

It is universally acknowledged that the most important therapeutic intervention in DKA is the immediate administration of fluids. Crystalloid is the fluid of choice (0.9% sodium chloride) even in the hypotensive individual. Fluids are required to:

- *Restore circulatory volume:* the required rate of fluid infusion will vary depending on the age of the patient (children and young adults appear to be at increased risk of cerebral oedema from over-exuberant fluid resuscitation, while otherwise previously fit adults generally tolerate rapid initial fluid replacement, e.g. first 1 litre of 0.9% sodium chloride over 1 h, with the second and third litres over 2 h each, increasing to 4-hourly bags for the fourth and fifth litres, and then 6-hourly, with reassessment of cardiovascular status on a regular basis). Care must also be exercised in the elderly, during pregnancy and in patients with pre-existing renal or cardiac failure or other serious comorbidities.
- *Enable clearance of ketones:* with lower glucose levels at presentation, administration of intravenous insulin can lead to hypoglycaemia well before ketogenesis is fully suppressed; as it is imperative to continue the insulin infusion until the latter has been achieved, the administration of 10% glucose, often concurrently with 0.9% sodium chloride, is often required (most units would start intravenous glucose when blood glucose levels fall below 14 mmol/l).
- *Correct electrolyte imbalance:* potassium is the predominant intracellular cation and is actively transported into cells through a glucose/insulin-dependent channel; at presentation hyperkalaemia is common in DKA, as potassium cannot enter the cells in the absence of insulin; however, total body potassium is low and following the administration of intravenous insulin serum potassium levels plummet and regular monitoring is therefore mandatory.

NB: Hypo- and hyperkalaemia are important causes of mortality in DKA.

The JBDS IP Group also provides simple guidance for the addition of potassium to intravenous fluids during the first 24 h of treatment:

- serum potassium > 5.5 mmol/l – none
- serum potassium 3.5–5.5 mmol/l – add 40 mmol/l
- serum potassium < 3.5 mmol/l – senior review as additional potassium is required and the patient may require transfer to a higher care setting to allow this to be given safely.

NB: Caution must be exercised in patients with suspected renal failure, especially in those with poor/no urine output despite initial fluid resuscitation.

Insulin replacement

The most significant change in the new guidance is the replacement of the traditional insulin sliding scale (variable rate intravenous insulin infusion [VRIII]) with a fixed rate intravenous insulin infusion (FRIII). The predominant rationale for this change is the increasing prevalence of obesity, an insulin-resistant state. Hence, the fixed rate is calculated per kilogram of body weight – initially 0.1 unit/kg/h. The previous recommendation for a 'priming bolus' has also been dropped, given that evidence has proven no benefit, providing the insulin infusion is started promptly, and in reality, it was often omitted.

Continuation of a subcutaneous long-acting analogue insulin alongside the insulin infusion is now recommended (it facilitates a smoother transition back to the individual's normal subcutaneous regimen, without rebound hyperglycaemia). Most units would recommend those using CSIII (i.e. insulin pump therapy) if *compos mentis* – should continue CSII running on basal rate as an alternative to subcutaneous long-acting analogue.

Metabolic treatment targets

- Reduction of blood ketone concentration by ≥0.5 mmol/l/h: generally measured hourly for the first 6 h; if ketonaemia is not responding adequately, reassess patient and increase FRIII by 1 unit/h, until adequate rate of resolution achieved.
- If blood ketone measurement is not available, aim to increase the venous bicarbonate by ≥3 mmol/l/h: again, if there is an inadequate response to treatment, increase FRIII as above.

NB: However, after 6 h, venous bicarbonate may become unreliable, particularly in the presence of hyperchloraemia as a consequence of the 0.9% sodium chloride infused.

- Alternatively, aim for a reduction in capillary blood glucose (CBG) of ≥3 mmol/l/h: again, this is an alternative to ketone analysis; however, falling CBG is not an accurate indicator of the resolution of acidosis (especially in 'euglycaemic acidosis'), which should be confirmed on venous gas analysis.

NB: If ketones and glucose are not falling as expected, check that the insulin infusion pump is working and connected and that the expected amount of insulin has been infused.

- Maintenance of serum potassium between 4.0 and 5.0 mmol/l: serum potassium should be measured at least 2-hourly for the first 6 h, and at regular intervals thereafter.

Additional measures

- Screen for infection: mid-stream urine sample, chest radiograph, blood cultures.

NB: A moderate rise in CRP may be seen in DKA without intercurrent infection.

- ECG: screen for silent myocardial ischaemia, but also to assess the impact of hypo-/hyperkalaemia on the myocardium.
- Urethral catheterisation: accurate fluid assessment is critical to effective management; placement of a urinary catheter is not mandatory, but if accurate urine volume assessment is not possible without a catheter, then one is required.
- A nasogastric tube should be placed if the conscious level is depressed, as acidosis predisposes to gastric stasis and the individual is therefore at high risk of aspiration.
- Adequate fluid and insulin therapy should produce prompt resolution of acidosis, and intravenous bicarbonate is therefore not routinely required and indeed may worsen the metabolic situation – acidosis promotes a right shift in the oxygen dissociation curve which may be an adaptive response; rapid correction of acidosis with bicarbonate leads to a rise in arterial $PaCO_2$ and a paradoxical fall in cerebrospinal fluid pH, exacerbating central nervous system depression.
- Whilst it is recognised that whole body deficit of phosphate is high, routine phosphate supplementation has no proven benefit. However, in the case of respiratory and muscular weakness it may be considered.

Resolution of DKA is defined as a blood ketone level of <0.3 mmol/l and venous pH > 7.3. If/when the individual is tolerating normal dietary intake they should be converted back to an appropriate subcutaneous insulin regimen. Trace/mild ketonuria may persist for a short time post-resolution of the acidosis.

However, an intermediate step down from a FRIII to VRIII is often needed if DKA has resolved but 'normal' eating has not resumed.

The diabetes specialist team should be involved in the care of all DKA episodes, in particular the diabetes specialist nurse who will be required to check education/understanding of possible DKA precipitants and the required actions to deal with these, as well as to facilitate follow-up post-discharge.

In the UK, DKA management attracts a BPT – best practice tariff.

Hyperosmolar hyperglyceamic state (HHS)

This typically occurs in the elderly, often previously undiagnosed, patient with type 2 DM. The onset may be drawn out, with polyuria precipitating dehydration over several days or even weeks. Precipitating factors include myocardial infarction, stroke and intercurrent infection. Unlike DKA, there is sufficient residual endogenous insulin to prevent ketogenesis, and hence no acidosis. Hyperosmolality is the predominant biochemical feature, in association with marked hyperglycaemia (blood glucose can exceed 100 mmol/l in extreme cases).

These patients are profoundly dehydrated and are at high risk of thrombosis (both arterial and venous), which is a significant contributor to the high mortality of this condition (30–50%). Low molecular weight heparin is therefore recommended unless there is a contraindication to its use (e.g. haemorrhagic stroke). The JBDS have produced a management guideline, 2013. Again, normalization of blood glucose is not the primary goal, but correction of the osmolality. Patients require rehydration to replace the massive fluid deficit, but this must be undertaken in a controlled manner (often with the aid of central venous pressure monitoring) especially where there is significant comorbidity (e.g. cardiac disease). In addition, overzealous rehydration may cause rapid osmotic shifts, precipitating cerebral oedema. Paradoxically these patients are often very insulin sensitive and may need only small amounts of insulin to lower their blood glucose satisfactorily – aim for a fall of 3 mmol/l/h. Reduction in glucose levels will occur automatically as osmolality is corrected so insulin is not recommended immediately unless significant ketonaemia (>1) is present. A FRIII is recommended, but at reduced dose (0.05 units/kg) compared to DKA management.

As with DKA, close monitoring of cardiovascular, renal and metabolic status, with regular checking of electrolytes, glucose, and osmolality is mandatory. Unlike DKA, insulin therapy is not always subsequently required once the acute episode has subsided, and survivors may manage on diet and oral hypoglycaemic agents.

Long-term diabetic complications

Long-term complications occur in all forms of DM and are broadly classified as microvascular or macrovascular in origin (Table 17.8).

Macrovascular complications

Diabetes is a major risk factor for the development of atherosclerotic vascular disease.

Attention to other cardiovascular risk factors in the patient with diabetes mellitus

Hypertension

With time, blood pressure targets in the context of diabetes have progressively fallen as data have emerged to show that in most cases 'the lower the better.' Combination therapy is often required to achieve a blood pressure of ≤135/85 mmHg, or even lower in those with concomitant renal involvement (130/80 mmHg). Angiotensin-converting enzyme (ACE) inhibitors and angiotensin receptor blockers (ARBs) are usually the preferred first-line agents, especially when there is evidence of microalbuminuria (see later). Calcium antagonists, α-adrenoceptor blockers and diuretics are useful adjuncts.

Dyslipidaemia

Several large-scale trials have shown that statins reduce both non-fatal and fatal cardiovascular events in patients with DM, when used in both primary and secondary prevention settings. Targets continue to be refined, but in general a total cholesterol level <4 mmol/l with low-density lipoprotein cholesterol (LDL-C) < 2 mmol/l are considered desirable. NICE Clinical guideline CG 181: Cardiovascular Disease: for those with type 2 diabetes with a >10% 10-year CVS risk (calculated using the QRISK2 tool) atorvastatin 20 mg should be commenced as primary prevention. For those with type 1 diabetes, the QRISK2 is not validated so atorvastatin 20 mg should be considered

Table 17.8 Long-term complications of diabetes mellitus

Microvascular complications	Macrovascular complications
Retinopathy	Coronary heart disease
Neuropathy – peripheral and autonomic	Peripheral vascular disease
Nephropathy	Cerebrovascular disease (stroke, transient ischaemic attack)

in those aged over 40 years, with disease duration >10 years, nephropathy or other CVS risk factor.

Smoking: Various studies have shown that smokers have an increased risk of myocardial infarction or sudden death and those with diabetes should be strongly advised not to smoke.

Aspirin: Low-dose aspirin (75 mg) is recommended for patients with a 10-year CVD risk of 10% and without an increased risk of bleeding from the gut.

Microvascular complications

Retinopathy

- The most common cause of visual loss in adults of working age in the UK.
- Proliferative retinopathy is more common in type 1 DM, and maculopathy in type 2 DM.
- Good glycaemic control is the key factor in preventing the development of, or deterioration in, retinopathy.
- Other risk factors include hypertension, smoking and pregnancy.

Various classification schemes for diabetic retinopathy have been proposed based largely on ophthalmological findings or functional severity: Table 17.9 provides an example of a traditional classification scheme; however, others argue for a simplification to just 'non-proliferative' and 'proliferative' subgroups, but again with maculopathy considered as a separate entity.

Management

Modification of all treatable risk factors and annual screening (visual acuities and retinal photography) are the mainstay of prevention and early intervention. If background retinopathy is present, glycaemic control should be reviewed, microalbuminuria, hypertension and dyslipidaemia sought and actively treated, and the patient kept under close surveillance. The presence of pre-proliferative retinopathy requires prompt referral for formal ophthalmological review. Laser photocoagulation, in which laser therapy is applied to peripheral areas of the retina (thereby reducing total oxygen requirements across the retina, and ameliorating ischaemia in other areas that are critical for vision), may be indicated. Again, maintenance of good glycaemic, blood pressure and lipid control is of paramount importance. For proliferative retinopathy, laser photocoagulation can reduce visual loss: here laser therapy is used to induce

Table 17.9 Classification of diabetic eye disease	
Type	**Features**
Background	Microaneurysms
	Haemorrhages (dot and blot/flame-shaped)
	Hard exudates (lipid deposits)
	Occasional (<5) soft exudates ('cotton wool' spots)
Preproliferative	As above
	Soft exudates*
	Intraretinal microvascular abnormalities (IRMAs)
	Venous beading, venous reduplication
Proliferative	New vessel formation at the disc/within one disc diameter (NVD)
	New vessels elsewhere (NVE)
	Rubeosis iridis
Maculopathy	Focal or diffuse oedema at the macula
	Haemorrhages, exudates or other changes at the macula
Advanced eye disease	Preretinal or vitreous haemorrhage
	Retinal detachment
Cataract	

*Multiple cotton wool spots signify retinal ischaemia.

regression of new blood vessels (thus reducing the risk of haemorrhage), in addition to reducing oxygen requirements throughout the retina, thereby retarding further new vessel proliferation. Laser therapy can also improve maculopathy. Anti-VEGFA therapy (anti-vascular endothelial growth factor A, e.g. ranibizumab) is now NICE approved (TA274, 2013) via intravitreous injection for treatment of maculopathy. Afibercept (NICE TA346, 2015) is both an anti-VGFA and B inhibitor. Vitrectomy (surgical removal of the vitreous) may be used as a salvage procedure in those with vitreous haemorrhage. It aims to improve vision by removing any blood from in or behind the vitreous, reattaches detached areas of retina, and is combined with panretinal laser photocoagulation to reduce the stimulus for further neovascularisation.

Cataracts are more common and occur at an earlier age in patients with DM, and should therefore be actively sought and treated.

Microalbuminuria and diabetic nephropathy

- Data from the UK Renal Registry show that diabetic nephropathy is the most common single cause of end-stage renal failure amongst adults starting renal replacement therapy.
- Nephropathy, i.e. the development of macroalbuminuria and a progressive decline in renal function (with falling glomerular filtration rate [GFR] and rising serum creatinine), ultimately affects approximately 20–30% of patients with DM, although this percentage is falling as earlier and more aggressive management of DM and its complications is pursued.
- Microalbuminuria heralds the onset of diabetic renal disease and, if left unchecked, progresses to intermittent and then persistent proteinuria. Progression is associated with either localised (Kimmelstiel–Wilson nodules) or diffuse fibrotic thickening of afferent and efferent arterioles. Proteinuria, hypertension and oedema become clinically apparent. Serum creatinine only rises after significant renal damage has occurred.
- Incipient nephropathy is synonymous with microalbuminuria. Normal urinary albumin excretion is <20 mg/l. Microalbuminuria is present when the urine albumin concentration is in the range 20–200 mg/l (30–300 mg/24 h), and macroalbuminuria when levels exceed this. Nephrotic syndrome is usually associated with urinary protein loss of >3 g/24 h.
- Screening for microalbuminuria is most commonly undertaken through estimation of the urine albumin to creatinine ratio (ACR) on a spot urine sample; values >2.5 mg/mmol in men and >3.5 mg/mmol in women signify the presence of microalbuminuria if confirmed on at least one further independent sample during the next few months. In practice, 24-hour urine collections are now rarely performed.
- The presence of microalbuminuria is also indicative of progressive generalised vascular disease, and attention must be paid to the management of other cardiovascular risk factors (e.g. hypertension, dyslipidaemia, smoking history).
- Other causes of renal impairment may coexist (e.g. hypertension, renal artery stenosis) and should be sought if there are specific clinical pointers or atypical features (e.g. development of renal disease in the absence of retinopathy).

NB: Intravenous contrast studies can precipitate acute renal failure in those with pre-existing renal impairment – adequate hydration and temporary withdrawal of agents such as metformin and ACE inhibitors/ARBs help reduce the risk in susceptible individuals – if in doubt, discuss with radiology and/or nephrology.

Management

The attainment of good glycaemic and, in particular, good blood pressure control is essential for the prevention and treatment of microalbuminuria. There is a large amount of data showing that ACE inhibitors are particularly effective in this setting, with ARBs an alternative in patients intolerant of the former. Both classes of agent appear to reduce proteinuria at levels above and beyond their antihypertensive effects.

Good blood pressure control remains the mainstay of treatment in those with established nephropathy, and again ACE inhibitors/ARBs are the preferred option(s), although additional antihypertensive therapy is often required, and diuretics may be helpful in treating fluid overload. Oral hypoglycaemiac agents that are long-acting and/or renally excreted (including insulin) should be reviewed on a regular basis and dosages adjusted or alternatives substituted where necessary.

NB: Metformin should be avoided in those with established renal impairment (eGFR < 30 ml/min) because of the risk of inducing lactic acidosis.

Early referral to a renal specialist service is generally recommended to ensure appropriate management of complications (e.g. secondary hyperparathyroidism, anaemia) and for consideration of/preparation for renal replacement therapy (dialysis and/or transplantation).

Continued aggressive management of cardiovascular risk factors is mandatory, as this is the major cause of morbidity and mortality in this group of patients.

Neuropathy

- More common in patients with a long history of DM (males > females), especially in those with poor glycaemic control.
- Multifactorial, reflecting a combination of metabolic and vascular factors.

Distal symmetrical polyneuropathy ('sensory peripheral neuropathy')

This is the most common form of diabetic neuropathy (characterised by loss of both myelinated and unmyelinated nerve fibres) and typically affects the longest fibres first – hence the so-called 'glove and stocking' distribution. Symptoms include dysaesthesia (numbness and tingling), often worse at night, progressing to chronic pain (stabbing/burning/shooting) with time. Examination reveals absent ankle jerks, diminished vibration sense in the lower limbs, and an inability to feel the standard 10-g monofilament. Reduced pain and temperature sensation follow, with muscular wasting and weakness late features. Affected individuals are at high risk of developing diabetic foot complications (neuropathic/neuro-ischaemic ulcers, Charcot arthropathy).

Optimal diabetic control is central to the prevention of distal symmetrical polyneuropathy. Tricyclic antidepressants (e.g. amitriptyline), duloxetine (a serotonin and noradrenaline reuptake inhibitor) and various anticonvulsants (e.g. carbamazepine, gabapentin and pregabalin) may help with symptom relief. Topical capsaicin may also be tried.

Acute (painful) sensory neuropathy

This is predominantly seen in male patients and is associated with poor glycaemic control or rapid improvement in glycaemic control (e.g. following commencement of insulin therapy).

Acute mononeuropathies

These motor neuropathies are thought to result from ischaemia and occlusion of vasa nervorum. Various cranial nerves (e.g. third, fourth and sixth), the ulnar nerves and the lateral common peroneal nerves are most commonly affected, and more than one nerve can be involved at any given time (i.e. mononeuritis multiplex). It is often transient and spontaneous recovery of function usually occurs over a period of months, but can be variable.

Diabetic amyotrophy (proximal motor neuropathy)

This is a rare disorder, which usually occurs in middle-aged men who develop painful, asymmetric weakness and wasting of the quadriceps muscles, and is often associated with marked anorexia and weight loss. Insulin, even in those with apparently satisfactory glycaemic control, remains the mainstay of treatment.

Autonomic neuropathy

Autonomic neuropathy may manifest in a number of different ways, including:

- cardiovascular: postural hypotension, tachycardia, painless ischaemia

- gastrointestinal: constipation, diarrhoea (especially nocturnal), gastroparesis
- genitourinary: erectile dysfunction/impotence, atonic bladder
- others: hypoglycaemia unawareness, gustatory sweating, oedema.

Other complications

The diabetic foot

Foot problems are very common and give rise to significant morbidity and mortality. The most commonly encountered problems are:

- *Neuropathic ulceration* – typically painless and occurring at pressure points (e.g. under the first and fifth metatarsal heads); lack of pain sensation and build-up of callus are predisposing factors; may be complicated by abscess formation/osteomyelitis. Ulcers should be swabbed and plain radiographs performed; if there is any suggestion of more deep-seated infection/osteomyelitis, consider MRI scan of the foot. Depending on the absence or presence of infection and the extent of tissue involvement, treatment may involve removal of callus and debridement, oral or intravenous antimicrobials and surgical drainage/debridement/amputation. Specialist non-weight-bearing footwear/total contact casting (TCC) is also often recommended to facilitate healing.
- *Neuroischaemic ulceration* – here the situation is exacerbated by concomitant vascular insufficiency; patients may also complain of intermittent claudication and/or rest pain; ulcers also occur over the heel and dorsum of the foot/toes, and pre-gangrenous or frankly gangrenous changes may be present. Investigation and management is similar to that for neuropathic ulceration, but in addition the extent of vascular disease requires formal assessment, often with a combination of Doppler ultrasound studies and arteriography to determine the feasibility of attempted revascularisation.
- *Neuropathic joints (Charcot arthropathy)* – a less common but well-recognised complication, often affecting the tarsometatarsal joints (i.e. mid-foot) and/or the ankle; impaired sensation with abnormal mechanical stresses/load-bearing may contribute to its development/progression. Left unchecked, joint instability and trophic bone changes lead to major and severe deformities of the foot. MRI scanning can help to differentiate from

infection and, in combination with isotope bone scintigraphy, may reveal new bone formation. The mainstay of treatment is to prevent deformity and destruction of the foot by strict avoidance of weight bearing, e.g. through the use of a TCC (see above). Surgical reconstruction of affected joints may be indicated in refractory cases. There is no evidence that intravenous bisphosphonate therapy is of benefit, but it is often used.

Diabetes-related skin conditions

Skin changes in diabetes may reflect:

- an immediate consequence of hyperglycaemia, e.g. opportunistic infection including candidiasis (particularly genital, e.g. balanitis) and *S. aureus* folliculitis
- long-term changes resultant from chronic hyperglycaemia
- a consequence of treatment.

Necrobiosis lipoidica diabeticorum (pretibial diabetic dermopathy) is pathognomonic of DM. It is characterised by atrophy of subcutaneous collagen, usually over the shins. Lesions typically start as small, brownish, erythematous shiny patches and may evolve to develop a central yellow area with atrophy that can ulcerate. Unfortunately, no treatment has been shown to be of benefit – the most important management is to protect the lesions from trauma.

Granuloma annulare typically manifests as a cluster of small papules that form a ring on the back of the hands or feet. Although spontaneous resolution usually occurs, cryotherapy or intralesional corticosteroid therapy may hasten the process.

Skin changes associated with insulin resistance include acanthosis nigricans (pigmented velvety thickening of the skin, typically seen in the axillae and nape of the neck, and considered a marker of severe insulin resistance) and scleroderma diabeticorum (thickening of the skin on the upper back and neck).

Lipoatrophy is painless localised necrosis of subcutaneous fat tissue at the site of insulin injection therapy; it is now uncommon following the introduction of recombinant/analogue human insulins. In contrast, lipohypertrophy (localised accumulation of fat tissue at the site of multiple injections) is very common, as hypertrophied sites are relatively painless to inject into! However, the insulin absorption from these sites is erratic, leading to unpredictable glycaemic excursions.

Diabetes and pregnancy

Pregestational DM

Commissioned in 2002, and reporting in 2007, the UK Confidential Enquiry into Maternal and Child Health (CEMACH) quantified the risks of diabetic pregnancy: perinatal mortality was 3–5 times higher and congenital malformation rate 4–10 times higher than in the general population; 'suboptimal care' was highlighted as a major factor in those cases with poor outcomes.

Prepregnancy counselling

The importance of optimal diabetic control before conception should be strongly emphasised. Women should be given realistic information regarding the effects of diabetes on pregnancy (miscarriage, congenital malformation, stillbirth and neonatal death) and advised that these risks can be reduced (but not eliminated) with good preconceptual and antenatal glycaemic control. Counselling should also discuss the potential effects of pregnancy on the progression of diabetic complications.

Antenatal care

Daily oral folic acid supplements (5 mg) should be taken from 3 months prior to conception, and for at least the first 12 weeks of gestation, to reduce the risk of neural tube defects. Tight glycaemic control must be maintained throughout pregnancy. To facilitate this, women should undergo an early antenatal assessment (as soon as pregnancy is confirmed) and antenatal care should be provided by a multidisciplinary team (as described earlier). Women with pregestational DM have a higher risk of pre-eclampsia and should be offered 75 mg aspirin daily post-viability scan.

Glycaemic control

Targets for home self-monitoring of blood glucose (HBGM) should be agreed with the individual woman. Where possible, aim to keep fasting blood glucose levels between 3.5 and 5.3 mmol/l. HBGM should be performed 1 h after each meal, with the aim, where safe, of keeping levels below 7.8 mmol/l. HBGM should also be performed before retiring to bed each night.

NB: HbA_{1c} is less reliable in the second and third trimester to gauge the adequacy of control.

Women should have regular contact with the diabetes centre, ideally on a weekly basis (and no less than fortnightly), for regular reassessment. They must be advised of the increased risk of hypoglycaemia in pregnancy, particularly during the first and early second trimester and that hypoglycaemia unawareness is also more common – this is particularly important with respect to driving.

It is also important to warn of the increased risk of ketogenesis and the particular hazards to the fetus/pregnancy of ketosis. Clear guidance should be offered regarding testing for ketosis and the '*sick day rules*' (see later) reiterated. Blood ketone testing strips (ketonaemia) should be prescribed.

Medication

All oral hypoglycaemics with the exception of metformin, should be discontinued prior to conception or as soon as pregnancy is confirmed. Metformin can be offered as a first-line agent where glycaemic control has not been achieved through lifestyle measures alone.

NB: Although the use of metformin is supported by NICE, it is not currently licensed in pregnancy and women should therefore be appropriately counselled.

If glycaemic control is not achieved rapidly, i.e. within 10–14 days, insulin therapy should be commenced. A multiple dose injection (MDI) ('*basal-bolus*') regimen is preferred for all women requiring insulin therapy. Although NICE does not currently recommend the routine use of basal analogue insulin preparations in pregnancy, most units will continue their use if started preconceptually, and indeed many diabetologists would also initiate treatment with them when required, because of their favourable hypoglycaemic profile.

Drugs affecting the renin-angiotensin system (e.g. ACE inhibitors, ARBs) should be stopped as soon as possible as they are potentially fetotoxic. Alternative antihypertensive agents (e.g. methyldopa, labetalol, nifedipine) can be substituted where necessary.

Where an ACE inhibitor/ARB has been used prior to pregnancy for the purpose of renoprotection, close surveillance for nephropathy must be observed. Statins should be discontinued, and the risk to benefit ratios of all other medications must be carefully discussed.

Retinal assessment

Women should be advised of the importance of retinal assessment in the preconception period, and during and after pregnancy.

Renal assessment

Renal assessment is important both in the preconception period and during pregnancy. Diabetic nephropathy is a progressive disease that can significantly adversely affect the outcome of the pregnancy; in addition, pregnancy can accelerate the progression of nephropathy. Early involvement of the renal team is advisable in any patient in whom there is concern regarding renal status. Nephropathy is a risk factor for intrauterine growth retardation and pre-eclampsia.

NB: eGFR is not validated for use in pregnancy and should not therefore be used as an indicator of renal function.

Fetal growth and well-being

Women should have all aspects of routine fetal monitoring and well-being offered. In addition a four-chamber view of the fetal heart and outflow tracts should be offered at 18–20 weeks' gestation. Assessment of fetal growth and amniotic fluid volume by ultrasonography every 4 weeks is recommended between 28 and 38 weeks' gestation. Routine monitoring of fetal well-being (e.g. cardiotocography) prior to 38 weeks is not generally recommended; however, in women at risk of intrauterine growth retardation (IUGR; i.e. those with macrovascular disease/nephropathy) an individualised approach should be tailored to assess fetal growth and well-being, including fetal Doppler.

Women with DM in pregnancy should be advised of the possibility of fetal macrosomia and its associated risks (e.g. birth trauma, and an increased requirement for induction of labour and/or caesarean section, increased risk of neonatal hypoglycaemia).

Intrapartum care

Delivery should be completed by 39 weeks' gestation; every woman should have an individualised care plan for her glycaemic control during the intrapartum and immediate postpartum period, and this should be clearly documented in her notes. During labour, blood glucose must be monitored hourly, aiming to keep levels between 4 and 7 mmol/l; if this cannot be achieved using the patient's standard diabetes treatment, then a variable rate intravenous insulin infusion (i.e. sliding scale) should be initiated. The JBDS inpatient guidelines would recommend a VRIII as soon as active labour is established for all using MDI therapy.

Neonatal care

Blood glucose testing is carried out routinely in all off-spring of mothers with DM, and babies should remain in hospital for 24-h post-delivery to ensure maintenance of adequate glucose levels.

Preterm labour

In the case of threatened or actual preterm labour, women with DM receiving corticosteroids antenatally require admission for blood glucose monitoring. If glycaemic control is not maintained between 4 and 7 mmol/l on the patient's regular treatment regimen, then a variable rate intravenous insulin infusion should be initiated and continued for 24 h after the last dose of steroids.

Gestational diabetes mellitus

Gestational diabetes mellitus (GDM) is diabetes that develops or is first recognised in pregnancy. In the UK, the prevalence varies from 1 in 220 to 1 in 330 depending on the ethnicity of the region. Both IADPSG and NICE have recently issued guidance on the definition of, and screening for, GDM (see classification, earlier).

Management is along similar lines as for pregestational DM, with a particular emphasis on diet and HBGM; target glycaemic levels and fetal surveillance strategies are the same. Glucose tolerance often returns to normal after delivery. NICE recommends that a fasting venous plasma glucose level be checked at 5–6 weeks postnatally, repeated on an annual basis thereafter, as it is well recognised that a substantial proportion of women affected with GDM go on to develop type 2 DM in later life, with estimates varying from 20–50% depending on the population under study.

Other important information for patients with diabetes

Diabetes and intercurrent illness

'Sick day rules'

During times of illness, particularly when oral intake is poor, many insulin-dependent/treated patients with DM become concerned regarding the risk of developing hypoglycaemia; however, in reality hepatic glycogenolysis provides sufficient glucose to prevent the development of hypoglycaemia during most intercurrent illnesses, even when calorie intake is markedly reduced. In fact, the main risk with intercurrent illness is of developing hyperglycaemia, precipitated by relative insulin resistance, which may lead to DKA/HHS, particularly if insulin doses are inappropriately omitted or reduced. It is important therefore that patients are educated to:

- never stop insulin during intercurrent illness
- perform HBGM frequently
- check for ketones regularly
- maintain a high fluid intake wherever possible.

Most patients require frequent small doses of rapid-acting insulin to avoid developing hyperglycaemia and, in the case of type 1 DM, ketoacidosis. If in doubt, patients should be advised to seek early medical advice. This information should be provided in written format, as well as verbally, and reinforced at each annual review.

Diabetes and surgery

Most hospitals have protocols for the management of individuals with DM undergoing procedures that require a period of fasting, e.g. colonoscopy through to major abdominal surgery. Again the JBDS have produced consensus guidelines 'Management of adults with diabetes undergoing surgery and elective procedures: Improving standards Revised September 2015'. It is recommended that routine elective surgery should not be routinely scheduled if a patients HbA_{1c} is >69 mmol/l. Ideally, patients should be given written as well as verbal instructions on medication adjustments at their preprocedural/preoperative assessment. To facilitate optimal glycaemic control, those with DM should be scheduled as early on the operative/procedure list as is practical, and a variable rate intravenous insulin infusion instituted to maintain euglycaemia as the stress of surgery (cortisol, glucagon, growth hormone and catecholamine surges) predispose to hyperglycaemia. Once the patient is eating and drinking normally postoperatively, it is usually possible to return to his/her regular therapy.

Diabetes and driving in the UK

In the UK, patients with DM treated with tablets and/or diet may hold a 'car/motorcycle' group 1 license and need not inform the DVLA unless they have complications (see later for specific rules relating to hypoglycaemia); however, they must inform their insurance company. The DVLA (and insurance company) must be notified once a patient commences insulin therapy. Those treated with insulin will be given a group 1 entitlement licence for 1, 2 or 3 years depending upon the quality of their glycaemic control, the regularity of medical surveillance and the extent of complications. Patients with type 2 DM not requiring insulin may be issued with a 'till 70' license, unless they have complications of their DM. Recent changes to DVLA regulations mean that it is now possible for a patient receiving insulin to hold a group 2 (LGV, PCV) license with review on an annual basis; however, a series of strict medical criteria must be met (in particular with respect to hypoglycaemia (preserved awareness, regular recorded testing, no episodes requiring third-party rescue, etc.), absence of complications, and annual review by an independent Consultant Diabetologist).

The onus is on the driver to prove they are fit to drive and should test at times relevant to driving, a capillary blood glucose should be recorded on a memory meter, with time and date set correctly, within 2 hours of driving. CBG must be 5 mmol/l or above. 'Five to drive'.

Hypoglycaemia is the major factor that impacts on driving in all categories. Patients must be able to effectively recognise and treat hypoglycaemia. The DVLA advises that patients should check their blood glucose at times relevant to driving. Patients must carry glucose tablets (or equivalent) to treat hypoglycaemia, as well as their glucometer; they are expected to stop and test their glucose level every 2 h on a long journey. If a hypoglycaemic episode occurs whilst driving, they should pull over, remove the keys from the ignition and move to the passenger side, so they are no longer in charge of the vehicle. They must wait an appropriate time (45 min) after correcting the hypoglycaemia before recommencing their journey. Hypoglycaemia requiring third-party rescue is considered a major concern and will lead to even a group 1 licence being revoked if it has occurred on more than one occasion in the preceding 12 months.

Dyslipidaemia

The major importance of dyslipidaemia lies in its close relationship with cardiovascular disease. At a simplistic level, LDL-C is potentially 'deleterious', as small dense LDL particles are capable of penetrating the endothelial barrier and are taken up by macrophages before undergoing oxidation to give rise to 'foam cells'. The latter contribute to atheromatous plaque formation and instability, e.g. in coronary blood vessels. In contrast, HDL particles predominantly work to remove excess cholesterol from cells for transport back to the liver in a process known as reverse cholesterol transport. Hence, LDL-C is sometimes referred to as 'bad cholesterol' and HDL-C as 'good cholesterol'. Hypertriglyceridaemia is also considered an independent risk factor for vascular disease, and predisposes to pancreatitis.

Classification

A practical classification is shown in Table 17.10.

Primary dyslipidaemias

Familial hypercholesterolaemia
Familial hypercholesterolaemia (autosomal dominant) is caused by mutations in the LDL receptor gene, which results in reduced LDL-C clearance and consequent hypercholesterolaemia (severe in the homozygous form, less marked in heterozygotes) leading to premature atherosclerosis. Affected individuals are often asymptomatic but manifest clinical signs including corneal arcus, xanthelasmata and tendon xanthomata. Left untreated, premature cardiovascular death is common. Heterozygotes respond to pharmacological management of their hypercholesterolaemia and modification of other cardiovascular risk factors. Liver transplantation can correct the metabolic abnormality in homozygotes. Family screening is strongly recommended.

Familial defective apolipoprotein B-100
This is caused by a single amino-acid substitution in apolipoprotein B, resulting in defective binding of LDL to its receptor. It is clinically indistinguishable from familial hypercholesterolaemia and treated in the same way.

Polygenic hypercholesterolaemia
Often considered a diagnosis of exclusion in which there is isolated LDL-C elevation without peripheral stigmata, but premature ischaemic heart disease within a family. Variants in Apo E4 alleles have been implicated in some instances. Statins are the preferred treatment option.

Familial hypertriglyceridaemia
This may be caused by either increased hepatic VLDL production or a failure of triglycerides to be cleared from chylomicrons by lipoprotein lipase. Inheritance is autosomal dominant. Marked hypertriglyceridaemia is

Table 17.10 Classification of dyslipidaemia

	Lipoprotein class	Fredrickson type	Primary causes	Secondary causes
Hypercholesterolaemia (predominant)	↑ LDL	IIa	Familial hypercholesterolaemia Polygenic hypercholesterolaemia	Hypothyroidism Obstructive jaundice Corticosteroids Anorexia nervosa
Hypertriglyceridaemia (predominant)	↑ CM	I	Lipoprotein lipase deficiency Apo CII deficiency	Diabetes mellitus Oral contraceptive pill
	↑ VLDL	IV	Familial combined hyperlipidaemia Familial hypertriglyceridaemia	Alcohol excess Thiazide diuretics
	↑ CM and VLDL	V	Lipoprotein lipase deficiency Apo CII deficiency	
Mixed dyslipidaemia	↑ Remnants	III	Familial dysbetalipoproteinaemia	Diabetes mellitus Obesity
	↑ VLDL and LDL	IIb	Familial combined hyperlipidaemia	Nephrotic syndrome Renal failure Paraproteinaemia

CM, chylomicron; HDL, high-density lipoprotein; IDL, intermediate-density lipoprotein; LDL, low-density lipoprotein; VLDL, very low-density lipoprotein.

associated with eruptive xanthomata, lipaemia retinalis and acute pancreatitis. Management involves avoiding/treating potential exacerbating conditions such as obesity, hypothyroidism and diabetes mellitus, together with pharmacotherapy aimed at reducing the hypertriglyceridaemia (e.g. fibrates and nicotinic acid).

Familial combined hyperlipidaemia

This condition is inherited as an autosomal dominant trait and affects ~1% of the general population but up to 15% of patients suffering myocardial infarction who present before 60 years of age. It is characterised by an overproduction of hepatic-derived Apo B100 (genetic basis unknown). Cholesterol and triglycerides are classically both increased (with increases in LDL and/or VLDL cholesterol; HDL-C is typically low), but one or other may be normal. Clinical signs include corneal arcus and xanthelasmata, but not tendon xanthomata. The risk of atherosclerosis is increased. Treatment often requires combination statin (targeting LDL-C) and fibrate (triglyceride lowering) therapy, with the attendant increased risks of rhabdomyolysis and hepatic upset.

Familial dysbetalipoproteinaemia

This is a rare (autosomal recessive) disorder characterised by elevations in triglyceride and total cholesterol levels. The disease develops in individuals who are homozygous for apolipoprotein E2 (Apo E2) variants. There is a reduced ability to convert VLDL and IDL to LDL particles in the blood and decreased clearance of chylomicron remnants. Affected individuals are at increased risk of atherosclerotic cardiovascular disease and peripheral vascular disease. Linear xanthomata of the palmar creases are considered pathognomonic. The condition responds well to avoidance/treatment of other disorders that predispose to hypertriglyceridaemia, and to medications that reduce blood triglyceride concentrations (e.g. fibrates, nicotinic acid).

Secondary dyslipidaemias

Secondary dyslipidaemias are very common, and treatment of the underlying cause generally improves the dyslipidaemia. Common secondary causes include endocrine disorders (e.g. hypothyroidism, Cushing syndrome, acromegaly), renal failure/nephrotic syndrome, drugs (e.g. oral oestrogen, thiazide diuretic or retinoid therapy), alcohol excess, obstructive liver disease, diabetes mellitus and obesity.

Associations between lipids and vascular disease

Epidemiological studies such as the Multiple Risk Factor Intervention Trial (MRFIT) and Prospective Cardiovascular Munster study (PROCAM) have examined the potential links between dyslipidaemia and ischaemic heart disease. In general, most have shown a strong curvilinear association between plasma total cholesterol or LDL-C and ischaemic heart disease (IHD), whereas there is an inverse relationship with HDL-C. For example, a 10% increase in total/LDL-C increases the IHD risk by 20%. (As 60–70% of plasma cholesterol is present in LDL, total cholesterol is often used as a surrogate measure of LDL-C.) Raised levels of lipoprotein A also predict the risk of ischaemic heart disease. In contrast, studies have given variable results with regard to the association of hypertriglyceridaemia and IHD, although on balance it appears that raised plasma triglyceride levels are a risk factor.

Clinical presentation

Dyslipidaemia is typically identified in the context of cardiovascular disorders or other related metabolic conditions (e.g. diabetes mellitus). Occasionally the clinical stigmata of dyslipidaemia trigger screening (xanthelasmata, corneal arcus and tendon xanthomata are associated with hypercholesterolaemia, and eruptive or tuberous xanthomata and lipaemia retinalis with hypertriglyceridaemia). Screening should also be offered to asymptomatic individuals with a positive family history. Patients with more marked hypertriglyceridaemia (>10 mmol/l) are prone to pancreatitis.

Investigation

Total cholesterol

Fasting samples are not strictly necessary, although should be requested when patients record non-fasting cholesterol levels that would require treatment, and in those suspected of having dyslipidaemia.

NB: A mild or moderate elevation in LDL-C with an associated reduction in HDL-C can result in a normal total cholesterol level, which can therefore be misleading with respect to cardiovascular risk.

LDL cholesterol

A fasting sample is required for an accurate result. However, the assay is difficult and expensive to run and the majority of laboratories actually calculate/estimate the LDL level, from the Friedewald equation (LDL cholesterol = Total cholesterol – HDL cholesterol – [triglycerides/2.2]) (all values in mmol/l).

NB: The Friedewald equation should not be used when chylomicrons are present, when plasma triglycerides exceed 4.5 mmol/l or in patients with known dysbetalipoproteinaemia.

HDL cholesterol

Measurement is not standardised and there are generally only small differences between normal and abnormal levels. However, the ratio of total serum cholesterol to HDL cholesterol is commonly used in coronary risk prediction charts.

Triglycerides

Plasma triglycerides rise dramatically after a meal so a fasting sample, preferably overnight, is required.

Other investigations

- *Fasting blood glucose:* to exclude dyslipidaemia secondary to DM.
- *Renal function:* to exclude chronic kidney disease.
- *Liver function tests (transaminases):* to exclude intrinsic liver disease, and as a baseline for monitoring while on statin therapy.
- *Creatine kinase:* some advocate measuring at baseline prior to statin therapy, while others suggest checking only in those complaining of muscle symptoms while on treatment.
- *Thyroid function tests:* to exclude hypothyroidism.
- *Genetic testing/screening:* as clinically indicated (see earlier).

Management

The primary purpose of treating dyslipidaemia is to prevent or reduce the risk and complications of cardiovascular disease. There is a large volume of powerful clinical trial data to show that lipid-lowering therapy reduces the risk of cardiovascular morbidity and mortality in at-risk individuals – both in the context of primary and secondary prevention.

The decision to initiate treatment in those without a prior history of vascular disease is often based on an assessment of overall risk of coronary heart disease. Risk assessment calculators are recommended by both NICE (Clinical guideline [CG181], July 2014 and

JBS3 (Joint British Societies' consensus recommendations for the prevention of cardiovascular disease 2014). They should not be used in patients at high cardiovascular risk. Both calculators are unsuitable for assessing risk in those aged 85 years and over. The QRISK®2 risk calculator is recommended by NICE CG181, and the JBS3 risk calculator is endorsed by JBS3. Cardiovascular disease risk is underestimated in those who are already taking antihypertensive or lipid-regulating drugs, and in those who have recently stopped smoking.

Non-drug therapy

Diet
Dietary modification may lower cholesterol and triglyceride levels, but typically only by 5–10% (remember, <15% of cholesterol is dietary in origin). Longer chain saturated fatty acids raise and mono and polyunsaturated fatty acids lower LDL-C.

In general, individuals should aim for:

- total fat intake ≤ 30% of total energy intake
- saturated fats ≤ 10% of total energy intake
- dietary cholesterol < 300 mg/day
- replacement of saturated fats with mono- or polyunsaturated fats
- five portions of fruit and vegetables per day
- two portions of fish per week, including one portion of oily fish.

Other lifestyle measures

- weight reduction
- regular physical exercise
- smoking cessation
- avoidance of excess alcohol ingestion
- good blood pressure and glycaemic control

Drug therapy

Statins
Statins are competitive inhibitors of HMG CoA reductase. They are potent in lowering LDL-C, but less effective than fibrates in reducing triglycerides or raising HDL-C levels. They reduce cardiovascular disease events irrespective of the starting cholesterol concentration, although patients with a total serum-cholesterol concentration of ≥5 mmol/l are likely to derive most benefit. In diabetes mellitus it is generally advised that all patients >40 years of age be considered for statin therapy, which may also be indicated in younger subjects with complications (however, statins should be avoided in females desiring pregnancy owing to risk of fetal anomalies).

Myositis (which can lead to rhabdomyolysis) is a rare, but potentially serious, adverse effect of statin therapy – patients should be warned to promptly report unexplained muscle pain, tenderness or weakness. Liver function should be monitored during treatment.

For primary prevention, NICE (CG181, 2014) currently recommends atorvastatin 20 mg/day in those with a 10-year cardiovascular risk of ≥10%. For secondary prevention, atorvastatin is also recommended. Patients taking a low- or medium-intensity statin should discuss the benefits and risks of switching to a high-intensity statin (e.g. atorvastatin 80 mg/day) at their next medication review.

Other options include simvastatin, pravastatin, fluvastatin and rosuvastatin.

Dose reduction or temporary cessation of treatment may need to be considered in cases where there is a 'temporary' drug interaction or intercurrent illness that predisposes to statin toxicity.

Fibrates
Fibrates (which are high affinity ligands for the nuclear receptor peroxisome proliferator-activated receptor α [PPARα]) act mainly by decreasing serum triglycerides; they also tend to raise HDL-C levels, but have variable effects on LDL-C. They are generally considered first-line therapy only in those who have marked hypertriglyceridaemia (>10 mmol/l) or in those who cannot tolerate a statin.

The fibrates may also cause a myositis-like syndrome (particularly in those with chronic renal impairment), and this risk is significantly increased when used in conjunction with statins. Dual therapy should therefore only be initiated under expert supervision.

Bile acid sequestrants
These agents bind bile acids in the small intestine, preventing their reabsorption, which in turn promotes hepatic conversion of cholesterol into bile acids; the resultant increase in hepatic LDL receptor expression/activity increases LDL-C clearance from plasma. Colestyramine, colestipol and colesevelam are all effective in reducing hypercholesterolaemia, but may worsen hypertriglyceridaemia and cause malabsorption of fat-soluble vitamins.

Nicotinic acid derivatives
Agents in this category (e.g. niacin, Niaspan®) reduce the synthesis of both cholesterol and triglycerides; they also increase HDL-C. However, their use is limited by side effects, particularly vasodilatation leading to flushing. Nicotinic acid is licensed for use with a statin or in those intolerant of statins.

Ezetimibe

Ezetimibe inhibits the intestinal absorption of cholesterol. It is used as an adjunct to dietary manipulation in patients with primary hypercholesterolaemia in combination with a statin (or alone if a statin is inappropriate or not tolerated), and in patients with homozygous familial hypercholesterolaemia in combination with a statin. Side effects include gastrointestinal upset, and there is an increased risk of myositis/rhabdomyolysis when used in conjunction with a statin.

Omega-3 fatty acid compounds (commonly known as fish oils)

These may be used as an adjunct to reduce serum triglycerides; however, there is little evidence that they reduce cardiovascular risk.

Microsomal triglyceride transfer protein (MTP) inhibitors

These prevent the assembly of apo B-containing lipoproteins thus inhibiting the synthesis of chylomicrons and VLDL and leading to decrease in plasma levels of LDL-C. Lomitapide may confer benefits in familial hypercholesterolaemia.

Proprotein convertase subtilisin/kexin type 9 (PCSK9) inhibitors

These agents increase LDL receptor availability through inhibition of the PCSK9 protein, which normally binds to the LDL receptor and targets it for degradation. Current PCSK9 inhibitors available in clinical practice are the monoclonal antibodies alirocumab and evolocumab. In the UK, NICE (Technology Appraisals 393 and 394, June 2016) currently allow their use in primary heterozygous familial hypercholesterolaemia and in patients with atherosclerotic cardiovascular disease who require further LDL-lowering therapy.

Obesity

Traditionally, body mass index (BMI = weight in kilograms divided by height in metres squared) has been used to categorise body weight: <18.5 = underweight; 18.5–24.9 = normal; >25 = overweight; >30 = obese; >40 = severe/morbid obesity. However, BMI takes no account of body composition, overestimating obesity in muscular individuals and failing to discriminate between central (visceral) and peripheral (gluteal, limb) adipose tissue accumulation. The former (i.e. central obesity) is particularly associated with metabolic dysfunction (and the metabolic syndrome) and increased cardiovascular risk. In addition, obesity predisposes to sleep apnoea, joint failure (especially hips and knees) and cancer.

The prevalence of overweight/obesity has been estimated to be as high as 50% or more in Western societies, and childhood/adolescent obesity is an increasing problem. Sadly, the developing world is also catching up as the 'obesity epidemic' becomes truly global.

Aetiology

In most instances, obesity is the result of complex interactions between genetic, environmental and behavioural factors. Although a sedentary lifestyle and excess caloric intake are major predisposing factors, there is increasing evidence to suggest that not only extreme forms of obesity but also more common variants are linked to genetic predisposition, i.e. put simply, some individuals are genetically more prone to weight gain than others. Table 17.11 lists some of the recognised factors that contribute to being overweight/obese.

Clinical features

Age at onset, previous success/failure in attempts to lose weight, family history, diet/alcohol consumption and physical activity should all be enquired about when assessing patients who are overweight/obese. Specific features of conditions that predispose to obesity (e.g. hypothyroidism, Cushing syndrome) should also be sought and a careful drug history taken. Clinical examination is important in determining the pattern of obesity (e.g. global versus central) and identifying specific markers of insulin resistance (e.g. acanthosis nigricans) or other disorders.

Investigation

If there is suspicion of an underlying predisposing condition (e.g. hypothyroidism, Cushing syndrome, monogenic form of obesity), then investigations should be tailored accordingly. In all other cases, investigations are directed towards assessment of cardiovascular risk and other comorbidities.

Management

Wherever possible, underlying predisposing disorders should be treated and offending drugs withdrawn/substituted. Care of the obese patient is best provided by a multidisciplinary team, which usually includes a

Table 17.11 Factors implicated in weight gain/obesity

Type	Example(s)
Diet	Simple over-eating (especially energy dense foods)
Exercise	Sedentary work/lifestyle Enforced inactivity (e.g. following surgery/injury) Ageing
Social/behavioural	Habitual eating Binge-eating
Genetic variation	
• Common variants	FTO gene polymorphisms
• Rare conditions	Leptin and leptin receptor gene defects, melanocortin 4-receptor gene defects; Prader–Willi syndrome; Laurence–Moon–Biedl syndrome
Drugs	Glucocorticoids, oral contraceptive preparations, sulfonylureas, insulin, TCAs, SSRIs, olanzapine, clozapine, lithium, sodium valproate
Endocrine disorders	Hypothyroidism Cushing syndrome Hypothalamic disorders
Others	Low birth weight ('fetal programming') Cardiac/renal/hepatic failure – with fluid retention

FTO, fat mass and obesity-associated gene; SSRIs, selective serotonin reuptake inhibitors; TCAs, tricyclic antidepressants.

physician trained in obesity medicine, a nurse specialist, obesity dietitian and a psychologist. The treatment strategy typically involves five elements:

- Dietary modification: a variety of regimes exist, which in general involve three phases: (1) a screening phase, (2) an intensive weight loss phase, and (3) a weight maintenance phase. Specialist advice should be sought if considering the use of more calorie-restricted regimes, to minimise the risk of adverse effects.
- Exercise programme: in particular, aerobic exercise.
- Behavioural modification: a core feature of any weight reduction programme; may involve goal setting, meal planning, self-monitoring and group work.
- Medical therapy: considered if dietary/behavioural modification/exercise in combination are ineffective. The gastric/pancreatic lipase inhibitor orlistat facilitates mild to moderate weight loss when used in combination with lifestyle measures, but may be associated with malabsorption of fat-soluble vitamins. Although initially introduced to improve glycaemic control in type 2 DM, GLP-1 agonists/analogues (e.g. exenatide and liraglutide – see *diabetes mellitus*) have shown great potential to promote weight loss, and liraglutide (Saxenda™) has recently been licensed in the UK as an adjunct to a reduced calorie diet and physical activity for weight management in adult patients with an initial BMI of $\geq 30\,\text{kg/m}^2$ or from 27 to $<30\,\text{kg/m}^2$ in the presence of at least one weight-related comorbidity (e.g. prediabetes/DM, hypertension, dyslipidaemia, obstructive sleep apnoea).

- Bariatric surgery: two main forms exist – gastric banding or stapling and malabsorptive (i.e. bypassing the small bowel) – the latter tends to be more effective in promoting sustained weight loss, but long-term outcomes/adverse effects are still under review.

Prognosis

- Data from prospectively followed cohorts, such as the Framingham study, indicate that morbidity and mortality are substantially increased in obese individuals.
- Common complications of obesity include hypertension, diabetes mellitus, ischaemic heart disease, osteoarthritis/joint failure, herniae, gallstones and varicose veins. In women there is an increased incidence of hirsutism/menstrual disturbance and breast and endometrial carcinoma. Obese subjects also present an increased surgical risk.

Under(mal)nutrition

Undernutrition is a major problem of the developing world. *Marasmus* refers to severe protein-energy malnutrition. Children are grossly underweight with muscle wasting and markedly diminished fat. There is no oedema. In *kwashiorkor* there is protein deficiency, but with adequate calorie intake. There is oedema from hypoproteinaemia, and lipids accumulate in the liver, causing hepatomegaly.

In industrialised countries, undernutrition may be seen during any acute illness, but particularly those involving the gastrointestinal tract. Protein loss may also be substantial following burns (due to cutaneous loss), and can arise postoperatively (reflecting reduced intake and increased catabolism).

Vitamin deficiencies

Vitamins are organic substances, each with specific biochemical functions. They are mostly found in food and typically only required in small amounts.

Fat-soluble vitamins

- *Vitamin A* (retinol): found in liver, fish and dairy products; it is also produced in the intestine by cleavage of β-carotene (found in carrots and other vegetables); it is required for night vision (11-*cis*-retinaldehyde combines with rhodopsin in retinal rods) and is important for epithelial keratinisation; deficiency is rarely seen in industrialised countries, but it is associated with night blindness, xerophthalmia (a relatively common cause of blindness in the developing world) and increased susceptibility to infections. Over-dosage reduces keratinisation of skin and sebum production (causing rough, dry skin and hair, but explaining the efficacy of agents such as isotretinoin in the treatment of conditions such as acne) and liver enlargement. Vitamin A and its derivatives should be avoided in pregnancy (teratogenic).
- *Vitamin D* (see metabolic bone disorders).
- *Vitamin E* (α-tocopherol and related compounds) is found in vegetable oils. It is antioxidant and present in all cell membranes. Severe deficiency, especially in childhood, may predispose to haemolytic anaemia, and muscular and neurological disorders.
- *Vitamin K* is found in green vegetables. It is a cofactor for the synthesis of several clotting factors (II, VII, IX and X), and deficiency causes a prolonged prothrombin time and bleeding tendency. Oral coumarin anticoagulants (e.g. warfarin) act by interfering with vitamin K metabolism in hepatocytes.

Water-soluble vitamins

- *Vitamin B_1* (thiamine): found in many foods, including wheat, cereals and meat. Deficiency rapidly occurs if dietary intake is low as body stores are small. It is a cofactor in many metabolic pathways. Deficiency causes:
  - *Wernicke–Korsakoff syndrome:* typically occurs in chronic alcoholics; there is ataxia, nystagmus and ophthalmoplegia, and confusion; the inability to retain new memories is accompanied by confabulation (Korsakoff's psychosis); ischaemia and capillary haemorrhages occur in the mammillary bodies and around the aqueduct in the midbrain; red cell transketolase levels are reduced; the disorder usually responds to parenteral thiamine (50–100 mg), although the memory defect often persists.
  - *Beriberi:* now rare outside Asia; in addition to Wernicke's encephalopathy, there is cardiomyopathy and peripheral neuropathy.
- *Vitamin B_2* (riboflavin): found in most foods (rich sources are dairy products, liver and cereals); it is a cofactor for cellular oxidation; deficiency causes angular stomatitis, atrophic glossitis and seborrhoeic dermatitis, and usually occurs in the context of other B vitamin deficiencies.
- *Nicotinamide:* found in many foods, including liver, meat, fish and cereals; it can also be synthesised from the amino acid tryptophan; it forms part of the coenzymes nicotinamide adenine dinucleotide (NAD) and nicotinamide dinucleotide phosphate (NADP); deficiency causes pellagra with dermatitis, diarrhoea and dementia.
- *Vitamin B_6* (pyridoxine): found in many foods, including liver, meat, fish and cereals. Dietary deficiency is rare, but a number of drugs, including isoniazid, penicillamine and hydralazine, antagonise its effects. Isoniazid peripheral neuropathy is preventable by co-treatment with pyridoxine.
- *Vitamin B_{12}* and *folic acid* (see haematology, Chapter 20).
- *Vitamin C* (ascorbic acid): main sources are fresh fruits and vegetables; it is an antioxidant; one of its many roles is the reduction of proline to hydroxyproline, which is necessary for collagen formation, and impaired collagen production is the principal defect in scurvy, which is characterised by swollen, spongy gums, spontaneous bleeding/bruising,

perifollicular haemorrhages, subperiosteal haemorrhages, anaemia and hair follicle keratosis with 'corkscrew hairs'.

Enteral feeding

Indications

Patients who are unable/unwilling to eat sufficient food but who have a functioning gut may be subjected to enteral feeding. Potential indications include:

- unconsciousness
- dysphagia: neurological; oesophageal obstruction; following head and neck surgery
- loss of nutrients from fistulas or stomas
- any major illness, e.g. postoperatively, following radiotherapy or chemotherapy, with moderate/ severe burns.

Administration

A fine-bore nasogastric (NG) tube is usually well tolerated. If there is oesophageal obstruction or prolonged feeding is necessary, a tube can be inserted directly into the stomach via the abdominal wall (percutaneous endoscopic gastrostomy – PEG).

Requirements

Average adult daily requirements include:

- 2000–3000 kcal
- 10–15 g nitrogen (60–90 g protein)
- vitamins (see earlier) and trace elements.

A number of commercial preparations are available. Most contain milk or soya proteins. Protein hydrolysates or free amino acids are only necessary if the ability to break down protein is limited by pancreatic or bowel disease.

Complications

- vomiting/aspiration
- diarrhoea
- electrolyte and metabolic disturbances

Parenteral nutrition

Parenteral nutrition is indicated when feeding via the gut is not possible because of:

- a reduction in functioning gut mass, either because of parenchymal disease or loss of small intestine
- ileus (usually postoperatively)
- loss of intestinal contents via fistulas.

It may supplement oral or enteral feeding, or be the only source of nutrition (= total parenteral nutrition).

Administration

The tendency for peripheral veins to thrombose makes administration through a tunnelled central venous catheter necessary. Patients requiring long-term parenteral nutrition can be taught to administer infusions overnight at home.

Requirements

Protein is provided as essential and non-essential L-amino acids. Energy is given as 150–250 kcal/g nitrogen. Glucose is the usual source of carbohydrate. Insulin may be necessary, particularly if more than 180 g of glucose is given daily. Some 30–40% of required energy is provided as fat. Fat emulsions provide essential fatty acids and have a high energy to volume ratio. The mixture of amino acids, glucose and fat together with trace elements and vitamins is prepared under sterile conditions by pharmacy, e.g. in a 3-l bag.

Complications

- catheter-related infection, blockage or venous thrombosis
- air embolism
- metabolic disorders, e.g. hyperglycaemia, electrolyte imbalance, trace element or vitamin deficiencies
- fluid overload if renal insufficiency or cardiac impairment

Anorexia nervosa

This is a challenging disorder (most commonly of young women) in which the patient fasts, vomits and/ or purges to maintain a markedly low weight. Bulimia nervosa is habitual vomiting or purging, with eating binges between. Anorexia nervosa is associated with extreme thinness, anovular amenorrhoea and fine hairs on the arms and legs (lanugo). Such patients have a markedly altered body image. There is often evidence of hypothalamic-pituitary dysfunction with low levels of luteinising hormone (LH), follicle-stimulating hormone (FSH) and oestradiol, related in part to low circulating levels of the adipose tissue-derived hormone leptin. More global hypothalamic-pituitary dysfunction may also be evident (e.g. thyroid function tests may show the pattern of 'non-thyroidal illness', while the hypothalamic-pituitary-adrenal axis is 'activated'). Treatment requires expert psychiatric advice and often periods of hospitalisation with the aim of readjusting abnormal psychopathology and increasing weight/correcting nutritional deficiencies.

Porphyria

The porphyrias are a group of inherited or acquired metabolic disorders due to enzymatic defects in the haem biosynthetic pathway (Fig. 17.1). In most familial cases, inheritance occurs in an autosomal dominant fashion, but autosomal recessive and X-linked forms are also recognised. Porphyria cutanea tarda shows heritability in only a small number of cases.

Classification

The porphyrias may be classified as (1) hepatic or erythropoietic (according to the principal site of the enzyme defect and excess precursor production) or (2) acute or non-acute (Table 17.12).

Clinical presentation

Acute porphyrias

These disorders show autosomal dominant inheritance. The biosynthesis of haem (Fig. 17.1) involves eight stages and enzymes and is subject to negative feedback control by haem itself. Reduction in intermediary enzyme activity renders patients susceptible to an increased demand for haem, with reduced negative feedback such that excess toxic precursors (e.g. porphobilinogen and δ-aminolevulinic acid [d-ALA]) accumulate. Attacks may be triggered by a variety of agents including:

- drugs: e.g. sex steroids, enzyme inducers and many other commonly prescribed medications – hence, it is vital to check with either the *British National Formulary* (BNF) or another reliable source (see later) before prescribing treatment in a patient with known or suspected acute porphyria
- alcohol, prolonged fasting
- stress, including intercurrent infection
- electrolyte disturbances
- hormonal changes: e.g. during the menstrual cycle.

The clinical manifestations vary according to subtype, but in general the acute porphyrias predominantly exhibit neurovisceral symptoms, including:

- abdominal pain, vomiting, constipation (which may therefore mimic obstruction)
- sensorimotor neuropathy, seizures, confusion/coma, bulbar paralysis, quadriplegia, respiratory muscle weakness
- psychiatric disorders, including acute psychosis, depression
- sinus tachycardia, hypertension, postural hypotension and rarely left ventricular failure
- hyponatraemia (due to syndrome of inappropriate antidiuretic hormone) in acute intermittent porphyria.

Acute intermittent porphyria (AIP)
Presentation is typically between 15 and 35 years of age, with abdominal pain and vomiting the most common features. The skin is 'never' affected. There may be a positive family history.

Variegate porphyria (VP)
Clinical features overlap those of AIP, but cutaneous manifestations are also seen (the skin, photosensitised by porphyrins, is fragile, particularly on the back of the hands).

Hereditary coproporphyria (HCP)
Features are similar to variegate porphyria. HCP is extremely rare.

Non-acute porphyrias

The non-acute porphyrias are typically associated with photosensitivity due to activation by ultraviolet light of porphyrins deposited in the skin.

Porphyria cutanea tarda (PCT)
PCT is predominantly an acquired disorder and is sometimes seen in the context of liver disease (particularly alcoholic), although in this setting there may be a genetic predisposition. Patients are not usually susceptible to drug-induced attacks, although they can present following an alcoholic 'binge'. Manifestations are predominantly cutaneous with porphyrin-induced photosensitivity leading to bullae on sun-exposed areas (which heal by scarring) and hyperpigmentation. Other features can include hepatomegaly and an association with haemochromatosis.

Congenital erythropoetic porphyria (CEP)
CEP is characterised by marked skin manifestations which may develop at a very young age. Other features include nail dystrophy, red staining of dentition

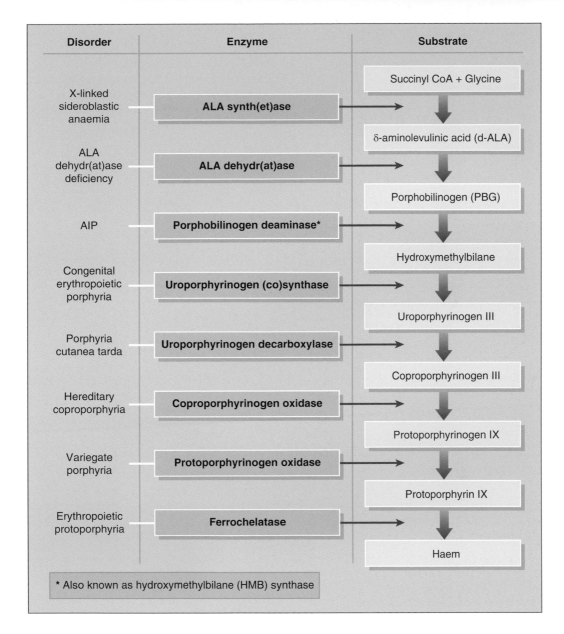

Disorder	Enzyme	Substrate
		Succinyl CoA + Glycine
X-linked sideroblastic anaemia	**ALA synth(et)ase**	
		δ-aminolevulinic acid (d-ALA)
ALA dehydr(at)ase deficiency	**ALA dehydr(at)ase**	
		Porphobilinogen (PBG)
AIP	**Porphobilinogen deaminase***	
		Hydroxymethylbilane
Congenital erythropoietic porphyria	**Uroporphyrinogen (co)synthase**	
		Uroporphyrinogen III
Porphyria cutanea tarda	**Uroporphyrinogen decarboxylase**	
		Coproporphyrinogen III
Hereditary coproporphyria	**Coproporphyrinogen oxidase**	
		Protoporphyrinogen IX
Variegate porphyria	**Protoporphyrinogen oxidase**	
		Protoporphyrin IX
Erythropoietic protoporphyria	**Ferrochelatase**	
		Haem

* Also known as hydroxymethylbilane (HMB) synthase

Figure 17.1 Schematic representation of the different steps in the haem biosynthetic pathway, showing the various enzyme defects in porphyria. AIP, acute intermittent porphyria; ALA, aminolevulinic acid.

and in some cases ocular and skin manifestations. CEP is extremely rare.

Erythropoietic protoporphyria (EPP)

This typically presents in childhood with cutaneous photosensitivity of varying severity. Unlike the other porphyrias, the rash is usually non-blistering. Hepatic dysfunction is a recognised association, especially in long-standing disease.

Investigation

The diagnosis of acute porphyria is readily established in patients who present during an acute episode by finding a substantial elevation of urinary porphyrins in a spot urine sample. Porphobilinogen (PBG) accumulation (Fig. 17.1) yields a red/brown colour due to production of porphobilin (a brownish auto-oxidation product of PBG) and porphyrins

Table 17.12 Classification of porphyria

Type	Enzyme defect	Inheritance	Key clinical features
Acute porphyrias			
Acute intermittent porphyria (AIP) (hepatic)	Porphobilinogen deaminase	AD	Neurovisceral symptoms Skin not affected
Hereditary coproporphyria (hepatic)	Coproporphyrinogen oxidase	AD	Neurovisceral symptoms Cutaneous features present Extremely rare
Variegate porphyria (hepatic)	Protoporphyrinogen oxidase	AD	Neurovisceral symptoms Cutaneous features present
Non-acute porphyrias			
Porphyria cutanea tarda (hepatic)	Uroporphyrinogen decarboxylase	AD	Chronic blistering skin lesions in sun-exposed areas Most common porphyria
Erythropoietic protoporphyria (erythropoietic)	Ferrochelatase	AD	Painful cutaneous photosensitivity, which may initially present in childhood Hepatic involvement may occur in long-standing disease
Congenital erythropoietic porphyria (erythropoietic)	Uroporphyrinogen (co)synthase	AR	Cutaneous features (may present in early childhood) Dystrophic nails; red staining of teeth Ocular and skeletal manifestations can also occur
X-linked sideroblastic anaemia (erythropoietic)	ALA-synth(et)ase	X	Pallor, fatigue, hepatosplenomegaly Microcytic (hypochromic) anaemia Ringed sideroblasts in bone marrow

AD, autosomal dominant; AR, autosomal recessive; X, X-linked.

(which are reddish). PBG in fresh urine can be detected by the development of a distinct pink/red colour on mixing with Ehrlich's reagent, which is not absorbed out by chloroform or other organic solvents.

AIP, VP and HCP all cause increases in PBG and can be differentiated from each other on the basis of profiling of blood, urinary and faecal porphyrins, together with assessment of enzymatic activity. For example, the identification of increased urinary excretion of both PBG and d-ALA in the context of reduced PBG deaminase activity is diagnostic of AIP.

NB: Biochemical testing must be carried out during an acute attack as profiling may be normal between episodes. Samples should be protected from light and sent urgently to the laboratory.

Abnormal liver function tests may be found during an acute episode

Genetic screening for mutations in specific enzymes is possible and permits easier family screening.

Management

Acute porphyrias

Wherever possible, triggers should be avoided and intercurrent infections and electrolyte disturbances promptly treated/corrected. During acute episodes, supportive measures remain the mainstay of treatment, including:

- fluids (with attention to electrolytes)
- antimicrobial therapy if infection suspected (avoid 'unsafe' drugs)
- analgesia/anti-emetics (avoid 'unsafe' drugs)
- ventilatory support if respiratory muscle involvement (can be monitored by using bedside spirometry)

- high carbohydrate intake (glucose polymer drinks or intravenous infusion of 10% dextrose) provides nourishment and rehydration and suppresses ALA synth(et)ase activity
- an infusion of haem arginate (3 mg/kg/day for 4 days) as haem replacement may help to restore 'negative feedback' and curtail severe/refractory attacks.

Once the acute attack has subsided patients should be (re)educated about future avoidance of drug precipitants and alcohol and advised to wear a medical bracelet.

Relatives should be offered screening.

NB: A list of drugs that are considered '**un**safe for use' in acute porphyrias is provided in the British National Formulary (BNF), while an up-to-date list of treatments that are considered 'safe' is available at https://www.wmic.wales.nhs.uk/specialist-services/drugs-in-porphyria/.

Non-acute porphyrias

Measures include:

- avoidance of sunlight in cutaneous porphyrias
- PCT may respond to iron reduction (e.g. through venesection) or low-dose hydroxychloroquine; avoidance of alcohol is also important
- beta-carotene may improve sunlight tolerance in EPP.

Metabolic bone disease

Physiology

Hormonal control of bone homeostasis involves three important hormones: parathyroid hormone (parathormone, PTH), calcitonin, and vitamin D.

- PTH secretion is predominantly controlled by the concentration of ionised calcium in extracellular fluid. PTH increases osteoclastic cell number and activity and thereby increases bone resorption, but at low and intermittent levels PTH increases bone formation. PTH decreases renal tubular phosphate reabsorption and increases renal tubular calcium reabsorption. It indirectly increases intestinal calcium absorption through increased formation of active (1,25-dihydroxy) vitamin D.
- Calcitonin is secreted by C cells of the thyroid. Its principal action is to inhibit osteoclastic bone resorption.
- Vitamin D is predominantly synthesised from 7-dehydrocholesterol in the skin in response to exposure to ultraviolet light. Dietary intake is only important when ultraviolet irradiation does not occur. The major circulating/storage form is 25-hydroxy-cholecalciferol ($25[OH]D_3$ = 25-hydroxyvitamin D_3), which is converted to either 1,25-dihydroxycholecalciferol ($1,25[OH]_2D_3$) or 24,25-dihydroxycholecalciferol in the kidney. 1,25-Dihydroxycholecalciferol is the most potent vitamin D metabolite. It decreases renal 1(α)-hydroxylase activity and increases 24(α)-hydroxylase activity, whereas PTH increases 1(α)-hydroxylase activity and decreases 24(α)-hydroxylase activity. The vitamin D receptor is a member of the steroid nuclear receptor superfamily.

Osteoporosis

- Osteoporosis is a condition characterised by loss of bone mass and alteration in the microarchitecture, leading to increased bone fragility and fracture risk. The most common fracture sites are the spine, femoral neck and radius.
- In clinical practice osteoporosis is considered to be present if bone mineral density (BMD) as determined by dual-energy X-ray absorptiometry (DXA – see later) is >2.5 standard deviations (SD) below peak bone mass, or if susceptibility fractures have occurred (e.g. low-impact hip or wrist fractures, non-traumatic vertebral fractures).

Aetiology

Broadly speaking, osteoporosis can be considered as primary (e.g. postmenopausal and age-related) or secondary (when occurring in the context of a predisposing condition) (Box 17.2).

Clinical features

Osteoporosis is often asymptomatic, only manifesting when the patient suffers a fracture:

- Vertebral fractures (wedge or crush) are most common in the mid-thoracic spine and at the thoracolumbar junction (T12 and L1). They may be asymptomatic, or cause sudden onset severe back pain. Spinal cord compression is rare, and other causes such as metastases should be sought. Multiple fractures cause loss of height and spinal deformity (e.g. kyphosis).
- Hip fractures invariably follow a fall.
- Colles' fracture usually follows a fall onto the outstretched hand.

Immobility and chronic pain (e.g. due to secondary osteoarthritis) may ensue in some cases.

Box 17.2 Recognised risk factors for osteoporosis

- History of fracture as adult
- History of fracture in first-degree relative
- Caucasian race
- Advanced age
- Female sex
- Poor health, frailty
- Reduced physical activity, immobility
- Low body weight
- Current cigarette smoking
- Chronic excess alcohol intake
- Drugs, e.g. corticosteroids, heparin, ciclosporin, certain anticonvulsants
- Endocrine disorders, e.g. thyrotoxicosis, hypogonadism, hyperparathyroidism, Cushing syndrome, growth hormone deficiency
- Gastrointestinal disorders, e.g. malabsorption states, chronic liver disease
- Chronic illness, e.g. renal failure, rheumatoid arthritis
- Others, e.g. haematological disorders (multiple myeloma, haemoglobinopathies), neoplastic disorders

Investigations

Biochemistry

The standard bone profile (serum calcium, phosphate and alkaline phosphatase) is normal.

NB: Alkaline phosphatase may be elevated following a fracture.

Other markers of bone turnover (e.g. procollagen type 1 N-terminal peptide [P1NP] for bone formation; N-terminal telopeptide [NTX] or C-terminal telopeptide [CTX] of collagen crosslinks for bone resorption) are available, and are finding increasing clinical use.

Radiology

Lateral X-rays of thoracic and lumbar spine may reveal wedging or concave deformities (codfishing) of the vertebral bodies.

Bone densitometry

Quantitative computed tomography (QCT), single and dual-photon absorptiometry (SPA/DPA), DXA and radiation absorptiometry (RA) assess bone density by measuring the absorption of γ- or X-rays at clinically relevant sites such as the radius, hip or spine. DXA is the most commonly applied method in clinical practice, providing a rapid method of assessment which is associated with low radiation exposure. Bone density can be reported as either T-scores (SD compared to young normal individuals, i.e. compared to peak bone mass) or Z-scores (SD above or below the mean age-matched BMD at that site). Z-scores are generally preferred in younger patients.

According to the WHO classification of BMD (based on T-scores), values above −1 SD are normal, values between −1 and −2.5 SD signify osteopenia and scores below −2.5 SD indicate osteoporosis.

Screening for secondary causes

This should be considered in all patients, and especially when there are atypical features, e.g. low-impact fracture at young age (Box 17.2).

Prevention and treatment

As always, prevention is better than cure and efforts should be directed towards prevention in those with identifiable risk factors (e.g. early menopause, long-term corticosteroid therapy, excess alcohol ingestion and smoking).

Risk calculators, e.g. QFracture® (http://www.qfracture.org) or FRAX® (www.shef.ac.uk/FRAX), which integrate clinical risk factors, with or without femoral neck BMD, can be used to calculate the 10-year probability of hip fracture or a major osteoporotic fracture (clinical spine, hip, forearm or proximal humerus). Postmenopausal women with a previous fragility fracture should be considered for treatment without further need for risk assessment. For other groups QFracture and FRAX are useful tools in helping to determine who should receive intervention.

Current NICE recommendations for the treatment of osteoporosis can be found at www.nice.org.uk and typically involve one or more of the following strategies/agents.

Exercise

Physical activity (especially weight-bearing) helps to maximise BMD during childhood, adolescence and early adulthood, maintain bone mass through mid-life, diminish bone loss with ageing, and improve stability and strength to minimise falls and fractures in the elderly.

Calcium

A daily calcium intake of 0.5–1 g is recommended.

Vitamin D

Various studies have shown that small doses of vitamin D (400–800 IU/day) can reduce bone loss and prevent fractures in women with postmenopausal osteoporosis.

Hormone replacement therapy (HRT)

HRT slows bone loss and reduces the occurrence of fractures when started at the menopause. However, the results of several studies have linked HRT to an increase in the risk of breast cancer, cardiovascular disease and thromboembolic disorders. Accordingly, HRT is no longer routinely recommended for prophylaxis against bone loss in postmenopausal women, although it may offer positive benefits in those women taking HRT (e.g. as treatment for vasomotor symptoms), and in whom a careful risk to benefit assessment has been undertaken.

NB: In contrast, hypogonadism in males and in premenopausal females should be corrected wherever possible.

Selective oestrogen receptor modulators (SERMs)

Raloxifene exhibits variable effects depending on the tissue, e.g. oestrogen-like effect in bone, but anti-oestrogen effects in breast and uterus. It has also been linked to venous thromboembolism.

Bisphosphonates

Bisphosphonates, which are synthetic analogues of inorganic pyrophosphate, are a mainstay of prophylaxis and treatment of osteoporosis in many settings, and are potent inhibitors of bone resorption. Commonly used preparations range from those given once weekly, to monthly or even annually. Oral preparations can cause oesophageal irritation and should be taken before breakfast on an empty stomach with the patient upright for 30 min. In addition, concern has arisen recently that prolonged use may be linked to atypical fractures of the femur. Accordingly, the need for continued use should be re-evaluated on a regular basis and treatment duration is typically restricted to <5 yr. Osteonecrosis of the jaw is a rare but potentially serious complication most commonly seen in those with pre-existing dental disease receiving intravenous therapy.

Strontium ranelate

This acts by increasing bone formation and decreasing bone resorption. However, following various safety alerts, and with diminishing clinical use, the major manufacturer of this drug ceased production in the UK and worldwide in 2017.

Teriparatide (recombinant parathyroid hormone)

This is very effective but currently very expensive and is generally reserved for severe/refractory osteoporosis.

Denosumab

Recently introduced monoclonal antibody targeting RANK ligand (inhibits osteoclast formation/function).

Treatment of underlying cause

Wherever possible predisposing factors/conditions should be actively addressed.

Osteomalacia

In osteomalacia ('soft bones') there is inadequate mineralisation of bone, resulting in weakness, with propensity to fracture and subsequent deformity. If this occurs during childhood before fusion of the epiphyseal growth plates, then it is referred to as rickets.

Causes

The most common cause is vitamin D deficiency. Other causes are shown in Table 17.13.

Clinical features

Adult osteomalacia

Patients may be aymptomatic or can present with:

- generalised muscle aches and pain – worse with activity

Table 17.13 Causes of osteomalacia

Type	Mechanism	Example
Vitamin D deficiency/altered metabolism	Reduced substrate	Limited sunlight exposure
		Inadequate dietary intake
		Small bowel malabsorption
		Liver disease (e.g. PBC)
	Enhanced clearance	Enzyme-inducing agents (e.g. phenytoin, carbamazepine)
	Reduced hydroxylation	Renal disease (1α hydroxylation)[a]
		Vitamin D-dependent rickets type I (AR)[a]
		Impaired 25α-hydroxylation (very rare)[b]
	Impaired action	Vitamin D-dependent rickets type II (AR)[b]
Hypophosphataemia	Reduced intake	Phosphate-binding medication (e.g. antacids)
	Increased loss	X-linked hypophosphataemia (vitamin D-resistant rickets, XLD)
		Fanconi syndrome and/or RTA
		Oncogenic osteomalacia

AR, autosomal recessive; PBC, primary biliary cirrhosis; RTA, renal tubular acidosis; XLD, X-linked dominant.
[a] 25-hydroxycholecalciferol 1α-hydroxylase deficiency.
[b] Defective vitamin D receptor signalling.

- bone pain and tenderness
- pathological fractures
- proximal myopathy
- features of underlying disease (e.g. malabsorption)
- very rarely hypocalcaemia may be evident.

Childhood rickets

- deformities in the legs (bow-legs, knock-knees)
- deformities in the chest (prominent costochondral junctions = 'ricketic rosary')
- deformities in the skull (craniotabes, open fontanelles and delayed eruption of the teeth)
- hypotonia, weakness, tetany.

Investigation

Biochemistry

- Serum calcium is usually low/low normal (maintained by secondary hyperparathyroidism).
- Serum phosphate is low (except in the presence of renal failure).
- Serum alkaline phosphatase is raised.
- Serum vitamin D levels: 25-hydroxycholecalciferol is low in vitamin D deficiency, but otherwise often normal. In contrast, 1,25-dihydroxycholecalciferol may be low (vitamin D deficiency, renal failure, vitamin D-dependent rickets type 1), elevated (vitamin D-dependent rickets type II) or inappropriately normal.
- Plasma PTH is commonly raised (secondary hyperparathyroidism).

X-ray

- Generalised osteopenia with cortical thinning may be associated with multiple fractures, particularly in the ribs.
- Pseudofractures ('Looser's zones') are translucent bands perpendicular to the surface of the bone, extending from the surface inwards (best seen in the pubic ramus, femoral or humeral neck, and outer borders of the scapula).
- *In rickets,* in addition to bone deformities there are widened and irregular metaphyses ('cupping, splaying and fraying').

Bone scan

There is a generalised diffuse increase in uptake, although routine scanning is not required. Occasionally, Looser's zones show multiple areas of increased uptake (c.f. in osteoporosis bone scanning is normal, whereas in Paget's disease there is typically strong focal uptake).

Investigation of underlying disease (malabsorption, uraemia) may be required.

Treatment

Vitamin D

The dosage and formulation depend on the underlying aetiology. Serum calcium must always be monitored, especially in those receiving larger (pharmacological) doses and activated forms.

NB: Ergocalciferol=calciferol=vitamin D_2; c(h)olecalciferol=vitamin D_3; alfacalcidol=1α-hydroxycholecalciferol; calcitriol=1,25-dihydroxycholecalciferol – both alfacalcidol and calcitriol are considered 'activated' forms of vitamin D.

- For vitamin D insufficiency, 400–800 units (IU)/day (of simple ergocalciferol or colecalciferol) may suffice.
- For those with clear evidence of deficiency, the recommended treatment is based on fixed loading doses of vitamin D (ergocalciferol or colecalciferol – up to a total of 300 000 IU) given either as weekly or as daily split doses, followed by lifelong maintenance treatment (typically 800 IU/day).
- In severe malabsorption states/chronic liver disease, pharmacological doses (e.g. 40–50 000 units/day of ergocalciferol) may be required.
- Vitamin D-resistant states: in familial vitamin D-resistant (hypophosphataemic) rickets treatment is with oral phosphate supplements and calcitriol. Type II vitamin D-dependent rickets (end-organ resistance) responds poorly to treatment, although huge doses of calcitriol with calcium supplements are sometimes effective.
- In uraemia there is failure of 1α-hydroxylation: treatment is with 1α-hydroxycholecalciferol or 1,25-dihydroxycholecalciferol (i.e. activated forms).
- Calcium supplements are not usually required unless there is severe osteomalacia or poor dietary intake.
- Clinical and biochemical improvement takes weeks to months.

Paget's disease (osteitis deformans)

This is a localised disorder of bone remodelling, in which excessive bone resorption is followed by excessive bone formation, leading to hypertrophic osteosclerotic bone formation with deformity and fragility. It is a disease chiefly of the elderly, and shows geographical variation, being more common in North America and Europe, but rare in Asia. Only 5–10% of those with radiological evidence of bone involvement manifest clinical features.

Aetiology

Familial clustering and the finding of viral inclusions in osteoclastic nuclei has been taken to suggest that the disease may be triggered by viral infection in genetically predisposed individuals.

Clinical features

- Many patients are asymptomatic.
- Pain is the most common symptom, sometimes with a rise in temperature over the site of the lesion.
- Bone deformity is most obvious when there is enlargement of the skull with frontal bossing or bowing of the legs.

Complications

- Fractures: up to 15% of patients suffer pathological fractures in abnormal bone.
- Deafness is common in patients with skull involvement; it may result from involvement of the ossicles or compression of the cochlea or internal auditory canal.
- Occlusion of other foramina of the skull leading to compression of other cranial nerves occurs less often; platybasia or flattening of the base of the skull may, rarely, lead to brainstem compression or obstructive hydrocephalus.
- Spinal involvement may cause cord compression, particularly in the cervical and thoracic regions.
- Less than 1% of patients develop osteogenic sarcoma in Pagetic bone (the pelvis and femur are the most common sites); it may be heralded by increasing pain.
- High-output cardiac failure is a rare complication of extensive disease.

Investigations

Biochemistry

- Bone profile: increased osteoblastic activity is reflected in increased levels of serum alkaline phosphatase; serum calcium levels are usually normal.
- Markers of increased bone activity.

Radiology

- Expansion and disorganisation of bone with both lytic and sclerotic lesions are characteristic; there is cortical thickening and coarsening of trabeculae; the pelvis and lumbar spine are most frequently affected, followed by the sacrum, thoracic spine, skull, lower limbs and upper limbs.

- Bowing deformity occurs in weight-bearing long bones, and osteoarthritis is common in adjacent joints.
- Bone scintigraphy shows increased uptake at affected sites and helps to define the full extent of the disease.

Treatment

- Pain may be controlled with analgesics and NSAIDs.
- Physiotherapy maintains mobility.

A number of specific treatments are now available. These agents are effective in relieving symptoms.

- *Bisphosphonates:* the mainstay of treatment in symptomatic patients; their role in asymptomatic patients remains controversial, but should be considered if complications due to hypervascularity or disease progression are likely (e.g. fractures, nerve entrapment).
- *Calcitonin:* can be given subcutaneously in those who are intolerant to bisphosphonates.

Serum alkaline phosphatase and 24-h urinary hydroxyproline measurement can be used to monitor response to treatment. Urinary hydroxyproline levels reflect bone resorption and give a more rapid indication of response and an earlier warning of relapse.

Hypercalcaemia

True hypercalcaemia is defined as an elevation in free ionised serum calcium. However, ionised calcium is not always measured/available, and for practical purposes total calcium is therefore used in most clinical settings. Calcium is bound to albumin and 'correction' should be performed when albumin levels are abnormal. For every 1 g/l that the serum albumin level is lower than 40 g/l, add 0.02 mmol/l to the serum calcium (or subtract if serum calcium is raised above 40 g/l). Most laboratories routinely provide a corrected calcium value.

NB: Acidotic states increase ionised calcium by decreasing binding of calcium ions to albumin, whereas alkalosis has the reverse effect.

Aetiology

Primary hyperparathyroidism (see later) and malignancy are the commonest causes of hypercalcaemia. A variety of mechanisms may underlie malignant hypercalcaemia, including: tumour secretion of parathyroid hormone-related peptide/protein (PTHrP); osteolytic metastases with local release of osteoclast-activating cytokines; systemic production of cytokines that promote bone resorption; local production/activation of vitamin D). Other causes of hypercalcaemia are listed in Table 17.14.

Clinical features

The clinical features depend predominantly on the rapidity of onset and, to a lesser extent, on the magnitude of the rise in serum calcium levels. Slow-onset, mild hypercalcaemia (<3.0 mmol/l) is usually asymptomatic. Severe hypercalcaemia, usually caused by malignant disease, with an onset over only a few weeks or months, may produce significant symptoms.

Table 17.14 Causes of hypercalcaemia

Type	Example
Parathyroid-dependent	Primary hyperparathyroidism – adenoma or hyperplasia of parathyroid
	Tertiary hyperparathyroidism
	Familial hypocalciuric hypercalcaemia
Parathyroid-independent	Malignancy
	Vitamin D-related: e.g. excess ingestion; granulomatous disorders, Williams syndrome
	Endocrine disorders: e.g. thyrotoxicosis; adrenal failure; phaeochromocytoma Iatrogenic: e.g. thiazide diuretics; total parenteral nutrition
	Milk-alkali syndrome (excess ingestion of calcium and absorbable alkali)
	Prolonged immobilisation
	Vitamin A intoxication
	Jansen's metaphyseal chondrodysplasia

Remember the old adage – '*bones, stones, moans and groans*'!

- musculoskeletal ('*bones*') – muscle weakness, bone pain, arthritis
- renal ('*stones*') – polyuria (nephrogenic diabetes insipidus), nephrolithiasis, nephrocalcinosis, acute or chronic renal impairment
- neuropsychiatric ('*moans*') – anxiety, depression, cognitive dysfunction and hypotonicity; lethargy, confusion stupor and coma may occur in severe cases
- gastrointestinal ('*groans*') – anorexia, nausea/vomiting, constipation, dyspepsia/peptic ulceration, pancreatitis

Cardiovascular complications include bradycardia, shortened QT interval and cardiomyopathy.

Investigation

After excluding iatrogenic causes, paired measurement of serum parathyroid hormone and serum calcium is the first key step in elucidating the underlying cause:

- If PTH is elevated or inappropriately normal in the presence of raised serum calcium, then the diagnosis is usually one of primary hyperparathyroidism. Tertiary hyperparathyroidism is normally easily distinguishable based on the clinical context, as is hyperparathyroidism due to lithium therapy. However, familial hypocalciuric hypercalcaemia (FHH) must be excluded before considering treatment for presumed primary hyperparathyroidism (see section on primary hyperparathyroidism for further investigation to distinguish these two entities).
- If PTH is low/suppressed, then PTH-independent causes should be considered. Further investigations will be determined by the clinical context, but may include:
- full blood count, ESR, electrolytes, renal/liver function, serum electrophoresis/urinary Bence Jones protein, serum angiotensin-converting enzyme (ACE)
- chest radiograph/cross-sectional imaging; isotope bone scintigraphy, skeletal survey
- endocrine testing (thyroid function, Synacthen®, plasma/urinary metanephrines)
- PTHrP measurement (but not routinely available).

NB: As vitamin D metabolism is intricately linked with PTH and calcium metabolism, many endocrinologists recommend routinely assessing vitamin D status in all patients with hypercalcaemia. Typically, vitamin D excess is associated with a suppressed PTH level, but less commonly recognised is that vitamin D deficiency can be associated with a mild elevation in PTH and serum calcium.

In addition, consideration should be given to screening for secondary complications of long-standing hypercalcaemia, e.g. nephrolithiasis/nephrocalcinosis.

Management

Mild hypercalcaemia (<3.0 mmol/l)

This rarely requires urgent treatment. Advice should be given to avoid factors that can aggravate hypercalcaemia (predominantly dehydration and medications). Further investigation should be undertaken to determine the cause, and then treatment targeted as appropriate.

Moderate hypercalcaemia (3.0–3.5 mmol/l)

Although chronic hypercalcaemia of this magnitude may not outwardly appear to be associated with significant symptomatology in all cases, these patients are at significant risk of developing more severe hypercalcaemia, e.g. during intercurrent illness, and treatment is therefore required – however, the extent and aggressiveness of the intervention should be determined based on symptoms, comorbidities, magnitude of hypercalcaemia and underlying cause (see later for management options).

Severe hypercalcaemia (>3.5 mmol/l)

This requires urgent treatment regardless of whether the patient is symptomatic or not as there is a significant risk of cardiac dysrhythmias.

Principles of treatment

- Rehydrate with intravenous 0.9% sodium chloride – typically 4–6 l over the first 24 h, aiming to achieve a high urine output (100–150 ml/h).

NB: Caution should be exercised in those with renal and/or cardiac impairment.

NB: Furosemide is no longer routinely recommended – the risk of exacerbating intravascular depletion largely outweighs any potential benefit of enhancing renal calcium excretion – however, it may still be useful in those at risk of fluid overload.

- Following adequate rehydration, intravenous bisphosphonate (e.g. zoledronic acid (4 mg over 15 min) or pamidronate (30–90 mg as an infusion at 20 mg/h)) inhibits osteoclast-mediated bone resorption; the hypocalcaemic effect develops over 24–72 h and typically lasts for several weeks, at which point further courses can be considered if the underlying cause is not amenable to correction.

- Corticosteroids (e.g. prednisolone 40–60 mg/day) can be used to suppress hypercalcaemia associated with haematological malignancy (myeloma, lymphoma), sarcoidosis and vitamin D toxicity.
- Calcitonin/denosumab/calcimimetics may also be considered, but should only be used under specialist supervision.
- Dialysis is reserved for severe hypercalcaemia or those with renal impairment/fluid balance problems.

The UK Society for Endocrinology has recently published concise guidelines: https://www.endocrinology.org/clinical-practice/clinical-guidelines/.

Hyperparathyroidism

Parathyroid hormone (PTH) is secreted from the four parathyroid glands in response to a fall in serum calcium. PTH exerts its effects by:

- increasing calcium absorption from the gut through activation of vitamin D; PTH upregulates renal 1α-hydroxylase, which converts inactive 25-hydroxyvitamin D_3 to active 1,25-dihydroxyvitamin D_3.
- mobilising calcium from bone (through indirect activation of osteoclasts)
- reducing renal calcium clearance (PTH stimulates calcium and magnesium reabsorption from the distal tubule; at the same time, it also increases renal phosphate clearance and this may indirectly facilitate mobilisation of calcium from bone).

The term hyperparathyroidism simply denotes overproduction of PTH. It may be primary or secondary/tertiary in origin.

Primary hyperparathyroidism

Primary hyperparathyroidism shows a female preponderance (female to male ratio = 2–3 : 1) and is more common in the >45 years age group. In most cases this results from the development of a single autonomous parathyroid adenoma (90%); other causes include multiple adenomas (4%), hyperplasia of all four parathyroid glands (6%) and, rarely, parathyroid carcinoma (<1%).

In those with four-gland hyperplasia, consideration must be given to the possibility of multiple endocrine neoplasia (MEN), especially MEN 1.

Another rare cause of 'apparent' primary hyperparathyroidism is familial hypocalciuric hypercalcaemia (FHH), an autosomal dominant condition associated with loss-of-function mutations in the calcium-sensing receptor – it is important to distinguish this disorder from true primary hyperparathyroidism as parathyroidectomy is not indicated in FHH.

Secondary/tertiary hyperparathyroidism

Secondary hyperparathyroidism is a physiological response to hypocalcaemia caused by another disorder, e.g. chronic renal failure or hypovitaminosis D. Serum calcium may be normal (compensated), frankly low, or even occasionally raised (see later). Histologically, there is four-gland hyperplasia.

Tertiary hyperparathyroidism refers to the situation in which chronic secondary hyperparathyroidism ultimately progresses to autonomous adenoma/hyperplasia, with hypercalcaemia and elevated PTH levels.

High serum phosphate levels, due to renal failure, may be seen in both secondary and tertiary hyperparathyroidism (this is in contrast to primary hyperparathyroidism where phosphate levels are typically low).

Clinical presentation

Primary hyperparathyroidism is commonly associated with mild hypercalcaemia that develops slowly over many months or even years. Patients are often asymptomatic, and the hypercalcaemia is discovered incidentally during investigation for other reasons. Moderate to severe hypercalcaemia may result in a variety of symptoms (see hypercalcaemia, above). Chronic hypercalciuria predisposes to renal calculi, nephrocalcinosis and, eventually, renal failure. Classical skeletal changes of hyperparathyroidism (see later) are now rarely seen in the Western world; however, routine D(E)XA scanning frequently reveals previously unsuspected osteopaenia/osteoporosis. In addition, in patients presenting with fragility fractures, there is a relatively high prevalence of previously undiagnosed primary hyperparathyroidism.

Investigation

Biochemistry

Primary hyperparathyroidism
Classically:

- ↑ serum calcium
- ↓ or low normal serum phosphate

- serum alkaline phosphatase may be normal or raised (reflecting increased bone turnover)
- ↑ or inappropriately normal PTH.

NB: Most laboratories measure PTH using a two-site immunoassay, with antibodies directed against both ends of the PTH molecule, which therefore only detects intact full-length PTH and not the smaller fragment PTHrP.

- Twenty-four-hour urinary calcium excretion is high normal/raised (as opposed to low normal/low in FHH; measurement of a spot calcium : creatinine excretion ratio is another helpful way of distinguishing primary hyperparathyroidism and FHH).

Secondary hyperparathyroidism

Traditionally, secondary hyperparathyroidism in the context of renal impairment is characterised by:

- ↓ or low normal serum calcium
- ↑ serum phosphate
- ↑ PTH
- ↑ serum urea and creatinine/↓ eGFR.

Occasionally mildly elevated serum calcium, with raised PTH and alkaline phosphatase, may be seen in the context of vitamin D deficiency, with resolution of the biochemical abnormalities following replenishment of vitamin D stores (therefore arguing against autonomous adenoma/hyperplasia formation). However, this condition is difficult to distinguish clinically from true primary hyperparathyroidism with coincident vitamin D deficiency, and vitamin D supplementation in the latter setting can result in rapid development of moderate/severe hypercalcaemia – hence, referral to an endocrinologist is recommended for further assessment and trial of vitamin D therapy under close supervision.

Radiology

Screening for complications

The radiological hallmark of hyperparathyroidism is subperiosteal bone resorption, most easily seen in the distal phalanges of the hands; a similar process in the skull gives rise to the so-called 'pepper-pot' skull appearance. Other specific changes include loss of the lamina dura of the teeth (25%) and osteitis fibrosa cystica with bone cysts (rare).

DXA scanning typically reveals reduced BMD, which is more pronounced in the forearm (cortical bone) than in the spine (trabecular bone) and hip (mixed cortical and trabecular bone).

Abdominal ultrasound or plain radiographs may help identify/exclude nephrolithiasis/nephrocalcinosis.

Tumour localisation for operative planning

Although preoperative localisation may be deemed unnecessary for an experienced parathyroid surgeon undertaking a conventional neck exploration in a previously untreated patient with primary hyperparathyroidism, recently there has been a resurgence of interest in preoperative imaging. This has been driven in large part by the move towards minimally invasive parathyroidectomy, in which only unilateral neck exploration is performed. In addition, preoperative localising strategies may be helpful in cases requiring surgical re-exploration.

NB: In MEN, four-gland hyperplasia is common, and full neck exploration is therefore required in virtually all cases, thus rendering preoperative imaging of limited value.

- [99m] Technetium-sestamibi scanning: early phase images typically show both thyroid and parathyroid tissue, although asymmetric foci of increased radiotracer uptake may be seen in the presence of abnormal parathyroid tissue. Delayed images (≥2 h after radiotracer administration) are acquired to look for foci of retained radiotracer, characteristic of hyperfunctioning parathyroid tissue (the use of SPECT can increase sensitivity). If doubt remains as to whether an abnormality resides within parathyroid or thyroid tissue, then thyroid scintigraphy (using a radioisotope not taken up by the parathyroids), with subsequent overlay and subtraction of the superimposed images may help.
- Neck ultrasound: non-invasive, but requires a skilled operator; most adenomas are greater than 1 cm in size and homogeneously hypoechoic; hyperplastic glands are generally smaller and more difficult to detect.
- CT/MRI and/or selective venous sampling: generally reserved for cases who have previously undergone parathyroid surgery, which has failed to control hyperparathyroidism; interpretation may be confounded by altered anatomy following surgery.

Management

Hypercalcaemia should be managed as outlined earlier.

Surgery

The definitive treatment for primary hyperparathyroidism is resection of the affected parathyroid gland(s). Most single/ipsilateral double adenomas can now be resected as a minimally invasive day-case procedure; however, patients with suspected bilateral disease should be considered for conventional full neck exploration.

The US National Institutes of Health (NIH), recognising (1) the changing presentation of primary hyperparathyroidism (with increasing numbers of younger patients being detected), (2) the potential for long-term adverse sequelae in untreated cases (especially renal, bone and cardiovascular [hypertension] complications), and (3) improved surgical techniques, has issued revised guidance as to which patients with 'apparently asymptomatic disease' should be referred for surgery (those with symptoms should be automatically referred):

- all patients who are <50 years of age
- when the serum corrected calcium level is >0.25 mmol/l above the upper limit of the reference range
- when the 24-h urine calcium excretion is persistently >10 mmol/day
- in the presence of impaired renal function (30% reduction in creatinine clearance, age-matched)
- in the presence of nephrolithiasis or nephrocalcinosis
- in the presence of osteoporosis as defined by WHO DXA criteria
- in hyperparathyroidism complicated by osteitis fibrosa cystica
- in patients with demonstrable proximal weakness, hyperreflexia or ataxia.

The more complex issue of surgical intervention and its effects on psychiatric function/performance is not fully addressed by the NIH guidance, but some studies have shown benefits in cognition and well-being in asymptomatic patients postoperatively.

Surgical complications include haematoma and wound infection (as with any surgical procedure) and hypocalcaemia, producing hypocalcaemic tetany in severe cases (including the so-called 'hungry bones syndrome', which is more common in those with significant hypercalcaemia and multigland involvement; a raised level of alkaline phosphatase preoperatively may provide an important clue as to the risk of this complication).

Routine prescription of activated vitamin D and calcium supplements followed by early postoperative review (at approximately day 14) facilitates early discharge following surgery.

Medical management

Calcimimetics (e.g. cinacalcet), which lower PTH and hence serum calcium levels through activation of the calcium-sensing receptor, may provide an alternative treatment strategy for selected cases, including in patients:

- with recurrent/relapsing disease
- deemed unsuitable for surgery
- with refractory secondary/tertiary hyperparathyroidism, especially if total parathyroidectomy is contraindicated
- with parathyroid carcinoma failing primary surgery.

Hypocalcaemia

Symptomatic hypocalcaemia is rare but potentially life-threatening.

NB: During alkalosis there is a reduction in free ionised calcium, and hypocalcaemic symptoms may be present despite normal total serum calcium levels; the presence of other anions, particularly citrate following large-scale blood transfusion, can promote a similar picture.

Aetiology

The majority of cases of hypocalcaemia are related to abnormalities in PTH secretion/action and vitamin D deficiency/resistance (Table 17.15).

Clinical features

These are highly dependent upon the rapidity and severity of onset of the hypocalcaemia: rapid significant falls are classically associated with tetany, i.e. neuromuscular irritability. Symptoms range from mild to severe, from perioral paraesthesia through to laryngeal spasm and seizure activity. Trousseau's sign denotes carpopedal spasm induced by inflation of a sphygmomanometer cuff above systolic blood pressure (for 3 min) in a patient with hypocalcaemia. Chvostek's sign signifies contraction of the facial muscles in response to tapping over the facial nerve in the preauricular region. It may be seen in up to 10% of the normocalcaemic population.

Papilloedema, lethargy, malaise and rarely psychosis are features of chronic hypocalcaemia.

Dental abnormalities (e.g. enamel hypoplasia) may be evident if hypocalcaemia occurs during childhood/youth, as may other features of chronic/congenital hypoparathyroidism (e.g. candidiasis with the type 1 polyglandular syndrome [see endocrine disorders, Table 16.7], basal ganglia calcification with extrapyramidal features and cataracts).

Table 17.15 Causes of hypocalcaemia

Type	Examples
Low PTH	
hypoparathyroidism	Idiopathic parathyroid gland failure
	Post-surgery or neck irradiation
	Type 1 autoimmune polyglandular syndrome
	Infiltration (haemochromatosis, Wilson's disease, granulomatous disorders, neoplasia)
	Congenital (e.g. DiGeorge syndrome)
impaired PTH secretion	Hypomagnesaemia
	Treatment with cinacalcet (calcimimetic)
	Activating mutations of the calcium-sensing receptor
High PTH	
resistance to PTH action	Drugs: e.g. bisphosphonates, calcitonin
	Renal failure
	Pseudohypoparathyroidism
Vitamin D deficiency/resistance	See Table 17.13
Other causes	Drugs: e.g. chelators (citrate)
	Osteoblastic metastases
	Acute pancreatitis
	Alkalosis
	Severe hyperphosphataemia: e.g. acute renal failure, rhabdomyolysis, tumour lysis

Cardiac arrhythmias and conduction abnormalities may be seen, including prolongation of the QT interval.

Investigations

As with hypercalcaemia, paired measurement of PTH and calcium is invaluable in defining the cause of hypocalcaemia in the majority of individuals. Vitamin D measurement is also often useful (but check which form of vitamin D is routinely measured by your laboratory – see osteomalacia, above).

Other investigations will be determined by the clinical presentation but may include full blood count, electrolytes, renal/liver/bone function tests, serum magnesium, arterial blood gas (to check acid–base status and ionised calcium level) and vitamin D metabolites. A modified Ellsworth–Howard test can be used to demonstrate failure to increase urinary cAMP excretion in response to infused PTH in pseudohypoparathyroidism.

Management

Severe symptomatic hypocalcaemia

This requires urgent treatment:

- 10–20 ml of 10% calcium gluconate intravenously: this should be followed by a maintenance infusion (e.g. a further 40 ml infused over 24 h, with close monitoring of serum calcium).

NB: Calcium-containing solutions must be infused slowly (e.g. 10 ml of calcium gluconate given over a 10-min period); otherwise there is a risk of precipitating dysrhythmias. Cardiac monitoring is advised.

- Commence oral calcium and vitamin D replacement without delay.
- Wherever possible, attention should be paid to identifying/treating the underlying cause.

NB: Undetected/untreated concomitant hypomagnesaemia is likely to render the patient refractory to correction of hypocalcaemia.

The UK Society for Endocrinology has recently published concise guidelines: https://www.endocrinology.org/clinical-practice/clinical-guidelines/.

Chronic hypocalcaemia

Currently, long-term therapy for hypoparathyroidism involves the use of vitamin D analogues (alfacalcidol or calcitriol) ± calcium supplements to raise the serum calcium towards normal levels – in the majority of subjects with a normal dietary calcium intake additional exogenous calcium is not required and overtreatment predisposes to nephrocalcinosis and nephrolithiasis. Again, the underlying cause should be addressed where possible. Recombinant human PTH is increasingly being considered as an alternative, but is still largely limited to specialist centres.

Hypoparathyroidism

Decreased PTH leads to:

- increased renal loss of calcium and retention of phosphate
- reduced bone resorption
- reduced calcium absorption.

Aetiology

Table 17.15 outlines the common causes of hypoparathyroidism mediating hypocalcaemia.

NB: Pseudohypoparathyroidism (very rare) is caused by a failure of end-organ response in bone and kidney to endogenous PTH, which is thus present in excess amounts. Unlike patients with true idiopathic hypoparathyroidism, there is no increase in urinary cAMP excretion when PTH is injected.

Clinical presentation

This depends upon its speed of onset and its degree.

- Acute hypocalcaemia – see earlier.
- Ectodermal changes: teeth, nails, skin and hair; there is an excessive incidence of cutaneous moniliasis in primary hypoparathyroidism.
- Ocular changes: cataract and, occasionally, papilloedema.
- Calcification in the basal ganglia and, less commonly, other soft tissues.
- The hereditary syndrome of pseudohypoparathyroidism is caused by tissue resistance to PTH and usually presents in childhood. The patients have a moon face, short stature, reduced IQ, calcification of the basal ganglia and often short fourth or fifth metacarpals. The biochemistry is similar to idiopathic hypoparathyroidism.
- Pseudopseudohypoparathyroidism refers to patients who have the somatic manifestations of pseudohypoparathyroidism but normal biochemistry.

Investigation

- Typically, there is a low serum calcium and a high serum phosphate level with normal alkaline phosphatase.
- Investigation for other features depends on the clinical presentation.

Management

As per hypocalcaemia.

18

Rheumatology

Rheuma (greek – stream/flow) was historically one of the bodily humours characterized as a clear and watery discharge. The presence of such fluid within inflamed joints led to the characterization of rheumatic fever and subsequently rheumatoid arthritis. Rheumatology has come to encompass the spectrum of autoinflammatory/autoimmune disorders that have a propensity to present with musculoskeletal manifestations. Since autoinflammatory/autoimmune disorders are a differential diagnosis in patients who present with mechanical non-inflammatory musculoskeletal problems, rheumatology includes other common musculoskeletal problems such as osteoarthritis.

Osteoarthritis (OA)

OA is the commonest form of musculoskeletal presentation.It is a condition of wear, tear and repair of the joint. It is characterised by a metabolically active healing response within the periarticular bone following cartilage damage or injury, and should not be considered to be simply 'wear and tear'. Cartilage damage may occur as a result of biomechanical/occupational factors, due to structural damage or due to previous inflammatory effects. The metabolically active bony response to cartilage damage is twofold: a hypertrophic/osteophyte response and a subchondral sclerotic response. There is increasing evidence that although this healing response may be painful (the sclerotic response appears to be more strongly associated with pain), in a high proportion of patients the pain progressively resolves and the bony response results in healing with normal joint function (albeit with clinical and radiographic evidence of the previous healing response). OA management should therefore focus on optimizing the repair response to prevent joint failure; where characterized by recalcitrant pain and persistent impairment of function, surgical intervention and joint replacement should be considered. Radiological evidence of OA can be detected in a quarter of the population by their mid-40s, and in virtually everyone by their mid-60s. As would be predicted, radiological evidence of previous bony reaction correlates very poorly with current pain. There is some evidence that MRI or nuclear medicine evidence of active subchondral bone reaction is better correlated with current pain. Both sexes are affected, although severe disease and hand involvement are seen more frequently in women. The most common joints to be affected are the interphalangeal joints, the 1st carpometacarpal joint, cervical and lumbar spine, knees and hips.

Genetic factors play a role in the pathogenesis of OA It is likely that interacting polygenetic influences affect both cartilage strength and the subsequent bony reaction. Obesity increases the prevalence of OA in the weight-bearing joints of the lower limb, as do certain occupational factors (e.g. hip OA in farmers). Other predisposing factors include trauma, meniscectomy, congenital joint dysplasias, joint inflammation, neuropathic joints, acromegaly, haemochromatosis, haemoglobinopathies, alkaptonuria and Gaucher's disease. All of these predisposing factors cause premature cartilage wear and tear, which subsequently triggers the bony repair reaction.

Clinical presentation

Since OA is characterized by a repair response it may be asymptomatic (especially in the spine). Clinical features will vary depending on the joint(s) involved,

Clinical Medicine Lecture Notes, Eighth Edition. John R. Bradley, Mark Gurnell, and Diana F. Wood.
© 2019 John Wiley & Sons Ltd. Published 2019 by John Wiley & Sons Ltd.

and whether the response remains metabolically active. Symptoms include the following:

- joint pain, worse with activity and towards the end of the day. The pain is characteristically not associated with early morning stiffness beyond 10–15 min.
- bony swelling, e.g. of the distal and proximal interphalangeal joints with Heberden's and Bouchard's nodes, respectively.

On examination there is bony swelling (osteophyte formation), variable restriction of movement, crepitus and, if the patient has not been adequately using the affected joint, muscle wasting. In a metabolically active or failing joint there may be tenderness when palpating the joint and pain on movements. There may also occasionally be a cool synovial effusion

Functional impairment, immobility, deformity and occasionally nerve (e.g. carpal tunnel syndrome) or nerve root (cervical or lumbar spine) entrapment may all complicate OA.

NICE Clinical guideline 177 (CG177, Feb 2014) – Osteoarthritis: care and management.

Diagnose osteoarthritis clinically without investigations if a person:

- is 45 years or over *and*
- has activity-related joint pain *and*
- has either no morning joint-related stiffness or morning stiffness that lasts no longer than 30 min.

Be aware that atypical features, such as a history of trauma, prolonged morning joint-related stiffness, rapid worsening of symptoms or the presence of a hot swollen joint, may indicate alternative or additional diagnoses. Important differential diagnoses include gout, other inflammatory arthritides (e.g. rheumatoid arthritis), septic arthritis and malignancy (bone pain).

Investigation

Diagnosis (see earlier) can be made following clinical assessment and does not necessarily require radiological confirmation. Plain radiographs typically reveal:

- loss of joint space (cartilage loss)
- osteophytes
- sclerosis of subchondral bone
- ± bone cyst formation.

Management

OA requires a holistic approach to treatment. The key goal is maintenance of joint function during the painful repair phase and prevention of subsequent joint failure. This often requires a multiprofessional approach and includes assessment of patient goals relating to daily activities, hobbies, occupation, etc.

- Exercise/physical activity is the key intervention in OA. Physiotherapy and graded exercise help to maintain muscle bulk and strength, and patients often need to be reassured that there is no evidence that exercise will be harmful (OA is not simply a wear and tear process). With regular exercise, approximately one-third of people will have significantly less pain after 2 years.
- Weight loss in obese subjects improves patient function but does not improve pain.
- Smoking cessation is associated with a significant reduction in pain in patients with OA.
- Analgesia – initially paracetamol +/- weak opioids and occasionally NSAIDs (topical and oral). There is some evidence that treatments such as glucosamine can be used as additional pain relief.
- Walking aids and orthotics may offer effective symptomatic relief.
- Intra-articular corticosteroids can provide transient pain relief in approximately two-thirds of patients for up to 6 weeks.
- Joint replacement is indicated in those with evidence of joint failure where there is persistent pain (particularly nocturnal pain) associated with ongoing impairment of function.
- There is research interest in stem cell-based treatments to address the cartilage damage associated with the subsequent bony reaction.
- Domestic and mobility aids can help improve day-to-day function.

Prognosis

In the majority of patients symptoms can be controlled with conservative management approaches including regular exercise, and in approximately one-third of patients joints will become asymptomatic over time. The minority of patients have progressive OA resulting in joint failure requiring joint replacement. However, the outcome from surgery (for those in whom arthroplasty is indicated) is generally excellent.

Rheumatoid arthritis (RA)

The commonest cause of polyarticular joint inflammation, RA is characterised by a distinct pattern of joint involvement, predominantly involving the small joints of the hands, often accompanied by extra-articular disease manifestations. It occurs throughout the world, with an estimated prevalence of 1%. Women are more frequently affected than men (~3 : 1). RA can present at any age but there is a peak of disease incidence around the ages of 30–50, and then a progressive increase in disease incidence beyond the age of 60. RA is associated with certain HLA haplotypes, including HLA-DR4. HLA-DR4 positivity is associated with erosive seropositive disease. Environmental factors that have been implicated in the development of RA include cigarette smoking, diet, hormonal changes and infections. Although epidemiological studies have failed to establish a causal link with any specific organism there is increasing interest in changes in the microbiome, particularly *Porphyromonas gingivalis,* an oral mucosal organism, which is associated with gingivitis and periodontitis.

Antibodies directed against cyclic citrullinated peptides/proteins (CCP) are strongly associated with RA, and have been reported with increased prevalence in smokers. Anti-citrullinated peptide/protein antibodies (ACPAs) are detectable in the serum of a patient prior to the onset of clinical symptoms. Production of these ACPAs may therefore be key to the development of RA. There is interest in whether mucosal changes (particularly affecting the microbiome) may disrupt the process of immune tolerance and promote the development of these antibodies.

It is likely that RA is really a phenotypic syndrome with characteristic clinic features. Different subtypes of RA may include those with ACPAs, those with RhF, those with HLA-DR4 association, those with or without radiological erosive damage, those with or without extra-articular features.

Irrespective of the subtype of RA, synovial inflammation (synovitis) is the hallmark of musculoskeletal involvement. In the early stages there is disruption of the synovial microvasculature, followed by synovial thickening and heavy infiltration with lymphocytes, macrophages and plasma cells. The latter may secrete rheumatoid factors (RF; see later). Inflamed hypertrophied synovium (pannus) encroaches on the adjacent cartilaginous surface, resulting in thinning of the cartilage and erosion of the underlying bone. An array of cytokines (interleukin-1 [IL-1], IL-2, IL-4, IL-6 and tumour necrosis factor-α [TNF-α]) have been implicated in the pathogenesis of RA.

Clinical presentation

RA is a multisystem autoinflammatory disorder with a predilection for causing synovitis of the joints. Extra-articular disease is more likely in RF seropositive/ACPA positive patients and is associated with a worse prognosis. Figure 18.1 summarises the diverse array of clinical features associated with RA.

ACR/EULAR 2010 Classification Criteria for RA (Box 18.1)

Requirements:

1. Patient with at least one joint with definite clinical synovitis;
2. Synovitis is not better explained by 'another disease'.

Musculoskeletal system

Musculoskeletal manifestations are by far the commonest feature of RA and are usually the presenting problem at diagnosis. This is reflected in the ACR/EULAR 2010 classification criteria used for RA. Synovitis is symptomatically characterized by prolonged early morning stiffness of the affected joints (usually >30 min and frequently several hours) alongside pain and swelling. The small joints of the hands and feet are the most commonly affected, usually symmetrically, but large synovial joints (hips, knees, elbows) are often involved. The symptoms usually develop over a period of several weeks but can be more acute. Since RA is a systemic autoimmune disorder fatigue, fever and general malaise are also well recognized alongside the musculoskeletal symptoms.

Box 18.1 Joint distribution (0–5 points)

1 large joint	0
2–10 large joints	1
1–3 small joints (large joints not counted)	2
4–10 small joints (large joints not counted)	3
>10 joints (including at least one small joint)	5
Serology (0–3 points)	
Negative RF *and* negative ACPA	0
Low positive RF *or* low positive ACPA	2
High positive RF *or* high positive ACPA	3
Symptom duration (0–1)	
<6 weeks	0
≥6 weeks	1
Acute phase reactants (0–1 point)	
Normal CRP *and* normal ESR	0
Abnormal CRP *or* abnormal ESR	1

≥6 points = definite RA.

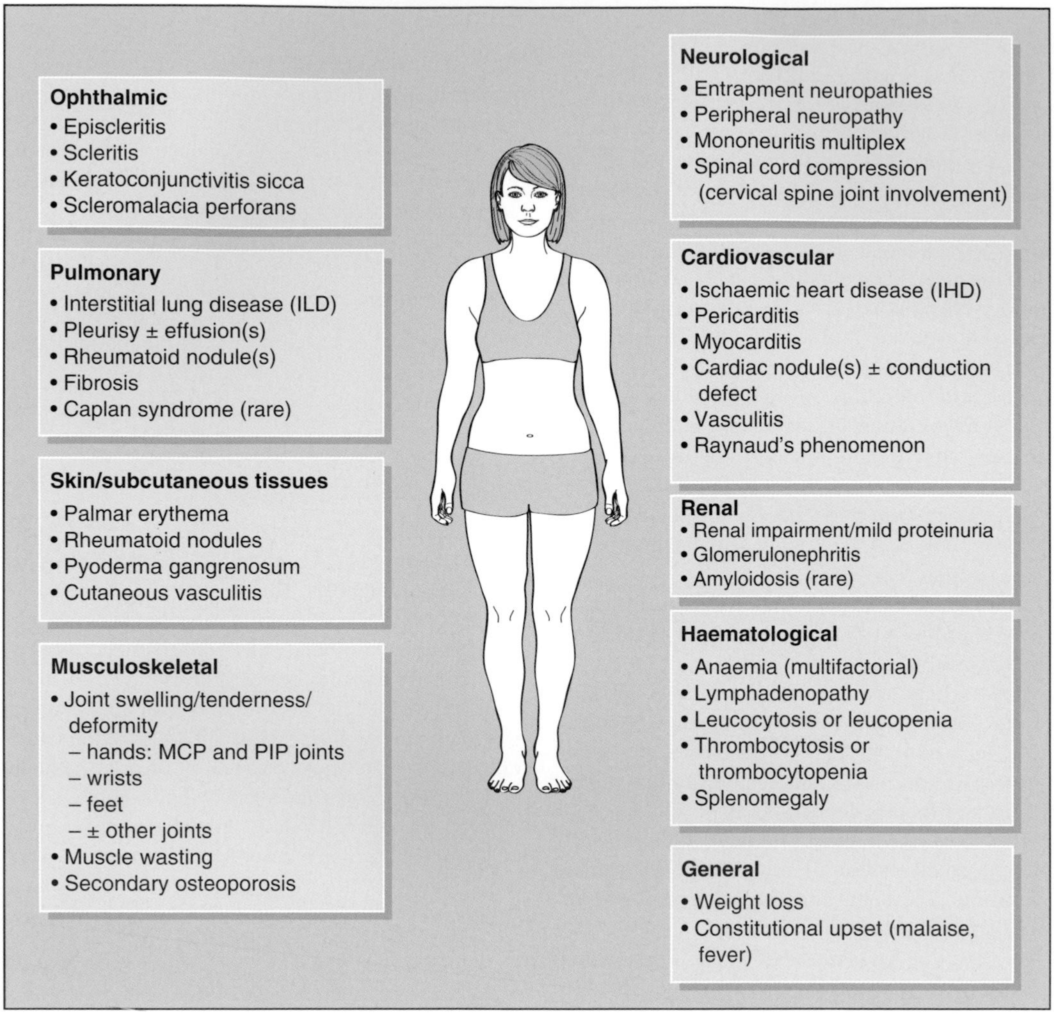

Ophthalmic
- Episcleritis
- Scleritis
- Keratoconjunctivitis sicca
- Scleromalacia perforans

Pulmonary
- Interstitial lung disease (ILD)
- Pleurisy ± effusion(s)
- Rheumatoid nodule(s)
- Fibrosis
- Caplan syndrome (rare)

Skin/subcutaneous tissues
- Palmar erythema
- Rheumatoid nodules
- Pyoderma gangrenosum
- Cutaneous vasculitis

Musculoskeletal
- Joint swelling/tenderness/
  deformity
  - hands: MCP and PIP joints
  - wrists
  - feet
  - ± other joints
- Muscle wasting
- Secondary osteoporosis

Neurological
- Entrapment neuropathies
- Peripheral neuropathy
- Mononeuritis multiplex
- Spinal cord compression
  (cervical spine joint involvement)

Cardiovascular
- Ischaemic heart disease (IHD)
- Pericarditis
- Myocarditis
- Cardiac nodule(s) ± conduction
  defect
- Vasculitis
- Raynaud's phenomenon

Renal
- Renal impairment/mild proteinuria
- Glomerulonephritis
- Amyloidosis (rare)

Haematological
- Anaemia (multifactorial)
- Lymphadenopathy
- Leucocytosis or leucopenia
- Thrombocytosis or
  thrombocytopenia
- Splenomegaly

General
- Weight loss
- Constitutional upset (malaise,
  fever)

Figure 18.1 Schematic representation of the major systems affected by rheumatoid arthritis.

Hands

- symmetrical polyarthropathy involving the wrists, the proximal interphalangeal (PIPJ) and the metacarpophalangeal (MCPJ) joints; most commonly the first joints involved are the wrists and the index and middle finger PIPJs and MCPJs
- *tenderness* and diminished movement of involved joints:
  - a positive metacarpal squeeze test is a particularly sensitive test for synovitis of the metacarpophalangeal joints
  - RA characteristically spares the terminal/distal interphalangeal joints
- *swelling:*
  - fusiform soft-tissue swelling of the metacarpophalangeal (MCP) and proximal interphalangeal (PIP) joints
  - soft tissue involvement causes swelling, tenosynovitis and tendon rupture
- *wasting:*
  - often due to a combination of disuse atrophy and reflex muscle wasting due to joint swelling (vasculitis and peripheral neuropathy can also contribute to wasting)
- *deformity* due to joint subluxation and tendon misalignment (this is a late manifestation and indicative of underlying damage to the joint due to poorly controlled inflammatory disease)

- o swan-neck
- o boutonnière
- o z-deformity of the thumb
- o metacarpophalangeal subluxation
- o ulnar deviation at the metacarpophalangeal joints
- *reduced function.*

Feet

- symmetrical polyarthropathy involving the meta-tarsophalangeal (MTPJ) joints.
- *tenderness* and diminished movement of involved joints:
  - o a positive metatarsal squeeze test is a particularly sensitive test for synovitis of the metatarsophalangeal joints
  - o RA characteristically spares the terminal/distal interphalangeal joints
- *swelling:*
  - o soft tissue swelling of the MTPJ
  - o soft tissue involvement causes swelling, tenosynovitis and tendon rupture
  - o abnormal biomechanics results in rapid development of callouses under the metatarsals that can be an indicator of underlying joint involvement.
- *wasting:*
  - o often due to a combination of disuse atrophy and reflex muscle wasting due to joint swelling
- *deformity* due to joint subluxation and tendon misalignment (this is a late manifestation and indicative of underlying damage to the joint due to poorly controlled inflammatory disease)
  - o metatarsophalangeal subluxation with clawing and lateral deviation.

Other joints

- Elbows, shoulders and knees commonly involved.
- Ankles, costovertebral, temporomandibular and the cricoarytenoid joints may be affected.
- Cervical spine: inflammation can cause laxity of the atlanto axial joint ligaments with erosion of the odontoid peg. This can result in instability of this joint complex and acute or chronic cord compression with paraplegia. Subluxation can be life-threatening and the stability of the cervical spine should therefore be considered if general anaesthesia is required – hyperextension of the cervical spine during intubation can induce subluxation.

Extra-articular manifestations

Extra-articular/systemic manifestations of RA are all seen more commonly in patients with positive ACPA or RhF. The presence of extra-articular features is normally indicative of a worse long-term prognosis.

Skin and subcutaneous tissues

- palmar erythema – frequently seen in patients with hand joint involvement
- rheumatoid nodules – typically overlying areas of pressure/friction. This is most frequently the ulnar border of the forearms. Nodules are seen more frequently in patients who are RhF or ACPA positive
- scars of previous surgery (e.g. metacarpophalangeal joint replacement, excision of the ulnar styloid process, extensor tendon repair, carpal tunnel release)
- pyoderma gangrenosum is a rare manifestation of systemic RA
- vasculitis including lower limb ulceration
- thin, fragile skin in those on long-term corticosteroid therapy with other features of iatrogenic Cushing syndrome

Ocular

- keratoconjunctivitis sicca is the commonest ocular manifestation of RA – seen in approximately 15% of patients
- episcleritis/scleritis
- scleromalacia perforans
- iatrogenic – retinal changes with antimalarial disease-modifying anti-rheumatic drug (DMARD) treatment (hydroxychloroquine)and cataracts from corticosteroid therapy

Pulmonary

- Although clinical symptoms of pulmonary involvement are relatively uncommon, lung function tests show changes in gas transfer in up to 50% of all patients with RhF positive or ACPA positive RA.
- Interstitial lung disease (ILD) is the most common pulmonary manifestation of RA with approximately 1/10 patients developing problems. ILD is a significant contributor to the increased mortality seen with RA. Usual interstitial pneumonia (UIP) and nonspecific interstitial pneumonia (NSIP) patterns are both seen and can progress to fibrotic lung disease.
- Symptomatic ILD can sometimes develop before the musculoskeletal manifestations of RA.

Other less common pulmonary presentations include:

- pleural effusion(s)
- rheumatoid nodules – single or multiple – RhF or ACPA positive.
- Caplan syndrome – an extremely rare syndrome characterized by the presence of multiple round well-defined nodules (typically 0.5–2 cm, but in some cases as large as 5 cm in diameter) in the lungs of miners (coal, silicosis, asbestos) with RA; they may calcify, cavitate or coalesce and be mistaken for tuberculosis.

Cardiovascular

All patients with RA are at increased risk of ischaemic heart disease (the magnitude of risk is comparable to having type 2 diabetes) and this risk is independent of other conventional cardiovascular risk factors (smoking, diet, lipid profile, etc.). Patients with RA can also develop more uncommon cardiovascular manifestations of their underlying disease:

- pericarditis (with or without effusion)
- myocarditis
- cardiac nodules.

Peripheral vascular manifestations include:
- arteritic lesions:
  - nail-fold infarcts
  - 'splinter' necrosis in the digital pulps
  - necrotising arteritis affecting larger vessels causing digital gangrene, bowel infarction or stroke
  - vasculitis
  - Raynaud's phenomenon.

Neurological

- entrapment neuropathies (e.g. carpal tunnel syndrome, ulnar neuropathy)
- peripheral neuropathy – predominantly sensory, secondary to arteritis or complicating drug therapy
- mononeuritis multiplex – usually digital, ulnar and lateral popliteal nerves
- spinal cord compression – secondary to cervical spine joint involvement (see earlier).

Haematological (Table 18.1)

- A normochromic normocytic anaemia is common and its severity generally correlates with the systemic inflammatory response (so-called anaemia of chronic disease).
- Iron deficiency can occur secondary to drug therapy (particularly NSAIDs).
- The ESR reflects the activity of the disease (it is an indirect measure of immunoglobulin levels and plasma viscosity). The CRP is an alternative measure of the systemic inflammatory response and reflects the levels of serum IL-6.
- Leucocytosis is unusual due to RA itself – it may signify intercurrent infection or corticosteroid therapy (which causes an elevation of the neutrophil count).

Reticuloendothelial system

- Generalised lymphadenopathy is present in up to 10% of cases.
- The spleen is enlarged in about 5% of patients and 1% develop leucopenia.

Table 18.1 Causes of anaemia in RA

Type	Cause
Normochromic normocytic	Anaemia of chronic disease
Hypochromic microcytic	Iron deficiency secondary to aspirin and other NSAIDs
Macrocytic	Folate deficiency secondary to methotrexate (or occasionally sulfasalazine); vitamin B_{12} deficiency (due to associated pernicious anaemia)
Haemolytic	Drug-induced (e.g. sulfasalazine, dapsone)
Bone marrow suppression	Drug-induced (e.g. methotrexate, sulfasalazine, gold, tocilizumab)
Hypersplenism	Felty syndrome

- Felty's syndrome: an unusual syndrome characterized by the triad of RA, splenomegaly with neutropenia and thrombocytopenia. Lymphadenopathy may also be present.

Renal

- Renal impairment and mild proteinuria are relatively common in RA (approximately 10% of patients). This has been shown to correlate more with the increased prevalence of hypertension and cardiovascular disease in patients with RA than with specific RA disease activity or severity.
- There is a slightly increased risk of glomerulonephritis in patients with RA compared to the normal population (particularly membranoproliferative glomerulonephritis).
- Serum amyloid A is an inflammatory marker (like CRP). Historically, persistently elevated levels of serum amyloid A resulted in development of AA amyloidosis. This is now extremely rare, reflecting improved disease control. Proteinuria or overt nephrotic syndrome complicated treatment with pencillamine and gold but these are rarely used in contemporary practice.

Iatrogenic

Clinical evidence of side effects of therapy may be observed (see later).

Investigation

As indicated in the ACR/EULAR 2010 classification criteria, the diagnosis of RA is largely clinical. A high index of suspicion and early onward referral for expert opinion are recommended as uncontrolled inflammation translates into joint damage and subsequent disability. Any patient reporting prolonged early morning stiffness (+/- pain or swelling) of the small joints of their hands, for more than 2–3 weeks, should be referred for further assessment (irrespective of blood test and radiological findings).

Serology

Rheumatoid factor (RF)

High titres of IgM RF correlate with more severe arthritis and with extra-articular disease. RF is not specific to RA, being found in low titres in ~5% of the general population (and does not predict disease in clinically normal individuals), in Sjögren's syndrome and in other connective tissue disorders. Although 75% of patients with RA will eventually develop a positive RF, the figure is nearer 25% at first presentation making it of low utility in initial diagnosis. Twenty-five percent of patients with RA remain seronegative throughout the course of their disease.

Anti-citrullinated peptide/protein antibodies (ACPAs)

ACPAs have similar sensitivity to RF (approximately 75%), but improved specificity. Furthermore they are more predictably present at first presentation and are therefore more useful than RF as a diagnostic test. The development of ACPA predates the onset of clinical symptoms and it has been shown that the presence of ACPA in asymptomatic individuals predicts the development of RA over the subsequent months.

Radiology

The joints are typically radiologically normal in the early disease stages. The characteristic sequence of abnormalities is:

- soft-tissue swelling and periarticular osteoporosis, reflective of local cytokine effects on the adjacent bone
- narrowing of joint space – due to damage to the articular cartilage from the inflammatory process
- periarticular erosions – these represent generally irreversible damage to the underlying joint and the development of erosive damage predicts functional disability. Erosive damage develops over the course of the disease and aggressive early intervention mitigates the risk
- subluxation due to disruption of the joint structure – this is generally irreversible
- secondary osteoarthritis – due to the cartilage damage (shown by joint space narrowing) there is a

healing osteoarthritic reaction in the periarticular bone (see osteoarthritis).

Management

Assessment of disease activity depends on both clinical and laboratory findings. The objectives of therapy are:

- suppression of active disease and symptom relief – in particular control of pain and stiffness
- arrest of disease progression and prevention of radiological damage
- restoration of joint function.

This requires a multiprofessional team approach involving rheumatologists, physiotherapists, occupational therapists, orthopaedic surgeons, specialist nurses and social services across primary and secondary care. Patient education is key and should involve information about the disease chronicity and tendency to cycle between exacerbations and remissions. Patients should have a named contact (usually a specialist nurse) who can ensure rapid access to the team in the event of a disease flare. The UK National Institute for Health and Clinical Excellence (NICE) issued guidelines in 2009 emphasising the importance of the MDT in ensuring high-quality care for patients with RA (Box 18.2).

Drug therapy

Symptom-relieving treatments

- Simple analgesics (paracetamol and weak opioids): can help some patients with very mild disease and patients with secondary osteoarthritic pain.
- NSAIDs: although they provide useful short-term symptom relief, NSAIDs do not alter the underlying disease process. They should not be used in isolation and long-term use is limited by side effects. Cyclo-oxygenase-2 specific (COX-2 specific) NSAIDs are an alternative to conventional NSAIDs. They significantly reduce gastrointestinal risks but, like all NSAIDs of any class (except naproxen) they are associated with an increased risk of ischaemic cardiovascular disease. All NSAIDs of any class have been associated with an increased risk of hypertension and of supraventricular dysrhythmias including atrial fibrillation.

Disease-modifying antirheumatic drugs (DMARDs) – conventional DMARDs

A heterogenous group of immunomodulatory drugs for use under expert supervision. Treatment should be commenced as soon as the diagnosis has been established, and not delayed until complications

Box 18.2 Summary of National Institute for Health and Clinical Excellence (NICE) 2009 guidance for the management of rheumatoid arthritis in adults*

- *Referral, diagnosis and investigations* – consider early serological and radiological screening and referral for expert review in all suspected cases
- *Communication and education* – offer verbal and written information to patients with RA; encourage involvement in self-management programmes
- *MDT* – ensure ongoing regular access to the individual members of the MDT (e.g. physiotherapist, occupational therapist, podiatrist); patients should have easy access to a named point-of-contact (e.g. nurse specialist)
- *Management of symptoms: analgesics and NSAIDS* – offer simple analgesics if pain control is inadequate; NSAIDs and COX-2 inhibitors should be used at the lowest effective dose for the shortest time possible (choice of agent should be decided on an individual basis), with co-prescription of a PPI to provide gastric protection; if symptom control is inadequate, review DMARDs/'biologics' regimens
- *Management of symptoms: DMARDs:*
  - *For newly diagnosed active disease* – offer a combination of DMARDs; ideally include methotrexate + at least one other agent + short-term corticosteroids
  - *For recent-onset disease (<2 years)* – once sustained and satisfactory disease control established, cautiously try to reduce dosages of DMARDs
  - *For established disease (>2 years)* – if disease is stable, cautiously reduce dosages of DMARDs or 'biologics', but return promptly to disease-controlling regimens at the first sign of a flare-up; when introducing new drugs to improve disease control, consider decreasing or discontinuing pre-existing agents
- *Management of symptoms: corticosteroids:*
  - *For recent-onset or established disease* – offer short-term courses for flare-ups

- *For established disease* – continue long-term therapy only after careful discussion with the patient regarding adverse effects, and after offering all other treatment options
- *Monitoring RA* – regularly monitor CRP and key components of disease activity (e.g. using a composite score such as DAS28 that includes assessment of 28 joints) to help guide treatment decisions; arrange regular clinic/specialist nurse follow-up; check for comorbidities (e.g. hypertension, ischaemic heart disease, osteoporosis, depression); assess for complications (e.g. ocular involvement, disease of the cervical spine)
- *Timing and referral for surgery* – offer early referral for specialist surgical opinion when there is persistent pain, worsening joint deformity/function or persistent synovitis despite medical therapy; urgent surgical review is also indicated when there is imminent/actual tendon rupture, nerve entrapment, stress fracture or evidence of cervical myelopathy
- *Diet and complementary therapies* – for patients wishing to experiment with their diet explain that currently there is no strong evidence that their arthritis will benefit; advice to follow a 'Mediterranean diet' is reasonable; advise that there is little or no evidence for complementary therapies offering long-term efficacy in RA, and therefore if tried these should not replace conventional treatment even if they yield short-term symptomatic benefit

*National Institute for Health and Clinical Excellence (2009) Rheumatoid arthritis in adults: management. Clinical guideline [CG79]; www.nice.org.uk/CG79. Reviewed in Deighton et al., *BMJ* 2009; **338**: 710–712. COX-2, cyclo-oxygenase 2; CRP, C-reactive protein; DMARDs, disease-modifying antirheumatic drugs; MDT, multidisciplinary team; NSAIDs, non-steroidal anti-inflammatory drugs; PPI, proton-pump inhibitors; RA, rheumatoid arthritis.

develop. Aggressive combination therapy (generally incorporating methotrexate) is usually favoured:

- Methotrexate: first-line DMARD provided there are no contraindications to its use. Given *weekly* with folic acid supplementation on a different day; adverse effects include gastrointestinal disturbance, bone marrow suppression, hepatotoxicity, pneumonitis, renal damage.

- Sulfasalazine: adverse effects include gastrointestinal upset, skin rashes, bone marrow suppression, hepatotoxicity.
- Hydroxychloroquine (chloroquine): adverse effects include ocular toxicity (particularly with chloroquine), gastrointestinal upset, skin reactions, seizures, myopathy and psychiatric disturbance.

- Azathioprine: adverse effects include gastrointestinal upset and bone marrow suppression.
- Leflunomide: adverse effects include gastrointestinal upset, raised blood pressure, bone marrow suppression, hepatotoxicity.
- Gold (intramuscular sodium aurothiomalate or oral auranofin): (now rarely used as a standard therapy) – adverse effects include oral ulceration/stomatitis, irreversible skin pigmentation in sun-exposed areas, gastrointestinal upset, hepatotoxicity, blood dyscrasias (may be sudden and fatal), nephrotic syndrome.
- Penicillamine: (now rarely used as a standard therapy) – adverse effects include gastrointestinal upset, transient loss of taste, skin disorders, bone marrow suppression, cholestatic jaundice.
- Ciclosporin and cyclophosphamide may be effective in severe disease refractory to other agents.

Biologic disease-modifying antirheumatic drugs (bDMARDs) or biologics

There are four currently available bDMARD classes, targeting different immunological pathways known to be important in RA. All are generally reserved for use in patients who have failed conventional DMARD therapy, have to be given by injection (either intravenous or subcutaneous), are expensive compared to conventional DMARDs, have similar efficacy to each other (for both symptom control and radiographic progression), are more effective as combination treatment with methotrexate, and are associated with an increased infection risk. There is no evidence of any benefit in using combinations of bDMARDs and a lack of response to one class does not predict response to another class. They are therefore generally used serially until one is identified that a patient responds to. These response characteristics suggest that there are different immunological disturbances in different patients with the diagnosis of RA. In the future it may be possible to predict which bDMARD would be most appropriate for an individual patient.

Tumour necrosis factor-α inhibitors (anti-TNF-α therapies)

Namely, infliximab (intravenous infusion treatment), golimumab, certolizumab and adalimumab (all self-injectable subcutaneous treatments) are monoclonal anti-TNF-α antibodies. Etanercept (self-injection subcutaneous treatment) is a soluble TNF receptor antagonist. Generally methotrexate is given in combination with these treatments, since it improves efficacy and reduces the risk of neutralizing antidrug antibodies developing. Adverse side effects include hypersensitivity reactions/anaphylaxis, gastrointestinal upset, increased susceptibility to infections including tuberculosis and hepatitis B reactivation, bone marrow suppression and cardiac failure.

Rituximab

Rituximab is an anti-B-cell monoclonal antibody targeting the B-cell marker CD20 and thereby reducing circulating B-cells. Like other bDMARDs it is used in patients who have not responded adequately to conventional DMARDs and is used in conjunction with methotrexate. It is more effective in patients with positive rheumatoid factor and positive ACPAs. It is administered by intravenous infusion and can be associated with infusion reactions and a cytokine-release syndrome with initial infusions. Like all bDMARDs it predisposes to infection and there is some evidence that it also increases the risk of progressive multifocal leukoencephalopathy through reactivation of the polyomavirus JC (JCV).

Tocilizumab

Tocilizumab is a monoclonal antibody targeting the IL-6 receptor, thus inhibiting the action of IL-6. Like other bDMARDs it is used in patients who have not responded adequately to conventional DMARDs. It has similar efficacy to anti-TNF bDMARDs and can be administered by either intravenous infusion or subcutaneous self-administration. Patients with significantly elevated levels of CRP (production of which is driven by IL-6) and more systemic symptoms, respond well to tocilizumab.

Abatacept

Abatacept is a synthetic fusion protein of the co-stimulatory molecule CTLA4 and an immunoglobulin Fc fragment. By binding to CD80 and CD86 on T-cells it interferes with the ability of antigen-presenting cells to activate T-cells. It has similar efficacy to anti-TNF bDMARDs and is administered by intravenous infusion.

Corticosteroids

Glucocortocoids are effective for both symptomatic relief and suppressing disease activity. Low-dose oral prednisolone (<10 mg) has been shown to reduce radiographic progression particularly in early disease. Systemic corticosteroids (either intramuscular or as intra-articular injections) are effective in controlling disease flares or while waiting for DMARDs to take effect. High-dose oral or pulsed intravenous therapy can be effective for systemic manifestations of RA.

Surgical management

Synovectomy, realignment and repair of tendons, joint prostheses and arthrodesis may be required for severe pain or, less commonly, for deformity that is impacting on function.

Prognosis

The ideal aim of treatment is drug-free disease remission. Although potentially possible for a small number of patients, with aggressive bDMARD treatment in early disease, a more realistic goal is drug-induced disease remission. Patients are therefore likely to require lifelong ongoing treatment with DMARDs (conventional and biologic). Nonetheless, remission is increasingly achievable with aggressive treatment strategies. Unfortunately, there are patients who do not respond adequately to DMARDs, and some of these will go on to develop severe disability.

Cardiovascular disease and infection are major causes of morbidity and mortality, although data suggest that the morbidity and mortality rates in RA are progressively improving as the inflammatory processes are brought more quickly under control with current treatment pathways.

Young age at onset, severe disease/disability at presentation, early radiographic erosive damage, early involvement of the feet, extra-articular manifestations and high RF or ACPA titres all predict a worse prognosis.

The spondyloarthropathies (SpA)

A group of rheumatological disorders (psoriatic arthritis, ankylosing spondylitis, reactive arthritis, enteropathic arthritis [associated with Crohn's/ulcerative colitis], undifferentiated spondyloarthritis) sharing common features:

- sacroiliitis and spinal involvement (spondylitis)
- entheseal involvement (enthesitis – see below)
- peripheral arthritis (typically medium and large joints, especially of the lower limbs)
- mucocutaneous inflammation
- familial aggregation with an association with HLA-B27
- lack of association with rheumatoid factor (hence historically termed 'seronegative').

Psoriatic arthritis

Psoriatic arthritis affects between 0.2–0.3% of the population, with a mean age of onset between 30 and 50 years and equal sex distribution. It is associated with HLA-B27 (spinal disease) haplotypes, and is more prevalent in HIV-positive subjects. A similar pathological process (increased vascularity with an inflammatory cell infiltrate) occurs in and around the joints as in the skin although, unlike RA, the inflammatory processes are initiated in the enthesis (the insertion of tendons and ligaments onto bone). Enthesitis most commonly affects the Achilles tendon and plantar fascia, the tendon insertions in the fingers (causing diffuse finger swelling [dactylitis – characterized by 'sausage digits']), and the multiple entheses in the spine and chest wall.

Clinical presentation

Approximately 10–15% of patients with psoriasis develop psoriatic arthritis. There is no correlation between the presence or severity of psoriatic skin changes and joint involvement. Furthermore, joint involvement precedes skin manifestations in about 10% of patients. There is, however, frequently a family history of psoriasis. The key clinical features of psoriatic arthritis are swelling and early morning stiffness of either the entheses and/or a few peripheral joints (most commonly the knees), inflammatory spinal pain (early morning stiffness, night pain, buttock pain and NSAID responsiveness) and dactylitis (diffuse swelling of a finger or toe). Several different (but not mutually exclusive) patterns are recognised:

- Asymmetric oligoarthritis (~30–50% of cases) typically affecting a few large or small joints. Diffuse swelling of the digits (dactylitis), in which one or two digits take on a 'sausage-like' appearance, is an associated feature.
- Symmetrical polyarthritis (~20–40%) in a rheumatoid pattern.
- Sacroiliitis and spondylitis (~5–30%) which may be associated with Achilles tendonitis and plantar fasciitis.
- Isolated distal interphalangeal joint involvement (~5–15%) which correlates with nail dystrophy.
- Arthritis mutilans (~5%) causes gross joint destruction in which resorption of terminal digits and juxta-articular bone results in 'telescoping' of the digits.

Psoriatic arthritis is often characterized by intermittent flares and periods of remission, irrespective of the pattern.

Nail changes (pitting and onycholysis) may be the only evidence of underlying psoriasis, but a careful search for skin changes (including the scalp, hairline, gluteal crease and behind the ears) should be performed.

Investigation

There is no single diagnostic test for psoriatic arthritis and a high index of clinical suspicion is required. The following may be useful:

- Elevated inflammatory markers (ESR and CRP) +/- a normochromic, normocytic anaemia
- Radiological changes
  - sacroiliitis
  - spondylitis (changes at the corners of vertebral bodies [Romanov changes])
  - erosive changes (less commonly than in RA)
  - new bone formation and extra-articular calcification (indicative of enthesitis)
  - distal interphalangeal joint involvement
  - digital juxta-articular bone resorption
- HLA-B27 positivity (~20% of all cases, and 50% of cases with spondylitis)

Management

- Patient education.
- Supportive measures – physiotherapy, aids, simple analgesics.
- NSAIDs and/or intra-articular corticosteroids for mono or oligo articular flares
- Conventional DMARDs – sulfasalazine, ciclosporin and lefunomide are the best evidence-based treatments for psoriatic arthritis but, with the exception of ciclosporin, are less efficacious than methotrexate for psoriatic skin disease. Apremilast is a newer DMARD (a phosphodiesterase 4 [PDE4] inhibitor) that has efficacy in both skin and joint disease. Methotrexate is the preferred option for patients with a rheumatoid pattern of joint involvement, although there is a lack of evidence for its efficacy in patients with other patterns of psoriatic arthritis, despite its benefits in skin psoriasis. Patients with psoriatic arthritis have an increased prevalence of hepatic abnormalities so all DMARDs require close monitoring of liver function tests.
- bDMARDs – indicated when conventional DMARD treatment has failed.
  - Anti-TNF-α therapies – (see earlier under rheumatoid arthritis) current NICE guidance recommends considering these treatments in those patients with ≥ three tender and swollen joints failing treatment with ≥ two DMARDs.
  - Anti-IL-12/IL-23 – ustekinumab is a monoclonal antibody that targets the p40 subunit of these two cytokines, preventing them from activating T-cells. Like other bDMARDs (see earlier under

rheumatoid arthritis) it is expensive, given by injection (subcutaneously) and is associated with an increased infection risk.
  - Anti-IL-17 – secukinumab is a monoclonal antibody that targets the IL-17A receptor, thereby inhibiting Th17 T-lymphocytes, known to have an important role in both psoriasis and psoriatic arthritis. It is given by subcutaneous injection and has been shown in trials to be effective in psoriasis and psoriatic arthritis.

Prognosis

Approximately 30–40% of patients with psoriatic arthritis have non-progressive good prognosis disease, which can be managed with NSAIDs and supportive measures. Features of poor prognosis disease, which is likely to be progressive and cause increasing functional problems and joint damage, include: polyarticular presentation, elevated ESR/CRP, and male sex. There is increasing evidence that aggressive early management (with conventional and biologic DMARDs) of patients with poor prognostic features improves subsequent disability. Psoriatic arthritis is associated with an increased mortality rate (largely due to cardiovascular disease and metabolic syndrome). This may be improved with more aggressive management strategies.

Ankylosing spondylitis

Ankylosing spondylitis (AS) is an inflammatory spondylarthritis, with a predeliction for the sacroiliac joints and the spine, associated with characteristic radiographic features (which are required for the diagnosis). It affects between 0.1% and 1% of Caucasians and is strongly associated with HLA-B27 (95% of patients with AS). It affects males and females similarly, but males are affected more severely. There may be a history of other systemic diseases that link with the spondyloarthropathies (inflammatory bowel disease, psoriasis [either in themselves or a family history] or reactive arthritis).

Enthesitis (inflammation of ligament or muscle tendon attachments to bone) is the cardinal pathological finding, as in other spondyloarthritides. Inflammation of the sacroiliac, facet and intervertebral joints is followed by ossification of spinal ligaments and intervertebral discs. Bony outgrowths from the vertebral margins extend vertically and coalesce. Eventually spinal fusion can occur.

Clinical presentation

Spinal symptoms (inflammatory back pain [IBP])

- pain (worse at night [in the second half of the night] and in the morning, improving with exercise) felt in the back and the buttock areas.
- stiffness (particularly in the morning [often lasting several hours] and after inactivity)
- reduced movement (especially the lumbosacral and cervical spine)

IBP itself does not equate to a diagnosis of AS. Inflammatory back pain may link with a diagnosis of spondyloarthritis, non-radiographic AS or AS. Approximately 15% of patients with IBP will go on to develop AS.

Advanced AS may result in a characteristic posture with cervical hyperextension, exaggerated thoracic kyphosis, loss of lumbar lordosis and compensatory knee flexion.

Systemic symptoms (linked with other spondyloarthritides)

- large joint involvement (lower limbs)
- plantar fasciitis
- achilles tendinitis
- anterior uveitis
- apical pulmonary fibrosis ± respiratory failure (fixed ribcage with kyphoscoliosis)
- aortitis with aortic incompetence
- amyloidosis

Investigation

The diagnosis of AS requires a history of inflammatory back pain plus evidence of characteristic plain radiographic changes in the sacroiliac joints. Increasingly, MRI findings are being used to diagnose AS (in the context of IBP) before these plain radiographic changes are identified. This cannot be diagnosed as 'true' AS but is termed non-radiographic AS. It is likely that non-radiographic AS is a precursor (in a proportion of patients) to AS.

Several different diagnostic criteria (e.g. Modified New York criteria; Assessment of Spondylitis International Society [ASAS] classification) have been proposed to help establish a diagnosis of AS.

Modified New York criteria for diagnosing AS:

- Clinical: low back pain, present for more than 3 months and improved by exercise but not relieved by rest; limitation of lumbar spine motion in both the sagittal and frontal planes; limitation of chest expansion relative to normal values for age and sex

- Radiological: sacroiliitis on X-ray
- Diagnosis: definite AS if radiological criterion plus at least one clinical criterion; probable AS if three clinical criteria present alone, or if radiological criterion met, but no clinical criteria

ASAS classification criteria for axial spondyloarthritis:

- Sacroiliitis on imaging plus one or more spondyloarthritis features* or
- HLA-B27 plus two or more other spondyloarthritis features*

*Inflammatory back pain; arthritis; enthesitis (heel); uveitis; dactylitis; psoriasis; Crohn's disease/ulcerative colitis; good response to NSAIDs; family history of spondyloarthritis; HLA-B27; elevated CRP.

Radiography: plain X-ray findings

- sacroiliitis (evidence of severe unilateral changes or mild bilateral changes are required for the diagnosis of AS)
- squaring of vertebrae
- syndesmophytes (bridging spurs of bone at the corners of adjacent vertebral bodies)
- facet joint involvement
- ossification ('bamboo spine')

Radiography: MRI findings

MRI changes are characteristically seen earlier than plain X-ray changes but, as indicated earlier, are inadequate in isolation to make the diagnosis. Inflammatory back pain with associated MRI findings is termed non-radiographic AS.

- Inflammatory changes (high signal on T2 or STIR sequencing of the sacroiliac joints)
- Inflammatory changes at the corners of vertebral bodies (Romanov lesions or 'shiny corners') – often seen first in the thoracic spine

Blood tests (supportive of the diagnosis but not required):

- ESR elevated (~80% of cases) and CRP raised
- HLA-B27 positivity (in 95% compared with 5–10% of the general population and 50% of asymptomatic relatives)
- Rheumatoid factor – characteristically negative

Management

- Physiotherapy (the cornerstone of AS treatment – short-term anti-inflammatory effects and long-term postural maintenance).

- NSAIDs are characteristically extremely effective and patients frequently require regular long-term NSAID treatment.
- Conventional DMARDs – sulfasalazine and leflunomide may be effective for peripheral joint involvement (as in other spondyloarthritides) but have no benefit for the spinal symptoms. There is no evidence of a true DMARD effect and no other conventional DMARDs (including methotrexate) are of benefit.
  - ○ Biological DMARDs – tumour necrosis factor-α inhibitors (anti-TNF-α therapies): current NICE guidance recommends considering anti-TNF treatments in patients with severe AS (with X-ray changes) with evidence of sustained active spinal disease and where treatment with two or more NSAIDs for 4 weeks has failed to control symptoms. There is some evidence that treatment of patients with non-radiographic AS with anti-TNF therapy may prevent progression to AS but more detail on which patients to treat is required before this is a recommended treatment strategy. The anti-IL-17 monoclonal antibody secukinumab is an alternative NICE approved bDMARD that is used in patients with ankylosing spondylitis.
- Corticosteroids are beneficial for their anti-inflammatory effects but patients with AS are at an increased vertebral osteoporotic fracture risk, and so caution must be exercised.

Prognosis

With expert care most individuals will maintain complete or almost complete activity. It is hoped that by identifying patients with non-radiographic AS early, that treatment may prevent progression to AS. In patients with more severe longstanding AS, moderate to severe bony ankylosis of the spine can produce fixation of mobility and rounded kyphosis of the cervical and thoracic spine, which may impair ventilation. In severe cases extreme rigidity of the spine may occur within 3–5 years. The inflammatory component of the disease may remit at any stage but recurrent episodes can occur. Bony ankylosis is irreversible. Poor prognostic indicators include onset in adolescence, high CRP and extraspinal joint involvement.

Reactive arthritis

The term *reactive arthritis* (historically referred to as Reiter's syndrome [initially described as a triad of post-shigella inflammatory oligoarthritis, conjunctivitis and sterile urethritis]) is a post-infectious (usually the infection has completely resolved) inflammatory arthritis with extra-articular features that link with other spondyloarthritides. The infective organism cannot be found within the joint itself, but results from an immune response to one or more bacterial antigens, following which activated T-lymphocytes and macrophages migrate to the synovium. Reactive arthritis is seen most commonly following infection with one of the following organisms:

- *Chlamydia trachomatis* – sexually associated reactive arthritis
- *Salmonella* species }
- *Shigella* species   } – gut-associated reactive
- *Campylobacter jejuni* }   arthritis
- *Yersinia enterocolitica* }

There is an increased incidence of reactive arthritis in populations where HLA-B27 is prevalent (HLA-B27 is involved in the presentation of bacterial antigens to $CD8^+$ T-cells) and the presence of HLA-B27 is associated with more severe and protracted disease. Notwithstanding this, the majority of patients are still HLA-B27 negative.

Clinical presentation

An episode of diarrhoea (gut-associated) or urethritis (sexually-associated) may precede the onset of arthritis by up to a month. In up to half of all cases no prior infective episode can be identified. Clinical features include:

- Arthritis: acute or subacute – this is usually oligoarticular and asymmetrical affecting medium/large joints of the lower limbs (especially the knees)
- Inflammatory back pain in up to 30% of cases
- Enthesitis (most commonly plantar fasciitis and Achilles tendinitis)
- Conjunctivitis: common in the acute phase
- Sterile urethritis (not due to the causative organism) can be a feature of both gut-associated and sexually-associated reactive arthritis
- Circinate balanitis is a penile rash seen in some patients with reactive arthritis
- Pustular hyperkeratotic lesions of the soles of the feet and palms of the hands (keratoderma blennorrhagica) occurs in ~15% of patients
- Distal interphalangeal joint swelling or dactylitis may be seen in chronic disease although should trigger consideration of an alternative spondyloarthritis
- Anterior uveitis can be a feature of chronic recurrent disease, but should trigger consideration of an alternative spondyloarthritis.

Investigation

There is no single diagnostic test for reactive arthritis and a high index of clinical suspicion is required. The following may be useful:

- Raised inflammatory markers
- Joint aspiration: fluid is turbid/inflammatory, but contains no organisms or crystals
- HLA-B27 positive (although more patients with reactive arthritis are HLA-B27 negative than positive)
- Radiological changes: MRI evidence of sacroiliitis may be seen
- All patients should be screened for *Chlamydia trachomatis* infection, which can be clinically silent.

Management

Acute phase

- simple analgesics are often of limited benefit
- NSAIDs are characteristically extremely effective, particularly for the enthesitis and inflammatory back pain
- joint aspiration and intra-articular injection of corticosteroids are particularly effective for the oligoarticular arthritis
- oral prednisolone can be effective (particularly if NSAIDs are contraindicated)

Chronic peripheral joint disease

- conventional DMARDs (e.g. sulfasalazine or leflunomide) may be required; as in other spondyloarthritis, methotrexate is ineffective
- treat underlying sexually transmitted infection (although this does not influence the course of joint disease)

Prognosis

Most patients recover within weeks or months. A small number may suffer recurrence at a later date. For 15–30% it becomes a chronic disorder requiring ongoing treatment. Persistence and recurrence are more likely in HLA-B27 positive individuals.

Enteric arthropathy

Around 20% of patients with inflammatory bowel disease (Crohn's disease, ulcerative colitis) develop an arthropathy, in the form of a peripheral mono- or oligoarticular arthritis or sacroiliitis. The condition overlaps with other spondylarthritides (psoriatic arthritis, ankylosing spondylitis and reactive arthritis) and shares the characteristic features:

- sacroiliitis and spinal involvement (spondylitis)
- entheseal involvement (enthesitis)
- peripheral arthritis (typically medium and large joints, especially of the lower limbs)
- mucocutaneous inflammation
- familial aggregation with an association with HLA-B27

Treatment is as with other spondyloarthritides:

- simple analgesics (frequently of limited benefit)
- NSAIDs are characteristically extremely effective (particularly if there is associated enthesitis and inflammatory back pain), but need to be used with caution due to the propensity to flare inflammatory bowel disease
- joint aspiration and intra-articular injection of corticosteroids are effective for the oligoarticular arthritis
- oral prednisolone can be effective (particularly if NSAIDs are contraindicated)
- conventional DMARDS (particularly sulfasalazine) may be effective for chronic peripheral joint symptoms and recalcitrant enthesitis

Autoimmune rheumatic disorders (connective tissue diseases)

The term 'connective tissue diseases' has generally been used to describe a group of conditions characterized by autoimmune systemic presentations and associated with autoantibody production (particularly antinuclear antibodies). The term 'connective tissue disease' is misleading and often causes confusion with 'true connective diseases' such as collagen vascular disorders (e.g. Ehlers–Danlos syndrome). The phrase autoimmune disorders is therefore increasingly preferred.

The autoimmune rheumatic disorders include: SLE, Sjogren's syndrome, antiphospholipid antibody syndrome, inflammatory myositis and systemic sclerosis. Although they are seen as separate diagnoses they are best considered as a group of syndromes that share common autoimmune features (fatigue/general malaise, Raynaud's phenomenon, photosensitive skin rashes, inflammatory joint and muscle pain [with early morning stiffness], mouth ulcers and positive antinuclear antibodies). Some patients may exhibit symptoms of different diagnoses at different times.

Systemic lupus erythematosus (SLE)

SLE is nine times more common in women than men and usually presents at age 20–40 years (90% of cases). It is exacerbated by exposure to ultraviolet radiation, infections, certain drugs, stress and pregnancy. In North America and Northern Europe the prevalence per 100 000 is estimated at 30–50 for white women, 100 for Asian women and 100–200 for African Caribbean women. Cause unknown, it seems likely that environmental triggers act, together with a genetic predisposition and dysregulated apoptotic processes, to breach the mechanisms of immunological tolerance and cause the disease. HLA-B8, DR2 and DR3 are associated with SLE, and other non-HLA loci have also been implicated. Congenital hypocomplementaemia (C3 and C4 complement), low CRP and serum amyloid A levels may contribute to inadequate clearance of autoantigens and engender a susceptibility to autoreactivity.

The development of antinuclear antibodies (ANA positivity) and antibodies to specific nuclear components (extractable nuclear antigens [ENAs]) are the key serological findings in patients with SLE. Histopathology commonly reveals lymphocytic infiltration and deposition of immunoglobulins and immune complexes in affected tissues/organs. Associated small-/medium-vessel vasculitis can then lead to ischaemic damage.

Hormonal factors are also important in SLE and SLE characteristically flares during pregnancy.

Clinical presentation

The commonest early manifestations of SLE are:

- tiredness and fatigue +/- fever and weight loss
- migratory arthritis/arthralgia with associated early morning stiffness
- mouth ulcers
- photosensitivity (not necessarily the classic malar butterfly rash).

Major organ involvement may be present at the outset or can evolve over time. The ACR classification criteria (see Box 18.3) provide an overview of the major clinical and laboratory manifestations. Typically, one or more of the following systems are involved (Fig. 18.2).

Musculoskeletal system (in 90% of cases)

- Migratory polyarthritis with early morning stiffness is common, and it can mimic rheumatoid arthritis, although swelling is less common.

Box 18.3 American College of Rheumatology (ACR) revised criteria for the diagnosis of SLE

To establish a diagnosis of SLE, ≥ four of the following criteria are required, serially or simultaneously, during any interval of observation:

- malar rash
- discoid rash
- photosensitivity
- oral ulcers
- arthritis (non-erosive)
- serositis (pleuritis, pericarditis)
- renal disease (persistent proteinuria/casts)
- neurological disorder (seizures or psychosis)
- haematological disorder (haemolytic anaemia, leucopenia or thrombocytopenia)
- antinuclear antibodies (ANA)
- immunological disorder (antibodies to double-stranded DNA/anti-ENA/antiphospholipid antibodies)

DNA, deoxyribonucleic acid; ENA, extractable nuclear antigens.
NB: Leonard's mnemonic for the diagnostic criteria for SLE: A RASH POINts MD. **A**rthritis **R**enal disease **A**NA **S**erositis **H**aematological disorders **P**hotosensitivity **O**ral ulcers **I**mmunological disorder **N**eurological disorders **M**alar rash **D**iscoid rash.
Source: *Annals of the Rheumatic Diseases* 2001; **60**: 638.

- Secondary fibromyalgia (see later) is common.
- Inflammatory myositis and myopathy are less common.
- Jaccoud's arthropathy: a non-deforming arthropathy caused by tendonitis rather than synovitis affecting the fingers, wrists, elbows, shoulders, knees and ankles is an uncommon late sequelae of chronic SLE arthritis.
- Avascular necrosis (most commonly of the hip) may follow prolonged corticosteroid therapy or can occur due to associated vasculitis or antiphospholipid antibody syndrome.

Skin and mucous membranes (in 80% of cases)

Lupus may be confined to the skin as discoid or subacute cutaneous lupus; typically a raised, scarring rash on the face, scalp or limbs.

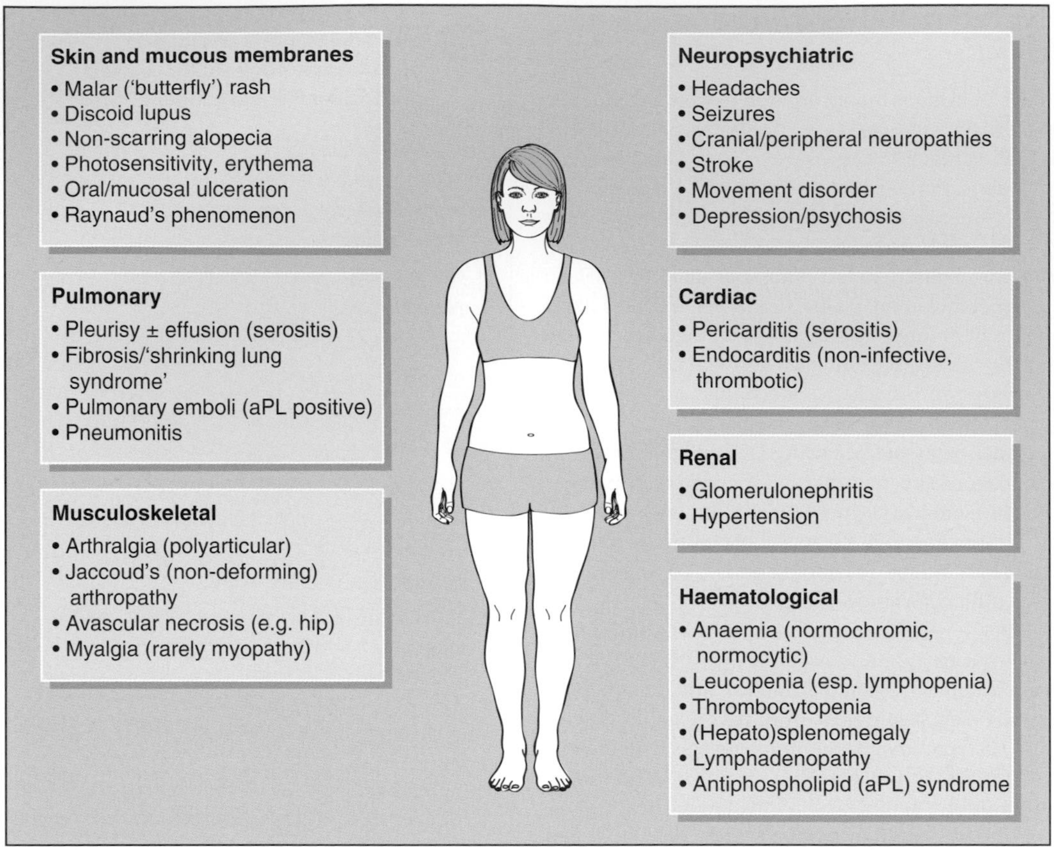

Skin and mucous membranes
- Malar ('butterfly') rash
- Discoid lupus
- Non-scarring alopecia
- Photosensitivity, erythema
- Oral/mucosal ulceration
- Raynaud's phenomenon

Neuropsychiatric
- Headaches
- Seizures
- Cranial/peripheral neuropathies
- Stroke
- Movement disorder
- Depression/psychosis

Pulmonary
- Pleurisy ± effusion (serositis)
- Fibrosis/'shrinking lung syndrome'
- Pulmonary emboli (aPL positive)
- Pneumonitis

Cardiac
- Pericarditis (serositis)
- Endocarditis (non-infective, thrombotic)

Renal
- Glomerulonephritis
- Hypertension

Musculoskeletal
- Arthralgia (polyarticular)
- Jaccoud's (non-deforming) arthropathy
- Avascular necrosis (e.g. hip)
- Myalgia (rarely myopathy)

Haematological
- Anaemia (normochromic, normocytic)
- Leucopenia (esp. lymphopenia)
- Thrombocytopenia
- (Hepato)splenomegaly
- Lymphadenopathy
- Antiphospholipid (aPL) syndrome

Figure 18.2 Schematic representation of the major systems affected by systemic lupus erythematosus.

Other features include:

- photosensitivity (the most common manifestation of SLE [up to 80% of patients] and frequently a precursor to the development of SLE)
- oral and mucosal ulceration (30%)
- Raynaud's phenomenon in between a quarter and half of all cases
- alopecia
- malar 'butterfly' rash – bridging the nose and cheeks in 30%
- nail-fold infarcts (10%)
- livedo reticularis
- panniculitis
- bullous eruptions.

Kidneys (in ~100% of cases)

SLE is associated with a range of glomerulonephritides. Almost all patients with SLE have histological abnormalities on renal biopsy but only 50% develop any overt renal involvement. When present, overt renal disease is associated with a worse prognosis. Significant renal involvement is more common in African Caribbean women. Clinical presentation includes:

- hypertension
- haematuria (dipstick positive/microscopic haematuria is more typical than visible/macroscopic haematuria)
- proteinuria (and occasionally nephrotic syndrome)
- acute kidney injury
- end-stage renal disease.

Neuropsychiatric manifestations (in 50–60% of cases)

Neurological involvement in SLE usually arises in the context of active systemic disease. Manifestations include:

- headache
- cognitive dysfunction
- peripheral neuropathy
- cranial nerve abnormalities

- mononeuritis multiplex
- tremor
- strokes
- seizures
- psychoses/depression
- limb weakness/numbness.

Although headaches, subclinical cognitive dysfunction, and mild depression are commonly seen, more severe neuropsychiatric manifestations of SLE occur in <10% of patients. Central nervous system (CNS) abnormalities are associated with a poorer prognosis.

Lungs (in 40–50% of cases)

Commonly:

- pleurisy, occasionally with effusion
- patchy consolidation and areas of collapse
- diffuse reticulonodular shadowing on chest X-ray.

Rarely:

- 'shrinking lung syndrome'
- lupus pneumonitis, which may be haemorrhagic, is rare but often fatal
- pulmonary emboli in patients with secondary antiphospholipid antibody syndrome.

Cardiovascular system (in 40% of cases)

- patients with SLE have a significantly increased risk of ischaemic cardiovascular disease (approximately 50 times increased risk compared to the general population)
- mild pericarditis: may be the first presenting feature of SLE
- non-infective thrombotic endocarditis (Libman–Sacks) – rare
- asymptomatic pericardial effusions may be detected on echocardiographic assessments performed for other reasons.
- hypertension is usually associated with renal involvement

Haematology

- anaemia – may be a mild normochromic normocytic anaemia or more rarely Coomb's test positive haemolytic anaemia
- leukopenia – mild lymphopenia is common; occasionally autoimmune neutropenia with antineutrophil antibodies
- thrombocytopenia (usually mild – occasionally severe)
- secondary antiphospholipid antibody syndrome (~20%) – may present with premature miscarriage or thromboembolic disease (recurrent DVT and PE)

- reactive lymphadenopathy (30–40%)
- splenomegaly (10%)

Investigation

- Routine blood tests:
  - full blood count: anaemia, normal or low white blood cell count (WBC), thrombocytopenia (see earlier under haematology)
  - elevated ESR with a relatively normal CRP and normal/low complement levels
  - renal function may be normal (but the urine dipstick may show subtle changes of renal disease) (see later)
  - liver function is usually normal although hypoalbuminaemia may be seen secondary to either chronic inflammation or nephrotic syndrome.
- Urinalysis:
  - proteinuria, haematuria (± casts).
- Antibodies to nuclear antigens (ANA): ANA positivity (by both immunofluorescent staining and by ELISA) is found in most but not all patients with active disease (NB: ANA positivity can be transiently found in patients with a variety of infections and can also be associated with chronic infections such as hepatitis and infective endocarditis).
- Antibodies to extractable nuclear antigens (ENAs) are also common in SLE, but are less commonly elevated than ANA in other infections. Of the ENAs (see Box 18.3) antibodies to double-stranded DNA (dsDNA) are specific for lupus or lupus overlap disorders. All the other ENAs may be found in SLE, but are also associated with other autoimmune conditions.
- Serum complement levels; low C3 and C4, especially in lupus nephritis.
- Antiphospholipid antibodies: anticardiolipin antibodies and lupus anticoagulant occur in up to one-third of cases of SLE
- Further investigations depending on presentation include: e.g.
  - renal or skin biopsy
  - pulmonary function tests/CT chest
  - CT/MRI of the head.

Disease activity can be assessed by monitoring complement levels and ESR. dsDNA titres frequently change with disease activity but less reliably than the ESR. Patients with SLE frequently have an inability to drive CRP production (which may be important in pathogenesis) and therefore a rise in CRP should trigger assessment for intercurrent infection.

The American College of Rheumatology has proposed criteria for the diagnosis of SLE based on a combination of clinical and laboratory features (Box 18.3).

Management

Patient education and support are vital – SLE is a chronic relapsing condition with potentially life-threatening complications.

General measures:

- Avoidance of UV light and high-factor sunscreen protection since UV light can flare not only skin disease but also the more systemic manifestations.
- Vitamin D supplementation (800–1000 IU/day) – there is an increased risk of SLE in patients with low Vitamin D and a tendency to low vitamin D in patients with SLE due to sunlight avoidance.
- Warm socks and gloves for Raynaud's phenomenon.
- NSAIDs – may be sufficient to relieve joint symptoms.
- Topical steroids for skin rashes.
- Management of conventional cardiovascular risk factors – smoking cessation, aggressive management of dyslipidaemia.

Disease-specific measures

- Antimalarials (e.g. hydroxychloroquine) are particularly efficacious for skin and joint disease but can also maintain remission. They may cause lens opacities and more rarely maculopathy – both generally resolve on stopping treatment. Patients should be counselled about the ocular symptoms to be aware of and have regular eye examinations.
- Systemic corticosteroids (oral or pulsed intravenous) are frequently used when NSAIDs and antimalarials are insufficient to control symptoms. Sometimes low-dose oral steroids (e.g. prednisolone < 10 mg/day) are used for longer term treatment.
- Immunomodulatory, steroid-sparing agents (e.g. azathioprine, methotrexate) can be used, particularly in non-organ-threatening disease, to maintain disease remission. Cyclophosphamide, mycophenolate mofetil and ciclosporin are generally reserved for more severe cases with organ- or life-threatening disease.
- Biologic DMARDs: B-cell targeting treatments such as rituximab (anti-CD20) and belimumab (anti-B-cell activating factor [BAFF or BLyS]) have

both been tried with limited success but their role remains uncertain.

- Patients with the antiphospholipid syndrome (see later) require appropriate antithrombotic therapy.

Prognosis

The natural history of SLE is of episodic relapses and remissions lasting months to years. Five-year survival is >95%. There is an overall increase in mortality in patients with SLE (largely due to infection and disease complications in younger patients and premature cardiovascular disease in older patients). Patients with renal involvement have a higher mortality rate than those without.

Antiphospholipid syndrome (APS)

APS is an autoimmune disorder characterised by:

- venous thrombosis (deep vein thrombosis, DVT) and pulmonary embolism (PE) and/or arterial thromboses (TIA, stroke); and/or
- obstetric morbidity (recurrent spontaneous miscarriage, usually in the second or third trimester);
- thrombocytopenia, and abnormalities of the CNS, skin (livedo reticularis) and heart valves.

Although first described in SLE, patients can have primary antiphospholipid syndrome (unrelated to any underlying autoimmune syndrome) or secondary to conditions such as SLE. Antiphospholipid antibodies (aPL, e.g. anticardiolipin, 'lupus anticoagulant') bind to plasma proteins or charged phospholipids in cell membranes. These antibodies bind phospholipids used in coagulation tests, paradoxically causing an anticoagulant effect *in vitro* with prolongation of the activated partial thromboplastin time (APTT), hence the term lupus anticoagulant.

IgG anticardiolipin antibodies are of more pathological significance; IgM anticardiolipin antibodies can be found incidentally and are less strongly associated with significant thrombotic disease.

Management involves anticoagulation (with warfarin, newer oral anticoagulants or LMW heparin) and antiplatelet therapy with aspirin. The choice of therapy is determined by the serotype of the antibodies, the pattern of thrombotic disease and whether the condition is primary or secondary (see Box 18.4).

There is evidence that an anticoagulant/antiplatelet management strategy not only reduces the risk of thrombosis but also improves constitutional symptoms such as headache and general malaise.

Box 18.4 Clinical trials/recommendations in antiphospholipid syndrome

In a retrospective study of 147 patients with APS and a history of thrombosis, treatment with high-intensity warfarin (INR > 3), with or without low-dose aspirin, was more effective in preventing thrombosis than treatment with low-intensity warfarin (INR < 3), with or without low-dose aspirin, or treatment with aspirin alone. Source: Khamashta et al., *New England Journal of Medicine* 1995; **322**: 993–997.

Recently several authors have proposed a more targeted/personalised approach for patients with aPL or different manifestations of APS. For example, it has been argued that those with asymptomatic aPL should only be treated with aspirin if they have persistently positive aPL, obstetric APS or coexistent SLE. For those with APS, lower risk patients (i.e. first venous thrombosis) should be treated with warfarin to an INR 2.0–3.0. Those at higher risk (i.e. arterial thrombosis or recurrent events) should be treated with warfarin to an INR > 3.0. During pregnancy in APS, low-molecular weight heparin (LMWH) and aspirin should be used under the care of a specialist team. Additional vascular and thrombotic risk factors should be actively reduced in all groups. Source: Tuthill and Khamashta, *Journal of Autoimmunity* 2009; **33**: 92–98.

aPL, antiphospholipid antibodies; APS, antiphospholipid syndrome; INR, international normalised ratio.

Systemic sclerosis (scleroderma)

Systemic sclerosis (SSc) is rare (estimated incidence of 1–2 per million in the UK), with females more commonly affected than males (~3–4 : 1). It is an autoimmune disorder characterised by the excessive deposition of collagen and other matrix proteins in various organs, including the skin. Initial inflammatory and endothelial changes are followed by progressive fibrosis with narrowing of blood vessels, which exhibit vasomotor instability (Raynaud's phenomenon is virtually universal in SSc), and subsequent intimal thickening leading to ischaemia.

There are two subtypes of SSc: limited cutaneous systemic sclerosis (LCSSc), which has a better long-term prognosis and is associated with anti-centromere pattern ENA; and diffuse cutaneous systemic sclerosis (DCSSc), which characteristically has a more aggressive course and is associated with anti-SCL-70 pattern ENA.

The aetiology of systemic sclerosis remains unclear and no reproducible environmental trigger or genetic predisposition has been identified, although associations with certain HLA-DR subtypes have been noted. Pathologically various immunological changes have been reported, including infiltration of skin and other affected organs by activated CD4+ and CD8+ T-cells, increased production of cytokines (including interleukin [IL]-1, IL-2, IL-6, TNF and transforming growth factor [TGF]-β), increased expression of adhesion molecules (e.g. selectins, integrins) and polyclonal B-cell activation (with associated hypergammaglobulinaemia).

Although skin involvement is the most characteristic feature of SSc it is important to recognize that it is a systemic autoimmune disease which can present with symptoms secondary to involvement of other organ systems.

Clinical presentation (Fig. 18.3)

- Raynaud's phenomenon is seen in virtually all patients with SSc and is frequently the first symptom noted. However, primary Raynaud's is common in the general population and only about 1% of patients with Raynaud's have an underlying autoimmune problem such as SSc.
- Limited cutaneous systemic sclerosis (LCSSc) – formerly known as *CREST* syndrome (calcinosis, Raynaud's phenomenon, oesophageal dysmotility, sclerodactyly and telangiectasia). Usually seen in females aged 30–50 years with a long history of Raynaud's phenomenon, LCSSc is characterised by limited skin involvement (typically face, hands and feet) and late appearance of visceral complications often limited to pulmonary hypertension.
- Diffuse cutaneous systemic sclerosis (DCSSc): a more extensive form of the disease often with abrupt onset. Skin involvement is both truncal and acral; visceral involvement may include the heart, lungs, kidneys, gastrointestinal tract, all of which show evidence of significant fibrotic changes. It can be associated with scleroderma renal crisis.
- Systemic sclerosis without scleroderma: a small number of patients have visceral disease without cutaneous involvement.
- Morphoea: changes are limited to the skin and may be localised or generalised.

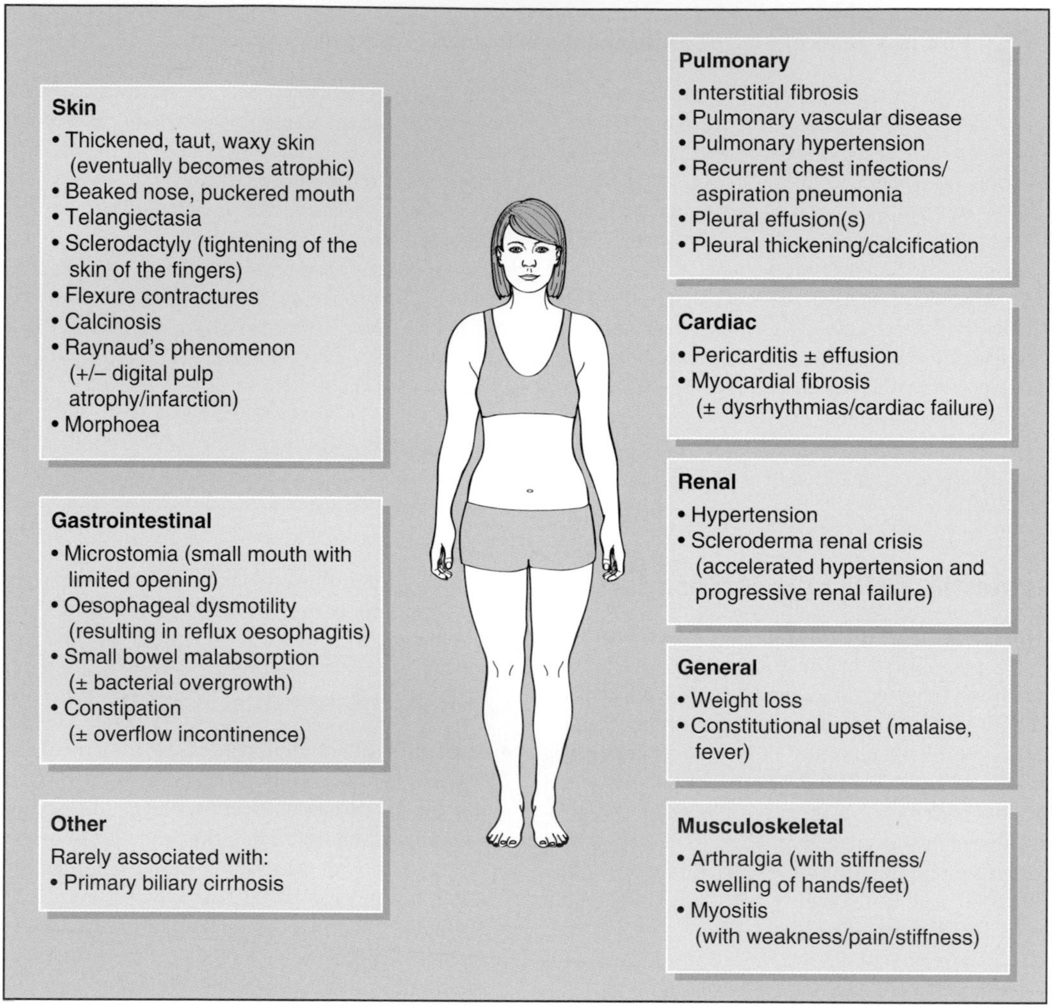

Skin
- Thickened, taut, waxy skin (eventually becomes atrophic)
- Beaked nose, puckered mouth
- Telangiectasia
- Sclerodactyly (tightening of the skin of the fingers)
- Flexure contractures
- Calcinosis
- Raynaud's phenomenon (+/− digital pulp atrophy/infarction)
- Morphoea

Gastrointestinal
- Microstomia (small mouth with limited opening)
- Oesophageal dysmotility (resulting in reflux oesophagitis)
- Small bowel malabsorption (± bacterial overgrowth)
- Constipation (± overflow incontinence)

Other
Rarely associated with:
- Primary biliary cirrhosis

Pulmonary
- Interstitial fibrosis
- Pulmonary vascular disease
- Pulmonary hypertension
- Recurrent chest infections/ aspiration pneumonia
- Pleural effusion(s)
- Pleural thickening/calcification

Cardiac
- Pericarditis ± effusion
- Myocardial fibrosis (± dysrhythmias/cardiac failure)

Renal
- Hypertension
- Scleroderma renal crisis (accelerated hypertension and progressive renal failure)

General
- Weight loss
- Constitutional upset (malaise, fever)

Musculoskeletal
- Arthralgia (with stiffness/ swelling of hands/feet)
- Myositis (with weakness/pain/stiffness)

Figure 18.3 Schematic representation of the major systems affected by scleroderma (systemic sclerosis).

- Systemic sclerosis is an autoimmune syndrome and in addition to the specific cutaneous features and fibrotic organ disease, patients often exhibit other features associated with autoimmune syndromes – inflammatory joint and muscle pain, mouth ulcers, cutaneous photosensitivity and general malaise.
- Pulmonary arterial hypertension – this is seen more commonly in LCSSc and can present with exertional breathlessness.

Investigation

- Elevated ESR +/- CRP
- Blood pressure/renal biochemistry/urinalysis: early detection of renal involvement in DCSSc

- Antinuclear antibodies:
  - anti-centromere antibodies in LCSSc
  - anti-DNA topoisomerase-1 (anti-Scl-70) antibodies in DCSSc associated with pulmonary fibrosis and peripheral vasculopathy
  - anti-RNA polymerase I/II/III may also occur in DCSSc where they are associated with renal involvement
- Radiography:
  - hand X-ray: soft tissue calcification (calcinosis), loss of terminal phalangeal tufts
  - chest X-ray
  - HRCT imaging if pulmonary function testing is abnormal

- Pulmonary function testing – looking for either:
  - reduced diffusion capacity with normal lung volume (PAH)
  - reduced diffusion capacity and reduced lung volume (fibrosis)
- Doppler echocardiography
- Gastrointestinal endoscopy ± contrast studies/ oesophageal manometry/malabsorption screen

Monitoring

Patients should be monitored regularly for development of pulmonary arterial hypertension (echocardiography and PFTs), since symptoms can develop relatively late. There is potential for early treatment of PAH (see later).

Management

No treatment has been proven to alter the course of the disease although early use of ACE inhibitors (ACE-I) has been shown to reduce the morbidity and mortality associated with scleroderma renal crisis in DCSSc, and there is some evidence for early treatment of PAH.

Symptomatic treatment of SSc includes:

- Calcium-channel antagonists, vasodilators, cold avoidance/use of thermal gloves and abstinence from smoking reduce the symptoms of Raynaud's phenomenon
- Antacid therapy/PPIs and sleeping upright help alleviate the symptoms of oesophageal reflux; antibiotics may assist in bacterial overgrowth
- NSAIDs can help with inflammatory joint and muscle symptoms (particularly the early morning stiffness) but are generally avoided due to the risks of exacerbating oesophageal symptoms
- Physiotherapy relieves joint pain/stiffness and helps maintain muscle strength/function
- Prostaglandins, phosphodiesterase type 5 inhibitors and endothelin antagonists may help reduce progression of pulmonary hypertension and digital ulceration
- Penicillamine may be of value; trials of other immunomodulators and alkylating agents are ongoing
- Corticosteroids and other immunomodulatory/ immunosuppressant treatments are often tried empirically in patients with significant end-organ involvement
- Endothelin 1 (ET-1) receptor blockade (e.g bosentan) and 5′-phosphodiesterase inhibitors (e.g sildenafil and tadalafil) are increasingly used in patients with pulmonary arterial hypertension.

Prognosis

The extent of skin involvement, and cardiac, pulmonary and renal disease dictate the outcome in DCSSc. The overall 5-year survival rates for DCSSc are approximately 85–90%. LCSS has a more favourable prognosis with 5–10-year survival rates >95%.

Sjögren's syndrome

Sjögren's syndrome is a chronic autoimmune disorder characterised by keratoconjunctivitis sicca (KCS) and xerostomia (dryness of the eyes and mouth ± other mucosal surfaces), due to inflammation and fibrosis of the lacrimal and salivary glands (which are infiltrated by CD4+ T-lymphocytes). The aetiology remains unclear but is probably very similar to that of SLE. It likely reflects a combination of genetic (particularly HLA-DR52, HLA-DR3 and HLA-DQ2) and environmental factors including Epstein–Barr virus, cytomegalovirus, HIV and hepatitis C driving dysregulated apoptosis and allowing breaching of immunological tolerance. B-lymphocyte hyper-reactivity, as part of this process, with a polyclonal hypergammaglobulinaemia, is a characteristic feature of Sjögren's syndrome.

Sjögren's syndrome may occur in isolation (primary Sjögren's syndrome) or in association with other autoimmune syndromes including SLE and rheumatoid arthritis (secondary Sjögren's syndrome). It is most commonly seen in middle-aged women (male to female ~1 : 10).

There is significant overlap between patients with Sjögren's syndrome and other autoimmune syndromes, particularly SLE. Patients with Sjögren's syndrome often exhibit other features associated with autoimmune syndromes – inflammatory joint and muscle pain, Raynaud's phenomena, mouth ulcers, alopecia, cutaneous photosensitivity and general malaise. This can make differentiation of 'primary' and 'secondary' Sjögren's syndrome difficult. Some clinicians will diagnose such patients with 'an autoimmune syndrome in the SLE/Sjögren's spectrum'.

Clinical presentation

- dry, gritty eyes which may lead to corneal ulceration (keratoconjunctivitis sicca)
- dry mouth (xerostomia), with dysphagia for dry foods, and predisposition to oral candidiasis and accelerated dental caries
- salivary gland enlargement – particularly the parotid glands

Diagnostic criteria

It can be difficult to differentiate Sjögren's syndrome from age-related sicca symptoms; the 2012 ACR/SICCA classification criteria can be used to guide appropriate investigation of patients with symptoms and signs suggestive of Sjögren's syndrome.

A diagnosis of Sjögren's syndrome can be made in patients who have at least two of the following objective features:

- positive serum anti-SSA/Ro and/or anti-SSB/La or (positive rheumatoid factor and antinuclear antibody titer ≥ 1 : 320);
- labial salivary gland biopsy exhibiting focal lymphocytic sialadenitis, and
- keratoconjunctivitis sicca with ocular staining score ≥3 (assuming that the individual is not currently using daily eye drops for glaucoma and has not had corneal surgery or cosmetic eyelid surgery in the last 5 years).

Less commonly, other exocrine glands may be affected leading to sinusitis, vaginal dryness and dyspareunia.

Extraglandular features may include:

- dry skin with urticaria (approximately 50% of cases)
- non-erosive inflammatory arthritis/arthralgia with early morning stiffness (up to 60–70% of cases)
- fibromyalgia (seen in a higher frequency in patients with Sjögren's syndrome)
- Raynaud's phenomenon
- cutaneous leukocytoclastic vasculitis
- purpura (occasionally secondary to mixed cryoglobulinaemia)
- interstitial lung disease
- interstitial nephritis
- distal renal tubular acidosis
- peripheral neuropathy/mononeuritis multiplex.

Due to the B-cell hyperreactivity, Sjögren's syndrome is associated with a significantly increased risk of B-cell non-Hodgkin's lymphoma (approximately 5% risk in patients with Sjögren's syndrome [15–20 times increased relative to the general population]). The risk is greatest in those with hypergammaglobulinaemia (particularly if associated with a monoclonal band), cryoglobulinaemia or hypocomplementaemia. MALT lymphomas (Chapter 12) are the most common type. All patients should be monitored for developing lymphadenopathy.

Babies born to mothers with Sjögren's syndrome who are anti-SSA/Ro antibody positive are at risk of neonatal lupus and congenital heart block.

Investigation

- Schirmer's test: a small strip of filter paper is hooked over the lower eyelid; wetting of <10 mm in 5 min is considered abnormal.
- Ocular slip lamp examination – allows measurement of the tear break-up time. With specific staining (fluorescein [cornea], lissamine [conjunctive], and rose bengal) the severity of dryness can be ascertained and corneal damage identified. An ocular staining score ≥3 is required to satisfy the ACR/SICCA diagnositic criteria (see earlier).
- Assessment of saliva flow rates and salivary gland scintigraphy can be used to assess the severity of oral involvement.
- ESR is raised (due to the polyclonal hypergammaglobulinaemia), but CRP is often normal.
- Serum protein electrophoresis will frequently show a polyclonal hypergammaglobulinaemia.
- Rheumatoid factor is typically detected (>90% of cases), particularly in those with hypergammaglobulinaemia.
- ANA is frequently present (~70%).
- Anti-Ro (anti-SSA) and anti-La (anti-SSB) antibodies are found in approximately 70% of cases. Anti-La is more specific for Sjögren's syndrome (anti-Ro is frequently found in other autoinflammatory syndromes, particularly SLE).
- Biopsy of minor salivary glands in the lip shows a focal T-cell infiltrate and a positive salivary gland biopsy is one of the three ACR/SICCA diagnostic criteria (see earlier).
- Other investigations are dictated by the clinical presentation.

Management

Treatment of the sicca symptoms is predominantly symptomatic with artificial tears and saliva and meticulous oral hygiene. Diuretics and anticholinergic agents are best avoided since these tend to exacerbate the sicca symptoms. Corticosteroids and other immunosuppressive agents may be required for extraglandular complications. Hydroxychloroquine is frequently used in patients with overlap symptoms with SLE. Regular supplementary vitamin D (800–1000 IU/day) is recommended. Due to the increased prevalence of ischaemic cardiovascular disease aggressive management of conventional cardiovascular risk factors is required.

Prognosis

Like patients with other autoimmune syndromes, there is an increased mortality rate, largely secondary to an increased incidence of ischaemic cardiovascular disease.

In addition, in Sjögren's syndrome, awareness of the possible development of lymphoma is important for long-term surveillance.

Idiopathic inflammatory myopathies

Polymyositis and dermatomyositis

These are rare autoimmune disorders with an incidence of ~1 per million per year; peak onset is in middle age with a male to female ratio of ~1 : 2. Several forms include:

- polymyositis (primary idiopathic)
- dermatomyositis (primary idiopathic)
- antisynthetase syndrome – polymyositis or dermatomyositis associated with interstitial lung disease and anti-tRNA synthetase antibodies
- polymyositis or dermatomyositis with malignancy (~10% of cases, e.g. bronchus, breast, stomach, ovary, lymphoma)
- polymyositis or dermatomyositis with another autoinflammatory disease (SLE, Sjögren's syndrome, systemic sclerosis)
- juvenile dermatomyositis
- inclusion body myositis
- other rare forms of idiopathic myositis (e.g. eosinophilic, focal).

In polymyositis and inclusion body myositis muscle damage appears to be driven predominantly via $CD8^+$ T-cells, whereas in dermatomyositis it is antibody/complement-mediated.

Clinical presentation

The onset may be acute or chronic. In dermatomyositis, skin and muscle changes occur in any order, or together. General ill health and fever are common.

Muscle involvement

- Proximal muscle weakness and associated early morning stiffness are common; mild pain and muscle tenderness may occur. Patients report difficulty climbing stairs and undertaking tasks of daily living.
- Involvement of other striated and smooth muscle groups may result in cardiac and/or respiratory failure, oropharyngeal dysfunction and dysphagia.

Skin involvement in dermatomyositis

- Classically, a purple photosensitive rash occurs around the eyes (termed heliotrope after the purple heliotrope flower); the remainder of the face, neck, shoulders and extensor surfaces of the fingers and forearms may be involved – seen more frequently in patients with anti-Mi2 antibodies.
- Raised scaly nodules over the dorsum of the small joints of the hands (Gottron's papules) – seen more frequently in those with anti-Mi2 antibodies.
- Mechanics hands – fissuring and cracking of the distal finger pulps – seen more frequently in patients with antisynthetase syndrome/anti-Jo-1 antibodies.
- Nail-fold infarcts.
- Generalised telangiectasia and/or angio-oedematous changes, especially of the face, chest and arms.

Other systems

- Lungs – interstitial disease with fibrosis (~20% of cases) – more commonly associated with antisynthetase antibodies (most commonly anti-Jo-1) and termed the antisynthetase syndrome.
- Joints – inflammatory arthritis with additional pain and stiffness of the joints with associated tenderness (less commonly swelling).

Investigation

- Serum creatine kinase (CK) levels: although CK levels can be normal they are usually markedly raised and are a marker of response to treatment; alanine transaminase levels (muscle rather than hepatic origin) can also be elevated.
- Electromyography (EMG) – confirms myopathy and excludes denervation.
- Muscle biopsy for definitive diagnosis.
- MRI – increasingly the sensitivity of MRI is adequate to confirm the diagnosis. It can also be used to identify a suitable site for biopsy if the myositis is patchy.
- Autoantibody profile: these can be divided into myositis-associated antibodies (also associated with other autoinflammatory syndromes) and myositis-specific antibodies (MSAs; linked with particular clinical phenotypes of myositis). However, one-third of all patients with polymyositis or dermatomyositis do not have any detectable autoantibodies.
- *Myositis-associated autoantibodies*: positive ANA and anti-ENA antibodies are common but do not reliably distinguish from other autoimmune diseases, since there is overlap in the clinical

presentations; anti-U1 RNP (uridine-rich ribo-nucleoprotein) and anti-PM-Scl antibodies are associated with overlap autoimmune syndromes that include myositis, lung disease and scleroderma-like changes.

- *Myositis-specific autoantibodies (MSAs)*: antibodies to aminoacyl tRNA synthetase (ARS; most commonly anti-Jo-1) identifies a subgroup of patients (approximately 20% of patients with inflammatory myositis) with antisynthetase syndrome (fever, myositis, interstitial lung disease, Raynaud's phenomenon and symmetrical non-erosive arthritis); antibodies to the nucleosome remodeling complex (most commonly anti-Mi-2 antibodies) – identifies patients more likely to have cutaneous manifestations alongside inflammatory myositis (20% of patients with dermatomyositis have anti-Mi-2 antibodies); antibodies to the signal recognition particle (anti-SRP) – identifies patients more likely to have acute-onset severe disease with cardiac and severe oesophageal involvement.

The extent of investigation for underlying malignancy is determined by clinical suspicion and the patient's age but should be considered in all patients.

Management

- Corticosteroids (oral or intravenous – initially at high dosages).
- Steroid-sparing immunomodulatory agents, e.g. azathioprine, methotrexate, and ciclosporin, are substituted as the corticosteroid dose is lowered.
- Immunosuppressive treatments (cyclophosphamide, tacrolimus or mycophenolate) can also be used to induce or maintain remission, particularly when there is associated pulmonary involvement.
- Intravenous immunoglobulin may help, especially if the initial response to treatment is poor and/or there is evidence of respiratory compromise.
- Physiotherapy is important in restoring muscle strength/function.

Prognosis

This is variable but generally worse in older patients. The disease may remit spontaneously, particularly in younger subjects, but relapse/progression is a feature in at least half of all cases. Underlying malignancy determines the outcome if polymyositis or dermatomyositis is associated with malignant disease. In this case the inflammatory muscle disease can resolve with successful treatment of the underlying malignancy.

Overlap autoimmune syndromes and mixed connective tissue disease (MCTD)

Patients with one specific autoimmune condition frequently exhibit symptoms that overlap with other conditions. These patients are often described as having an overlap autoimmune syndrome or connective tissue disease. One specific rare disorder, in which patients present with features that resemble elements of SLE, scleroderma and poly-/dermatomyositis, is termed mixed connective tissue disease. In mixed connective tissue disease affected individuals exhibit high titres of specific autoantibodies to a uridine-rich ribonucleoprotein (U1-RNP).

Despite the specific antibody profile patients with MCTD often show features that overalap other autoimmune syndromes such as:

- dermatomyositis or scleroderma, in which skin manifestations are a dominant feature
- polymyositis, in which muscle weakness is marked
- SLE.

Investigations and treatment are generally along the lines of the individual component disorders.

Vasculitides

These are a heterogeneous group of disorders characterised by vascular inflammation. Several classifications have been proposed, but currently the most useful are those based on (1) vessel size (the Chapel Hill Criteria), and (2) serological markers, in particular antineutrophil cytoplasmic antibodies (ANCA) (Fig. 18.4). The vasculitides may occur as idiopathic or secondary phenomena. The cause remains unknown, although flare-up of disease is often associated with intercurrent infection. Various organs can be affected including skin, lungs, ears, nose, kidneys, joints, eyes and the nervous system.

Clinical features

- General: malaise, fever, rashes, uveitis
- Renal: haematuria, renal failure (glomerulonephritis)
- Lung: dyspnoea, cough, haemoptysis (pulmonary haemorrhage), late-onset asthma
- Skin: vasculitic rashes – petechial, purpura and gangrene
- Nasopharangeal: nose bleeds, nasal crusting, deafness, septal perforation and nasal bridge collapse

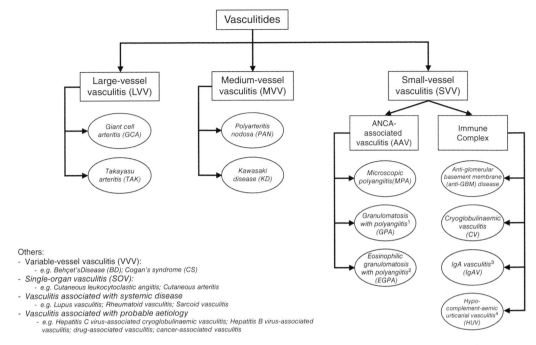

Figure 18.4 Classification of the vasculitides.

Others:
- Variable-vessel vasculitis (VVV):
  - e.g. Behçet'sDisease (BD); Cogan's syndrome (CS)
- *Single-organ vasculitis (SOV):*
  - e.g. Cutaneous leukocytoclastic angiitis; Cutaneous arteritis
- *Vasculitis associated with systemic disease*
  - e.g. Lupus vasculitis; Rheumatoid vasculitis; Sarcoid vasculitis
- *Vasculitis associated with probable aetiology*
  - e.g. Hepatitis C virus-associated cryoglobulinaemic vasculitis; Hepatitis B virus-associated vasculitis; drug-associated vasculitis; cancer-associated vasculitis

Key: [1]GPA, formerly known as Wegener's; [2]EGPA, formerly known as Churg-Strauss; [3]IgAV, formerly known as Henoch-Schönlein; [4]HUV is also known as anti-C1q vasculitis

- Ears: deafness
- Musculoskeletal: inflammatory stiffness, arthritis and myositis
- Neuropsychiatric: epilepsy, stroke, peripheral neuropathy, psychiatric disturbance
- Gastrointestinal: acute abdominal pain, gastrointestinal bleeding and perforation (ischaemic)
- Eyes: uveitis

Large-vessel vasculitis

Giant-cell arteritis (GCA; temporal arteritis, cranial arteritis) and polymyalgia rheumatica (PMR)

Giant-cell arteritis (GCA) is the most common of all the vasculitides and in view of the risk to eyesight, it is a medical emergency. The aetiology of GCA and PMR remains unclear. GCA is a granulomatous large-vessel vasculitis, whereas PMR is an inflammatory articular disorder classically manifesting with shoulder and pelvic girdle muscular pain and

stiffness in the absence of weakness. Nonetheless both share common epidemiological, clinical and serological features, with significant elevations of circulating IL-6 levels in both conditions. The cellular infiltrate (macrophages, T-cells, giant cells) in the synovium in PMR is similar to that found in the vascular lesions of GCA, where thickening of the arterial intima may be associated with luminal thrombosis. Associations with HLA-DR4 and HLA-DRB1 suggest a genetic predisposition. Both conditions are more common in women than men and tend to occur in patients over the age of 50 years. GCA and PMR are probably best considered as part of an overlapping spectrum – approximately 15% of patients with PMR will develop GCA (approximately 30% have evidence of vascular inflammation on FDG-PET imaging) whilst >50% of patients with GCA have associated PMR.

Clinical presentation

Giant-cell arteritis (GCA)

The large-vessel vascular inflammation of GCA has a predisposition for the extracranial blood vessels but can occur in any large vessels (including the aorta – aortitis is found in >50% of patients with GCA on FDG-PET imaging). It is important to be aware that headaches and scalp pain are not always present at first presentation. The symptoms of GCA usually include the following:

- mild or severe unilateral, temporal headaches, often of abrupt onset
- burning sensation and tenderness over the scalp
- claudication of the jaw (± tongue) muscles, producing pain on chewing in 33–50% of cases
- blurring of vision, diplopia or amaurosis fugax: initially often transient, ultimately progressing to complete visual loss if not recognised and treated. Occurring in up to 20% of patients they reflect involvement of the arteries supplying the retina and/or optic nerve
- systemic manifestations: fatigue, fever and weight loss
- features of other large vessel involvement: limb claudication
- symptoms of PMR (see later).

Examination

- ipsilateral temporal artery tenderness, thickening and irregularity with reduced or absent pulsation
- scalp tenderness
- visual field defect
- relative afferent pupillary defect
- anterior ischaemic optic neuritis (pale swollen optic disc with haemorrhages); occasionally central retinal artery occlusion
- asymmetry of pulses and blood pressure
- arterial or aortic bruits

Polymyalgia rheumatica (PMR)

FDG-PET imaging suggests that PMR is predominantly an inflammatory periarticular syndrome with inflammatory changes in periarticular bursae and tendons with or without associated synovial involvement. There is no evidence of muscle inflammation on either imaging or biopsy studies.

Clinical features

- Relatively abrupt onset of pain and prolonged early morning stiffness in the shoulder and/or pelvic girdles
- Symptoms are typically worse after periods of inactivity and first thing in the morning
- Few physical signs

Restricted movement, objective synovitis, muscle weakness and muscle tenderness are not features of PMR and should prompt consideration of other diagnoses, e.g. frozen shoulder, inflammatory arthritis or inflammatory myositis.

Investigation

There is no specific serological test for either GCA or PMR. ESR and CRP are typically markedly raised (e.g. ESR > 90 mm/h), although GCA may be diagnosed in the presence of normal inflammatory markers. A mild normochromic normocytic anaemia is often present. ANCA and ANA are characteristically negative.

- *Temporal artery biopsy:* classical pathological appearances of arterial wall thickening with mononuclear cell infiltration or granulomatous inflammation with giant cells throughout the vessel wall causing luminal occlusion confirms the diagnosis of GCA. Although steroid treatment rapidly alters the histological appearances the biopsy often remains positive for several weeks after treatment is started, so institution of corticosteroid therapy must not be delayed. Normal biopsy appearances do not exclude the condition, as the inflammatory changes with the artery are often patchy and skip lesions may occur. Patients with negative biopsies should therefore be managed as having GCA if the clinical and biochemical picture are consistent with the diagnosis, especially if there is a rapid response to corticosteroid therapy.
- *Duplex ultrasonography:* may detect a characteristic 'hypoechoic halo', vessel occlusions and stenosis. The ultrasound findings resolve more rapidly than biopsy changes following institution of treatment.
- *MRI and PET imaging:* show promise for diagnosis and monitoring of response to treatment in GCA, especially in the context of large vessel involvement. Imaging findings may resolve more rapidly than biopsy changes following institution of treatment.
- *Muscle enzymes, radiology, electromyography, muscle biopsy:* normal in PMR; may be undertaken to exclude other diagnoses.
- The American College of Rheumatology (1990 classification criteria) has proposed that a patient should be deemed to have GCA if he/she exhibits ≥ three of the following: age at disease onset ≥50 years; new headache; temporal artery abnormality; ESR ≥ 50 mm/h; abnormal artery biopsy.

Management

Both GCA and PMR are very sensitive to corticosteroid therapy.

- GCA: high-dose prednisolone (generally 1 mg/kg/day [40–80 mg] prednisolone reducing progressively by titration against symptoms and inflammatory markers)
  - Treatment should be started without delay, and intravenous methylprednisolone may be used in the early stages if there is visual involvement – in the case of evolving visual disturbance IV methylprednisolone 500 mg–1 g/day for 3 days is recommended.
  - Treatment should continue for at least 12–24 months.
  - Monitor response by clinical review and serial monitoring of ESR/CRP.
  - Low-dose aspirin may reduce the rate of visual loss and cerebrovascular accidents in GCA and is generally given concurrently with prednisolone – but consider gastric protection.
- PMR: prednisolone 10–20 mg/day is usually sufficient. Again this is then reduced progressively, titrated against symptoms and inflammatory markers.
- Good evidence for other immunomodulatory steroid-sparing agents in GCA/PMR is limited. Despite this methotrexate is frequently used. Other options include azathioprine, ciclosporin and sometimes cyclophosphamide. These treatments tend to be reserved for those who develop significant steroid-related side effects.
- There is increasing interest in the use of biological DMARDs in GCA – particularly anti-IL-6 treatments.

Prognosis

The prognosis in GCA is determined by the extent of visual involvement. Most patients with PMR can discontinue steroid therapy within 3–5 years, although some require long-term low-dose maintenance therapy.

Takayasu's arteritis ('pulseless disease')

This is a rare disorder affecting the aorta and its major branches; sometimes the pulmonary arteries. Its aetiology remains unknown, but the pathology is similar to GCA with focal granulomatous arteritis and >50% of patients with GCA have an associated aortitis. In contrast to GCA, Takayasu's arteritis is most common in young (<40 years of age) females (most commonly of Asian and South American origin). Differentiation from GCA can be difficult – age of onset is the key differentiating factor.

Clinical presentation

- systemic features: fever, arthralgia, myalgia, anaemia
- symptoms of arterial insufficiency/ischaemia: typically upper limbs but may also result in TIA/stroke
- bruits: aortic, carotid and subclavian
- hypertension: in the majority of cases

Investigation

- ESR and CRP are typically elevated, with anaemia and leucocytosis.
- ANCA and ANA are characteristically negative.
- Aortic arch angiography: reveals diffuse narrowing of the aorta and main arteries.
- MR angiography: increasingly used to monitor disease activity and lesion progression.
- Although PET imaging is also effective in demonstrating the extent of arterial involvement, its utility for serial monitoring is limited by radiation exposure.

Management

- High-dose corticosteroids (generally 1 mg/kg/day [40–80 mg] prednisolone reducing progressively by titration against symptoms and inflammatory markers)
- Additional immunosuppression (e.g. azathioprine, methotrexate or cyclophosphamide) may be required in some cases.
- Hypertension is managed conventionally.
- Surgical intervention may be required for critical carotid or renal artery stenosis, or significant aortic regurgitation.

Prognosis

The prognosis is generally good, although relapse is common.

Medium-sized vessel vasculitis

Polyarteritis nodosa (PAN) (also known as classical PAN)

Polyarteritis nodosa is characterised by necrotising inflammation of medium-sized arteries, leading to the formation of small aneurysms. It is an immune-complex-mediated vasculitis of unknown aetiology, although some cases (approximately 1/3) are associated with hepatitis B virus (HBV) infection. It has an estimated annual incidence of between 1 and 10 cases per 10 million population.

Clinical presentation

Clinical features of PAN are shown in Fig. 18.5. Skin manifestations should include tender nodules and skin ulceration.

Investigation

- marked inflammatory response, raised ESR and CRP with anaemia and leucocytosis
- renal and liver function tests
- HBV status
- urinalysis – proteinuria and microscopic haematuria
- renal/visceral angiography: reveals vessel narrowing, pruning of the peripheral vasculature and aneurysms. Characteristically the appearance of multiple microaneurysms on vascular imaging is likened to the appearance of a 'rosary bead'
- biopsy of involved tissue (e.g. muscle, nerve, skin, kidney): vasculitic changes with segmental fibrinoid necrosis of the walls of medium-sized arteries and arterioles and cellular infiltration
- ANCA is not associated with classical PAN. However, perinuclear ANCA (pANCA) is found in a proportion of patients with PAN who have an associated microscopic polyangiitis (MPA) (see later). This is more correctly classified as microscopic polyangiitis.

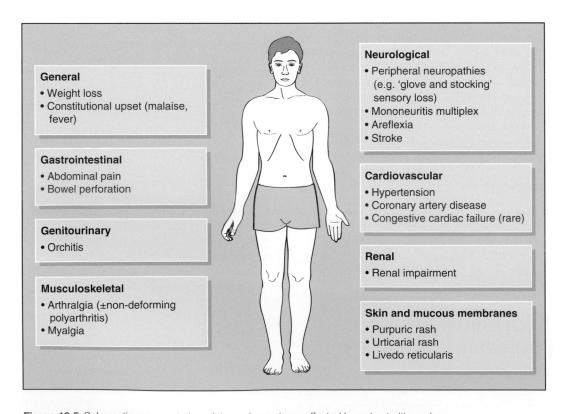

General
- Weight loss
- Constitutional upset (malaise, fever)

Gastrointestinal
- Abdominal pain
- Bowel perforation

Genitourinary
- Orchitis

Musculoskeletal
- Arthralgia (±non-deforming polyarthritis)
- Myalgia

Neurological
- Peripheral neuropathies (e.g. 'glove and stocking' sensory loss)
- Mononeuritis multiplex
- Areflexia
- Stroke

Cardiovascular
- Hypertension
- Coronary artery disease
- Congestive cardiac failure (rare)

Renal
- Renal impairment

Skin and mucous membranes
- Purpuric rash
- Urticarial rash
- Livedo reticularis

Figure 18.5 Schematic representation of the major systems affected by polyarteritis nodosa.

Management

- Systemic disease is treated with a combination of corticosteroid and cytotoxic chemotherapy. PAN confined to the skin may be treated with corticosteroids alone.
- HBV infection should be treated appropriately and complications (hypertension, bowel infarction or perforation) managed along conventional lines.
- Renal impairment, proteinuria > 1 g per 24 h and visceral involvement are adverse prognostic markers.

Kawasaki disease

This rare medium-vessel vasculitis typically affects children, causing fever, mucocutaneous features (e.g. conjunctival infection, fissuring of the lips, erythema and desquamation of the hands) and lymphadenopathy. Various organs may be affected, including the coronary vasculature. Treatment is with aspirin and intravenous immunoglobulin therapy.

Small-vessel vasculitides

ANCA associated vasculitides (AAVs): these constitute:

- Granulomatosis with polyangiitis (GPA) – historically termed Wegener's granulomatosis
- Eosinophilic granulomatosis with polyangiitis (EGPA)/allergic granulomatosis – historically termed Churg–Strauss syndrome
- Microscopic polyangiitis (MPA).

These conditions are all associated with characteristic immunofluorescent staining of the neutrophilic cytoplasm (ANCA). Different patterns of staining (and different antigenic targets help the classification of this group of disorders):

- cytoplasmic staining (classical or cANCA; usually PR3-ANCA directed against proteinase 3) is seen in GPA/Wegener's granulomatosis
- perinuclear staining (perinuclear or pANCA; usually MPO-ANCA (directed against myeloperoxidase) is seen in microscopic polyangiitis, also in a subset of patients with EGPA/allergic granulomatosis/Churg–Strauss syndrome.

ANCA negative vasculitides: these include hypersensitivity vasculitis, Henoch–Schönlein purpura, and cryoglobulinaemic vasculitis.

Granulomatosis with polyangiitis (GPA)/Wegener's granulomatosis

GPA is characterised by necrotising granulomatous vasculitis with few or no immune deposits. Localised inflammation, usually in the upper or lower respiratory tract, is followed by the development of a systemic vasculitis and glomerulonephritis. It affects both sexes equally, can occur at any age (commonly in older middle age [peak incidence 65–75]) and has an estimated annual incidence of approximately 10 per million population with a prevalence of approximately 150 per million population in Northern European populations (less common in other populations). The aetiology of GPA is unknown although some infections (e.g. nasal carriage of *Staphylococcus aureus*) are associated with disease relapse.

Clinical presentation

The key clinical features are shown in Fig. 18.6. Typically GPA involves the upper and lower airways and the kidneys, although rarely, other organ systems including the gastrointestinal tract, heart, central nervous system and pituitary gland are involved. There is frequently significant overlap of clinical features with the other AAVs.

Investigation

- ESR and CRP: typically raised in proportion to disease activity
- renal function: requires close monitoring
- urinalysis: for proteinuria, microscopic haematuria and casts – anything to suggest glomerulonephritis
- cANCA (usually PR3-ANCA): positive in the majority (80–90%) of cases
- plain chest X-ray, CT chest and CT/MRI of the nasal sinuses: elucidate respiratory tract involvement
- biopsy of affected tissue (nasal, lung or renal [renal biopsy is the most diagnostically productive]): shows necrotising vasculitis with granuloma formation

Management

Remission induction

High-dose corticosteroids and pulsed intravenous cyclophosphamide are the first-line therapy for patients with GPA with renal involvement. Mycophenolate mofetil and rituximab (an anti-CD20 monoclonal antibody, which depletes B-cells) can also be effective in inducing remission. Methotrexate can be used in

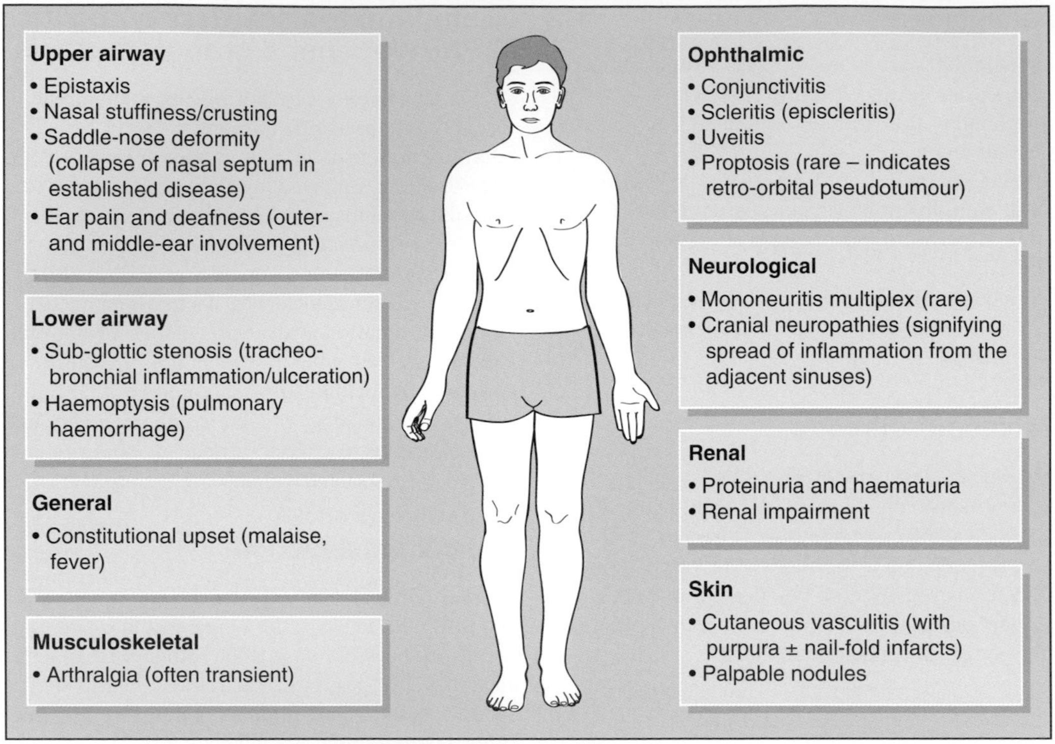

Upper airway
- Epistaxis
- Nasal stuffiness/crusting
- Saddle-nose deformity (collapse of nasal septum in established disease)
- Ear pain and deafness (outer- and middle-ear involvement)

Lower airway
- Sub-glottic stenosis (tracheo-bronchial inflammation/ulceration)
- Haemoptysis (pulmonary haemorrhage)

General
- Constitutional upset (malaise, fever)

Musculoskeletal
- Arthralgia (often transient)

Ophthalmic
- Conjunctivitis
- Scleritis (episcleritis)
- Uveitis
- Proptosis (rare – indicates retro-orbital pseudotumour)

Neurological
- Mononeuritis multiplex (rare)
- Cranial neuropathies (signifying spread of inflammation from the adjacent sinuses)

Renal
- Proteinuria and haematuria
- Renal impairment

Skin
- Cutaneous vasculitis (with purpura ± nail-fold infarcts)
- Palpable nodules

Figure 18.6 Schematic representation of the major systems affected by granulomatosis with polyangiitis (GPA).

patients with non-renal GPA. Adjunctive treatments with IV immunoglobulin or plasma exchange are sometimes used in severe cases.

Maintenance treatment

Lower dose oral corticosteroids and cyclophospha-mide-sparing therapy (e.g. azathioprine, methotrex-ate, mycophenolate and rituximab) are used for maintenance therapy.

Prognosis

The 5-year survival rate is >80%, although up to 50% of patients will suffer one or more relapses during this time. Superadded infection and renal and respiratory failure are major causes of long-term morbidity.

Microscopic polyangiitis (MPA)

Clinical presentation

This necrotising vasculitis predominantly affects the kidneys, causing rapidly progressive glomerulone-phritis. Approximately 50% of patients have associ-ated lung involvement presenting as haemoptysis,

pleurisy or asthma. Frank pulmonary haemorrhage is rare but potentially fatal. Other features include arthralgia, vasculitic or purpuric rashes, hyperten-sion, mononeuritis multiplex and peripheral neuropathy. The aetiology is unknown but is thought to be different to GPA, due to variation in epidemio-logical patterns. Like GPA, MPA affects both sexes equally, tends to present in those in older middle age, with a peak incidence between 65 and 75. However, the incidence rates for MPA are lower than GPA in Northern European populations (incidence of MPA approximately 6 per million population). By contrast MPA appears to be more common than GPA in other populations (Southern Europe, India and Asia), despite a similar overall incidence of AAV (approximately 20 per million population). Whether these differences are due to genetic or environmental factors is unknown.

Investigation and management

As for GPA and EGPA, MPA is characterised by elevated titres of ANCA – for MPA (like EGPA) this is more characteristically a perinuclear pattern (pANCA [usually MPO-ANCA]). There is an absence of both eosinophilic infiltration and granulomas on biopsy.

Management

The management of MPA is comparable with that of GPA and EGPA with remission induction and maintenance treatment:

Remission induction

High-dose corticosteroids and pulsed intravenous cyclophosphamide are the first-line therapy for patients with GPA with renal involvement. Mycophenolate mofetil and rituximab (an anti-CD20 monoclonal antibody, which depletes B-cells) can also be effective in inducing remission. Methotrexate can be used in patients with non-renal GPA. Adjunctive treatments with IV immunoglobulin or plasma exchange are sometimes used in severe cases.

Maintenance treatment

Lower dose oral corticosteroids and cyclophosphamide-sparing therapy (e.g. azathioprine, methotrexate, mycophenolate and rituximab) are used for maintenance therapy.

Eosinophilic granulomatosis with polyangiitis (EGPA)/allergic granulomatosis/Churg–Strauss syndrome

EGPA patients often present with late-onset asthma and allergic rhinitis that precedes the development of vasculitis. Subsequently there is frequently a peripheral eosinophilia on the full blood count (>10% of the peripheral white cells) which can again precede the development of vasculitis. In the vasculitic phase of disease eosinophils predominate in the inflammatory infiltrates, which are often granulomatous. Perinuclear ANCA staining (pANCA [MPO-ANCA]) positivity is seen in approximately 70% of patients with EGPA. EGPA appears to be less common in all populations than either MPA or GPA (incidence 1–5 per million population). It tends to affect younger patients than MPA or GPA (peak incidence approximately 40 years). Men and women are equally affected. Again the aetiology is unknown.

Like GPA and MPA, EGPA can affect multiple organs and the clinical presentation of all AAVs frequently show overlapping clinic features.

- peripheral nerves: mononeuritis multiplex or peripheral neuropathy*
- lungs: infiltrates (may be transient) and haemorrhage*

- ENT: paranasal sinusitis*
- GI tract: pain, diarrhoea, bleeding, perforation
- heart: myocardial infarction
- brain: stroke
- skin: purpura
- kidneys: focal segmental necrotising glomerulo-nephritis.

*most diagnostically suggestive of EGPA (alongside late-onset asthma, peripheral eosinophilia and histology showing eosinophilic infiltrates).

Management

The management of EGPA is comparable with that of GPA and MPA with remission induction and maintenance treatment:

Remission induction

High-dose corticosteroids and pulsed intravenous cyclophosphamide are the first-line therapy for patients with significant organ involvement. Mycophenolate mofetil and rituximab (an anti-CD20 monoclonal antibody, which depletes B-cells) can also be effective in inducing remission. Methotrexate can be used in patients with non-renal GPA. Adjunctive treatments with IV immunoglobulin or plasma exchange are sometimes used in severe cases.

Maintenance treatment

Lower dose oral corticosteroids and cyclophosphamide-sparing therapy (e.g. azathioprine, methotrexate, mycophenolate and rituximab) are used for maintenance therapy.

Non-AAV small-vessel vasculitides

Hypersensitivity (leucocytoclastic) vasculitis

This is characterised by inflammation of small vessels, resulting in palpable purpuric skin lesions that coalesce to form plaques or ecchymoses, especially on the lower limbs. There may be joint, renal or gastrointestinal involvement. Usually idiopathic, it is associated with autoimmune/connective tissue diseases (RA, SLE, Sjögren's syndrome), infections (hepatitis B/C, HIV), drugs (penicillin, sulfonamides, thiazides) and lympho- and myeloproliferative disorders.

Henoch–Schönlein purpura (HSP)

This is a systemic vasculitis characterised by deposition of immunoglobulin A (IgA)-containing immune complexes, usually following an upper respiratory tract infection. It typically occurs between the ages of 3 and 15 years, more commonly affects males and is rare in adults, in whom the prognosis is worse. A palpable purpuric rash develops over the buttocks and legs, with arthritis, abdominal pain with bloody diarrhoea and glomerulonephritis which is indistinguishable from IgA nephropathy. A leucocytoclastic necrotising vasculitis with IgA deposition is demonstrable at the dermo-epidermal junction in skin biopsies, and there is mesangial IgA deposition in the kidneys. Episodes are usually self-limiting (days or weeks) but relapses may occur, especially in the elderly and those with nephritis. Evidence of progressive renal involvement is an indication for high-dose corticosteroid/immunosuppressive therapy.

Cryoglobulinaemic vasculitis

Cryoglobulinaemic vasculitis/mixed cryoglobulinaemia syndrome

This rare small-vessel vasculitis typically affects patients with hepatitis C (HCV) infection (>80% of cases) and is one of the extrahepatic manifestations of HCV. Cryoglobulins are immunoglobulins that precipitate from the serum in the cold – HCV is associated with polyclonal or monoclonal IgG or IgM types (type II/type III mixed cryoglobulins). Vasculitis is not an inevitable consequence of the cryoglobulinamia – only about 10% of HCV patients with documented cryoglobulinaemia develop vasculitis.

Clinical presentation

The vasculitis causes fever, vasculitic rashes with palpable purpura on the lower extremities, acute neuropathies, inflammatory arthritis, abdominal pain, renal impairment (secondary to glomerulonephritis) and Raynaud's.

Investigation

- ESR/CRP are raised
- HCV serology is positive in 90% of cases. HCV RNA may be detected in the cryoprecipitate
- Rheumatoid factor (RhF) is generally positive (RhF is positive in the majority of patients with chronic HCV)
- Low complement (C4) levels are characteristically seen

- Cryoglobulin detection – correct sample collection and transport to the laboratory (at 37 °C) is essential if cryoglobulinaemia is suspected to avoid cryoprecipitation occurring in transit
- Biopsy of affected tissues (skin and/or renal biopsy): vasculitic changes with neutrophil infiltration of small- and medium-sized vessels
- MRI brain: high-signal white matter changes
- Lumbar puncture: raised protein level with lymphocytes and neutrophils

Management

- asymptomatic cryoglobulinaemia merely requires treatment of the underlying HCV infection
- antiviral treatments should be initiated if HCV is present
- corticosteroids – high-dose therapy is often required
- immunosuppressants – methotrexate, azathioprine, mycophenolate mofetil and cyclophosphamide are all used particularly if there is progressive renal disease
- plasma exchange can be used as an adjunctive treatment

Other vasculitides

Behçet's disease

Behçet's disease is a rare condition of unknown aetiology characterised by disordered regulation of the inflammatory response with vasculitis of veins and arteries of all sizes, hypercoagulability and neutrophil dysfunction. It therefore sits outside the conventional Chapel Hill Criteria (see Fig. 18.4). It occurs with greater prevalence in the Middle East and Central Asia but is not restricted to these areas. Globally, males are more commonly affected than females, with a peak age of onset in the 20s. There is an association with HLA-B51 which is found in greater frequency in patients of Middle Eastern or Central Asian origin (traditionally a geographical area referred to as the 'silk route').

Clinical presentation

The diagnosis remains predominantly clinical (see Box 18.5). Common manifestations include:

- mucocutaneous
  - oral aphthous ulcers
  - anogenital ulcers

Box 18.5 International Study Group for Behçet's Disease diagnostic criteria

To establish a diagnosis of Behçet's disease the following criteria are required:

- oral ulceration – occurring on ≥ three occasions during a 12-month period together with ≥ two of the following 'hallmark' features:
  - ○ genital ulceration (majority of cases)
  - ○ skin lesions (> two-thirds of cases)
  - ○ eye lesions (half to three-quarters of cases)
  - ○ pathergy

NB: In addition, alternative diagnoses (see text) should be excluded.

- ○ erythema nodosum
- ○ acneiform lesions
- ○ vasculitic lesions
- ○ a papule or pustule may form at sites of minor trauma (pathergy)
- eyes
  - ○ relapsing anterior and posterior uveitis
  - ○ retinal vasculitis
- joints (50–60% of cases)
  - ○ arthralgia or non-deforming mono- or polyarthritis
- neuro (-psychiatric) (10–20% of cases)
  - ○ transient ischaemic attacks
  - ○ cerebrovascular accidents
  - ○ seizures
  - ○ dementia/psychosis reflecting involvement of cerebral vessels
- cardiovascular/respiratory
  - ○ dyspnoea, haemoptysis (pulmonary vasculitis), pulmonary embolism
  - ○ myocardial ischaemia/infarction
  - ○ thrombophlebitis, deep vein thrombosis
- gastrointestinal
  - ○ abdominal pain, constipation, bloody diarrhoea (intestinal vasculitis with mesenteric ischaemia).

Differential diagnosis

- herpes simplex: recurrent orogenital ulceration
- sarcoidosis: erythema nodosum, uveitis, pulmonary involvement
- inflammatory bowel disease: oral/perianal ulceration, gastrointestinal involvement
- seronegative arthritis: arthritis, uveitis

Investigation

- ESR/CRP are raised in active disease
- biopsy of affected tissues: vasculitic changes with neutrophil infiltration of small- and medium-sized vessels
- MRI brain: high-signal white matter changes
- lumbar puncture: raised protein level with lymphocytes and neutrophils

Management

- corticosteroids: topical therapy may be tried for local ulceration, but systemic high dose therapy is often required
- cytotoxics: methotrexate, cyclophosphamide, chlorambucil
- thalidomide, colchicine, interferon-α have all been tried with variable response
- azathioprine and ciclosporin: especially for eye involvement
- antitumour necrosis factor-α (anti-TNF-α) therapy may be useful
- anticoagulation to treat thrombosis

Crystal arthropathies

Gout

Gout is a disorder of uric acid metabolism. Chronic hyperuricaemia leads to deposition of monosodium urate (MSU) crystals in soft tissues, especially cartilage/synovium, skin and renal tubules. Humans and great apes are susceptible to hyperuricaemia and subsequent gout due to mutation of the enzyme uricase, which breaks down uric acid to the more soluble breakdown product allantoin in other species. The deposition of crystals frequently occurs over several years before the first presentation.

Joint involvement initially results in an intermittent mono- or oligoarticular inflammatory arthropathy (less commonly a chronic polyarticular inflammatory arthritis in untreated chronic hyperuricaemia). Skin involvement results in tophi (cutaneous deposits of uric acid) and renal involvement results in uric acid stones.

Gout is common, affecting 1% of the UK population. Its prevalence varies according to social and geographical factors, being more common in affluent societies. It is found more commonly in men (uric acid levels are higher in men than women due to the effects on oestradiol on uric acid excertion).

Postmenopausal women are affected more frequently (when uric acid levels rise) and in the elderly there is a similar incidence of gout in men and women.

Hyperuricaemia can result from overproduction/increased intake, inefficient renal excretion or a combination of the two. Overproduction/increased intake may be caused by:

- excess alcohol ingestion (particularly beers which are high in purines)
- consumption of purine-rich foods (e.g. red meat).
- increased cell turnover states: haematological disorders (myeloid leukaemia, myelofibrosis, polycythaemia rubra vera, multiple myeloma, Hodgkin's disease), antimetabolite chemotherapy and psoriasis (all associated with enhanced purine production due to increased rates of DNA breakdown)
- genetic factors may very rarely contribute to a predisposition to gout due to overproduction; an X-linked disorder of the purine salvage enzyme hypoxanthine guanine phosphoribosyltransferase (HPRT) results in hyperuricaemia and gout in childhood/adolescence (Lesch–Nyhan syndrome).

Renal excretion of uric acid is via specific transport channels in the renal tubules. Impaired renal excretion may be the result of:

- metabolic syndrome with obesity and hyperinsulinaemia, which inhibits uric acid excretion
- alcohol
- diuretics (thiazide more commonly than loop diuretics)
- dehydration
- renal failure for whatever causes.

Any process that results in sudden changes in uric acid concentration can cause instability of the deposited crystals, resulting in their release and an acute attack. Alcohol/dietary excess or sudden abstinence/starvation, surgery, infection and initiation of uric acid-lowering treatment may all trigger an acute attack.

MSU crystals shed into the joint cavity from microtophi on the joint lining provoke an intense inflammatory reaction, via innate immune system pattern recognition receptors, activation of the intracellular inflammasome and cleavage of IL-1 to its active form. This response is identical to the mechanism by which the inate immune system recognizes bacterial infections such as *Staphylococcus aureus*. The innate immune response causes acute vasodilatation (hence redness of the affected area), activation of synovial macrophages, and recruitment of neutrophils.

Clinical presentation

Acute and chronic gout

In men, the first attack effects the first metatarsophalangeal joint in 75% of cases, the ankle or tarsus in 35%, the knee in 20%, with polyarticular involvement at presentation in 10% of cases (generally patients with underlying renal disorders). In women, the knee and ankle are more frequently the first affected joints. The initial onset of gout is usually sudden and reaches maximum intensity by 8–12 h. The affected joint is red, hot, swollen and exquisitely tender and there may be fever with systemic upset due to the neutrophil activation. Initially monoarticular in most patients, attacks tend to entirely resolve within 7–10 days. During the subsequent intercurrent period there is usually a complete resolution of symptoms. However, without treatment gout becomes recurrent and can become polyarticular, also involving the upper limbs. As chronic gout evolves the severity of attacks become less prominent but the patients often describe ongoing inflammatory joint pain and stiffness during intercurrent periods.

Tophaceous gout

Uric acid deposition in the skin produces *tophi* (well-demarcated crystal aggregates that can rupture, releasing a chalky substance), commonly on the pinna of the ear, the fingers and toes and over pressure sites. They are a feature of chronic gout and may occasionally be confused with rheumatoid nodules and nodular OA.

Nephrolithiasis and urate nephropathy

Uric acid-containing stones account for 5–10% of all cases of renal/ureteric calculi. Deposition of urate crystals in the renal interstitium or collecting ducts can lead to progressive renal impairment.

Investigation of gout

- Joint aspiration: definitive test, excludes septic arthritis. The aspirated fluid is turbid, containing MSU crystals which are needle-shaped and exhibit negative birefringence under polarised light microscopy. Crystals can also be identified in material aspirated from bursae or tophi.
- Serum uric acid levels: ideally this is measured during the intercurrent period since 10% of patients with acute gout have normal serum uric acid levels. Nonetheless an elevated serum uric acid level during an attack is highly suggestive of gout.

- Routine blood tests: neutrophil leucocytosis is common and the ESR and CRP are often markedly raised. Renal function and evidence of comorbidities (hypertension, dyslipidaemia, glucose intolerance/type 2 diabetes mellitus) should be investigated.
- Radiology:
  - Plain radiographs
    - asymmetrical soft-tissue swelling may be the only visible abnormality on plain radiographs in acute gout
    - irregular punched-out bony erosions near the articular margins (seen in chronic disease)
    - calcified tophi
    - osteoarthritic reactive healing changes may develop in chronic disease
    - uric acid renal/ureteric stones are radiolucent and cannot be visualized on plain radiographs.
  - Ultrasound
    - A characteristic double contour sign is seen on ultrasound of joints – an echogenic line (due to the uric acid crystals) parallel to the echogenic bony margin.

Management

Acute episodes

- *NSAIDs:* the treatment of choice in those with no contraindications.
- *Corticosteroids:* in patients for whom NSAIDs are contraindicated. Intra-articular injection is effective; alternatively, oral prednisolone (up to 40 mg/day, with or without dose tapering, for a total of 7–10 days).

Prophylactic treatment

- *Colchicine* (500 µg b.d./t.d.s.) is an effective prophylactic treatment to reduce the frequency and severity of attacks of gout during initiation of definitive uric acid-lowering treatment (see later)

Long-term control of gout and hyperuricaemia

Potential precipitating factors should be sought and addressed, e.g. promotion of weight loss, reduction in/abstinence from alcohol consumption, dietary modification (calorie restriction [to reduce hyperinsulinaemia] is more effective than purine-restricted diets), withdrawal of offending drugs (particularly thiazide diuretics).

Medical therapy should be considered for:

- recurrent acute attacks
- chronic tophaceous gout
- renal involvement
- patients with haematological malignancy/high cell turnover states/inherited defects in purine metabolism.

Treatment should aim to reduce the serum uric acid level below the levels required for crystal resorption (serum uric acid levels < 6 mg/dl [360 µmol/l] – European League against Rheumatism [EULAR] guidance). Effective treatment can cure gout with resolution of attacks and dissolution of tophi.

Treatment options include:

- *Xanthine oxidase inhibitors (XOIs):* these block conversion of hypoxanthine to xanthine, and xanthine to uric acid. Allopurinol and febuxostat are the two most commonly used xanthine oxidase inhibitors.
  - *Allopurinol:* (initially 100 mg/day titrated by 100 mg/month to a maximum of 900 mg/day or until uric acid levels are <360 µmol)). Convention suggests allopurinol should be started 1–2 weeks after an acute attack has settled, as the inititation of treatment may precipitate an acute attack. An NSAID or colchicine (see earlier) should be used as a prophylactic and continued for 3–4 weeks after the hyperuricaemia has resolved. In tumour lysis syndrome it should be commenced in advance of cytotoxic chemotherapy. Allopurinol is generally well tolerated but may cause rashes and rarely a hypersensitivity syndrome.
  - *Febuxostat:* 40–80 mg/day – like allopurinol is conventionally started 1–2 weeks after an acute attack. It is more rapid acting than allopurinol in reducing serum uric acid levels.

NB: it is important to be aware of several potentially serious adverse interactions between xanthine oxidase inhibitors and other drugs that may be co-prescribed, including azathioprine (which is metabolised by xanthine oxidase, thus predisposing to bone marrow toxicity), ciclosporin (risk of nephrotoxicity), ACE-I and diuretics (increased risk of hypersensitivity reaction).

- *Uricosuric agents:*
  - sulfinpyrazone and probenecid both block renal tubular reabsorption of uric acid; benzbromarone is an alternative for use in patients with mild renal impairment.
  - *Rasburicase:* a recombinant urate oxidase, which catalyses the conversion of uric acid to allantoin. It is licensed for the prophylaxis and treatment of

acute hyperuricaemia, before and during initiation of chemotherapy in patients at risk of tumour lysis syndrome.

○ Lesinurad is a selective uric acid reabsorption inhibitor (SURI) that inhibits urate transporter 1 (URAT1), thereby normalizing uric acid excretion. It is yet to be licensed for general use.

Prognosis

Acute gout is self-limiting even without treatment. Recurrences are common and may occur even in the face of successful biochemical control of hyperuricaemia, until the crystals have been resorbed (can take several years in recalcitrant cases).

Pseudogout (calcium pyrophosphate deposition disease; chondrocalcinosis)

Calcium pyrophosphate dihydrate (CPPD) crystals form in articular cartilage and are shed into the joint cavity to provoke an inflammatory response similar to that seen in gout. Calcification of the joint cartilage (chondrocalcinosis) commonly occurs in association with the CPPD crystal deposition. Pseudogout is mainly seen in elderly subjects, with a slight female preponderance, and is often associated with osteoarthritis (possibly due to the hypertrophic response component since it is most closely associated with patients with prominent osteophyte formation in generalized nodal OA [see earlier]). In younger patients predisposing factors to CPPD deposition include:

- previous joint trauma/surgery/intra-articular bleeding
- primary hyperparathyroidism
- hereditary haemochromatosis
- hypophosphatasia
- Wilson's disease.

Clinical presentation

Chondrocalcinosis itself is asymptomatic and is frequently seen on plain radiographs of the knees. Acute attacks of pseudogout present as pain and effusion in larger joint (knees, wrists, elbows and shoulders) frequently triggered by intercurrent infections causing destabilization of the crystal structure. It may thus mimic gout, although the big toe is seldom affected. Symptoms may be less acute in onset than acute gout, less severe in intensity but attacks may be more prolonged (often lasting several weeks). Systemic upset and fever may similarly occur.

Chronic calcium pyrophosphate arthropathy mimics other inflammatory arthritides such as spondyoarthritis and rheumatoid arthritis.

Investigation

- Joint aspiration: for confirmation of diagnosis and exclusion of gout and septic arthritis. Aspirated fluid is turbid and CPPD crystals are found which are rhomboid or oblong with blunt ends and exhibit positive birefringence under polarised light microscopy.
- Routine blood tests: neutrophil leucocytosis is common and the ESR and CRP are markedly raised.
- Radiology: chondrocalcinosis is typically evident in affected joints ± changes of osteoarthritis.
- Screening for predisposing causes: e.g. serum calcium and parathyroid hormone, serum ferritin/transferrin saturation, serum caeruloplasmin (particularly in younger patients).

Management

Acute episodes

In addition to joint aspiration, treatment options include:

- *NSAIDs*
- *corticosteroids:* in patients in whom NSAIDs are contraindicated. Intra-articular injection is appropriate in most cases, but a short course of oral prednisolone is an alternative.

Long-term control

Underlying metabolic disorders should be treated. There is no specific therapy for pseudogout, although long-term low-dose colchicine (see under gout) may be tried in patients with recurrent attacks.

Prognosis

Most acute episodes resolve within 2–3 weeks, although low-grade inflammation may persist, as may the background pain of osteoarthritis.

Septic arthritis

Septic arthritis is a rheumatological/orthopaedic emergency. Although it may occur in patients of any age or gender, it is more common in the very young, the elderly, those with pre-existing abnormal/damaged joint(s), immunocompromised individuals and intravenous drug users.

Bacteria reach the joint through one of three routes:

- direct innoculation, e.g. following a penetrating injury, joint injection or surgery
- haematogenous spread during an episode of bacteraemia
- spread from neighbouring soft tissue (cellulitis) or bone (osteomyelitis) infection.

The most commonly implicated organisms include *Staphylococcus aureus*, β-haemolytic streptococci, Gram-negative bacilli (e.g. *Escherichia coli, Pseudomonas*) and *Neisseria gonorrhoea*.

Clinical presentation

The sudden development of a painful/swollen joint in the context of pre-existing infection or in a patient with otherwise quiescent chronic joint disease should be assumed to be septic arthritis until proven otherwise.

Usually a single joint is affected (most commonly the knee), but several sites may be involved. Septic joints are very painful and are often held immobile to minimise discomfort. Systemic upset with pyrexia ± rigors is common, but occasionally the patient may appear otherwise well.

Gonococcal infection may present with typical monoarthritic septic arthritis but can also present with polyarthralgia and a migratory inflammatory arthritis, associated with a pustular rash and teno-synovitis – clinically apparent genital infection is not always present.

Investigation

- Joint aspiration: joint fluid is turbid and microscopy excludes crystal arthropathy; a Gram stain may confirm the presence of bacteria, although the results of formal culture are required to confirm a bacterial origin and identify the organism.
- Routine blood tests: neutrophil leucocytosis is common and the ESR and CRP are significantly raised.
- Blood cultures: may confirm bacteraemia and identify an organism.
- Radiology: narrowing of the joint space is non-specific but can signify destruction of cartilage. Early radiographic assessment is key to subsequent monitoring.

Management

Following joint aspiration, empiric intravenous antibiotic therapy should be commenced, pending definitive identification of an organism. The initial choice of antibiotics must cover the most likely organisms, *Staphylococcus aureus* and β-haemolytic streptococci. The intravenous route should be continued for 7–14 days depending on local microbiological and rheumatological/orthopaedic advice. Oral antibiotics are normally required for a further 3–4 weeks and sometimes up to 12 weeks.

Repeated joint aspiration ± surgical drainage/lavage may be indicated, particularly during the acute phase of treatment

Prognosis

Early recognition and treatment are critical to preventing joint damage and destruction. Osteomyelitis and septicaemia may complicate cases in which the diagnosis is delayed. Even with best current treatments the mortality from septic arthritis is 10% and it is imperative to consider the diagnosis in any patient with a hot red swollen joint.

Miscellaneous inflammatory rheumatological disorders

Adult-onset Still's disease (AOSD)

Juvenile-onset Still's disease is a form of juvenile idiopathic arthritis (systemic onset JIA) characterized by

- constitutional upset
- fever
- skin rashes
- joint pain (75% of cases) at onset, which may be monoarticular (30%)
- eye changes: chronic iridocyclitis (10%), corneal band opacity and cataracts
- lymphadenopathy, splenomegaly and pericarditis.

The adult form of Still's disease shares some of these clinical features and is a rare acute systemic inflammatory disorder of unknown aetiology, onset is typically between 16 and 35 years of age, with both sexes affected equally. It is characterised by:

- high spiking fever
- evanescent rash
- arthralgia/arthritis
- sore throat
- generalised myalgia
- weight loss

- lymphadenopathy
- splenomegaly
- pleurisy
- pericarditis
- neutrophil leucocytosis
- renal/hepatic abnormalities.

Investigation

In the absence of a specific disease marker, the diagnosis is based on clinical features: the presence of five or more criteria, including at least two major, has a diagnostic sensitivity of >95% and specificity of >90%:

- *major:* spiking fever (≥39 °C for ≥1 week), arthralgia (≥2 weeks), typical rash, leucocytosis (>10 × 10⁹/l, with >80% neutrophilia)
- *minor:* sore throat, lymphadenopathy and/or splenomegaly, liver dysfunction, negative antinuclear antibody and rheumatoid factor screens
- *exclude:* infections, malignancies and other rheumatological disorders.

Marked elevation of serum ferritin is a key finding in most patients and correlates with disease activity. The ESR and CRP are also normally significantly elevated.

Management

Aspirin and NSAIDs may help as first-line therapy, but long-term treatment with corticosteroids is required in the majority of patients.

Conventional DMARDs such as methotrexate can be beneficial. TNF-α inhibitors, anti-IL-1 treatments (e.g anakinra) or anti-IL-6 treatments (e.g tocilizumab) may be required.

Acute rheumatic fever

This acute febrile systemic disorder affects mainly the heart and joints following a streptococcal infection (group A, β-haemolytic) and usually occurs between the ages of 5 and 15 years. The diagnosis is made when there is evidence of previous streptococcal infection plus one major and two minor or two major (Jones) criteria. In the section below, double asterisks denote major criteria, single asterisks minor criteria.

Clinical presentation

Symptoms

The disease usually presents with:

- flitting polyarthropathy**: common in adults

- carditis**: common in children
- arthralgia*: exquisitely tender joints and history of streptococcal infection of the throat or skin 10–20 days previously
- chorea**: Sydenham's chorea; usually in children.

Signs

The dominant features are:

- fever*
- flitting arthropathy of large joints (small joints may be ffected in the elderly)
- erythema nodosum and erythema marginatum** : more common in children
- symmetrical subcutaneous nodules** : over bony prominences and extensor surfaces in children correlating with severe carditis
- myocarditis: tachycardia, cardiomegaly, heart failure
- endocarditis: any valve may be involved and cause transient murmurs. A transient mitral diastolic murmur (Carey Coombs) is the most common. Mitral systolic and aortic murmurs also occur
- percarditis: friction rub or small effusion.

Investigation

- raised or rising antistreptolysin (ASO) or DNAase titre: evidence of preceding group A streptococcal infection
- throat swab: haemolytic streptococci may be isolated
- leucocytosis and hypochromic normocytic anaemia ESR and CRP elevated*
- ECG: may show first-degree heart block* or other rhythm disorder
- chest X-ray: progressive cardiac enlargement

Management

- *Anti-inflammatory therapy:* aspirin or other NSAIDs can be tried.
- *Corticosteroids* may be required, especially if there is evidence of cardiac involvement.
- *Antistreptococcal therapy:* intravenous benzylpenicillin during the acute phase and oral phenoxymethylpenicillin continued in those with cardiac involvement for at least 5 years and preferably until 20 years of age to prevent recurrence. Erythromycin may be used for patients sensitive to penicillin.
- *Neuroleptics:* may help with chorea.

Sarcoidosis

Sarcoidosis (or sarcoid) is considered in more detail under the respiratory section. However, in approximately 10% of cases it can present with musculoskeletal symptoms.

Clinical presentation

Acute sarcoid (Lofgren's syndrome)

This characteristically presents with acute inflammatory pain, swelling and stiffness of the ankles, erythema nodosum (most characteristically overlying the anterior tibial region) and bilateral hilar lymphadenopathy. Other medium/large joints can be involved (wrists, elbows, shoulders and knees) and patients frequently develop enthesitis, similar to patient with spondyloarthritis (see earlier). The syndrome tends to be self-resolving.

Chronic sarcoid arthritis

This characteristically presents with a more polyarticular distribution of arthritis (involving small, medium and large joints) with associated enthesitis and tendonitis, which can make it difficult to differentiate from spondyloarthritis, on solely clinical grounds.

Investigation

- Radiology – chest imaging (see under respiratory)
- Serum ACE – characteristically elevated
- ESR/CRP – elevated
- RhF and anti-CCP – negative

Management

- NSAIDs
- Steroids (initially at moderate/high doses and tapering according to symptoms) are frequently required in both acute and chronic sarcoidosis
- DMARDs – methotrexate, azathioprine, mycophenolate and leflunomide are all used as steroid-sparing treatments

Lyme disease

Lyme Disease (Lyme borreliosis) is an infectious disease caused by the spirochete *Borrelia burgdorferi* and is transmitted to humans by tick bites (most commonly from the Ixodes tick). It was first described in Lyme, Connecticut, USA.

Clinical presentation

The infection has three phases:

Early local infection/Stage 1

- Erythema chronicum migrans (EM) is seen (between a few days and 1 month post initial tick bite)
- Fever/general malaise
- Myalgic pain

Early disseminated Lyme disease/Stage 2

- General malaise/fevers
- Lymphadenopathy
- Cutaneous features
  - multiple EM lesions
  - Borrelia lymphocytoma
- Acute neurolopsychiatric presentations (neuroborreliosis)
  - meningitis
  - encephalitis
  - depression
  - mononeuritis
- Cardiac
  - AV block
  - dysrhythmias
- Arthritis
  - intermittent migratory mono or oligoarticular inflammatory arthritis (50%)
  - enthesitis, tendonitis and bursitis

Management of the early disseminated disease is with oral or IV antibiotics (often for several months).

Chronic/late Lyme disease/Stage 3

Characteristically patients do not give a history of EM but present with the late features months or years after the initial infection

- Inflammatory arthritis
  - mono or oligoarticular inflammatory arthritis (most commonly the knee)
- Cutaneous features
  - acrodermatitis chronica atrophicans
- Chronic neurological presentations
  - encephalopathy/encephalomyelitis
  - peripheral neuropathy

Investigation

ESR/CRP elevated

RhF and anti-CCP – negative

ANA – negative

Borrelia serology – usually a screening ELISA and subsequent Western immunoblotting

- serology generally positive from 2–4 weeks post EM
- serology remains positive for many years

Management

Initial management of all stages of Lyme disease is with oral antibiotics (usually doxycycline 100 mg b.d. or amoxicillin 500 mg t.d.s. for 28 days). Those with later stages of Lyme disease, with neuroborreliosis or with disease that has not responded may benefit from more prolonged courses of antibiotic treatment or to treatments such as IV ceftriaxone. Patients at all stages respond to antibiotic treatment.

Symptomatic management of musculoskeletal symptoms with NSAIDs.

Antibiotic-resistant chronic Lyme arthritis has been managed successfully with local steroid injections, arthroscopic synovectomy and hydroxy-chloroquine.

Viral-associated arthritis

A transient polyarticular peripheral small joint inflammatory arthritis characterized by early morning stiffness and swelling of the joints is recognized following most viral infections (including HIV, viral hepatitis, echovirus, enterovirus, parvovirus B19 and EBV). The symptoms characteristically develop during the initial viral infection but may not resolve for several weeks (or occasionally months) after the viral infection has resolved. Viral-associated arthritis is an important differential diagnosis for patients with new-onset rheumatoid arthritis.

Miscellaneous non-inflammatory rheumatological disorders

Fibromyalgia syndrome (FMS)

Fibromyalgia/fibromyalgia syndrome (FMS) is a common condition affecting 1–5% of the population (female > male) characterized by chronic widespread non-inflammatory pain (fibromyalgia), generalized tiredness/fatigue and poor/unrefreshing sleep. Current aetiological models suggest interactions of physical (particularly inadequate stage 3/stage 4 sleep patterns), neurobiological (changes in the dopaminergic and serotonergic systems) and psychological factors resulting in disturbance of central pain processing. This disturbed central pain processing becomes fixed over time resulting in chronic diffuse pain.

Clinical presentation

The core clinical features of the fibromyalgia syndrome are:

- chronic widespread musculoskeletal pain – see ACR criteria later
- tiredness/fatigue
- poor/unrefreshing sleep pattern.

Multiple additional symptoms are often found, in addition to the core symptoms, on systems review:

- Neurological
  - headaches
  - dizziness
  - poor memory/reduced concentration
  - paraesthesia
  - numbness
  - restless legs
- Psychiatric
  - anxiety
  - tearfulness
  - irritability
  - mood disturbance
- Gastroenterological
  - nausea
  - abdominal pain
  - irritable bowel symptoms
- Cardiovascular/respiratory
  - chest wall pain
  - shortness of breath
- Urogenital
  - urgency of urination/nocturia
  - gynaecological symptoms

ACR 1990 Classification Criteria for Fibromyalgia
Fibromyalgia is defined as the presence of chronic pain (i.e., pain for more than 3 months) in multiple parts of the body, i.e.,

- pain in the axial skeleton (cervical spine or anterior chest or thoracic spine or lumbar spine), and
- pain in the right and left sides of the body, and
- pain above and below the waist, and
- pain on palpation of at least 11 of 18 defined tender points (see Fig. 18.7)

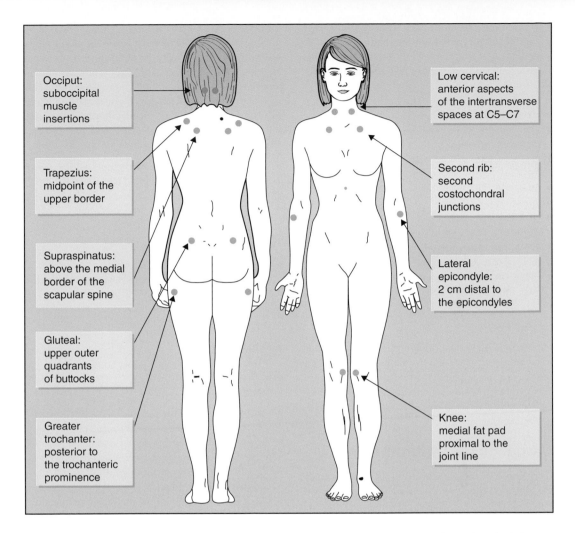

Figure 18.7 Fibromyalgia Tender Points. General locations of the 18 tender points that make up the criteria for identifying fibromyalgia.

Investigation

The lack of a specific diagnostic test means that fibromyalgia is often a diagnosis of exclusion, based on the clinical features described earlier. However, it is reasonable to arrange a simple panel of tests to exclude other causes including: full blood count, ESR, CRP, renal and liver biochemistry, creatine kinase, thyroid function tests, vitamin D levels, antinuclear antibodies, myeloma screen (in those >50 years of age) and a plain chest X-ray (especially in smokers).

NB: Beware the so-called 'red flag' markers for patients presenting with widespread pain, i.e. age >50 years, recent onset, associated with weight loss or fever, past history of malignancy or immunosuppressive therapy, areas of focal bony pain, abnormal physical signs other than tenderness, abnormalities in screening investigations – if any of these are present, then a diagnosis of fibromyalgia should not be made and other causes pursued.

Management

Non-pharmacological therapies

- Patient education – patient understanding of FMS and self-motivated engagement with individualized treatment approaches is key to management

- Programmes to improve physical fitness with aerobic endurance training (hydrotherapy and swimming are often helpful) – sometimes review with a physiotherapist can be beneficial
- Cognitive behavioural therapy
- Mindfulness
- Sleep hygiene approaches
- Involvement of the liaison psychiatry and pain management teams.

Pharmacological therapies

- Analgesics (paracetamol, codeine and moderate opiates [e.g. tramadol])
- Low-dose tricyclic antidepressants (e.g amitryptilline [25–50 mg/day]) – improve sleep and improve pain
- Serotonin norepinephrine reuptake inhibitors (SNRIs) (e.g. duloxetine 60–120 mg/day)
- Gabapentinoids (e.g. gabapentin or pregabalin) – improve sleep and improve pain.

Prognosis

Most patients experience ongoing long-term fluctuating symptoms but the severity of these symptoms and the impact on quality of life can be significantly improved with the management strategies mentioned earlier. There is no increased mortality associated with fibromyalgia.

Carpal tunnel syndrome

Entrapment of the median nerve as it passes under the flexor retinaculum causes carpal tunnel syndrome. Although it may occur spontaneously, recognised associations include pregnancy, inflammatory arthritis of the wrist, osteoarthritis of the wrist, previous wrist trauma/fracture, hypothyroidism, acromegaly and amyloidosis. Bilateral disease is relatively common, especially in the presence of an underlying systemic disorder, although symptoms are usually worse on one side than the other.

Clinical presentation

- Sensory disturbance (pain and paraesthesia) affecting the radial three-and-a-half digits, worse at night. Some patients report symptoms in the whole hand and extending up the forearm.
- Impaired function with clumsiness may be a feature.
- Symptoms may be relieved by hanging the arm out of bed at night or shaking the hand.

Physical examination can be normal, especially if symptoms are intermittent. When present, sensory disturbance is evident over the thumb, index and middle fingers, while the ring finger shows a loss of sensation on its radial border with preservation on the ulnar aspect; sensation in the little finger is also normal. In long-standing cases, there may be wasting and weakness of the muscles of the thenar eminence and motor involvement suggests the need for more aggressive intervention. Two additional clinical tests that are often employed to reproduce the patient's symptoms are:

- Tinel's test: percussion over the median nerve as it passes under the flexor retinaculum
- Phalen's test: in which the wrist is maintained in a fixed flexion position.

Investigation

- Nerve conduction studies: confirm compression of the median nerve at the wrist and can indicate the severity of the changes
- Perform investigation of underlying causes as indicated clinically.

Management

Treatment is dictated by the severity of the condition but may involve:

- splinting of the wrists at night (useful for mild symptoms)
- local injection of corticosteroids (can resolve problems of a mild to moderate severity [with or without objective neurological findings] but less effective with motor involvement)
- surgical decompression of the flexor retinaculum (likely to be required in patients in whom a local injection has failed or in whom there is evidence of motor involvement on examination).

Prognosis

Complete resolution of symptoms often occurs spontaneously in patients without objective neurological findings on examination. Resolution of symptoms is still achievable with injection treatment or surgical decompression, except in the most long-standing cases when permanent nerve damage has occurred.

Shoulder pain
Frozen shoulder

This is a relatively common and potentially disabling condition affecting 1–2% of the middle-aged and elderly population. It is of unknown aetiology but may reflect an abnormal local pain response. It results in progressive restriction of capsular movements at the glenohumeral joint typically unilaterally. It is seen more commonly in patients with type II diabetes and any patient with bilateral frozen shoulder should be screened for this.

Clinical presentation

Frozen shoulder is characterized by three phases

1. 'Freezing' phase – associated with significant pain around the anterior shoulder and the upper outer aspect of the arm that can be clinically indistinguishable from rotator cuff problems. This phase generally lasts 3–6 months.
2. 'Frozen' phase – the patient develops associated restriction of glenohumeral movements but the pain gradually resolves. Examination reveals a globally restrictive range of movements in all planes. This phase lasts up to 12 months.
3. 'Thawing' phase – there is progressive resolution of the restriction, although patients are often left with some mild/non-significant restriction of internal rotation. This phase lasts up to 2 years.

Management

Frozen shoulder spontaneously improves with time and there is no evidence that any treatment alters the time-course of this improvement. Analgesia and local nerve blocks can improve the pain during the painful phases. Regular shoulder exercises can help to restore movement during the resolution phase

Rotator cuff tendonopathy

Clinical presentation

Repetitive or unaccustomed movements of the shoulder may result in problems with one or more of the rotator cuff muscle tendons, most commonly the supraspinatus tendon, which is vulnerable due to its course through the subacromial space. The pain is characteristically felt over the upper outer aspect of the arm, is worse during abduction and is often accompanied by pain when lying on the affected side at night. Examination reveals a painful arc of abduction and pain on isolation of supraspinatus (with associated weakness when there is an associated tear).

Investigation

- Plain radiology may show tendon calcification.
- Ultrasound or MRI scanning may demonstrate oedema or tears within the tendon.

Management

- Pharmacological treatments include analgesics and NSAIDs.
- Physiotherapy for the rotator cuff is the key management strategy and frequently resolves the problem.
- Local injection of corticosteroids into the subacromial space can give short-term pain relief.
- Surgery is used in recalcitrant cases – arthroscopic subacromial decompression.

Mechanical spinal pain

Mechanical spinal pain (lumbar or cervical spine) is extremely common (affecting 80% of the population at some time in their lives). Mechanical spinal pain may be secondary to muscular pain, intervertebral disc prolapse (with or without osteoarthritic reactive changes in the adjacent vertebrae) or facet joint osteoarthritis. It may or may not be associated with peripheral radicular neuropathic pain (where a prolapsed intervertebral disc is the cause of the problem and is impinging on an exiting nerve root).

Intervertebral disc prolapse occurs following dehydration of the intervertebral disc – there is bulging of the gelatinous central nucleus pulposus through the annulus fibrosus of the intervertebral disc. Imaging evidence of intervertebral disc changes (in both the cervical and lumbar spine) is, like mechanical spinal pain, an extremely common finding. However, the correlation between imaging appearances and symptoms is limited (much as is the case in radiographic changes of osteoarthritis [see earlier]). Nonetheless it is likely that a significant proportion of self-resolving mechanical spinal pain is secondary to local intervertebral disc effects. If an intervertebral disc protrudes in a postero-lateral direction, it may lead to impingement of the nerve roots as they emerge from the spinal cord (e.g. sciatica). Less commonly, direct posterior protrusion of a large disc can threaten the cord itself (e.g. lumbar disc protrusion can result in spinal stenosis and the cauda equina syndrome) – see page 220, Chapter 15.

Clinical presentation

Mechanical lumbar spinal pain is characteristically felt across the lumbar spinal region radiating into the buttock area or down the top of the legs. Mechanical cervical spinal pain is generally felt across the neck and scapula regions into the tops of the arms. The symptoms are generally worse with activity/exercise, worse in particular positions and worse towards the end of the day. Patients do not generally describe symptoms of early morning stiffness; this would suggest inflammatory spinal problems (see spondyloarthritis section). Mechanical spinal pain may come on suddenly or gradually and not infrequently a precipitating episode is readily identified by the patient (e.g. lifting a heavy object). If there is intervertebral disc-related nerve impingement it may be associated with peripheral radicular neuropathic pain with or without numbness or weakness.

Examination generally reveals localised tenderness (particularly in the paraspinal musculature), usually with restricted movements of the lumbar or cervical spine. Smaller discs may also be associated with normal peripheral neurological assessments but with progressively increasing postero-lateral disc protrusion there may be evidence of either dermatomal sensory disturbance or myotomal motor effects (+/- reduction in the relevant deep tendon reflexes).

Investigation

Investigation should only be considered if symptoms persist or if there are features of inflammatory spinal pain or red flag symptoms. MRI scanning of the spine is the preferred modality for demonstrating disc protrusion and nerve root/spinal cord impingement. MRI (or other imaging) is only indicated where there is a likelihood of surgical intervention since it otherwise will not alter the management strategy.

Management

Patients should be advised that in the vast majority of cases their symptoms will self-resolve over a few weeks/months (whether or not there are associated neurological symptoms/signs). Patients should be encouraged to continue with normal activities.

- Simple analgesia (+/- low-dose diazepam if significant local muscle spasm acutely)
- Weight reduction and smoking cessation
- Regular aerobic exercise (group exercise is suggested for a specific flare of back pain +/- sciatica) and maintenance of daily activities
- Specific pelvic stabilizing exercises (e.g. Pilates for lumbar spinal pain)
- If radicular neuropathic pain low-dose tricyclic antidepressants and gabapentinoids (e.g. gabapentin or pregabalin) can be helpful adjuncts

- Local/epidural injection of corticosteroids/local anaesthetic may give short-term symptom relief of acute severe radicular neuropathic pain
- Radiofrequency denervation can be considered in patients with severe recalcitrant low back pain
- Advice on posture and lifting techniques, avoidance of bending, adjustments to work/leisure activities, may be considered
- There is some evidence for short-term benefit from manual therapy/manipulation techniques (e.g. osteopathy and chiropractic treatments)
- Psychological therapy – CBT can be useful but needs to be part of a treatment package
- Surgical decompression – consider in patients with objective neurological signs and symptoms (particularly motor weakness) failing to resolve with conservative approaches.

NB: Cauda equine syndrome (page 220, Chapter 15) is a surgical emergency and should be aggressively investigated and treated.

Useful reference on mechanical spinal pain: 'Low back pain and sciatica in over 16s: assessment and management' – NICE Guideline 59 [NG59], November 2016.

Vertebral crush fracture

This is most commonly seen in postmenopausal/elderly females in the context of osteoporosis of the thoracic spine. Sudden vertebral collapse results in abrupt onset of severe pain at the level of the fracture. Pain characteristically lasts for 6–8 weeks before gradually resolving. The subsequent biomechanical changes in the spine can result in ongoing mechanical back pain or further osteoporotic vertebral fractures at other levels.

Plain radiographs confirm the extent of vertebral involvement. Further investigation is geared towards excluding other underlying conditions (e.g. malignant infiltration), screening for osteoporosis and identifying potentially reversible causes of the latter. Achieving adequate pain control can be challenging and may require opioid analgesia. Osteoporosis is treated along conventional lines and any patient with a single vertebral fracture should be considered for a course of bisphosphonate treatment to prevent further fractures. If there are neurological symptoms/signs, then MRI scanning should be undertaken urgently (osteoporotic fractures are not generally associated with neurological impingement).

19

Dermatology

Skin disorders are common and a frequent mode of presentation to general practitioners. They are often associated with not only physical, but also significant psychological effects due to their visibility. In some instances, they may be indicative of underlying systemic disease.

Psoriasis

Psoriasis is a relatively common disorder affecting 1–2% of the population. Classically it presents with red, raised, scaly patches or plaques, which reflect increased keratinocyte proliferation within the epidermis, associated with an inflammatory cell infiltrate (including polymorph microabscesses). There is also increased vascularity within the upper dermis.

The aetiology of psoriasis is multifactorial. Although there is clearly a genetic component, with younger patients often reporting a positive family history, patterns of inheritance vary and several genes may be involved in affected individuals and families. In addition, it remains unclear why some areas of skin are affected, but others remain normal in the presence of an underlying genetic predisposition. Triggers that can be associated with the development of/flare-up/persistence of psoriasis in susceptible individuals include infections and trauma, and possibly stress.

Clinical presentation

Several different patterns of psoriasis are recognised, some of which are common, while others are only rarely seen. The key clinical features of each subtype are shown in Table 19.1 and Figs. 19.1–19.4.

Psoriatic arthropathy

Arthropathy occurs in 5–10% of patients with psoriasis and may take one of several forms:

- predominant distal interphalangeal joint involvement
- symmetric polyarthritis (seronegative rheumatoid-like changes)
- asymmetric oligo/pauciarticular arthritis
- spondylitis (± sacro-ileitis) with stiffness in the back/neck; HLA B27 positive
- arthritis mutilans, a severe deforming destructive arthritis.

Nail changes are common in patients with psoriatic arthropathy, but not all cases are associated with skin disease.

Treatment

Topical agents

- *Emollients* help to control scaling.
- *Salicylic acid* reduces hyperkeratotic, scaling lesions; often used in combination with coal tar, dithranol or topical corticosteroids.
- *(Coal) tar* is effective but unpleasant to use; typically reserved for scalp involvement; sometimes used in combination with ultraviolet (UV) radiation therapy (see later).
- *Dithranol* is effective for chronic plaque psoriasis; applied directly to lesions (may be covered with a dressing) and left for up to an hour (occasionally longer, but only under supervision); dithranol is irritant (start with 0.1% and gradually increase as required/tolerated) and stains skin, hair and bedding/clothes brown; avoid use on the

Clinical Medicine Lecture Notes, Eighth Edition. John R. Bradley, Mark Gurnell, and Diana F. Wood.
© 2019 John Wiley & Sons Ltd. Published 2019 by John Wiley & Sons Ltd.

Table 19.1 Clinical features and specific treatments for different types of psoriasis

Type	Clinical features	Specific treatment(s)
Classical plaque psoriasis (Fig. 19.1)	• Single or multiple red plaques, ranging from a few millimetres to several centimetres in diameter • Scaly surface – gentle scraping yields a silvery appearance; more vigorous rubbing may result in focal haemorrhage (Auspitz sign) • Plaques most commonly develop on extensor surfaces – elbows, knees – but may affect any part of the body – typically in a symmetrical manner • Most plaques are chronic and stable, although some will evolve/coalesce slowly over time, while others may disappear. New lesions may develop at sites of trauma (Köbner phenomenon) • The scalp and nails are also commonly involved (see below)	• First-choice options include vitamin D analogues, dithranol, topical corticosteroids (± tar or salicylic acid) • UV radiation therapy may be helpful • For more severe cases consider PUVA, cytotoxics, retinoids or biological agents
Scalp psoriasis (Fig. 19.2)	• Commonly coexists with classical plaque psoriasis, but may occur in isolation • Varies from one or two isolated plaques to a thick scaly sheet covering the whole scalp	• Tar shampoos/gels may be effective (± salicylic acid) • Topical corticosteroids (± salicylic acid) can also be used
Nail psoriasis (Fig. 19.3)	• Pitting – typically large/irregular • Onycholysis – separation of the nail plate from the nail bed; often begins as a small area of red/brown discolouration, but may spread to involve the whole nail. Subungual hyperkeratosis develops beneath the nail plate	• Often difficult to treat with topical agents; however, use of systemic agents is seldom justified
Guttate psoriasis (Fig. 19.4)	• Typically presents suddenly with a 'shower' of small round plaques, often on the trunk • May develop after an infective episode (especially streptococcal sore throat) • More likely to be itchy than other forms of psoriasis • Lesions may regress rapidly even without treatment	• First-choice therapy is UV radiation (± tar, emollients) • Topical vitamin D analogues and corticosteroid therapy (often in combination) may be effective
Flexural psoriasis	• May accompany plaque, scalp or nail psoriasis or occur in isolation • Affects groin, axillae, natal cleft, submammary folds • Maceration of the skin can result in marked redness and loss of the typical scaly appearance • Often itchy	• Difficult to treat: tar-based therapies and topical corticosteroids may help, but long-term use can lead to skin atrophy/striae • Low-strength dithranol or vitamin D analogues can be tried but often cause local stinging/irritation
Brittle or unstable psoriasis	• Thinner scales • May develop in a patient with previously stable plaque psoriasis • Rapid generalisation/coalescence of lesions leads to erythroderma or acute pustular psoriasis (see below) • Episodes may be triggered by use of potent topical or systemic corticosteroid therapy	• Requires careful management under expert supervision • Emollients may be tried, but PUVA or systemic therapy (e.g. methotrexate or retinoids) is often required

(Continued)

Table 19.1 *(Continued)*

Type	Clinical features	Specific treatment(s)
Erythrodermic psoriasis	• Occurs when plaques merge to involve most or all the skin • May develop rapidly and occasionally arises de novo	• Requires urgent dermatological review; may become life-threatening if treatment is delayed • Methotrexate or ciclosporin are effective • Biological agents are finding increasing use
Acute pustular psoriasis	• Characterised by widespread erythema with sterile pustules, which may coalesce • Associated with systemic upset, including fever • Secondary bacterial infections may be life-threatening if not treated promptly	• As for erythrodermic psoriasis
Chronic palmoplantar pustulosis	• Erythematous patches with multiple pustules, which dry to form circumscribed brown areas that eventually peel off • May affect only a small area of one hand or foot or involve the entire surface of both palms and soles • Associated with smoking	• Difficult to treat; topical measures are usually ineffective • PUVA or oral retinoid therapy may be tried, but relapses are common

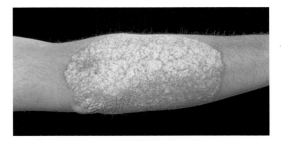

Figure 19.1 Psoriatic plaque on the elbow.

face or in flexures; may be combined with tar and UV radiation.

• *Topical corticosteroids* may suppress (although not eradicate) lesions (e.g. scalp, flexures), but should be used with care (risk of precipitating brittle or erythrodermic psoriasis) (Table 19.1).

• *Vitamin D analogues (e.g. calcipotriol, tacalcitol) and activated vitamin D (e.g. calcitriol)* are useful in mild to moderate psoriasis; serum calcium levels must be monitored in those using larger doses.

• *Tazarotene* is a retinoid; irritant, especially if applied to normal skin.

Phototherapy

• *UVB radiation* is effective in the treatment of chronic stable psoriasis and guttate psoriasis, especially

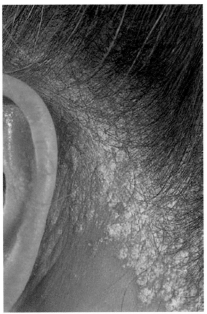

Figure 19.2 Scalp psoriasis.

when topical agents have proved ineffective; must be used with care due to risk of sunburn; typically given as short courses, e.g. 2–3 times per week until clearance is achieved; combination with coal tar, dithranol or vitamin D analogues increases efficacy.

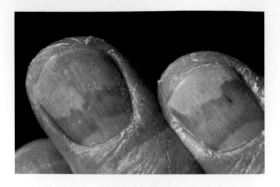

Figure 19.3 Psoriatic onycholysis.

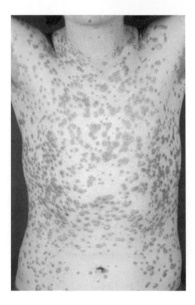

Figure 19.4 Guttate psoriasis.

- *Photochemotherapy (psoralens and ultraviolet A phototherapy [PUVA])*. Psoralens (given either by mouth or topically) enhance the effect of UV radiation; treatment is typically given twice weekly, and protective glasses are required to avoid ocular damage. Higher cumulative doses exaggerate skin ageing and are associated with an increased risk of keratoses and neoplastic lesions (especially squamous carcinoma).

Systemic therapy

- *Methotrexate*. Once-weekly dosing, together with folic acid; effective in severe psoriasis refractory to topical therapy; patients should be advised of potential adverse effects including myelosuppression

(sore throat, mouth ulceration, easy bruising), hepatotoxicity (nausea/vomiting, abdominal pain, dark urine), respiratory effects (shortness of breath), inhibition of spermatogenesis and teratogenicity (effective contraceptive measures must be in place before treatment is commenced).
- *Retinoids (e.g. acitretin)* are reserved for severe, resistant psoriasis. Side effects include dryness and cracking of skin and lips, epistaxis, transient hair loss, myalgia, hepatotoxicity, hyperlipidaemia and teratogenicity (effective contraceptive measures must be in place before treatment is commenced).
- *Ciclosporin (cyclosporin)* is effective even in very severe psoriasis; nephrotoxic and requires close monitoring of renal function, especially in the early stages of treatment; avoid concomitant UVB/PUVA therapy.
- *Biological agents*. Anti-TNF-α therapies (e.g. etanercept, adalimumab, infliximab) may be used in very severe plaque psoriasis that has failed to respond to systemic treatments and to photo(chemo)therapy, or in cases where standard treatments are not tolerated/contraindicated. Ustekinumab (targeting interleukins 12 and 23) and secukinumab (targeting IL-17A) are also of benefit.
- *Others*. Systemic corticosteroids are only rarely indicated and must be given under expert supervision. Mycophenylate mofetil and fumaric acid esters are rarely used.

Table 19.1 shows preferred treatment options for each subtype of psoriasis. Psoriatic arthropathy often responds to simple anti-inflammatory agents. In more severe cases, methotrexate or biological agents can be tried.

Eczema/dermatitis

Although the term 'dermatitis' is sometimes used specifically to describe skin inflammation caused by an exogenous agent, it is in fact synonymous with the term 'eczema' (Greek, meaning 'boiling over'). Eczema is common, affecting approximately 10% of the population at some stage during life.

Clinical presentation

In acute eczema the skin is erythematous and oedematous, with papules/vesicles and weeping (i.e. 'boiling over'). In chronic eczema, oedema is absent and the epidermis becomes thickened/hyperplastic, with exaggeration of the skin markings (so-called lichenification) (Fig. 19.6). Itching may be the dominant symptom. Secondary infection is common: bacterial (commonly staphylococcal) or viral (herpes simplex). Healed lesions do not scar, but may pigment.

Secondary spread to involve other areas is a well-recognised phenomenon of acute eczema and may even involve areas that have not been directly exposed to a particular allergen in cases of contact dermatitis. Rarely, the whole of the body may be affected by a generalised exfoliative dermatitis.

Several different patterns of eczema are recognised; the key clinical features of each subtype are shown in Table 19.2 and Figs. 19.5–19.7.

Treatment

Wherever possible, the local irritant or sensitiser should be removed. Many commercial soaps contain such irritants and washing with water ± soap substitutes is advised. If the lesion is weeping, local soaks, e.g. potassium permanganate (antiseptic and astringent) may aid healing; if dry, emollients should be applied liberally and regularly to the affected areas – bath/shower oils may further help. Continued emollient use is required even when the acute episode has subsided. Sedative antihistamines by mouth may relieve pruritus and allow sleep. Bandages (including those containing zinc oxide and ichthammol) may be applied over topical corticosteroids (see later) or emollients to treat eczema of the limbs. Systemic antibiotics are required for secondary bacterial infections and antiviral therapy for cases complicated by herpes simplex infection. Antifungal therapy may be useful in cases of seborrhoeic dermatitis where the yeast *Malassezia* is implicated.

Topical corticosteroids remain the mainstay of treatment for most patients with eczema. The potency of the corticosteroid should be appropriate for the site and severity of the condition, e.g. weaker preparations are preferred for the face and on flexures, while more potent preparations may be required on the limbs/trunk, especially if there is associated lichenification.

In more severe/refractory cases immunomodulatory agents can be tried, including topical tacrolimus or pimecrolimus and oral ciclosporin. The oral retinoid alitretinoin is also licensed for the treatment of severe chronic hand eczema refractory to potent topical corticosteroids (cautions and adverse effects are similar to those of other retinoid preparations; pregnancy must be excluded and effective contraception practised).

Table 19.2 shows preferred treatment options for each subtype of eczema.

Acne vulgaris

Acne vulgaris is a disease chiefly of puberty (but onset can occur up to 40 years of age, and even at later ages if there is an underlying endocrine disorder, e.g. Cushing syndrome) in which androgens (typically in normal amounts) promote increased sebaceous gland activity, leading to greasy skin. Hyperkeratosis results in plugging of hair follicles, and subsequent secondary infection with the obligate anaerobe *Propionibacterium acnes* leads to release of chemicals into the surrounding dermis, which provoke an intense inflammatory response.

Clinical presentation

Several different lesions may be seen:

- Comedones – closed ('whitehead') or open ('blackhead')
- Papules and pustules – spots or pustules on a red base; may recur repeatedly in the same locations
- Nodules and cysts – seen in more severe cases, as inflammation extends deeper; if these are numerous they are referred to as 'acne conglobata'; very rarely nodulocystic acne is associated with fever, malaise and systemic upset ('acne fulminans')
- Scars – these may be pitting and disfiguring, and in extreme cases associated with keloid formation.

Investigation

In the majority of patients investigation is not required, but disorders associated with hyperandrogenism should be considered in female subjects with later onset disease or in the presence of virilising features (e.g. Cushing syndrome, androgen-secreting tumours).

Treatment

Options include:

- over-the-counter preparations – effective in milder cases and work mainly as astringents/keratolytics, drying the skin and unblocking hair follicles
- topical benzoyl peroxide – astringent, keratolytic and delivers oxygen locally, reducing bacterial proliferation without inducing resistance; may cause local skin irritation

Table 19.2 Causes, clinical features and specific treatments for different types of eczema (dermatitis)

Type	Subtype	Epidemiology/ aetiopathogenesis	Clinical features/ investigation	Specific treatment(s)
Exogenous eczema	*Primary irritant dermatitis* (Fig. 19.5)	• Direct exposure of the skin to water and soaps/detergents or other solvents (e.g. petroleum products), removes the protective lipid layer and provokes an inflammatory response from keratinocytes	• Most commonly affects the hands, which are often repeatedly immersed in the irritant • Characterised by dryness and painful fissures	• Remove from contact with irritant or protect skin (e.g. use of gloves) • Liberal use of emollients

	Allergic contact dermatitis	• Delayed (type IV) hypersensitivity reaction to an external antigen
		• Examples include:
		  – nickel (in jewellery and metal clips/studs in clothing)
		  – perfumes, hair dyes
		  – latex, rubber chemicals, epoxy resin
		  – chromate (used in industrial processes)
		  – plants (e.g. hogweed)
		  – medicaments (e.g. antibiotics, antihistamines, topical corticosteroids, vehicle/preservatives)
		  – fungal, viral, parasitic infections
			• A detailed history should be taken including occupation (past and present), hobbies, use of perfumes/skin creams and medications
			• Distribution/pattern may suggest a specific allergen (e.g. at sites of earrings, metal clips on underwear, on scalp)
			• Patch testing may be required with a battery of standard allergens and/or specific suspected allergens (e.g. occupational)
				• Avoidance of the offending allergen is crucial to successful prevention/treatment
				• Emollients and topical corticosteroids may be used to settle a patch of eczema

Endogenous eczema	*Atopic eczema* (Fig. 19.6)	• Typically presents in infancy or early childhood; may resolve in later childhood/adulthood • Genetic predisposition coupled with environmental trigger(s) • Altered immune function with antigen responses diverted down the Th2 pathway, leading to enhanced IgE production	• Positive family history in many cases • Associated features include tendency to asthma and rhinitis/conjunctivitis • Eczema may be generalised in early stages but usually settles into a pattern involving flexural surfaces (e.g. wrists, antecubital and popliteal fossae, dorsal surfaces of feet)	• Provision of information/explanatory leaflets • Reduce exposure to soap and water • Liberal use of emollients (soap substitutes, bath oils, emollient creams)

Condition	Aetiology/pathogenesis	Clinical features	Treatment
(continued)	• Associated with disordered epidermal barrier function with reduced filaggrin expression in some patients • Colonisation with exotoxin-producing staphylococci may also contribute to pathogenesis	• Skin is dry and itchy • Repeated scratching leads to skin thickening (= lichenification) • Clinical course is often characterised by episodic exacerbations • May be complicated by secondary bacterial (folliculitis, impetigo) or viral (herpes simplex) infections, which can be life-threatening • Serum IgE levels are often raised	• Topical corticosteroids: aim to use the lowest strength preparation that is sufficient to control the condition; combination preparations including an antibacterial may be useful in those prone to secondary bacterial infection • Systemic antibacterial and/or antiviral therapy when obvious secondary infection is present • Topical tacrolimus or pimecrolimus may help in more refractory cases, while oral ciclosporin can be used for severe eczema. Short courses of systemic corticosteroids may also be helpful in poorly controlled eczema, but prolonged/repeated courses should be avoided • Wet wraps and antihistamines help with itchiness
• *Seborrhoeic dermatitis* (Fig. 19.7)	• Affects 1–2% of the population; more common in fairer-skinned individuals • Onset in young adulthood or middle age • Postulated to be a response to an antigen of the yeast *Malassezia* • More common and severe in the presence of HIV/AIDS	• Three patterns of involvement: – scalp, face (nasolabial folds, forehead, eyebrows) – sternum, upper back – flexures (axillae, groin, submammary areas) • Chronic condition requiring long-term treatment	• Topical antifungal therapy ± topical hydrocortisone cream • Ketoconazole-containing shampoo for scalp involvement • Treatment of secondary bacterial infection • Very occasionally systemic corticosteroids are required for widespread involvement
• *Venous (varicose) eczema*		• Typically seen in the context of chronic venous hypertension	• Affects lower legs/gaiter area; initially may be unilateral, but often spreads to involve other leg, upper limbs and even the trunk • Wet or weeping patches	• Topical corticosteroids • Compression therapy (check ankle-brachial pressure index first to exclude vascular insufficiency)

(Continued)

Table 19.2 (*Continued*)

Type	Subtype	Epidemiology/ aetiopathogenesis	Clinical features/ investigation	Specific treatment(s)
	• *Discoid eczema*		• Well-demarcated patches of eczema on the limbs and trunk • Tends to wax and wane	• Exclude ringworm • Topical corticosteroids control the condition
	• *Hand and foot eczema*	• In the absence of atopy, and with negative patch testing/mycology, a diagnosis of pompholyx (idiopathic vesicular eczema of the palms and soles) should be considered	• Typically symmetrical • Bullae formation may occur in pompholyx	• Topical corticosteroids • Alitretinoin reserved for severe/refractory hyperkeratotic hand eczema • Treatment of secondary bacterial infection • Potassium permanganate soaks may also help in pompholyx
	• *Asteatotic eczema*	• A consequence of normal ageing, with reduced lipid content in the stratum corneum resulting in reduced water retention • Exacerbated by dry/warm environments and excessive bathing	• 'Crazy-paving' pattern as the skin cracks • Common on the lower limbs (shins), but may also affect arms and trunk • Itchy	• Minimise triggers • Emollients • Mild topical corticosteroids occasionally required

AIDS, acquired immune deficiency syndrome; HIV, human immunodeficiency virus; IgE, immunoglobulin subtype E; Th2, T-helper 2 cell.

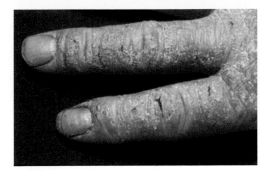

Figure 19.5 Hand dermatitis in a machine-tool operator.

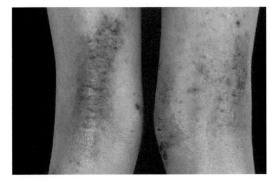

Figure 19.6 Flexural involvement in atopic eczema.

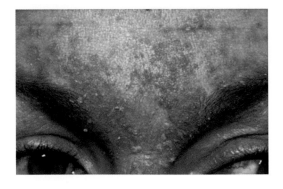

Figure 19.7 Seborrhoeic dermatitis.

- topical antibiotics – e.g. tetracyclines, erythromycin, clindamycin; effective in the early stages of treatment, but resistance often develops
- topical retinoids – e.g. isotretinoin, adapalene; reduce sebum production and follicular plugging, and attenuate inflammation
- oral antibiotics – e.g. tetracyclines, erythromycin; both antibacterial and anti-inflammatory

- oral isotretinoin – shrinks sebaceous glands, dramatically reducing sebum production; side effects are common, including facial erythema, dry skin and lips, nose bleeds, myalgia, hyperlipidaemia and abnormal liver function tests. It is teratogenic: pregnancy must be excluded and reliable contraception established before commencing treatment.

Patients should be warned that most treatments take several months of continued use before benefits become apparent.

It is important to tackle underlying disorders when present (e.g. promoting weight loss in overweight/obese females with polycystic ovarian syndrome; treating Cushing syndrome).

The role of UV light therapy in treating active acne and healing scar tissue is currently under investigation.

Rosacea

This is a disorder, more common in women, beginning usually after 30 years of age, with erythema, papules, pustules and telangiectasia over the cheeks, nose, chin and forehead. It may be mistaken for acne, but there are no comedones. Flushing is common, especially in warm environments or in response to alcohol. In men, sebaceous hyperplasia on the nose leads to the condition 'rhinophyma'.

Oral tetracyclines are preferred for treatment but as with acne take several months to produce maximum benefits. Topical metronidazole may also be added. Oral isotretinoin can be effective in more resistant/severe cases. Plastic surgery may be required for rhinophyma. Precipitating factors should be avoided (e.g. hot drinks, warm environments, alcohol, sunlight, topical corticosteroids).

Hidradenitis suppurativa

A rare disorder characterised by relapsing suppurative infection in the axillae and groins – sites at which apocrine glands open into pilosebaceous follicles. It is more commonly seen in females, and flare-ups may correlate with changes in hormonal levels, e.g. in the menstrual cycle. Obesity exacerbates, but does not cause, the condition. Recurrent painful abscesses and sinus tracks develop, which discharge pus, blood and serous fluid. Although oral antibiotics and oral isotretinoin can be tried, success is usually limited and surgical intervention is often required to lay open the sinus tracks and excise chronically inflamed and infected areas.

Bacterial, viral, fungal and parasitic skin infections

Several different organisms can cause primary cutaneous infections/infestations. The more commonly encountered pathogens and their associated clinical sequelae are shown in Tables 19.3–19.6 and Fig. 19.8.

Cutaneous drug reactions

Cutaneous drug reactions are relatively common and may arise through one of several different mechanisms:

- intolerance or idiosyncrasy
- hypersensitivity (types I, II, III and IV)
- interactions with other drugs
- interactions with other environmental or host factors (e.g. sunlight exposure)
- pharmacokinetic disturbances

Table 19.7 shows the different types of eruption that may be encountered. Drugs that are particularly prone to causing cutaneous reactions include antibiotics (e.g. sulfonamides, penicillins), NSAIDs and hypnotics/tranquillisers.

Key features of the major types of drug reaction are described in the following section.

Clinical features/causative agents

Exanthematous eruptions

- variable speed of onset – typically starts within the first few days of treatment, but may develop more quickly (e.g. within hours of exposure) or appearance may be delayed (e.g. several weeks, making the link more difficult to establish)
- usually widespread, symmetrical, erythematous maculopapular rash, often resembling a viral exanthem (Fig. 19.9)
- itchy
- examples: penicillins, sulfonamides, NSAIDs

Urticaria and anaphylaxis

- secondary either to direct effect on mast cells or type I or type III hypersensitivity reaction
- eruption usually occurs 3–7 days after therapy is started
- rarely, rapid onset anaphylactic reactions (with fever, wheezing, arthralgia and hypotension) occur and are potentially fatal if not rapidly recognised and treated
- examples: penicillins, cephalosporins, aspirin, opioids, certain vaccines

Eczema

- type IV hypersensitivity reaction
- typically in response to a topical agent
- examples: lanolin, preservatives, topical antibiotics (especially aminoglycosides), topical antihistamines, topical local anaesthetics (although not lignocaine), topical corticosteroids

Exfoliative dermatitis (erythroderma)

- widespread reddening/inflammation of the skin ± scaling
- in more severe cases may be associated with loss of temperature regulation, dehydration, superadded infection, hyperdynamic circulation (± cardiac failure in the elderly)
- examples: phenytoin, sulfonylureas, sulfonamides, allopurinol, gold, barbiturates

Fixed drug eruptions

- typically manifests as a circular/oval patch of erythema with central purple discolouration ± bullous change
- single or multiple sites
- often initially misdiagnosed as ringworm infection
- usually affects the same area(s) of skin each time the patient is exposed to the offending drug
- postinflammatory pigmentation
- examples: phenolphthalein-containing laxatives, tetracyclines, sulfonamides, dapsone

Vasculitis (see Chapter 18)

- typically a cutaneous small vessel vasculitis (leukocytoclastic vasculitis)
- numerous palpable, purpuric lesions (often on the lower limbs); occasionally developing into haemorrhagic vesicles/bullae
- may be associated with systemic involvement (e.g. renal)
- examples: thiazide diuretics, sulfonamides

Table 19.3 Bacterial infections involving the skin

Bacterium	Condition	Epidemiology/ pathogenesis	Clinical features/ investigation	Specific treatment(s)
Streptococcus pyogenes (Group A streptococcus)	Cellulitis	• Bacteria enter via minor abrasions, fissures or pre-existing ulcers	• Affected area is red, hot and swollen	• Oral or intravenous penicillin remains the treatment of choice for streptococcal infection depending on severity
	'Erysipelas' is the term used to describe a well-demarcated superficial rash without oedema	• More common in the presence of tinea pedis or peripheral oedema	• Systemic upset is common • Blood cultures should be taken in all patients with pyrexia/systemic features • Positive antistreptolysin O (ASO) titre	• Elevate lower limbs • Treat predisposing factors • Surgical debridement if extensive tissue necrosis • Consider prophylactic oral penicillin for prevention of recurrent episodes
	Necrotising fasciitis	• Exotoxin-mediated tissue destruction • Exuberant host inflammatory response may also be contributory	• Pain, which may initially appear disproportionate • Rapid progression to extensive tissue necrosis • Marked systemic upset • Blood cultures may identify the underlying organism and direct more specific therapy	• Broad-spectrum intravenous antibiotics to cover all potential pathogens • Early and aggressive tissue debridement
Staphylococcus aureus (S. aureus)	Folliculitis	• Superficial infection of hair follicle(s)	• Small pustule(s) centred on follicle	• Topical or systemic antibiotic depending on extent
	Furuncle (boil)	• Deep infection of hair follicle	• Painful abscess	• Often resolve spontaneously • Systemic antibiotic (e.g. flucloxacillin or erythromycin) ±drainage occasionally required
	Carbuncle	• Deep infection of a group of adjacent hair follicles	• Common on back/neck • Erythema and suppuration with discharge from several follicles	• Systemic antibiotic (e.g. flucloxacillin or erythromycin) • ± drainage

(Continued)

Table 19.3 (Continued)

Bacterium	Condition	Epidemiology/ pathogenesis	Clinical features/ investigation	Specific treatment(s)
	Impetigo	• Non-bullous impetigo is caused by *S. aureus*, streptococci or both organisms together • Bullous impetigo is caused by *S. aureus* • May complicate atopic eczema	• Non-bullous form is characterised by small pustules, which rupture with crusting exudates • In the bullous form large superficial blisters form, which rupture with exudation and crusting	• Topical antibiotic (e.g. mupirocin) for localised infection • Systemic antibiotic (e.g. flucloxacillin, erythromycin) for more extensive infection
	Scalded skin syndrome	• Caused by epidermolytic exotoxins produced by certain *S. aureus* phage types	• Extensive peeling of superficial epidermis, leaving a 'scalded skin' appearance	• Intravenous flucloxacillin • Supportive measures (e.g. correction of fluid and electrolyte imbalances)
Mycobacterium	Scrofuloderma	• Spread to involve the skin overlying a tuberculous focus, e.g. lymph node	• Multiple fistulae • Scar tissue	• Full screening to determine extent of tuberculous spread/involvement • Treatment with antituberculous chemotherapy
	Lupus vulgaris	• Slow but progressive spread • Typically affecting head and neck with eventual destruction of cartilaginous structures if left unchecked	• Reddish-brown nodular plaque • Destruction of cartilage of nose and ears	• Full screening to determine extent of tuberculous spread/involvement • Treatment with antituberculous chemotherapy
	Atypical mycobacteria	• e.g. *Mycobacterium marinum* in 'swimming pool' or 'fish tank' granuloma; direct inoculation into the skin	• Solitary granulomatous nodule at site of inoculation • Secondary spread along line of lymphatics	• Treatment with antituberculous chemotherapy
	Leprosy	• Acquired through close physical contact or nasal spray • Clinical pattern of disease is determined by the host's immune response to the organism: tuberculoid (good), borderline (intermediate), lepromatous (poor response)	• Tuberculoid: one or two skin lesions only • Borderline: scattered skin lesions • Lepromatous: extensive skin lesions	• Tuberculoid: rifampicin and dapsone for 6 months • Lepromatous: rifampicin, dapsone and clofazimine for at least 24 months

Table 19.4 Viral infections involving the skin

Virus	Condition	Epidemiology/ pathogenesis	Clinical features/ investigation	Specific treatment(s)
Human papillomavirus (HPV) family	Common warts	• Common in childhood and early adulthood	• Raised 'cauliflower-like' lesions • Single or multiple • Most commonly on the hands or plantar surfaces of feet (the latter are commonly referred to as 'verrucae' and are often painful)	• 'Wart paints' (typically containing salicylic acid); prolonged treatment is required • Cryotherapy for resistant lesions
A poxvirus	Molluscum contagiosum	• Common in childhood	• Pearly pink papules with central keratin plug • Commonly seen on the head, neck and trunk	• Usually resolve spontaneously • Cryotherapy can be used
A parapoxvirus	Orf	• Transmitted from sheep to man	• Solitary inflammatory papule/ nodule • Usually on a finger	• Usually resolve spontaneously
Herpes simplex types 1 and 2 (HSV)	Primary herpes simplex • Type 1 HSV classically causes cold sores • Genital herpes may result from sexual transmission of type 2 HSV or orogenital transmission of type 1 HSV	• Primary infection occurs by direct contact, e.g. with a cold sore • Following primary infection, the virus settles in sensory ganglia, where it lies dormant until it is reactivated	• Cold sores • Genital herpes • May run prolonged/more severe course in immunocompromised individuals	• Normally resolves spontaneously • Oral aciclovir may shorten duration of genital herpes • Intravenous aciclovir for severe genital herpes and in immunocompromised patients
	Recurrent herpes simplex	• Triggers for reactivation include intercurrent illness, strong sunlight, stress	• A prodrome of itching/tingling typically precedes appearance of small vesicles, which subsequently crust	• Resolves spontaneously, but topical aciclovir may be of benefit if used in the early stages of a cold sore • Systemic aciclovir may be used for recurrent genital herpes
	Eczema herpeticum	• Widespread herpes simplex infection complicating atopic eczema	• Commonly affects head and neck, but may spread rapidly to other areas • Associated with systemic upset, fever	• Stop topical corticosteroid therapy • Oral aciclovir for mild/early cases, intravenous for more widespread involvement/systemic upset

(Continued)

Table 19.4 (Continued)

Virus	Condition	Epidemiology/ pathogenesis	Clinical features/ investigation	Specific treatment(s)
(Herpes) Varicella zoster	Chickenpox	• Airborne droplet transmission; 2- to 3-week incubation period • Common in childhood, but may affect all ages • Following primary infection, the virus settles in sensory ganglia, where it lies dormant until it is reactivated	• Prodromal symptoms including fever precede the appearance of the characteristic vesicles and pustules • Lesions appear in crops, which crust; removal of the crusts may result in long-term scarring • Varies from mild illness with relatively few lesions in young children to a more debilitating condition with widespread rash in adults or immune-compromised patients • Chickenpox pneumonia can be a severe life-threatening disorder	• Resolves spontaneously • Systemic aciclovir for immunocompromised patients, pregnant mothers, chickenpox pneumonia • Avoid contact with immunocompromised individuals
	Shingles (herpes zoster)	• Triggers for reactivation include intercurrent illness, stress, local trauma • Consider possible immunocompromise (including HIV infection) • May affect any of the divisions of the trigeminal nerve, although ophthalmic zoster is the most common	• Appearance of rash is preceded by an aching/burning pain • Subsequently, erythema and vesicles appear within a given dermatome • Lesions typically resolve over 2–3 weeks • May run a more severe protracted course in the elderly with subsequent post-herpetic neuralgia • Ophthalmic zoster may be associated with conjunctivitis, keratitis and iridocyclitis	• Many cases do not require specific treatment • Oral aciclovir* may be used in more severe cases and may reduce the likelihood/severity of post-herpetic neuralgia • Ophthalmic zoster requires formal ophthalmic assessment • Avoid contact with immunocompromised individuals

*Famciclovir and valaciclovir are alternatives to aciclovir for the treatment of herpes zoster, acute genital herpes and recurrent genital herpes where oral therapy will suffice.

Table 19.5 Fungal infections involving the skin

Fungus	Condition	Epidemiology/ pathogenesis	Clinical features/ investigation	Specific treatment(s)
Candida albicans (yeast)	Candidiasis	• Normal commensal of the gastrointestinal tract • Pathogenicity is related to the development of conditions favourable to its multiplication, e.g. warm moist skin, poorly controlled diabetes mellitus, pregnancy, use of broad-spectrum antibiotics, corticosteroid therapy, immunocompromise (e.g. lymphoma, AIDS)	• Buccal mucosal candidiasis: white curd-like plaques and mucosal erythema • Balanitis: white patches on the foreskin and glans with erythema • Vulvovaginitis: creamy vaginal discharge; pruritus • Intertrigo • Angular cheilitis • Chronic paronychia • Diagnosis can be confirmed on swabs/skin scrapings taken from affected areas • Screen for diabetes mellitus and/or other underlying conditions	• Wherever possible, underlying predisposing factors should be corrected/treated • Nystatin (oral suspension), amphotericin (lozenges) or miconazole (gel) for oral candidiasis • Topical imidazole-containing preparations usually suffice for the treatment of balanitis, vulvitis, intertrigo, angular cheilitis and chronic paronychia • Combination anti-*Candida* therapy and corticosteroids (e.g. hydrocortisone) may confer additional benefits in intertrigo and angular cheilitis • Systemic antifungal therapy can be used in recurrent/refractory disease • Do not forget to treat the partner if appropriate!
Malassezia (yeast)	Pityriasis versicolor (Fig. 19.8)	• Commonly affects younger adults, especially in warmer climates • Corticosteroid therapy and immunocompromise may be associated with more extensive disease • Fungal hyphae interfere with melanin production/ deposition	• Light brown macules • Fine scaly surface • Common sites: trunk, upper arms • Patches of hypopigmentation in those with pigmented skin • Diagnosis is confirmed through skin scrapings	• Options include: selenium sulphide shampoo (used as a lotion); topical imidazole creams and ketoconazole shampoo; topical terbinafine • Recurrence is common and retreatment often necessary; pigmentary changes resolve over months

(Continued)

Table 19.5 (*Continued*)

Fungus	Condition	Epidemiology/ pathogenesis	Clinical features/ investigation	Specific treatment(s)
Dermatophytes (*Microsporum*, *Trichophyton*, *Epidermophyton*)	Tinea ('ringworm')	• Non-yeast fungi which live and multiply in the outermost layer of the epidermis (i.e. in dead keratin) • Infection typically occurs through direct contact with infected material	• Tinea pedis ('athlete's foot'): scaling/peeling skin, typically between the toes and on the soles of the feet; itchy • Tinea cruris: scaly, reddened margins, usually on the medial aspects of the thighs • Tinea corporis: erythematous, scaling, with central clearing • Tinea manuum (palmar or dorsal surface, usually of one hand) • Tinea unguium: toenail involvement is common in adults and often associated with tinea pedis • Tinea capitis: scaly patch of scalp with broken hairs ± papules/pustules • Diagnosis is confirmed by sending skin scrapings, nail clippings and hairs for mycological assessment	• Topical antifungal agents including imidazoles and terbinafine may be tried when small areas of skin are involved • For larger areas, and in cases of scalp ringworm, oral therapy is preferred, e.g. griseofulvin (preferred in children), itraconazole, terbinafine • Prolonged courses of treatment (weeks/months) are often required • Wherever possible, underlying predisposing factors should be corrected, e.g. foot hygiene

Table 19.6 Parasitic infections involving the skin

Parasite	Condition	Epidemiology/pathogenesis	Clinical features/ investigation	Specific treatment(s)
Sarcoptes scabiei	Scabies	• Transmitted by close/prolonged physical contact • Affects all ages • Female mite burrows in the epidermis, laying eggs behind her • Several weeks after initial infection, the development of host hypersensitivity (type IV) to the mite and/or its products heralds the onset of pruritus	• Pruritus, especially nocturnal • Burrows: especially on hands and feet, but may be widespread • Rash: eruption of tiny inflammatory papules, commonly seen around the umbilicus, in the axillae and on the thighs (represents allergic response) • Secondary changes including excoriation, eczema and secondary bacterial infection may also be present • Skin scrapings from a burrow allows identification of the mite and eggs	• Treatment consists of a cream or lotion applied to the whole body except the scalp and central part of the face • Options include 5% permethrin, 0.5% malathion, benzyl benzoate (rarely used now) • Topical application of crotamiton and use of sedative antihistamines at night may help with itching • All members of the family and close contacts should also be treated
	Crusted ('Norwegian') scabies	• Large-scale infestation, with crusting • Secondary to altered host response (e.g. lack of itching/scratching with failure to destroy burrows/dislodge mites; immunocompromise)	• Multiple crusting lesions (burrows may be difficult to see due to the crusting) • Thickened nails	• Barrier nursing/isolation • Repeated topical applications of 5% permethrin are often required • Oral ivermectin (available on named patient basis) aids clearance
Pediculus	Pediculosis ('lice')	• The head louse (*Pediculus capitis*) is a wingless insect that lives on the scalp and feeds on blood. It is transmitted by head-to-head contact. Females lay eggs, which are 'cemented' to hair shafts.	• Itching is the main symptom • Lice may be visible in heavier infestations	• Application of shampoo and conditioner and then combing with fine-toothed comb is an effective means of removing lice. The process should be repeated every 4–5 days for 2–3 weeks • Topical permethrin, malathion and other pediculicides may be used, but resistance is common; repeat application after 7 days is required
		• Crab/pubic lice (*Pthirus pubis*) are transmitted by close physical contact; as with head lice, females 'cement' eggs to hair shafts	• Itching • May also infest axillary and beard hair and eyelashes	• The whole body should be treated with an aqueous preparation of permethrin or malathion, repeated after 7 days • Sexual contacts should be traced and treated

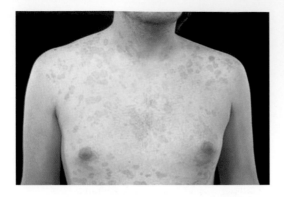

Figure 19.8 Pityriasis versicolor.

Table 19.7 Patterns of cutaneous drug reactions

- Exanthematous eruptions
- Urticaria/anaphylaxis
- Eczema
- Exfoliative dermatitis
- Fixed drug eruptions
- Vasculitis
- Erythema multiforme / Stevens–Johnson syndrome / toxic epidermal necrolysis
- Erythema nodosum
- Pigmentary changes
- Bullous/blistering reactions
- Photosensitivity
- Acneiform eruptions
- Pustular eruptions
- Hair loss or hair growth
- Lupus erythematosus-like syndrome
- Lichen planus-like eruptions
- Purpura
- Exacerbation of pre-existing skin disorder (e.g. acne, psoriasis, systemic lupus erythematosus, porphyria)

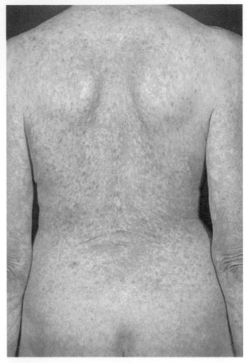

Figure 19.9 A typical exanthematic eruption due to an antibiotic.

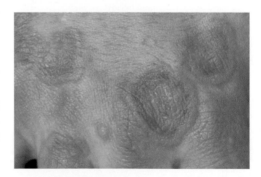

Figure 19.10 Target lesions of erythema multiforme.

Erythema multiforme (Fig. 19.10)

- target lesions
- examples: sulfonamides, cephalosporins, cotrimoxazole, rifampicin, barbiturates

Erythema nodosum

- tender, red, raised lesions (Fig. 19.11)
- typically on the shins, but may also affect upper limbs
- examples: sulfonamides, salicylates

Pigmentary changes

- various drugs can be associated with different pigmentary skin changes
- examples: blue-black (chloroquine, amiodarone [in sun-exposed areas]); brown (oestrogens causing melasma [chloasma])

Bullous/blistering reactions

- may be seen in the context of a fixed drug eruption or with drug-induced pemphigus, pemphigoid or porphyria cutanea tarda
- toxic epidermal necrolysis is the severe end of the erythema multiforme/Stevens–Johnson syndrome

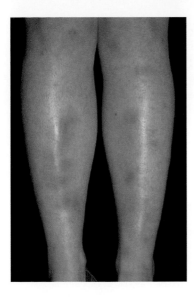

Figure 19.11 Erythema nodosum.

and has a significant mortality; examples: allopurinol, anti-convulsants, sulfhonamides

Photosensitivity

- direct phototoxic effect or exacerbation of a pre-existing condition
- in phototoxic reactions, the dose of the drug and the degree of ultraviolet radiation exposure determine the extent of the reaction; characterised by erythema, swelling ± eczematous changes
- examples: tetracyclines, sulfonamides, phenothiazines, thiazide diuretics

Acneiform eruptions

- papules/pustules
- examples: corticosteroids, androgenic drugs, lithium

Lupus-erythematosus-like syndrome

- rare
- examples: hydralazine, isoniazid, minocycline

Lichen planus-like eruptions

- rare
- may be indistinguishable from idiopathic lichen planus, although eczematous/scaly changes are more common
- examples: antimalarials, sulfonylureas, gold, thiazide diuretics (in sun-exposed areas)

Purpura

- may be a feature of any severe drug reaction and typically results from capillary damage and/or thrombocytopenia

Management

- Wherever possible discontinue suspected offending drug.
- Minimise other potential provoking factors, e.g. UV radiation exposure.
- Oral antihistamines for urticaria.
- Mild topical steroids may help itching.
- Adrenaline (epinephrine) may be life-saving in acute hypersensitivity reactions including shock and angioedema (see Respiratory Disease, page 129, Chapter 11), and systemic steroids may be required in severe but less acute cases.

Skin manifestations of systemic disease

Skin involvement in systemic disease is not uncommon and can be the presenting feature, e.g. erythema nodosum in sarcoidosis (see page 136, Chapter 11). In some instances, several different underlying disorders can give rise to the same skin condition (Table 19.8), while other cutaneous manifestations are more specific. Some disorders (e.g. diabetes mellitus) are associated with a wide array of cutaneous features.

Infections

- haemolytic streptococcal infection – erythema nodosum (Table 19.8, Fig. 19.11), erythema multiforme (Table 19.8, Fig. 19.10), erythema marginatum
- acquired immune deficiency syndrome (AIDS) – oral/oesophageal candidiasis, 'hairy leukoplakia' (Epstein–Barr virus), seborrhoeic dermatitis, warts, ano-genital intraepithelial neoplasia, recurrent/severe herpes simplex, Kaposi's sarcoma, lipodystrophy (in those on highly active antiretroviral therapy)
- Lyme disease (due to infection with the spirochaete *Borrelia burgdorferi*; transmitted by Ixodid tick bite) – erythema chronicum migrans

Diabetes mellitus

Skin manifestations include:

- neuropathic and neuroischaemic ulcers
- xanthomata – signifying hyperlipidaemia

Table 19.8 Skin conditions associated with a variety of systemic diseases

Cutaneous manifestation	Associated systemic disease(s)	Clinical features/treatment
Erythema nodosum (Fig. 19.11)	• Sarcoidosis • Streptococcal infection • Tuberculosis • Inflammatory bowel disease • Systemic fungal infections	• Tender, red, raised areas, typically on the shins but occasionally on the forearms • With time the lesions pass through the colour changes of a bruise before resolving • Simple analgesia usually suffices in the acute phase
Erythema multiforme (Fig. 19.10)	• Herpes simplex infection • Mycoplasma infection • Less commonly: connective tissue disorders; malignancy	• Target lesions, typically over extensor surfaces of arms and legs, but may spread to involve other areas of the body; dusky purplish centre which may blister • Self-limiting in most cases • Occasionally associated with major systemic upset (Stevens–Johnson syndrome), with lesions in the mouth, conjunctiva and anogenital regions; treatment is supportive (the role of systemic corticosteroids remains controversial)
Pyoderma gangrenosum (Fig. 19.14)	• Inflammatory bowel disease • Rheumatoid arthritis • Seronegative arthritis • Paraproteinaemia	• Necrotic ulceration with characteristic bluish/purplish undermined edge • Single or multiple lesions, usually on the lower limb • Painful • Treatment of the underlying condition, with judicious use of systemic corticosteroids; azathioprine and ciclosporin may also be effective

- lipohypertrophy (rarely lipoatrophy)
- necrobiosis lipoidica – typically occurs on the shins; initially erythematous, but becomes yellowish brown and atrophic with visible vessels beneath the skin; occasionally ulcerates (Fig. 19.12)
- diabetic dermopathy – small brown scar-like lesions, often on the shins
- acanthosis nigricans – indicating the presence of severe insulin resistance (Fig. 19.13)
- cheiroarthropathy – thickening of the skin of the hands
- mucosal candidiasis (e.g. balanitis, vulvovaginitis)
- granuloma annulare.

Endocrine disorders

- thyrotoxicosis/hyperthyroidism – palmar erythema, alopecia, urticaria; Graves' disease is specifically associated with acropachy (digital clubbing), onycholysis, pretibial myxoedema
- hypothyroidism – pallor, malar flush (which together may lead to the classical 'strawberries and cream' appearance), thinning of scalp hair, loss of

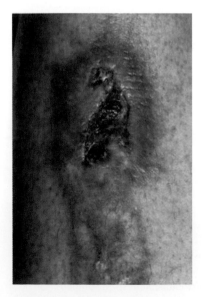

Figure 19.12 Necrobiosis lipoidica with a small ulcerated area.

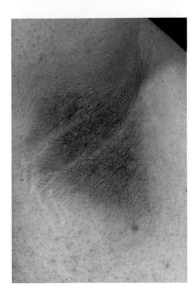

Figure 19.13 Acanthosis nigricans.

outer part of eyebrows, thickened/dry skin (myxo-edema)

- Cushing syndrome – thinning of skin, spontaneous/easy bruising, acne, hirsutism, violaceous striae
- Addison's disease – hyperpigmentation (especially palmar creases, buccal mucosa, scars); may be associated with vitiligo

Hyperlipidaemia

Both primary and secondary hyperlipidaemia may be associated with lipid deposits in the skin (xanthomata), which are yellow/orange in colour and may occur as:

- xanthelasma(ta) – eyelids
- tendon xanthomata – extensor tendons of the hands, Achilles tendons
- palmar xanthomata – creases of the palms
- tuberous xanthomata – over bony prominences
- eruptive xanthomata – crops of papules (indicative of hypertriglyceridaemia).

Rheumatological disorders

- gout – tophaceous deposits
- rheumatoid arthritis – palmar erythema, rheumatoid nodules, vasculitic lesions, pyoderma gangrenosum
- systemic lupus erythematosus – facial erythema ('butterfly rash'), photosensitivity, alopecia, Raynaud's phenomenon

- discoid lupus erythematosus – principally affects light-exposed areas, with scaling and erythematous plaques; healed areas show scarring and hypopigmentation
- dermatomyositis – purple heliotrope discolouration, classically around the eyes, but may involve other areas, especially sun-exposed; periorbital oedema; vasculitic lesions in the childhood variant
- systemic sclerosis – tight, shiny appearance of the skin over the face, with beaked nose and restriction of mouth-opening; facial telangiectasia; sclerodactyly, digital infarcts, calcinosis, Raynaud's phenomenon
- Reiter syndrome – keratoderma blennorrhagicum, buccal mucosal ulceration, circinate balanitis

Sarcoidosis

Skin manifestations include:

- erythema nodosum (Table 19.8, Fig. 19.11)
- lupus pernio – purplish discolouration of the skin of the nose and ears
- papules, nodules, plaques, sarcoid granulomas.

Malignancy

Skin manifestations of malignancy include:

- cutaneous deposits, e.g. breast, bronchus, renal, ovarian (including 'Sister Joseph's nodule', an umbilical metastatic nodule)
- generalised pruritus (associated with a wide array of systemic malignancies, especially lymphoma)
- acanthosis nigricans (Fig. 19.13) (gastrointestinal adenocarcinoma)
- dermatomyositis (bronchus, breast, stomach, ovary)
- thrombophlebitis migrans (pancreatic carcinoma)
- flushing (carcinoid syndrome)
- necrolytic migratory erythema (glucagonoma)
- pyoderma gangrenosum (Table 19.8, Fig. 19.14) (myeloma)
- acquired ichthyosis (lymphoma).

Miscellaneous disorders

- liver disease – pruritus, palmar erythema, spider naevi, xanthelasma(ta)
- inflammatory bowel disease – erythema nodosum, pyoderma gangrenosum (Table 19.8, Fig. 19.14), buccal mucosal and perianal ulceration
- amyloidosis – yellow waxy periorbital and perianal plaques

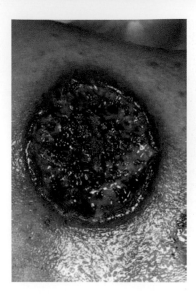

Figure 19.14 Pyoderma gangrenosum.

- scurvy (due to vitamin C deficiency) – perifollicular purpura, easy bruising, bleeding gums, poor wound healing
- pellagra (due to nicotinic acid deficiency) – triad of dermatitis (in sun-exposed areas, e.g. 'Casal's necklace'), diarrhoea and dementia
- neurofibromatosis – *café-au-lait* spots, axillary freckling, neurofibromas
- porphyria – photosensitive rash/blistering in certain types of porphyria (see page 286, Chapter 17)
- Ehlers–Danlos syndrome – skin hyperextensibility and fragility
- tuberous sclerosis complex (*Epiloia*) – hamartomas, angiofibromas, *shagreen patch,* periungual fibromas, hypopigmented (*ash leaf*) macules
- Peutz–Jeghers syndrome – pigmented macules (lentigines) in the mouth, on the lips, hands and feet
- hereditary haemorrhagic telangiectasia – facial telangiectasia
- pseudoxanthoma elasticum – 'plucked chicken' skin appearance

Bullous disorders

Blisters and bullae can be caused by a wide variety of disorders including physical injury (e.g. friction, extremes of temperature, chemicals, insect bites), infection (e.g. impetigo, varicella zoster), drugs (e.g. sulfonamides, barbiturates), systemic disease (e.g. porphyria) and primary skin conditions. The latter may be congenital (e.g. epidermolysis bullosa) or acquired (e.g. pemphigus, pemphigoid, dermatitis herpetiformis).

Epidermolysis bullosa

A rare disorder, which presents in the newborn with fragile skin that blisters on minimal contact; may be fatal.

Pemphigus

In pemphigus, splits occur within the epidermis above the basal layer, with degeneration of epidermal cells (acantholysis). Pemphigus vulgaris is the most commonly encountered variant.

Clinical presentation

Pemphigus is a relatively rare disorder usually of middle age, some of the characteristics of which are explained by the very superficial site of the lesions: clinically, it presents with widespread erosions and relatively few bullae (because they rupture so easily, leaving flaccid blisters), which are located over the limbs and trunk (Fig. 19.15). Most patients have lesions in the mouth and these may be the only visible lesions in the early stages. The surrounding skin is normal. The superficial skin layer at the edge of a blister can be moved over the deeper layers (Nikolsky's sign) and tends to disintegrate. Lesions appear at sites of pressure and trauma and are painful. Secondary bacterial infection may complicate the primary condition.

Investigation

- skin biopsy – for histopathology (to confirm superficial nature of the blister/bulla) and direct immunofluorescence on perilesional tissue (which

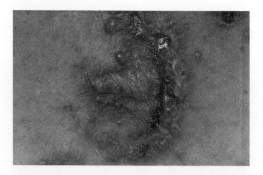

Figure 19.15 Pemphigus vulgaris: flaccid blisters and erosions.

shows staining around epidermal cells with antibodies directed against immunoglobulin G [IgG])
- serum for detection of anti-desmoglein antibody

Management

Aggressive management is required including:

- High-dose systemic corticosteroids (e.g. prednisolone initially 60–120 mg/day), with gradual dose tapering as blistering settles. Steroid-sparing agents (e.g. azathioprine, cyclophosphamide, methotrexate) are often substituted after the acute phase has subsided.
- Secondary bacterial infection is common and should be treated promptly.
- Significant fluid and protein loss may occur from weeping skin, and supportive treatment (including enteral/parenteral feeding in cases of severe oral involvement) may be required.

Pemphigoid

In contrast to pemphigus, blisters are subepidermal.

Clinical presentation

Bullous pemphigoid affects those >60 years of age. Clinically, it often presents with prodromal itch ± areas of erythema with eczematous or urticarial features, which may predate the appearance of bullae by several weeks. Numerous tense, subepidermal bullae then form, ranging in size from a few millimetres to several centimetres (Fig. 19.16). They are less likely to rupture than in pemphigus, but this can be provoked by trauma. Nikolsky's sign is negative. Scarring is rare and only a small number of cases develop mucosal ulceration.

Cicatricial or mucous membrane pemphigoid is a distinct variant in which the mouth and conjunctivae are involved and scarring can occur and be pronounced.

Investigation

- Skin biopsy – for histopathology (to confirm subepidermal blister/bulla). Immunofluorescence shows linear IgG and C3 at the basement membrane.
- Circulating IgG against antigen in the basement membrane is detectable in the serum of approximately two-thirds of patients with bullous pemphigoid.

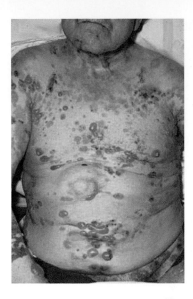

Figure 19.16 Bullous pemphigoid: numerous tense blisters.

Management

- Moderate dose systemic corticosteroids (e.g. prednisolone initially 40–60 mg/day) are required, with dose tapering as blistering settles, which usually occurs quite rapidly in bullous pemphigoid.
- Long-term low-dose maintenance therapy is often required; azathioprine may be substituted after the acute phase has subsided.

Dermatitis herpetiformis

A rare disorder associated with subepidermal blisters. It is classically seen in the context of coeliac disease.

Clinical presentation

Dermatitis herpetiformis is characterised by itchy erythematous papules and vesicles, which are common on the elbows and other extensor surfaces. Blisters/bullae may be burst by scratching, with marked excoriation.

Investigation

- Skin biopsy – for histopathology (to confirm subepidermal blister/bulla and 'microabscesses' at the edge of vesicles) and direct immunofluorescence (which shows granular deposits of IgA in dermal papillae)

Management

- gluten-free diet
- dapsone

Benign and malignant skin tumours

Skin tumours are common. Most are benign, but it is important to identify malignant or potentially malignant lesions. They may arise within the epidermis or the dermis. Clinical features and treatments for the more commonly encountered/important skin tumours are shown in Table 19.9 and Figs. 19.17–19.21.

Miscellaneous skin conditions

Skin pigmentation

Abnormalities of skin pigmentation are seen in a variety of settings and may be localised to small areas or more generalised. Table 19.10 lists some of the more common causes of hypo- and hyperpigmentation.

Urticaria

Urticaria describes a group of disorders that are characterised by weals, which typically appear and then disappear spontaneously in a matter of hours. Mast cell degranulation leads to vasodilatation with consequent dermal oedema. Often itching is the first symptom, followed shortly afterwards by the development of pink weals over a variable-sized area, e.g. localised in response to a nettle sting or more generalised as part of an allergic reaction (e.g. food or drug allergies). When part of a more systemic anaphylactic reaction, urticaria may be accompanied by angioedema, with swelling/oedema of the subcutaneous tissues, especially around the eyes, mouth and upper airway. A chronic relapsing form, in which attacks last for weeks, months or even years, is believed to be of autoimmune origin.

If possible, triggers should be identified and avoided. Aspirin is best avoided. Most types of urticaria respond to antihistamines (both H_1 and H_2 antagonists may be helpful). Angioedema/anaphylaxis are medical emergencies (see Respiratory Disease, page 129, Chapter 11).

Lichen planus

Lichen planus is uncommon, usually presenting in middle age with an irritating rash affecting the flexures of the wrist and forearms, lower back, mouth and genitalia. The rash consists of discrete, purple, shiny, polygonal papules with fine white lines ('Wickham's striae'), often occurring in scratch marks and other sites of injury (Köbner phenomenon). The papules may be widespread or confined to one or two sites. Lesions may arise on the buccal mucosa with a white, lacy network, or in the nails without other lesions on the skin. The disorder usually resolves within 6 months but can recur. The cause is unknown, but several drugs can produce an identical eruption, e.g. gold, antimalarials and antituberculous drugs. The epidermis is infiltrated with T-cells.

Topical corticosteroids are usually sufficient to suppress symptoms until resolution has occurred. Systemic corticosteroids or ciclosporin may be required for extensive/severe disease.

Pityriasis rosea

A self-limiting disorder, of unknown aetiology, commonest in children and young adults. Following a mild prodromal illness one or more 'herald patches' (red, oval, scaly) appear either on the trunk or arm. Several days later, multiple pink/red oval patches erupt over the trunk, upper arms and thighs, with the long axis of the oval appearing to follow individual dermatomes/spinal roots. It resolves spontaneously over 6–8 weeks.

Disorders of the hair and nails

Hair abnormalities

These generally fall into one or more of three categories:

- Changes in colour or texture (e.g. brittleness, coarseness).
- Thinning or loss of hair – may be congenital or, more commonly, acquired, e.g. *telogen effluvium* (in which large numbers of hairs suddenly stop growing and enter the 'telogen' phase simultaneously; often triggered by stress/intercurrent illness), *androgenetic alopecia, alopecia areata* (autoimmune disorder, with patchy loss of scalp hair [close inspection at the edge of the patch reveals

Table 19.9 Skin tumours

Tumour	Epidemiology/clinical features	Treatment
Benign		
Seborrhoeic keratoses (basal cell papillomas; seborrhoeic warts)	• Common, especially in the elderly • Solitary or multiple • Typically occurring on the head, neck, trunk, hands • Raised, flat-topped lesions, ranging in colour from light brown to deeply pigmented • May be associated with pruritus	• If required, treatment options range from cryotherapy for smaller lesions to curettage and surgical excision for larger ones
Keratoacanthoma	• Typically seen in elderly people • Round with raised edges and characteristic central keratin plug ± reddened/inflamed base • Develops over a relatively short interval (2–3 months) and ultimately regresses spontaneously	• Surgical excision and histological examination should be considered for (1) all lesions that cannot be reliably differentiated clinically from a squamous cell carcinoma and (2) persistent lesions
Dermatofibroma	• Commonly seen as single or multiple lesions on the lower limbs, especially in females • May arise at sites of minor trauma or insect bites • Slightly raised, skin-coloured or pigmented	Usually none required; surgical excision can be considered but may leave scarring
Pyogenic granuloma (benign proliferation of blood vessels/fibroblasts)	• Polypoidal lesion, which may bleed profusely following minor trauma	• Curettage or surgical excision with histological examination
Dysplastic/malignant		
Actinic (solar) keratoses (Fig. 19.17)	• Areas of dysplastic squamous epithelium, which typically develop in UV radiation exposed areas (e.g. scalp, face, hands, lower legs) • Dry, rough, scaly lesions, with erythematous background • May undergo spontaneous involution	• Topical application of 5-fluorouracil, imiquimod or a non-steroidal anti-inflammatory cream is generally effective • Cryotherapy (if lesions limited in size and number)

(Continued)

Table 19.9 *(Continued)*

Tumour	Epidemiology/clinical features	Treatment
Basal cell carcinoma (BCC; 'rodent ulcer') (Fig. 19.18)	• Commonest skin cancer • UV radiation exposure is an important trigger, and lesions are most commonly seen in sun-exposed areas, e.g. on the face • Often begins as a nodule, which develops a central depression as the lesion extends outwards, leaving a 'rolled' edge appearance • Contact bleeding from overlying telangiectasia and central ulceration may be seen • Locally invasive, but may rarely metastasise	• For superficial tumours (usually <1 mm deep), curettage, topical imiquimod, cryotherapy or photo(dynamic) therapy may suffice • Surgical excision and/or radiotherapy are required for deeper lesions
Squamous cell carcinoma in situ (Bowen's disease)	• Confined to the epidermis, and typically arises in regions subjected to long-term UV radiation exposure (e.g. lower legs), but may also occur in non-exposed areas • Often presents as a single red, scaly patch, which may be mistaken for psoriasis	• Curettage, cryotherapy, photo(dynamic) therapy or surgical excision may be required
Squamous cell carcinoma (SCC) (Fig. 19.19)	• Aetiological factors include UV radiation exposure, smoking in perioral tumours, human papilloma virus infection in genital lesions and immunosuppression (e.g. in transplant recipients) • Locally invasive, with greater propensity to metastasise than BCCs • Varied appearance: ulcer, keratotic nodule, rapidly expanding polypoidal mass	• Surgical excision and/or radiotherapy
Lentigo maligna ('Hutchinson's malignant freckle') (Fig. 19.20)	• Patch of malignant melanocytes that have not yet become invasive • Typically develops in UV radiation-damaged skin • Flat, brown with variable pigmentation	• Biopsy to confirm diagnosis followed by surgical excision • Occasionally surveillance (e.g. in a very elderly patient) may be reasonable • Cryotherapy and topical therapies are associated with higher rates of local recurrence

Malignant melanoma
(Fig. 19.21)

- Worldwide incidence has risen in recent years, especially in younger age groups
- UV radiation damage to skin (e.g. repeated sunburn) significantly increases risk
- May arise de novo or in a long-standing mole
- Metastasise to loco-regional and then distant lymph nodes
- Different patterns are recognised:
  - *lentigo maligna melanoma*: malignant nodule developing within a patch of lentigo maligna
  - *superficial spreading melanoma*: irregularly pigmented patch with irregular margins; may itch or bleed
  - *nodular melanoma*: more rapidly growing; occasionally lacks pigment ('amelanotic melanoma')
  - *acral melanoma*: pigmented patch on the sole or palm or subungual (must be distinguished from a haematoma)

- 'Prevention is better than cure', e.g. avoidance of strong sunlight, use of 'sun-blocks'
- Patients should be advised to seek early medical advice about suspicious lesions, especially those that develop or enlarge in adult life, if there is an irregular margin or irregular pigmentation, itching or crusting/bleeding
- Prognosis is related to the 'Breslow thickness' (i.e. depth of tumour at first surgical excision); in essence the thinner the melanoma the better the prognosis (traditionally <1 mm, 95% 5-year survival; >3.5 mm, <45% 5-year survival)
- Surgical excision remains the mainstay of treatment
- Standard chemotherapy regimens show limited efficacy in advanced (unresectable or metastatic) melanoma, but several targeted antibody therapies (e.g. anti-BRAF, anti-PD-1 [nivolumab], anti-CTLA-4 [ipilimumab]) may produce tumour shrinkage and improved survival
- Radiotherapy may be used for local/distant spread, but generally does not improve prognosis

Kaposi's sarcoma

- Multicentric malignant vascular tumour, originally limited to those of Mediterranean and Jewish descent, but now recognised as an AIDS-defining condition
- Purple to brown/black plaques/nodules

- In the context of AIDS, lesions often resolve in response to HAART

CTLA-4, cytotoxic T-lymphocyte-associated antigen 4; HAART, highly active antiretroviral therapy; PD-1, programmed cell death-1 receptor.

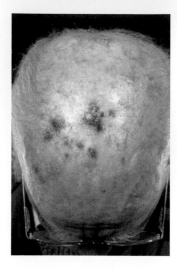

Figure 19.17 Multiple solar keratoses.

'exclamation mark hairs']); tends to run a relaps-ing/remitting course; occasionally involves the whole scalp (alopecia totalis) or whole body (alo-pecia universalis) and *trichotillomania* (compulsive plucking of the hair). It may also be seen in the con-text of skin conditions (e.g. psoriasis, seborrhoeic dermatitis, tinea capitis) and systemic disorders (e.g. hypothyroidism, hypopituitarism) and follow-ing drug therapy (e.g. cytotoxic agents)

- Excessive hair growth and development of hair in abnormal sites – hirsutism describes male-pattern hair growth in a female and is most commonly 'idi-opathic' or associated with the polycystic ovarian syndrome (page 254, Chapter 16), but occasionally can be a sign of a virilising tumour; hypertrichosis is excessive hair growth in a non-sexual distribu-tion and may occur in both sexes (e.g. in response to drugs such as minoxidil and ciclosporin).

Nail abnormalities

Nail disorders may occur in isolation or may be a sign of more generalised skin disease (e.g. psoriasis, fungal infections) or of an underlying systemic disorder (e.g. koilonychia in iron deficiency anaemia). They include:

- Beau's lines (horizontal lines following major ill-ness)

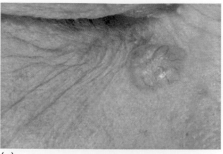

(a)

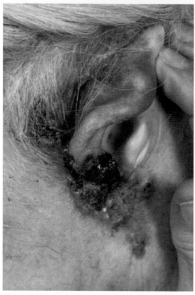

(b)

Figure 19.18 (a) Basal cell carcinoma: note the telangiectatic vessels. (b) Basal cell carcinoma: such destruction gives rise to the term 'rodent ulcer'.

- brittleness
- clubbing
- koilonychia ('spoon-shaped')
- onychogryphosis (gross thickening)
- onycholysis (lifting of the nail plate off the nail bed, e.g. in psoriasis, Graves' disease)
- paronychia (infection around the nail)
- pitting (e.g. in psoriasis)
- pterygium (e.g. in lichen planus).

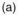
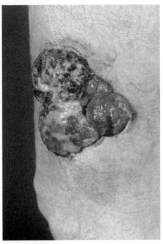
(a)

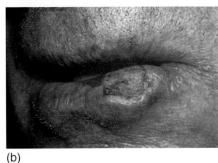
(b)

Figure 19.19 (a) A polypoid squamous cell carcinoma.
(b) Squamous cell carcinoma on the lip.

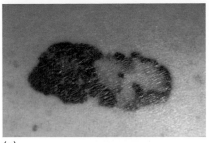
(a)

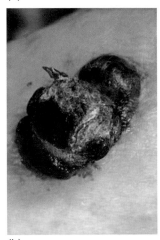
(b)

Figure 19.21 (a) Superficial spreading melanoma.
(b) Large nodular melanoma.

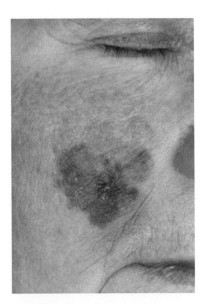

Figure 19.20 Lentigo maligna.

Table 19.10 Causes of hypo- and hyperpigmentation
Hypopigmentation
• Vitiligo • Postinflammatory • Pityriasis versicolor • Drug/chemical-induced • Leprosy • Lichen sclerosus • Congenital: albinism, phenylketonuria
Hyperpigmentation
• Addison's disease • Renal or liver failure • Haemochromatosis • Postinflammatory • Pityriasis versicolor • Drug/chemical-induced • Melasma (chloasma) • Acanthosis nigricans • Congenital: neurofibromatosis, Peutz–Jeghers syndrome

20

Haematology

Diagnosis of haematological disorders is made or confirmed on the basis of laboratory findings.

Peripheral blood film features (Fig. 20.1)

- reticulocytes (active marrow) – haemolysis or chronic blood loss
- anisocytes (variation in red cell size) or poikilocytes (variation in red cell shape) – iron deficiency
- target cells ('Mexican hat' cells) – thalassaemia
- rouleau formation (clumping together of red cells) – raised ESR (check for myeloma)
- burr cells (echinocytes with irregular 'crinkled' red cell membrane) – renal failure, carcinoma
- hypersegmented polymorphs – vitamin B_{12} or folic acid deficiency
- Howell–Jolly bodies (remnants of nuclear material) – splenectomy (or non-functioning spleen)
- blast cells (immature cells) – acute leukaemia
- eosinophilia – parasitic infection, allergy, occasionally systemic vasculitis or Hodgkin's disease

Reticulocytes

Normal range is $10–100 \times 10^9/l$. Reticulocytes are premature red cells in which traces of nucleoprotein remain as fine, reticular strands. They are larger than mature red cells and, if increased, may cause macrocytosis. An increase (reticulocytosis) suggests marrow hyperactivity because of:

- loss or destruction of red cells, e.g. bleeding
- a response to treatment of anaemia, e.g. of pernicious anaemia with vitamin B_{12}
- haemolysis.

Normocytic anaemia

Mean corpuscular volume (MCV) is normal. Usually anaemia is secondary to chronic disease. It is usually insidious, not progressive and fairly mild (>90 g/l) except in chronic kidney disease. The white cell count and platelets are normal. The serum transferrin is normal or low but, unlike iron deficiency, the serum iron and ferritin are normal.

Anaemia of chronic diseases occurs in:

- chronic kidney disease (Chapter 14) – check serum creatinine and estimated glomerular filtration rate (eGFR)
- chronic liver disease – check liver function tests, γ-glutamyl transferase, prothrombin time
- autoimmune disease (e.g. rheumatoid arthritis, systemic lupus erythematosus [SLE]) – check ESR, C-reactive protein and autoantibodies: rheumatoid factor, antinuclear antibodies and if positive specific tests for antibodies against nuclear antigens (Chapter 18), antineutrophil cytoplasm antibodies (ANCA; present in systemic vasculitis)
- chronic infection – abscesses, tuberculosis, bacterial endocarditis
- cancer.

NB: The anaemia of chronic kidney disease can be effectively reversed by treatment with recombinant human erythropoietin (Chapter 14). Erythropoietin can also reverse anaemia associated with cancer, although

Clinical Medicine Lecture Notes, Eighth Edition. John R. Bradley, Mark Gurnell, and Diana F. Wood.
© 2019 John Wiley & Sons Ltd. Published 2019 by John Wiley & Sons Ltd.

Red cell abnormalities	Causes	Red cell abnormalities	Causes
Normal		Spherocyte	Hereditary spherocytosis autoimmune haemolytic anaemia, septicaemia
Macrocyte	Liver disease, alcoholism. Oval in megaloblastic anaemia	Fragments	DIC, microangiopathy, HUS, TTP, burns, cardiac valves
Target cell	Iron deficiency, liver disease, haemoglobinopathies, post-splenectomy	Elliptocyte	Hereditary elliptocytosis
Stomatocyte	Liver disease, alcoholism	Tear drop poikilocyte	Myelofibrosis, extramedullary haemopoiesis
Pencil cell	Iron deficiency	Basket cell	Oxidant damage e.g. G6PD deficiency, unstable haemoglobin
Echinocyte	Renal failure, carcinoma	Howell–Jolly body	Hyposplenism, post-splenectomy
Acanthocyte	Liver disease, abetalipoprotein-aemia, renal failure	Basophilic stippling	Haemoglobinopathy, lead poisoning, myelodysplasia, haemolytic anaemia
Sickle cell	Sickle cell anaemia	Malarial parasite	Malaria. Other intra-erythrocytic parasites include Bartonella bacilliformis, babesiosis
Microcyte	Iron deficiency, haemoglobinopathy	Siderotic granules (Pappenheimer bodies)	Disordered iron metabolism e.g. sideroblastic anaemia, post-splenectomy

Figure 20.1 Morphology of red cells. *Source*: Mehta and Hoffbrand (2009) *Haematology at a Glance*, 3rd edn. Oxford: Wiley-Blackwell. DIC, disseminated intravascular coagulation; HUS, haemolytic uraemic syndrome; TTP, thrombotic thrombocytopaenic purpura.

concerns have been raised that erythropoietin may contribute to tumour progression.

Microcytic anaemia

MCV is low, e.g. <80 fl. The serum iron is either low (iron deficiency) or normal (haemoglobinopathies, usually thalassaemia minor, see later). The mean corpuscular haemoglobin (MCH) is usually low (hypochromic), i.e. <25 pg.

Iron deficiency is caused by poor intake, poor absorption, poor iron use by the marrow or increased blood loss (menstrually or from the gut). Check with serum iron (very low) and transferrin, which tends to be high. Serum ferritin is low and bone marrow demonstrate low iron stores.

Macrocytic anaemia

MCV is raised, often >100 fl.

- vitamin B_{12} deficiency (usually pernicious anaemia) – check serum B_{12}
- folic acid deficiency – check red cell folate
- hypothyroidism – check thyroid function tests
- liver disease (usually excess alcohol) – check liver function, including γ-glutamyl transferase

Pernicious anaemia is diagnosed by finding low serum vitamin B_{12} with parietal cell and intrinsic factor antibodies. Check the haemoglobin, and reticulocyte response to therapy. If in doubt, marrow examination may provide a definitive diagnosis (megaloblastic).

Pancytopenia

This is a rare combination of anaemia, leucopenia and thrombocytopenia. It is caused by either:

- reduced production of cells, caused by:
  - bone marrow infiltration (leukaemia, myeloma, carcinoma, myelofibrosis)
  - bone marrow aplasia: idiopathic or drug-induced (e.g. NSAIDs, chloramphenicol, chemotherapy for malignancy); severe vitamin B_{12} or folate deficiency
- increased destruction of cells, caused by hypersplenism; or autoimmune disease (e.g. SLE).

Bone marrow examination is the most important investigation in distinguishing these causes.

Marrow suppression

Secondary bone marrow failure may affect one or all of the formed elements of the blood – red cells, white cells or platelets. It may be idiopathic or secondary to infiltration, drugs, (gold, penicillamine, chloramphenicol, carbimazole), radiation, leukaemias, infections or other disorders such as uraemia, hypothyroidism and chronic disease.

Erythrocyte sedimentation rate (ESR)

ESR measures the rate of sedimentation (in millimetres per hour) of red cells in a column of anticoagulated blood. Rapid sedimentation (increased ESR) suggests increased levels of immunoglobulins or acute phase proteins, which cause the red cells to stick together. A raised ESR is therefore a non-specific indicator of inflammation or infection. The ESR is usually very high in myeloma.

A very high ESR (>100 mm/h) suggests:

- multiple myeloma
- SLE or vasculitis
- temporal arteritis
- polymyalgia rheumatica
- rarely, carcinoma or chronic infection, including tuberculosis.

Anaemia

There are three major types of anaemia, classified by cause: deficiency, haemolysis and marrow disorders. The symptoms are tiredness, physical fatigue and dyspnoea, with angina, heart failure and confusion in older people.

Anaemia can be caused by a deficiency in:

- iron
- vitamin B_{12}
- folic acid.

Iron-deficiency anaemia

Diagnosis

The cause of the iron deficiency must be identified and corrected. In premenopausal women, excess menstrual loss is often the cause, although this should not be accepted uncritically because other important causes may be present as well. Slow gastrointestinal loss is a common cause, with peptic ulceration, gastric carcinoma and carcinoma of the descending colon most common. Carcinoma of the ascending colon or caecum frequently produces no symptoms and its presence must be considered in all cases of iron-deficiency anaemia. In the elderly, dietary deficiencies remain an important cause, and remember that hypothyroidism can present as iron-deficient anaemia.

Examination

This includes assessment of pallor (very imprecise), glossitis, angular stomatitis, koilonychia and rectal examination. Investigate the gastrointestinal tract if no other cause is identified.

Laboratory investigation (Table 20.1)

The peripheral blood count shows hypochromia (MCH < 27 pg) and microcytosis (MCV < 80 fl), possibly with poikilocytosis (variation in shape) and anisocytosis (variation in size). The serum iron is low and the transferrin raised, with a low saturation. The serum iron can also be low in anaemia secondary to chronic disease, but normal in haemoglobinopathies and, usually, thalassaemia minor (see later). Serum ferritin reflects the state of the iron stores and is therefore low. There is a reduction in stainable iron in the marrow. The bone marrow shows adequate iron in macrophages but reduced amounts in developing erythroblasts. Thalassaemia also causes hypochromic, microcytic anaemia.

Table 20.1 Haematological reference values in anaemia. If you are attempting to analyse anaemia and are looking at a Coulter-style full blood count, first check the MCV. See if the cells are normal (normocytic), small (microcytic) or large (macrocytic)

Hb (male)	125–165 × g/l
Hb (female)	115–155 × g/l
An automated cell counter (e.g. Coulter counter) typically gives the following readings:	
Haematocrit (PCV; male)	0.42–0.53
Haematocrit (PCV; female)	0.39–0.45
Red cell count (male)	$4.5–6.5 × 10^{12}/l$
Red cell count (female)	$3.9–5.6 × 10^{12}/l$
MCV	80–96 fl[a]
RDW	11.1–13.7[b]
MCH	27–31 pg[c]
Transferrin (iron-binding plasma protein)	2–3 g/l Raised in iron deficiency (and pregnancy) Reduced in anaemia of chronic disease, acute inflammation and protein loss
Ferritin	Correlates with tissue iron stores (iron is stored in the tissues in two forms, ferritin and haemosiderin) Only low in iron-deficiency states

Hb, haemoglobin; MCH, mean corpuscular haemoglobin; MCV, mean corpuscular volume; PCV, packed cell volume; RDW, red cell distribution width.
[a] MCV is haematocrit/red cell count.
[b] This is an automated measure of anisocytosis: the variability of red cell size.
[c] MCH is Hb/red cell count.

Management

In the absence of active bleeding, ferrous sulphate 200 mg b.d. before food is usually all that is required. The reticulocyte count rises first and then the haemoglobin (at about 1 g/week), but iron should be continued for another 3 months to replenish the stores.

NB: *Hypochromic anaemia,* unresponsive to oral iron therapy, occurs in:

- incorrect diagnosis or mixed deficiency
- continued bleeding (reticulocytosis persists), e.g. microscopic from tumour of the bowel
- patients who do not take their tablets
- malabsorption (page 153, Chapter 12)
- thalassaemia (see later)
- myelodysplastic syndrome (see later) – refractory anaemia (if ringed sideroblasts present in marrow, sideroblastic anaemia).

Hazards of blood transfusion

- *Transfusion reaction* – minimise risk by cross-matching patient's serum with donor blood. If clinical manifestations of a transfusion reaction occur (fever, backache, hypotension and haemoglobinuria), stop the transfusion immediately and initiate supportive treatment to alleviate shock.
- *Transmission of infection* – blood is screened for viral infections, including hepatitis B and C and human immunodeficiency virus (HIV).
- *Circulatory overload* – give furosemide with transfusion in patients at risk of heart failure.
- *Coagulation defects and electrolyte abnormalities* – particularly hyperkalaemia (red cell breakdown releases potassium) where large volumes are transfused.

Vitamin B_{12} deficiency (usually pernicious anaemia)

Vitamin B_{12} is present in liver, and small amounts also in milk and dairy products, and requires intrinsic factor for absorption. The most common cause of vitamin B_{12} deficiency in the UK is lack of intrinsic factor as a result of parietal cell and intrinsic factor antibodies. It is associated with other organ-specific autoimmune disorders. Achlorhydria is invariably present. Rare causes of B_{12} deficiency include gastrectomy, intestinal blind loops (in which bacteria multiply using up B_{12}), a vegan diet, Crohn's disease involving the absorbing surface in the terminal ileum, other causes of malabsorption are *Diphyllobothrium latum,* a Finnish tapeworm that consumes B_{12}. Stores of B_{12} last 3–4 years.

Clinical features

Pernicious anaemia occurs in the middle-aged and elderly and is more common in women. Exhaustion and lethargy are the most common presenting complaints, although pallor may be noticed incidentally, or the blood picture noticed in the laboratory.

In chronic, severe B_{12} deficiency, which is uncommon, the skin typically has a pale lemon tint, the hair is snow white and the sclera may be slightly jaundiced as a result of mild haemolysis. The tongue may be tender, smooth and red because of atrophy of the mucosa. Peripheral neuropathy may be the presenting feature with pain, soreness or numbness of the feet on walking. Later, features of subacute combined degeneration of the cord may develop. Cardiac failure is common if the anaemia is marked. The spleen is sometimes palpable. There is an increased incidence of gastric carcinoma.

Diagnosis

The haemoglobin may be very low. The blood film shows macrocytes usually with anisocytosis and poikilocytosis, and the MCV is usually >100 fl. The total white blood cell (WBC) count may fall because of reduced numbers of both lymphocytes and neutrophils (Table 20.2). Some neutrophils may show hypersegmentation of the nuclei (>5 lobes). There may also be a moderate fall in the platelet count. Reticulocytes are generally not increased until treatment is started.

The marrow is hypercellular, with giant metamyelocytes and megaloblasts present – evidence that anaemia is in part caused by suppression of cell release. *Megaloblasts* (Fig. 20.2) are found only rarely in the peripheral blood. They are characterised by a large and inactive nucleus (maturation arrest) in a relatively hypermature, and even haemoglobinised, cytoplasm. They are not present in normal marrow and their presence denotes vitamin B_{12} or folate deficiency, which may be secondary to antifolate or phenytoin therapy. If sufficiently severe, vitamin B_{12}

Table 20.2 White cells. Normal white cell count: 4–10 × 10⁹/l

Neutrophils – normal range: $2.0–7.5 \times 10^9/l$ (40–75% of total white cells)
Causes of neutrophilia (raised neutrophil count)
- Acute bacterial infections
- Inflammation, e.g. arteritis
- Acute tissue necrosis, e.g. myocardial infarction, large pressure sores, burns
- Acute haemorrhages
- Leukaemias

Causes of neutropenia (low neutrophil count)
Viral infections, e.g. glandular fever, measles, acquired immunodeficiency syndrome (AIDS)
Drug reactions, e.g. carbimazole, chemotherapy
Blood diseases, e.g. leukaemias, pernicious anaemia, aplastic anaemia

Lymphocytes – normal adult range: $1.5–4.0 \times 10^9/l$ (20–45% of total)
There are two main subpopulations of T-lymphocytes, which bear different surface markers, or cluster of differentiation (CD) antigens. CD8 cells are 'cytotoxic' – their main function is to recognise and kill cells expressing foreign (usually viral) proteins. CD4 cells are 'helper' cells – they help B-lymphocytes to differentiate into plasma cells and produce antibodies. The normal ratio of CD4 : CD8 cells is 2 : 1.

Causes of lymphocytosis (raised lymphocyte count)
- Acute viral infections, e.g. glandular fever, chickenpox, rubella, mumps
- Lymphatic leukaemia
- Vasculitis and drug hypersensitivity

Causes of lymphopenia (low lymphocyte count)
- AIDS – a severely depressed CD4 count predicts the onset of opportunistic infections
- Ionising radiation (treatment for malignancy or accidental)
- Chemotherapy for malignancy
- Steroid therapy or Cushing syndrome

Eosinophils – normal range: $0.04–0.4 \times 10^9/l$
Causes of eosinophilia (raised eosinophil count)
- Allergies, e.g. bronchial asthma, urticaria, hay fever, drug reaction
- Parasitic infestation of gut or other tissues (muscles, subcutaneous tissues, liver, urinary tract)
- Systemic vasculitis (see Chapter 18 – polyarteritis nodosa; Churg–Strauss syndrome); Hodgkin's disease, see later

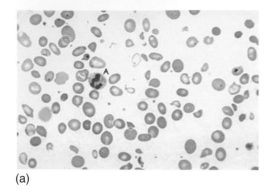

(a)

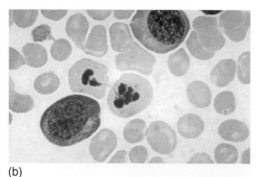

(b)

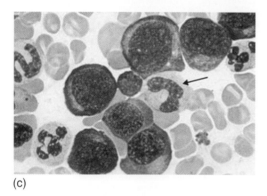

(c)

Figure 20.2 (a) Peripheral blood in megaloblastic anaemia, showing a hypersegmented neutrophil (A), oval macrocytes and poikilocytosis (variation in red cell shape). (b) Bone marrow in megaloblastic anaemia showing megaloblasts. (c) Megaloblasts with developing myeloid cells; the cell with a C-shaped nucleus (arrow) is a giant metamyelocyte. Source: Mehta and Hoffbrand (2009) *Haematology at a Glance*, 3rd edn. Oxford: Wiley-Blackwell.

and folate deficiencies produce depression of all the marrow elements, including neutrophils and platelets. There is usually some haemolysis with a raised unconjugated serum bilirubin. The haptoglobins are reduced. Urobilinogen is present in the urine as a result of reduced red cell survival and ineffective erythropoiesis. Antibodies to parietal cells are present in >90% of patients and to intrinsic factor in approximately 55%. Not all individuals who have parietal cell antibodies have pernicious anaemia.

Patients with pernicious anaemia treated with vitamin B_{12} usually have normal peripheral blood and a normal marrow within 24 h. The serum folates and B_{12} are normal. Parietal cell and intrinsic factor antibodies are still present.

Treatment

Vitamin B_{12} as hydroxocobalamin 1 mg is given five times at 2-day intervals and then every 3 months for life. The response of the marrow to therapy is very rapid with an early reticulocyte response maximal on the fourth to sixth day. The haemoglobin follows this and rises about 10 g/l every 1–2 weeks. The WBC and platelets are normal in about 7 days. The rapid production of cells with therapy may reveal an associated deficiency of, and demand for, iron, potassium or folic acid and supplements should be given where necessary.

Neurological features of B_{12} deficiency usually improve to some degree; sensory abnormalities more completely than motor, and peripheral neuropathy more than myelopathy. However, neurological features may remain static and occasionally even deteriorate.

NB: If folic acid alone is given to patients with pernicious anaemia the neurological features may become worse.

Blood transfusion contains enough B_{12} to make interpretation of serum B_{12} levels difficult. If anaemia is severe it may precipitate heart failure.

Folic acid deficiency

Folic acid is found in green vegetables and liver.

- *Dietary deficiency.* In the UK this is most commonly seen in chronic alcoholics, the poor and the elderly who eat no green vegetables. In the tropics it is often seen in association with multiple deficiencies and with gut infection and infestation.
- *Malabsorption* (page 153, Chapter 12).
- *Increased requirement.* Pregnancy and infancy. Haemolysis results in increased red cell formation, which requires folate more than B_{12}.
- *Folate metabolism.* Phenytoin therapy interferes with folate metabolism.

Haemolytic anaemia (Table 20.3)

Haemolytic anaemias are rare in the UK. Haemolysis is characterised by jaundice with a raised unconjugated serum bilirubin, increased urobilinogen in urine and stools, reticulocytosis and decreased haptoglobins. Haptoglobin binds free haemoglobin to form a hapto-globin-hemoglobin complex, which is removed by the reticuloendothelial system. Lactate dehydrogenase (LDH) is released by the lysed red cells, and serum levels are elevated. There is no bile pigment in the urine (the jaundice is acholuric). Splenomegaly and pigment stones may occur. The blood film may show polychromasia, spherocytes, and crenated and frag-mented red cells. There may be features of:

- rapid red cell destruction – increased plasma haemoglobin, methaemalbuminaemia, decreased haptoglobins, haemoglobinuria and haemosider-inuria;
- excess red cell formation – reticulocytosis, erythroid hyperplasia and increased folate requirements.

Hereditary haemolytic anaemias

These are caused by defects in the red cell membrane or specific red cell enzyme deficiencies.

Hereditary spherocytosis

An autosomal dominant disorder that causes increased osmotic fragility and produces spherocytes in the peripheral blood. Patients present with an intermittent jaundice, which may be confused with Gilbert's syn-drome or with recurrent hepatitis. Gallstones, leg ulcers, splenomegaly and haemolytic or aplastic crises during intercurrent infections may occur.

Splenectomy relieves the symptoms but does not cure the underlying defect.

Table 20.3 Classification of haemolytic anaemias

Intrinsic red cell disorders (abnormal RBCs) (all Coombs-negative)	Extrinsic disorders (normal RBCs)

Membrane disorder
 Hereditary spherocytosis; hereditary elliptocytosis
 Enzyme deficiency
 G6PD; pyruvate kinase
	Immune
	 Autoimmune (Coombs-positive)
	 Warm antibodies
	   Idiopathic
	   Secondary (SLE, CLL, lymphoma, Hodgkin's, carcinoma, drugs: methyldopa, mefenamic acid)
	   Cold-agglutinins
	   Idiopathic
	   Secondary (*Mycoplasma*, glandular fever, lymphoma)
	   Lysis

Haemoglobinopathy Sickle-cell anaemia; thalassaemia	*Isoimmune* (Coombs-negative) Mismatched transfusion Haemolytic disease of the newborn **Non-immune** (Coombs-negative) *Mechanical haemolytic anaemias*: disseminated intravascular coagulation, microangiopathic haemolytic anaemia (thrombotic thrombocytopenic purpura), haemolytic–uraemic syndrome, postcardiotomy – prosthetic heart valves (red-cell fragmentation), march haemoglobinuria, hypersplenism and burns *Infections*: malaria, *Clostridium perfringens*, viral infections *Paroxysmal nocturnal haemoglobinuria* *Drugs*: e.g. oxidative damage, dapsone, salazopyrine Secondary to renal or liver disease

CLL, chronic lymphoid leukaemia; G6PD, glucose-6-phosphate dehydrogenase; RBC, red blood cell; SLE, systemic lupus erythematosus.

Hereditary elliptocytosis

This is also inherited as an autosomal dominant trait and produces elliptical red blood cells, variable degrees of haemolysis and, rarely, splenomegaly.

Glucose-6-phosphate dehydrogenase deficiency

This is a disease found predominantly in Africa, the Mediterranean, the Middle and Far East. Inheritance is sex-linked on the X chromosome (affected males always show clinical manifestations but females will have variable degrees of haemolysis). Because of the phenomenon of random inactivation of the X chromosome, females will have two populations of red blood cells (RBCs), one normal and one glucose-6-phosphate dehydrogenase (G6PD) deficient: the susceptibility to haemolysis will be greater, the greater the size of the deficient population. In the UK, acute haemolytic episodes are usually drug-induced (sulfonamides, primaquine) or occur during acute infections. Attacks can be triggered by eating fava (broad) beans (favism). Neonatal jaundice is also a feature.

The diagnosis is confirmed by reduced or absent enzyme activity in the red cells.

Paroxysmal nocturnal haemoglobinuria (PNH)

This is an acquired clonal disorder of haematopoiesis in which cells have deficient production of the phospholipid glycosylphosphatidylinositol that anchors certain proteins to the cell surface. These include CD55 (delay accelerating factor) and CD59 (membrane inhibitor of reactive lysis), which protects cells from complement-mediated lysis. This accounts for the increased sensitivity of red cells to complement, which forms the basis of Ham's acid lysis test.

The clinical features occur usually in the over-30s, who develop paroxysmal haemolysis (with anaemia, macrocytosis, reticulocytosis, haemoglobinuria and haemosiderinuria) and life-threatening venous thromboses. Renal tubular iron deposition can be associated with renal failure, and gallstones are common. Patients may develop aplastic anaemia. Spontaneous remission can occur. Long-term anticoagulation should be considered.

Eculizumab, a monoclonal antibody that blocks the activation of terminal complement (page 176, Chapter 14) is licensed for the treatment of PNH.

Haemoglobinopathies

Clinical features

Normal adult haemoglobin is made up of two polypeptide chains, the alpha- and beta-chains, which are folded such that each chain can hold an oxygen-binding haem molecule. The haemoglobinopathies are a diverse group of disorders of haemoglobin synthesis which include sickle-cell anaemia (abnormal beta-chain synthesis) and the thalassaemias (deficient or absent alpha- or beta-chain synthesis). Together they form the most common group of single-gene disorders worldwide.

Genetic basis of haemoglobinopathies

Genes encoding five different beta-globin chains (beta, delta, gamma-A, gamma-C, epsilon) and three different α-globin chains are expressed in a precisely regulated manner during different stages of development. During fetal life the two β-globin variants called γ-globin combine with two α-globin chains to give rise to fetal haemoglobin (HbF). During adult life the β-globin variants combine with α-globin chains to form adult haemoglobin (HbA). HbA$_2$ is <3% of haemoglobin in adults and possesses two α- and two δ-chains.

The five β-globin chain genes are clustered on chromosome 11, whereas the α-globin chain genes occur together on chromosome 16. Numerous different mutations in the α-globin and β-globin genes have been described, which give rise to α- or β-thalassaemia, respectively. Sickle-cell anaemia is caused by a point mutation, which involves substitution of T for A in the second nucleotide of the sixth codon, changing the sixth amino acid from glutamine to valine in β-globin.

NB: HbA is 95% of haemoglobin in adults and possesses two α- and two β-chains ($\alpha_2\beta_2$.)

HbF is <0.5% of haemoglobin in adults and possesses two α- and two γ-chains ($\alpha_2\gamma_2$).

Sickle-cell haemoglobin (HbS) possesses two α- and two abnormal β-chains.

Haemoglobin A$_2$ (HbA$_2$) is <3% of haemoglobin in adults and possesses two α- and two δ-chains ($\alpha_2\delta_2$).

Sickle-cell disease

Sickle-cell disease is found predominantly in Africa, the Middle East, the Mediterranean and India and is transmitted as an autosomal dominant trait. Sickle-cell trait occurs in heterozygotes (HbA–HbS) whose haemoglobin contains characteristically 60% HbA and 40% HbS. Patients with the trait are usually symptom-free except when the oxygen tension is very low, e.g. through altitude and anoxic anaesthesia. The prevalence of the gene is probably because the HbS protects against the serious and occasionally lethal effects of falciparum malaria.

Sickle-cell disease occurs in homozygotes (HbS–HbS). The abnormal haemoglobin renders red blood cells susceptible to very small reductions in oxygen tension. This leads to the sickling phenomenon and to abnormal sequestration with thrombosis in small arterioles. The subsequent infarction may affect any part of the body.

Clinical features

In sickle-cell disease anaemia occurs within the first months of life as levels of HbF fall. Acute haemolytic crises begin after 6 months, causing bone infarcts, which are common, and children may present with pain and swelling in the fingers and toes (dactylitis). Infarcts may cause abdominal pain, haematuria or cerebrovascular accidents. Splenic infarction is common and by the age of 1 year children can be functionally asplenic. Repeated renal infarction causes chronic kidney disease.

Prognosis

Sickle-cell disease carries a high infant and child mortality from thrombosis to a vital organ or infection, with pneumococcus the most common as a result of hyposplenism. Children who survive beyond 4–5 years continue to have chronic ill health with anaemia, haemolytic and thrombotic crises, leg ulcers and infections (which may precipitate crises). Folate supplements are required throughout life. Pneumococcal vaccine should be given and penicillin prescribed to reduce mortality from pneumococcus. Hydroxyurea can help by increasing HbF production. Bone marrow transplantation is curative but limited by availability of well-matched donors.

Thalassaemia

Thalassaemia is found predominantly in the Middle and Far East and the Mediterranean and is caused by deficient alpha- or beta-chain synthesis. The deficiency is genetically determined and results in α- or β-thalassaemia. In the latter, gamma-chains continue to be produced in excess into adult life and excess HbF is present.

β-Thalassaemia minor (heterozygote)

This usually presents as a symptom-free, mild, microcytic, hypochromic anaemia which may be confused with iron deficiency. It is diagnosed by finding a raised HbA_2 level generally (4–7%). HbF levels may also be slightly raised (1–3%).

β-Thalassaemia major (homozygote)

Patients are relatively normal at birth (little beta-chain anyway) but develop severe anaemia later with failure to thrive and are prone to infection. The anaemia is hypochromic and the film contains target cells ('Mexican hat' cells) and stippling. Erythroid hyperplasia occurs in the marrow and chain precipitation appears as inclusion bodies on supravital staining. Infants who survive develop hepatosplenomegaly, bossing of the skull, brittle and overgrown long bones, gallstones and leg ulcers.

Transfusion can be used to maintain the haemoglobin at 100 g/l, but this, combined with increased iron absorption, results in iron overload. Desferrioxamine is given to reduce haemosiderosis with folic acid replacement, and splenectomy may be indicated if hypersplenism supervenes. Bone marrow transplantation has been used successfully.

Marrow disorders

Myeloproliferative disorders

Polycythemia vera (PV), essential thombocytosis (ET) and primary myelofibrosis (PMF) are related myeloproliferative disorders in which there is clonal expansion of haematopoietic progenitors. A somatic point mutation in the JAK2 (Janus kinase 2) non-receptor tyrosine kinase (JAK2V617F) was identified in most patients with PV and in about half of patients with ET and PMF. JAK2V617F has constitutive tyrosine kinase activity and is able to activate JAK-STAT signalling and transform hematopoietic cells. Median survival in both essential thrombocythaemia and polycythaemia vera exceeds 15 years and the 10-year risk of developing either myelofibrosis or acute myeloid leukaemia is relatively low. Prognosis is worse in primary myelofibrosis.

Polycythaemia vera usually presents in late middle age (50–60 years), most commonly as a chance haematological finding. If symptomatic, it presents usually with vascular occlusion, arterial or venous or, much less often, with gout, pruritus or a finding of

---

CASE STUDY Anaemia

A 73-year-old Caucasian male presents to his GP with tiredness. He had received treatment with lisinopril 10 mg o.d. for hypertension for 20 years, and had recently been taking lactulose 15 ml b.d. to alleviate constipation. He has smoked 20 cigarettes per day for 50 years, and drinks around 20 units of alcohol per week.

His blood pressure was 130/84, and further physical examination was unremarkable. Urinalysis was normal.

Investigations showed haemoglobin 76 g/l with MCV 76 fl and MCH 24 pg. White blood cell count was normal, but platelet count was elevated at 485×10^9/l. Serum creatinine was 126 μmol/l and electrolytes and blood glucose were normal. Liver function tests and bone profile were normal. One year previously haemoglobin was 145 g/l, and serum creatinine was 125 μmol/l.

The patient has a hypochromic microcytic anaemia, with an elevated platelet count. In addition *the patient has stable chronic kidney disease stage 3A. Calculated eGFR (Chapter 14) is 52 ml/min/1.73m², and was 53 ml/min/1.73m² 1 year previously. The absence of blood or protein on urinalysis make a primary glomerular disease unlikely, and his CKD is likely to be related to his hypertension or vascular disease. Although chronic kidney disease (CKD) is associated with anaemia, the level of haemoglobin is lower than would be expected at this stage of CKD and the hypochromic microcytic picture and elevated platelet count suggest bleeding. Iron deficiency was confirmed by finding a low serum iron with a high transferrin and low transferrin saturation. The recent alteration in bowel habit suggest a lower gastrointestinal source and colonoscopy revealed a carcinoma of the transverse colon. Smoking and drinking alcohol are associated with an increased risk of colorectal cancer.*

---

splenomegaly. Diagnosis is established by the presence of:

- a raised haemoglobin or red cell mass >25% above mean normal predicted value, *and* the presence of *JAK2*V617F or a similar mutation (major criteria);
- evidence of bone marrow trilineage myeloproliferation *or* subnormal erythropoietin levels *or* endogenous erythroid colony growth (minor criteria).

A diagnosis of polycythaemia vera can also be made if there is a raised haemoglobin or red cell mass and two minor criteria.

Secondary causes to be excluded include hypoxaemia and renal disease (ultrasound for polycystic disease and hypernephroma). Cerebellar haemangioblastoma and hepatoma are associated but very rare. Treatment is with repeated venesection, low-dose aspirin to reduce the incidence of intravascular coagulation and hydroxyurea in high-risk patients who are elderly or have a history of thrombosis.

NB: In polycythaemia vera, all cellular elements can be raised (RBCs, WBCs and platelets). In secondary polycythaemia (e.g. caused by increased erythropoietin production in hypoxia or renal disease) only the red cell count is raised.

Essential thrombocythaemia, if not found incidentally, presents with small vessel vascular occlusion.

Diagnosis depends on finding all four major criteria:

1. a platelet count $>450 \times 10^9 l^{-1}$ *and*
2. megakaryocyte proliferation with no or little granulocyte or erythroid proliferation *and*
3. presence of *JAK2*V617F or other clonal marker or no evidence of reactive thrombocytosis *and*
4. not meeting criteria for other myeloid neoplasms. Treatment is with low-dose aspirin and hydroxyurea in high-risk patients who are elderly or have a history of thrombosis.

Primary myelofibrosis typically presents with the finding of huge and increasing splenomegaly, and evidence of bone marrow failure: anaemia, infection, bleeding. Diagnosis depends on finding all three major criteria:

1. proliferation of atypical megakaryocytes with either reticulin and/or collagen fibrosis, or megakaryocyte changes accompanied by increased marrow cellularity, granulocytic proliferation and often decreased erythropoiesis;
2. presence of *JAK2*V617F or other clonal marker or no evidence of reactive marrow fibrosis *and*
3. not meeting criteria for other myeloid neoplasms.

In addition, two of the minor criteria should be met: leucoerythroblastosis, raised LDH, anaemia and splenomegaly.

Hydroxyurea, thalidomide and the thalidomide analogue lenalidomide have been used in therapy. Allogeneic hematopoietic stem cell transplantation is potentially curative.

Myelodysplastic syndromes

Myelodysplastic syndromes are a heterogeneous group of disorders that are characterised by clonal and ineffective hematopoiesis in the setting of a dysplastic bone marrow, peripheral blood cytopenias and progressive bone marrow failure. Transformation to acute myeloid leukaemia occurs in approximately 30% of cases. Survival following diagnosis varies from a few months to >10 years.

It is usually discovered on a routine peripheral blood film, usually as macrocytosis (with normal B_{12}, folates, liver and thyroid function tests, and γ-glutamyl transferase). Less commonly, patients may present with a refractory anaemia, pancytopenia, neutropenia or thrombocytopenia (Table 20.4).

Classification is continuously under review, but there are five major subgroups, which tend to have decreasingly satisfactory prognoses:

1. refractory anaemia
2. refractory anaemia with ringed sideroblasts
3. refractory anaemia with excess blasts
4. refractory anaemia with excess blasts in transformation
5. chronic myelomonocytic leukaemia.

NB: Sideroblasts are nucleated red cells that contain perinuclear rings of iron-containing granules. Although

---

Table 20.4 Causes of platelet disorders (normal range 150–400 × 10⁹/l)

Thrombocytosis (increased platelets)
- After haemorrhage, surgery or trauma
- Splenectomy or splenic atrophy
- Inflammation (as part of an inflammatory response)
- Malignancy
- Myeloproliferative disorders, e.g. megakaryocytic leukaemia (rare)

Thrombocytopenia (decreased platelets)
- Adverse drug reactions (e.g. NSAIDs, phenothiazines, gold, thiazides)
- Autoimmune thrombocytopenic purpura, in which circulating antiplatelet antibodies lead to premature platelet destruction
- Marrow aplasia

NB: If also anaemic, exclude disseminated intravascular coagulation (see later) and prosthetic valve dysfunction.

---

hereditary forms of sideroblastic anaemia exist, sideroblasts are most frequently seen in myelodysplastic syndromes.

Treatment

Haematinics (iron, folate, B_{12}) are ineffective. Blood transfusion is necessary and has to be repeated regularly. Chemotherapy, lenalidomide and allogenic bone marrow transplantation have all been used in therapy.

Complications

Anaemia (requiring the transfusion of about 1 unit blood/week), infection, haemorrhage and blast transformation.

Marrow failure

Marrow aplasia

Primary aplastic anaemia gives a pancytopenia with reduction in all the formed elements. It is rare. Patients present with:

- anaemia; and/or
- spontaneous bleeding because of lack of platelets; and/or
- infection caused by lack of polymorphonuclear leucocytes.

A peripheral blood film reveals a pancytopenia, although one cell line may be affected more than the others. A bone marrow aspiration is performed. If it is difficult to aspirate (possible myelofibrosis or malignancy), a trephine biopsy may be necessary to obtain a diagnostic specimen of marrow. The drugs that most commonly cause marrow suppression include cytotoxic drugs, gold, indometacin and chloramphenicol. Some marrow suppression is associated with uraemia, rheumatoid arthritis and hypothyroidism.

Bleeding disorders

Haemophilias

Haemophilia A (classical haemophilia) or haemophilia B (Christmas disease) results from defects in the clotting factor VIII (on chromosome Xq28) or factor IX (on chromosome Xq27), respectively. They are sex-linked recessive clotting disorders of men, carried by women, in which patients suffer mainly from spontaneous bleeding into joints and soft tissues and excessive bleeding in response to trauma or surgery. Carriers who wish to have children should be offered genetic counselling.

Treatment

Treatment is by replacement of the deficient clotting factor. As soon as possible after bleeding has started, purified factor VIII or IX is given as required. Purified factor VIII is also used to raise factor VIII levels in von Willebrand's disease (see later). Fresh frozen plasma contains both factors but is best reserved for when the single factors are not available. Aspirin-containing preparations should be avoided because they impair platelet function and may cause gastric erosion. Desmopressin can be used to increase factor VIII levels in mild to moderate haemophilia.

Von Willebrand's disease

This is a autosomal dominant disease of both sexes in which deficient or abnormal production of von Willebrand's factor causes abnormal bleeding. Factor VIII circulates bound to von Willebrand factor, which is a cofactor for platelet adhesion. There is a prolonged bleeding time, low factor VIII clotting activity and poor platelet adhesion

Skin haemorrhage

- Purpura refers to small areas of cutaneous bleeding. The purplish red spots do not fade on pressure. Ecchymosis refers to larger lesions (bruises).
- The most common causes of skin haemorrhage are senile purpura, therapy with corticosteroids or anticoagulants and, less commonly, thrombocytopenia caused by leukaemia and marrow aplasia.

Thrombocytopenia

This may result from decreased production (marrow aplasia, leukaemia or infiltration) or increased destruction (idiopathic thrombocytopenic purpura, hypersplenism and consumption coagulopathy).

Idiopathic thrombocytopenic purpura

Idiopathic thrombocytopenic purpura (ITP) is rare and not to be confused with thrombotic thrombocytopenic purpura (TTP), which is very rare. ITP occurs chiefly in children following a respiratory or gastrointestinal viral infection. Patients present with purpura

and a low platelet count. If the platelet count is very low, major bleeding may occur from the nose or gut or into the brain. The bleeding time is prolonged but coagulation times are normal. Spontaneous recovery is the rule. Steroids or intravenous immunoglobulin may be of benefit in the more severe cases, occasionally with lasting remission. Splenectomy should be avoided if possible, especially in children, in view of the risk of pneumococcal septicaemia in asplenic patients, but may be curative when medical management is unsuccessful.

Thrombotic thrombocytopenic purpura

Thrombotic thrombocytopenic purpura (TTP) is a rare disease that usually occurs in young adults and is characterised by microangiopathic haemolytic anaemia and thrombocytopenia, and microvascular thrombosis that causes variable tissue ischaemia and infarction. It typically occurs in patients with an acquired deficiency of the plasma metalloprotease ADAMTS13 (a disintegrin and metalloproteinase with a thrombospondin type 1 motif, member 13, also known as von Willebrand factor cleaving protease), which responds to plasma exchange in approximately 80% of cases. Prognosis is worse when it is associated with malignancy, drugs or transplantation. Familial TTP due to an inherited deficiency of ADAMTS13 can be treated with plasma infusions.

Henoch–Schönlein purpura

(See page 332, Chapter 18.)

Osler's disease (Osler–Weber–Rendu)

This is a hereditary haemorrhagic telangiectasia (autosomal dominant), which may present as intermittent bleeding, usually gastrointestinal. There are small capillary angiectases throughout the gastrointestinal tract, including the buccal mucosa and tongue. The majority of cases are caused by mutations in the genes coding endoglin or activin receptor-like kinase 1, which act as receptors for TGF-beta.

Disseminated intravascular coagulation (DIC)

This occurs in many severe insults including sepsis, trauma, malignancy, organ failure, obstetric practice (amniotic fluid embolism, placental abruption, pre-eclampsia), transplantation and mismatched blood transfusion. There is systemic activation of coagulation pathways that leads to formation of fibrin clots, which may cause organ failure, together with consumption of platelets and coagulation factors, which may result in bleeding. Diagnosis is based on finding a low platelet count and evidence of intravascular coagulation – prolonged clotting times with low fibrinogen and increased fibrin degradation products.

Treatment is of the underlying disease, usually septicaemia. Transfusions of platelet, plasma or factor concentrates may be used to prevent or stop bleeding. Heparin may be of value in cases where thrombosis predominates.

Leukaemia

This refers to malignant proliferation of blood-forming cells and is broadly classified according to:

- whether the disease, if untreated, is likely to follow an acute or more prolonged chronic course *and*
- whether lymphocytic or myeloid (marrow-related) cell lines are primarily involved.

Acute lymphatic leukaemia

This, the most common form of childhood leukaemia, accounts for 75–80% of all childhood leukaemias. Infiltration of bone marrow with lymphoblastic cells causes anaemia, bruising (thrombocytopenia) and infections (neutropenia). Lymphoblasts are usually present in the peripheral blood and always in the marrow. Lymphadenopathy, splenomegaly and hepatomegaly occur. Most children with acute lymphatic leukaemia can now be 'cured'.

Chronic lymphatic leukaemia

This occurs in the elderly with a generalised lymphadenopathy and a raised white cell count with lymphocytosis. It usually follows a benign course and treatment is only indicated if symptoms develop.

Acute myeloid leukaemia

This occurs at all ages but less commonly in childhood. Myeloblasts infiltrate the marrow and are found in the blood. Anaemia, bleeding or infections are common. Involvement of other organs is unusual.

Chronic myeloid leukaemia

This usually presents in middle age, often insidiously with anaemia, weight loss and fever. White cell count is markedly raised with myeloid precursors in the marrow and peripheral blood. The spleen, and in later stages the liver, are markedly enlarged. In over 90% of patients leucocytes contain the Philadelphia chromosome, a translocation of the breakpoint cluster region (*BCR*) gene on the long arm of chromosome 22 to a position adjacent to the *c-ABL* gene on chromosome 9. This results in formation of a *BCR-ABL* fusion gene, and the subsequent expression of the BCR-ABL fusion protein is involved in the malignant transformation of myeloid cells.

Lymphoma

These are solid tumours of the lymphoreticular system that are divided histologically into two main types: Hodgkin's disease, characterised by the presence of multinucleated giant cells (Reed–Sternberg cells); and non-Hodgkin's lymphoma (Fig. 20.3).

Clinical features

Patients may present with painless lymphadenopathy. Symptoms, if present, include lethargy, anorexia, weight loss, fever, night sweats and pruritus. Hepatomegaly and splenomegaly may occur.

Lymphomas are staged according to the extent of disease:

- Stage I: involvement of a single lymph node region.
- Stage II: two regions involved on the same side of the diaphragm.
- Stage III: disease on both sides of the diaphragm, but limited to nodes, spleen or a single extralymphatic organ or site.
- Stage IV: diffuse involvement of one or more extra-lymphatic sites, with or without lymph node involvement.

In Hodgkin's disease the suffix A (e.g. stage IIA) denotes the absence of symptoms, whereas the suffix B denotes the presence of >10% loss of body weight, fever or night sweats.

The diagnosis is usually made on lymph node biopsy. Staging requires careful examination for superficial nodes and computed tomographic (CT) scanning. Treatment is with chemotherapy, radiotherapy or a combination of the two depending on clinical, radiological and histological staging.

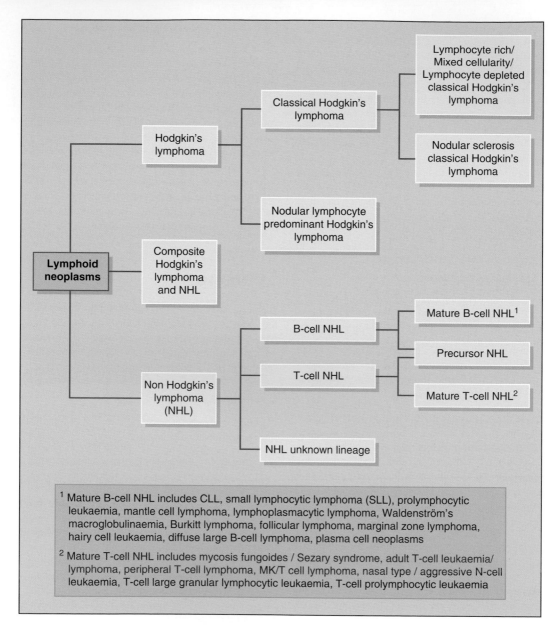

Figure 20.3 Classification of malignant lymphoid neoplasms.

Myeloma

There is malignant proliferation of a specific clone of plasma cells resulting in the production of a monoclonal immunoglobulin known as a paraprotein.

Clinical features

Most cases occur after the age of 50. Nonspecific symptoms include malaise, lethargy and weight loss. Bone destruction from the expanding plasma cell clone causes pain, fractures and hypercalcaemia. Normochromic anaemia, thrombocytopenia and leukopenia (infections are common) occur as the normal bone marrow is replaced. Renal failure may result from hypercalcaemia or the presence of light chains, which may be nephrotoxic or become precipitated in tubules.

The International Myeloma Working Group has produced a classification system for monoclonal gammopathies, multiple myeloma and related disorders:

Monoclonal gammopathy of undetermined significance (MGUS)

Low level of serum monoclonal protein (M-protein) present in serum *and*

bone marrow clonal cells < 10% *with*

no evidence of multiple myeloma, other B-cell proliferative disorders or amyloidosis.

Smouldering or indolent myeloma

M-protein ≥ 30 g/l *and/or*

bone marrow clonal cells ≥ 10% *but*

no related organ or tissue impairment (ROTI) (end-organ damage, see later).

Symptomatic myeloma

M-protein present in serum or urine *and*

bone marrow clonal cells ≥ 10% *and*

evidence of myeloma-related organ damage, which is typically manifested by increased calcium, renal insufficiency, anaemia, or bone lesions (CRAB) attributed to the plasma cell proliferative process.

Solitary plasmacytoma of bone

Biopsy-proven plasmacytoma of bone in a single site only, confirmed by X rays, MRI and/or FDG PET, which may be associated with a low serum and/or urine M-protein

No monoclonal plasma cells in the bone marrow

No other myeloma-related organ dysfunction.

Investigation

There is usually anaemia with a markedly raised ESR. The monoclonal antibody is detected as a discrete M band on plasma protein electrophoresis. Free immunoglobulin light chains may be detectable in the urine (Bence Jones proteins are urinary light chains that precipitate on heating to 56 °C and redissolve on boiling). There may be hypercalcaemia and renal failure. Osteolytic lesions are seen on X-ray. Alkaline phosphatase is usually normal (lesions are destructive without osteoclastic activity).

In *Waldenström's macroglobulinaemia* a monoclonal IgM paraprotein is produced. Radiological involvement of bone is rare, but anaemia and a bleeding tendency occur. Plasmapheresis is indicated if symptoms related to hyperviscosity are present.

Management of haematological malignancies

Management of haematological malignancies is under continuous review, and many patients are entered into multicentre trials. Patients should be treated in units with specialist experience of the drug regimens and supportive treatment, including transfusions and antibiotics.

Cytotoxics (to destroy rapidly dividing cells) are used alone or in combination with radiotherapy. In some cases induction of remission by intensive chemotherapy is followed by bone marrow transplantation. The following drugs are commonly used.

Alkylating agents

Alkylating agents transfer alkyl groups to DNA, interfering with its replication. They reduce fertility in males (consider sperm storage) and may be associated with premature menopause in females. They are teratogenic, but there does not appear to be an increase in fetal abnormalities in patients who are fertile after treatment. Bone marrow depression is common and prolonged use is associated with an increased incidence of acute non-lymphocytic leukaemia.

- *Cyclophosphamide* and the related drug *ifosfamide* for chronic lymphocytic leukaemia and lymphoma. Mesna is given if high intravenous doses are given to prevent haemorrhagic cystitis, which is caused by the urinary metabolite acrolein.
- *Chlorambucil* for chronic lymphatic leukaemia, lymphoma and Waldenström's macroglobulinaemia.
- *Melphalan* for myeloma.
- *Busulphan* for chronic myeloid leukaemia.
- *Lomustine (CCNU)* is a nitrosourea used for Hodgkin's disease.
- *Carmustine* is related to lomustine and used for multiple myeloma and non-Hodgkin's lymphoma.

Antimetabolites

Antimetabolites are usually competitive analogues of normal metabolites. They cause gastrointestinal upsets and bone marrow depression.

- *Mercaptopurine, cladribine, clofabrine, nelarabine* are purine analogues used in acute leukaemias.
- *Cladribine* is a purine analogue used for hairy cell leukaemia.

- *Cytarabine, fludarabine* and *fluorouracil* are pyrimidine analogues. Cytarabine is used in the induction of remission in acute myeloblastic leukaemia. Fludarabine is used in B-cell chronic lymphocytic leukaemia.
- *Tioguanine* (thioguanine) is a guanine analogue that it used for acute leukaemias and chronic myeloid leukaemia.
- *Methotrexate* inhibits dihydrofolate reductase, preventing synthesis of tetrahydrofolic acid that is needed as a coenzyme for synthesis of nucleic acids. It is used for childhood acute lymphoblastic leukaemia and non-Hodgkin's lymphoma. Folinic acid can help to prevent myelosuppression and mucositis. It is excreted by the kidneys.

Vinca alkaloids

The *vinca alkaloids* arrest the cell cycle in mitosis. They cause peripheral and autonomic neuropathy and alopecia. *Vincristine, vinblastine* and *vindesine* are used for lymphomas and acute leukaemias.

Cytotoxic antibiotics

Cytotoxic antibiotics interfere with DNA or RNA synthesis through various mechanisms. *Doxorubicin* is used to treat lymphomas and acute leukaemias. *Bleomycin* is used to treat lymphomas. Mucositis and skin pigmentation occur. Dose-related pulmonary fibrosis limits prolonged use.

Monoclonal antibodies

A number of monoclonal antibodies have been approved for the treatment of haematological malignancies. Examples include:

Anti-CD20 binds to CD20 on all B-cells, and is used for CLL (rituximab, ofatumumab and obinotuzumab) and B-cell lymphoma (rituximab).

Anti-CD52 binds to CD52 on the surface of mature lymphocytes. Alemtuzumab is indicated for B-cell chronic lymphocytic leukaemia in patients who have been treated with alkylating agents and have failed fludarabine therapy

Amyloidosis

Amyloidosis is characterised by the tissue deposition of fibrillar proteins that stain with Congo red. Excess κ and λ light chains, associated with abnormal plasma cell proliferation, can form AL-type amyloid. In reactive (secondary or AA-type) amyloidosis, amyloid A protein is deposited, usually after many years of an inflammatory response induced by chronic infection or rheumatic disease. Amyloid A is a 76-amino-acid polypeptide fragment of an acute-phase protein termed serum amyloid A.

Although any organ can be involved, proteinuria is the most common presenting feature. Other sites commonly involved are the gastrointestinal tract, heart and liver.

Treatment is aimed at reducing production of amyloid precursor proteins through immunosuppression or chemotherapy. Chemotherapy followed by autologous stem cell transplantation has been used in AL amyloidosis.

In long-term dialysis, the patient's β_2-microglobulin is deposited as amyloid in musculoskeletal tissue and the carpal tunnel. In Alzheimer's disease and Down syndrome amyloid plaques are found in the cerebral cortex.

21

Infectious diseases

Within the community, virus infections of the upper respiratory and gastrointestinal tract are the most common, followed by common virus infections usually of children such as chickenpox. Infections seen more frequently in hospitals usually relate to a single organ system and are dealt with in the relevant chapters.

Less frequent, but in diagnostic and management terms more difficult, are the imported diseases, septicaemia, pyrexia of unknown origin and infections of the immunosuppressed. The common infections, likely organisms and antibiotics of choice are shown in Table 21.1.

Imported diseases

The common diseases of travellers (Table 21.2) returning to temperate climates are malaria, acute gastroenteritis including typhoid, infectious hepatitis and worm infestation. Diarrhoea in returning travellers requires investigation for worms and parasites (especially *Giardia* and amoeba), but usually no organism is found and the symptoms settle spontaneously or with simple therapy. Other diseases in the tropics but rarely seen in returning travellers include tuberculosis, schistosomiasis, hydatid disease, tetanus, cholera, and trypanosomiasis. Multidrug treatment for leprosy is available free of charge through the World Health Organization, and the global registered prevalence of leprosy at the end of 2016 had fallen to 173,358 cases. There were just 22 reported cases of polio in 2017.

Malaria

Malaria is a disease of the subtropics and where the anopheline mosquito is found. Transmission is via the mosquito, which carries infected blood from infected to uninfected humans. The mosquito lives chiefly between latitude 15° North and South and not more than 1500 m (5000 ft) above sea level.

Clinical features

The patient may present with fever and rigors usually within 4 weeks of returning from or travelling through a malarial zone, but atypical presentations are common. Occasionally symptoms may not develop for 12 months or more. The patient has usually failed to take antimalarials regularly, not slept under mosquito nets or failed to continue prophylaxis for 6 weeks after returning. Diagnosis depends upon clinical awareness and then seeing the parasite in a blood film or detecting malaria antigens with a rapid diagnostic test. In the UK, *P. falciparum* and *P. vivax* are most frequently seen in travellers from Africa and Asia. Malignant tertian malaria refers to *P. falciparum* which, very occasionally, produces high levels of parasitaemia (only *P. falciparum* gives red blood cell parasitaemia of >1–2%), and serious complications of cerebral malaria or acute haemolysis and renal failure (blackwater fever).

Prophylaxis

Prophylaxis is by a combination of mosquito control, clothing cover, insect repellants, sleeping under mosquito nets and specific prophylaxis. Before advising travellers, check whether they are entering a malarial zone, and seek advice from the nearest centre for tropical diseases about the current recommended prophylaxis because drug resistance continually changes. Drugs used in prophylaxis include chloroquine, mefloquine, doxycycline and atovaquone-proguanil (Malarone®). Prophylaxis should be continued for 6 weeks after returning home, with the exception of Malarone, which only requires 1 week.

Table 21.1 Infections and antibiotics

Infection	Likely organism	Antibacterial of choice
Ear, nose and throat		
Sore throat	Viral (most commonly)	Nil
	Haemolytic streptococcus	Pencillin V or macrolide antibiotic (e.g. clarithromycin) if allergic to penicillin. Avoid amoxicillin if glandular fever possible
Sinusitis	*Streptococcus pneumoniae* (pneumococcus)	Amoxicillin or doxycycline or clarithromycin
	Haemophilus influenza	
Otitis media	Viral	Nil
	As above plus haemolytic streptococcus	Amoxicillin (or macrolide if penicillin allergy) in children
	Haemophilus influenzae	
Acute epiglottitis	*Haemophilus influenzae*	Maintain airway plus intravenous broad-spectrum cephalosporin
Urinary tract[a]		
Acute cystitis	*Escherichia coli*	Trimethoprim, or amoxicillin, or quinolone or cephalosporin
Acute pyelonephritis	*Escherichia coli*	Quinolone or cephalosporin
Prostatitis	*Escherichia coli*	Trimethoprim or quinolone
Bone and soft tissue		
Cellulitis	Haemolytic streptococcus *Staphylococcus aureus*	Flucloxacillin or penicillin if streptococcus confirmed (or macrolide if penicillin allergy)
Drip sites	*Staphylococcus aureus*	Flucloxacillin (or macrolide if penicillin allergy)
Erysipelas	Haemolytic streptococcus	Penicillin (by injection initially if severe; or macrolide if penicillin allergy)
Osteomyelitis	*Staphylococcus aureus*	Flucloxacillin (clindamycin if penicillin allergic) or vancomycin if meticillin-resistant staphylococcus. Add rifampicin or fusidic acid if prosthesis or severe infection. Prolonged treatment is needed
Gastrointestinal infections[b]		
Acute gastroenteritis	Viral	Nil
	Campylobacter	Macrolide or ciprofloxacin
Shigellosis	*Shigella* species	Ciprofloxacin or azithromycin
Amoebic	*Entamoeba histolytica*	Metronidazole
Typhoid fever	*Salmonella typhi*	Ciprofloxacin or cefotaxime
Salmonella	*Salmonella* species (>1000)	Nil (usually) unless invasive when ciprofloxacin or cefotaxime are used
Clostridium difficile	*Clostridium difficile*	Oral metronidazole or vancomycin Ciprofoxacin
Acute cholangitis	*Escherichia coli*	or gentamicin or cefotaxime (resistance to amoxicillin is common in biliary coliforms)
Chest infections (see Chap. 10)		
Acute bronchitis	Viral	Nil
Acute on chronic bronchitis	Bacterial (*H. influenzae*) (*Streptococcus pneumoniae*)	Amoxicillin or tetracycline or macrolide
Pneumonia (community-acquired)	*S. pneumoniae*	Amoxicillin or macrolide if penicillin allergic or atypical pathogen suspected. Add flucloxacillin or vancomycin if staphylococci suspected (e.g. complicating influenza)
	Mycoplasma pneumoniae *Legionella pneumoniae* (rarely *H. influenzae,* psittacosis)	

(Continued)

Table 21.1 (*Continued*)

Infection	Likely organism	Antibacterial of choice
In very unwell	Consider	Macrolide plus cephalosporin (cefotaxime, cefuroxime)
	Coliforms, *Klebsiella*, *Staphylococci* during influenza epidemics	
Meningitis (adult) – most are viral (90%)		
Viral		
Herpes simplex		Acyclovir
Bacterial	*Streptococcus pneumoniae*	Cefotaxime. Substitute penicillin if sensitive
Pneumococcal		Penicillin or cefotaxime / ceftriaxone
Meningococcal	*Neisseria meningitidis*	
Haemophilus (more common in children)	*Haemophilus influenzae*	Cefotaxime (chloramphenicol is an alternative)
Listeriosis	*Listeria monocytogenes*	Amoxicillin+gentamicin

[a] Recurrent infection or 'odd' organisms, e.g. *Klebsiella*, *Pseudomonas*, suggest an underlying abnormality such as stone or tumour and further investigation is required. It is rarely possible to clear infection if there is an indwelling catheter (only treat if systemically ill). Consider replacing the catheter before or when starting antibiotics. Antibiotic use encourages the development of resistant organisms.
[b] Patients with mild gastroenteritis without systemic illness or suspected systemic infection and who are excreting *Shigella* or *Salmonella* (including *S. typhi*) do not require antibiotics. The major problem is usually dehydration. Children in particular need fluid and electrolyte replacement.

Table 21.2 Diseases of the returning traveller

Incidence	Disease
Common	Malaria
	Typhoid
	Diarrhoea often viral as pathogens rarely found but consider:
	Giardia lamblia and worms
	Amoebic colitis, which must be distinguished from ulcerative colitis and Crohn's disease
	Salmonella and *Shigella* infection
	Tropical sprue
	Infectious hepatitis
Rare	Tuberculosis – usually not acute and more likely in Asian immigrants
	Amoebic liver abscess
	Hydatid liver cyst
Exceedingly rare	Rabies
	Cholera
	Exotic viruses
	Lassa fever
	Marburg
	Ebola

Treatment

See Table 21.3.

Acute attacks

Wherever possible diagnosis in patients with suspected malaria should be confirmed with microscopy or a rapid diagnostic test to detect malaria antigens before antimalarial treatment is started.

Uncomplicated *P. falciparum* malaria should be treated with an artemisinin combination therapy (e.g. artemether–lumefantrine (Riamet®) or dihydroartemisinin-piperaquine (Eurartesim®)). Quinine in combination with doxycycline or atovaquone–proguanil (Malarone®) are alternatives. Intravenous therapy should be initiated in severe falciparum malaria, or a high parasite count (>2% of red blood cells). Complications including acute respiratory distress syndrome (page 143, Chapter 11), haemolysis, disseminated intravascular coagulation (page 386, Chapter 20), acute kidney injury, seizures, and intercurrent infections may require intensive care.

Uncomplicated falciparum malaria in the first trimester of pregnancy is usually treated with quinine and clindamycin (seek specialist advice), and in the second and third trimester with artemether–lumefantrine.

Table 21.3 Antimalarial drugs

Drug	Important side effects	Comments
Chloroquine	GI upset, headache, retinal damage and cataracts, rarely myelotoxicity, psychosis. Contraindicated in epilepsy.* Reduce dose in renal failure	Resistance is widespread, but largely confined to *Plasmodium falciparum*. Not active against dormant hepatic forms (hypnozoites) of *Plasmodium vivax* and *Plasmodium ovale*
Eurartesim (dihydroartemisinin and piperaquine)	anaemia, QTc interval prolongation, arrythmia	Treatment of uncomplicated *Plasmodium falciparum*
Fansidar (pyrimethamine and sulfadoxine)	Skin rash, myelotoxicity	For eradication of *Plasmodium falciparum* infection
Maloprim (pyrimethamine and dapsone)		Prophylaxis only
Malarone (proguanil and atovaquone)	GI upset, mouth ulcers, insomnia, blood disorders, skin rash, hyponatraemia	Prophylaxis and treatment of uncomplicated *Plasmodium falciparum*
Mefloquine	Contraindicated in first trimester, breastfeeding, neurological disease, epilepsy* (including family history), liver disease, concurrent β-blocker therapy. Causes neuropsychiatric effects and GI upset. Avoid pregnancy for 3 months after stopping treatment. Treatment duration should not exceed 1 year	Prophylaxis and treatment of chloroquine-resistant *Plasmodium falciparum* malaria
Primaquine	GI upset, haemolysis, particularly in G6PD deficiency	Eradication of dormant hepatic forms (hypnozoites) of *Plasmodium vivax* and *Plasmodium ovale*
Proguanil	GI upset, rarely mouth ulcers. Reduce dose in renal failure	Prophylaxis only
Quinine	Tinnitus, hypoglycaemia, headaches, flushing, GI upset, rash, myelotoxicity	Agent of choice for treatment of chloroquine-resistant or severe *Plasmodium falciparum* malaria
Riamet (artemether and lumefantrine)	GI upset, skin rash, arthralgia, myalgia, arrhythmias (QT prolongation)	Treatment of uncomplicated *Plasmodium falciparum*

GI, gastrointestinal; G6PD, glucose-6-phosphate dehydrogenase.
*Doxycycline is an alternative in patients with epilepsy.

Either oral artemisinin combination therapy or chloroquine can be used for the treatment of non-falciparum malaria (usually *P. vivax,* but occasionally *P. ovale, P. malariae* or *P. knowlesi.*

Dormant parasites (hypnozoites) that persist in the liver after treatment of *P. vivax* or *P. ovale* infection require eradication with primaquine (check the glucose-6-phosphate dehydrogenase status first, and avoid in pregnancy).

Typhoid

Clinical features

Symptoms begin with malaise, headache, dry cough and vague abdominal pain, up to 21 days after returning from a typhoid area. Travellers to any area with poor sanitation are at risk and typhoid occasionally occurs in non-travellers. In the first week, fever is marked, with dry cough and constipation typical features.

CASE STUDY Malaria

A 26-year-old graduate student presented with headaches, myalgia and a fever 4 weeks after returning from a holiday in Indonesia. She had taken doxycline during her time in Indonesia, but had stopped this 2 weeks after her return.

> Malaria is endemic in Indonesia, where the predominant species is *P. falciparum* with a high incidence of chloroquine resistance. Doxycline is appropriate as prophylaxis, but should be continued for 6 weeks after return from an endemic area. A diagnosis of malaria was established by the identification of parasites in less than 1% of the patient's red cells on a Giemsa stained blood smear,

and the presence of *P. falciparum* was confirmed by antigen detection. Haemoglobin levels, liver function tests, blood glucose and serum creatinine and electrolytes were normal.

The patient was treated with artemether–lumefantrine using a 3-day treatment schedule as recommended by the World Health Organization; 4 tablets as a single initial dose, 4 tablets again after 8 h and then 4 tablets twice daily for the following 2 days. The patient was reminded of the importance of continuing malaria prophylaxis for 6 weeks after returning from an endemic area.

In the second week, the fever persists, the abdomen distends, diarrhoea may or may not occur and rose spots develop as crops of pale pink macules on the sides of the abdomen. Delirium and death may occur in untreated cases.

NB: Symptoms of dry cough, constipation and fever should be sufficient to alert the clinician, particularly in returning holiday-makers.

Investigation

Leukopenia and neutropenia may or may not be present. Blood culture is mandatory if typhoid is suspected and culture of urine and stool should also be performed.

Treatment

Salmonella typhi responds to ciprofloxacin. Cefotaxime is also effective.

NB:

- It is unnecessary to give antibiotics to patients who are clinically well but from whom *S. typhi* is grown from the stools. If these patients are given antibiotics, they are more likely to become chronic excretors of antibiotic-resistant *S. typhi*.
- Typhoid must be reported to the public health authorities in the UK.
- Excretors of *S. typhi* are not allowed to work in the food industry.

Dysentery

Bacillary dysentery (shigellosis)

Bacillary dysentery is caused by the genus *Shigella*. *S. sonnei* is the most common and occurs in outbreaks in close communities. It produces the most serious

clinical form of the disease, including septicaemia. It is transmitted by faecal contamination of food and water and 2–4 days after ingestion produces acute diarrhoea, sometimes accompanied by abdominal colic, vomiting and tenesmus. If severe, there is rectal blood, mucus and pus. Asymptomatic carriage can occur.

The disease is prevented by good sanitation, clean water supplies and good personal hygiene. Infected patients should be isolated and rehydrated. Ciprofloxacin (or amoxicillin or trimethoprim if sensitive) are required if the patient is unwell, but antibiotics are not indicated for mild cases. The public health service must be informed and patients and close contacts should not handle food until the stool cultures are negative.

Shigella dysentery can be confused with *Salmonella* food poisoning, and amoebic and ulcerative colitis (page 147, Chapter 12).

Amoebic dysentery

This is an infection of the colon by the protozoon *Entamoeba histolytica*. In the acute dysenteric form, the illness begins suddenly with fever, abdominal pain, nausea, vomiting and diarrhoea containing mucus and blood. More commonly, amoebic colitis presents less acutely with intermittent diarrhoea with or without abdominal pain, mucus and blood.

The major complications are hepatic abscesses and pericolic amoebomas, which can be confused with colonic carcinoma. The diagnosis is made by finding trophozoites or cysts in fresh faeces, rectal mucus or rectal biopsy and supported by a positive complement fixation test.

Metronidazole is the treatment of choice for all invasive forms of amoebiasis, but abscesses may have to be drained if they do not resolve on drug therapy.

Diloxanide furonate is used to eradicate chronic amoebic cysts.

Cyst excretors should not handle food, and contacts should be screened. Acute amoebiasis can be confused with bacillary dysentery, *Salmonella* food poisoning and ulcerative colitis, and chronic infection with *Giardia lamblia,* tropical sprue, ulcerative colitis and diverticular disease (Chapter 12).

Giardiasis

Giardia lamblia is a flagellate protozoon which infects the small intestinal wall but not the blood. Viable cysts are ingested with contaminated food and may be excreted asymptomatically, or produce diarrhoea and steatorrhoea. The diagnosis is confirmed by the presence of trophozoites or cysts in stools or duodenal aspirates. Metronidazole is the drugs of choice. Tinidazole or mepacrine are alternatives.

Pyrexia of unknown origin

There are many definitions of pyrexia of unknown origin. In practice, the difficulty arises when the cause is unidentified after the clear clinical possibilities have been excluded and a basic set of tests performed. It is usually a hospital problem. A broad-spectrum antibiotic has commonly been given. The causes are listed in Table 21.4.

Special points in the history

- exposure to infection (meals away from home, febrile illness in household contacts, unpasteurised milk or cheese, undercooked eggs and poultry)
- occupation: farmer, veterinary surgeon, sewer worker, forester (for *Brucella, Leptospira,* anthrax, cat scratch fever (Bartonellosis), Lyme disease)
- drug history, e.g. antibiotics, methyldopa, hydralazine, phenytoin, including non-prescribed preparations
- travel (malaria, amoebiasis) and sexual history
- pets, including dogs, cats and birds

Special points in examination

NB: Repeat regularly if the fever persists.

- *cardiovascular:* murmurs, especially if changing, suggest infective endocarditis; tender temporal arteries; Dressler syndrome
- *respiratory:* crackles for early pneumonia (e.g. Legionnaires' disease); sinuses; consider recurrent pulmonary thromboembolic disease
- *abdomen:* palpable liver, gall bladder or spleen (with or without tenderness)

Table 21.4 Causes of pyrexia of unknown origin (mnemonic – IMAGINE)

Infections	*Bacterial.* Endocarditis (including culture-negative)
	*Collections of pus
	  Subphrenic
	  Intrahepatic
	  Perirenal
	  Pelvic
	  Pleura
	Bone (osteomyelitis)
	Viral/rickettsial (including hepatitis B)
	Protozoal
	Malaria, amoeba, spirochaetes
	Specific
	Tuberculosis* (all sites), typhoid, *Brucella,* Lyme disease (*Borrelia burgdorferi*)

Malignancy	Kidney and liver (primary and secondary) Pancreas Micrometastases, lymphoma (Hodgkin's and non-Hodgkin's), leukaemia
Autoimmune diseases	*Systemic lupus erythematosus, polyarteritis nodosa, systemic vasculitis, chronic active hepatitis, rheumatoid disease, Still's disease (including adult Still's disease, Chapter 18)
Granulomas	Sarcoid Crohn's disease
Iatrogenic	Drug fever
Nurses, doctors and all paramedics, etc.	Factitious fever Consult exhaustive lists in big books, but remember that the cause is more often a rare manifestation of a common disease than a common manifestation of a rare disease

*Denotes a more likely cause of pyrexia of unknown origin; all are treatable and potentially curable.

- *musculoskeletal:* muscle stiffness and tenderness of inflammatory diseases, e.g. polymyalgia rheumatica
- *skin rashes* (drugs, rose spots of typhoid): splinter haemorrhages; Osler's nodes
- *lymph* nodes (all groups)
- *check all orifices:* mouth (teeth for apical abscesses), ears, perineum (anus and genitourinary tract)

Basic screening tests already performed (check)

May need to be repeated until a diagnosis has been achieved.

- *Haemoglobin*: if anaemia is present and considerable, it is usually relevant. If iron-deficient and there is no overt blood loss, exclude gut malignancy.
- *White blood cell* (WBC) count: neutrophilia is associated with pyogenic infection and neoplasia, and neutropenia with viral infection. Lymphocytosis may suggest tuberculosis. Leukaemia and infectious mononucleosis are usually associated with abnormal peripheral counts and cell types (remember direct tests for infectious mononucleosis). Eosinophilia may suggest parasites or polyarteritis nodosa.
- *Erythrocyte sedimentation rate:* if over 100 mm/h, check for myeloma and consider polymyalgia rheumatica or underlying malignancy.
- *Mid-stream urine*: haematuria, possibly microscopic, occurs with bacterial endocarditis, renal carcinoma, vasculitis and leptospirosis. WBCs in infection. Early morning urine for acid-fast bacillus (AFB).
- *Chest X-ray*: carcinoma (primary or secondary) in lungs, and bone metastases. Miliary shadowing in miliary tuberculosis and sarcoid. Hilar nodes in tuberculosis, lymphoma, sarcoid and carcinoma.
- *Sputum* for microorganisms, including AFB.
- *Liver function tests* (LFTs) for secondary or primary malignancy, abscess, biliary disease, hepatitis (Chapter 13).
- *Infectious mononucleosis* screening test.
- *Blood cultures.*

Further tests commonly required as determined by clinical leads

- viral, brucella, mycoplasma and coxiella antibody titres
- auto-antibody screen
- ultrasound or computed tomographic (CT) scan of abdomen for liver abscesses, and for secondaries, for renal tumours and abscesses, and for splenic enlargement, and of the pelvis for pelvic lesions
- echocardiography for vegetations
- CT scanning of chest for lymphadenopathy and infection

Invasive procedures as indicated

- temporal artery biopsy
- liver needle biopsy (tuberculosis, granulomas, neoplasm)
- muscle biopsy

Go back again and again to take a new history, to re-examine the relevant areas and to repeat selected investigations, especially those that might have been performed too early, i.e. before they could have become abnormal.

Other imported pathogens: nematodes, schistosomes

The worms listed in Table 21.5 are found worldwide and not uncommonly in travellers who live rough or enter areas of poor sanitation.

Table 21.5 Common worms

Worm	Major clinical features	Treatment
Threadworm	Anal itch	Piperazine
(*Enterobius vermicularis*)	Worm on stool	Thiabendazole (treat all household members to prevent reinfection)
Roundworm	Worm on stool	Piperazine
(*Ascaris lumbricoides*)		
Hookworm	Nil. If severe infection, iron-deficient anaemia; malnutrition in children	Bephenium (Alcopar)
(*Necator americanus*: *Ancylostoma duodenale*)		Pyrantel
	Eggs or worms in stools	Tetrachloroethylene
Schistosoma	Fever and eosinophilia	Praziquantel (for both)
S. mansoni (spur on side)	Initially diarrhoea	
S. haematobium (spur on tail)	Haematuria	

Septicaemia

Common organisms are *Staphylococcus aureus, Escherichia coli, Klebsiella pneumoniae* and *Enterococcus* species. Common sources include intravenous catheters, genitourinary and respiratory tract, and intra-abdominal foci. Coagulase-negative staphylococci isolated from blood cultures may be contaminants and not clinically significant, but they are a common cause of hospital-acquired bacteraemia related to intravenous catheters.

Management

General measures include good nursing care and fluid and electrolyte balance, and in severe cases intensive therapy, including treatment of shock and renal failure.

The key management points are:

1. Drain pus.
2. Antibiotics (see Table 21.6 for guidelines for appropriate choice).
3. Expert nursing care.
4. Fluid balance and monitor renal function.

Table 21.6 Antibiotics for septicaemia

Community-acquired septicaemia

Broad spectrum anti-pseudomonal penicillin (e.g. piperacillin with tazobactam, or ticarcillin with clavulanic acid)

Add
- vancomycin if meticillin-resistant *Staphylococcus aureus* suspected
- metronidazole if anaerobes suspected

Consider a more broad-spectrum beta-lactam antibacterial (e.g. meropenem) if resistant microorganisms suspected.

Hospital-acquired septicaemia

Broad spectrum anti-pseudomonal beta-lactam antibiotic* (e.g. piperacillin with tazobactam, ticarcillin with clavulanic acid, ceftazidime, or meropenem)

Add
- metronidazole if anaerobes suspected
- vancomycin if related to vascular catheter or meticillin-resistant *Staphylococcus aureus* suspected (remove or replace catheter)

*Beta-lactam antibiotics share a common structural feature, the beta-lactam ring, and include penicillins, cephalosporins, carbapenems, monobactams and beta-lactamase inhibitors.

TRIALS BOX 21.1 Fluid resuscitation in sepsis

A systematic review and meta-analysis with trial sequential analysis of all-cause mortality of randomised trials of human albumin solutions as part of fluid volume expansion and resuscitation for critically unwell adults with sepsis of any severity (with or without baseline hypoalbuminaemia) were not robustly effective at reducing all-cause mortality. Albumin seemed to be safe, but the analysis did not support a recommendation for use. Source: *BMJ* 2014; **349**: g4561. doi: 10.1136/bmj.g4561.

If the patient is shocked:

5. Treat hypovolaemia (Trials Box 21.1)
6. Intensive care monitoring of fluid balance
7. Consider use of vasopressors (norepinephrine/epinephrine) or inotropes
8. Treat disseminated intravascular coagulation (DIC, page 386, Chapter 20).

NB: Corticosteroids are not of proven value in septicaemic shock unless there is associated adrenal damage (consider performing a short Synacthen test).

Antibiotics

The choice of antibiotic depends upon the likely organism and local policies and knowledge of antibiotic sensitivities (Table 21.6).

Influenza

Influenza viruses are enveloped single-strand RNA viruses that require an RNA-dependent RNA polymerase of viral origin for replication. Their importance lies in their ability to cause epidemics (they occur more frequently than expected in a community or region) and pandemics (spread through populations). The virus escapes host immunity by mutation of surface antigens, and in particular haemaglutinin (HA), which is an important target for host antibodies. Vaccine development relies on worldwide surveillance to detect this process.

Influenza viruses primarily cause upper respiratory tract infection, typically with fever, headache, malaise and myalgia. Secondary bacterial pneumonia, particularly due to *Staphylococcus aureus,* is common in the elderly.

Oseltamivir and zanamivir reduce viral replication by inhibiting viral neuraminidase. They are licensed for use within the first 48 h of the onset of symptoms.

Human immunodeficiency virus infection

HIV-1 and HIV-2 are members of the Lentivirus family of retroviruses. The virus preferentially infects CD4$^+$ helper T-lymphocytes, leading to a decline in CD4 cell counts with impaired cell-mediated immunity. Eventually, the immune system becomes clinically compromised and the patient develops infectious, neurological and neoplastic complications.

HIV-2 shares 45% sequence homology with HIV-1, and is found mainly in West Africa. It is less pathogenic in vitro and transmission rates appear to be lower.

Viral transmission is through sexual contact (homo and heterosexual) or blood-borne (intravenous drug abuse or transfusion of blood or blood products). Blood for transfusion is routinely screened. Anti-retroviral prophylaxis taken by the HIV-infected mother or the breastfeeding HIV-exposed infant reduces mother-to-child transmission of HIV.

Clinical features

Half of cases develop a febrile illness with malaise, headache, pharyngitis, lymphadenopathy and maculopapular rash 2–4 weeks after infection. Antibody tests for HIV become positive 2–6 weeks after this illness. Patients then remain free from serious illness for a number of years. They may then develop symptoms of malaise, fever, weight loss with features of mild immunodeficiency (e.g. oral *Candida,* cutaneous herpes zoster or herpes simplex) or immune dysfunction (immune thrombocytopenia, drug allergies). There may be generalised lymphadenopathy.

Opportunistic infections

These remain the most frequent complications of HIV infection.

Candidiasis

Oral *Candida albicans* infection is common, presenting with typical white plaques or mucosal erythema or candidiasis. Topical treatments (nystatin or amphotericin lozenges) may be effective, but oesophageal or genital candidiasis are indications for systemic therapy with fluconazole.

Pneumocystis jiroveci pneumonia

Exposure is common in the general population, but clinical disease only occurs in severe immunodeficiency. Cough and progressive dyspnoea are accompanied by fever, cyanosis, tachycardia, tachypnoea and confusion. Auscultation of the chest may be normal.

Chest X-ray is normal early in the disease, but widespread, diffuse interstitial shadowing develops. There may be atypical features of lobar consolidation, upper zone shadowing or hilar lymphadenopathy. Pneumothorax is a recognised complication. Patients are usually hypoxic.

Diagnosis depends on identification of the organism by microscopy or PCR of sputum, bronchoalveolar lavage or transbronchial biopsy, although treatment is often commenced on clinical grounds.

Treatment is high-dose co-trimoxazole (100 mg/kg/day sulfamethoxazole and 20 mg/kg/day trimethoprim) in divided doses orally or intravenously for 21 days. Adverse reactions are common and intravenous pentamidine 4 mg/kg/day is an alternative. High-dose oxygen and mechanical ventilation may be required in severe disease. Steroids improve survival in HIV-infected patients with pneumocystis and hypoxia ($PaO_2 < 9.3$ kPa).

Prophylaxis is continued with co-trimoxazole 960 mg/day three times per week or monthly inhaled pentamidine.

Mycobacterial infections

Mycobacterium tuberculosis infection is the most frequent life-threatening opportunistic infection and the leading cause of death in people with HIV. It may occur as a result of reactivation or primary infection at any stage of HIV infection. Pulmonary presentation may be with typical apical cavitation and fibrosis or more generalised lung infiltrates. Extrapulmonary tuberculosis (lymph nodes, bone, bone marrow, genitourinary tract, liver, spleen, skin, peritoneum, central nervous system) occurs in 50% of patients. Antiretroviral therapy is the most important measure in reducing the incidence of TB. Standard treatment regimens (e.g. isoniazid with pyridoxine, rifampicin, pyrazinamide and ethambutol) are usually used (page 139, Chapter 11). Co-trimoxazole is usually given as prophylaxis against other infections. Multidrug-resistant TB is a major threat to individuals with HIV and public health, particularly in countries with a high prevalence of HIV.

Cytomegalovirus

Cytomegalovirus (CMV) retinitis usually presents as unilateral visual loss. Asymptomatic lesions may be detected as fluffy white areas of necrosis and haemorrhage on fundoscopy. Untreated progression to bilateral blindness occurs. Initial treatment is with intravenous ganciclovir. Maintenance therapy with oral or intravenous ganciclovir is continued. Slow-release ocular implants containing ganciclovir can treat immediate sight-threatening CMV retinitis. Valganciclovir, an ester of ganciclovir is an alternative. Foscarnet is often limited by toxicity, but can be used if there is ganciclovir resistance or intolerance.

CMV encephalitis presents with cognitive loss, and motor and behavioural abnormalities. It can be difficult to distinguish from other causes of AIDS dementia complex (direct effect of HIV infection, herpes simplex encephalitis, *Toxoplasma gondii*), although diagnosis can be established by brain biopsy. Response to ganciclovir is limited.

Cryptococcal infection

Cryptococcus neoformans is a capsulate yeast widely present in bird droppings. Infection occurs by inhalation. Meningitis is the most common manifestation in AIDS, although pneumonia and skin sepsis also occur.

Presentation of cryptococcal meningitis is usually non-specific, with prolonged fever, headache, malaise, nausea and vomiting. Diagnosis is confirmed by identification of capsulate yeasts or cryptococcal antigen in cerebrospinal fluid. Treatment is with intravenous amphotericin and flucytosine followed by oral fluconazole, continued indefinitely in the immunocompromised.

Toxoplasma

Primary infection with the protozoon *Toxoplasma gondii* is usually acquired during childhood by eating infected cat faeces or undercooked meat. An infectious mononucleosis-type illness is followed by persistence of *Toxoplasma* cysts in the central nervous system and elsewhere. Vertical transmission from mother to child also occurs and causes fetal abnormalities, including central nervous system abnormalities.

Reactivation of *T. gondii* in AIDS usually manifests with neurological features, including fever, confusion, fits and focal neurological deficit. Choroidoretinitis may precede encephalitis. Patients are seropositive for *T. gondii* and cranial CT reveals multiple hypodense lesions. Treatment is with pyrimethamine and folinic acid (to reduce haematological toxicity of pyrimethamine) and sulfadiazine. Pyrimethamine can also be used with clarithromycin or azithromycin or clindamycin.

Diarrhoea

Abdominal pain, diarrhoea and weight loss are common, and usually indicate infection, although a specific pathogen is often not identified. Bacterial pathogens such as *Salmonella*, *Shigella*, *Campylobacter jejuni*, *Giardia lamblia* and *Entamoeba histolytica* should be excluded by stool microscopy and culture. *Cryptosporidium parvum* usually causes a self-limiting illness in normal individuals, but causes severe, prolonged diarrhoea in AIDS patients who may also develop cholangitis and cholecystitis. It may respond to paromycin.

Herpes simplex

Recurrent oral, genital or perianal ulceration is common and usually responds to systemic (oral or intravenous) aciclovir. Herpes simplex encephalitis typically presents with headache, fever, confusion and temporal lobe abnormalities. Culture of cerebrospinal fluid is usually negative for herpes simplex. Diagnosis can be established by PCR of cerebrospinal fluid or brain biopsy, but treatment with intravenous aciclovir is usually started on clinical grounds.

Herpes zoster

Cutaneous dissemination of typical herpes zoster (Table 19.4) can occur. Treatment is with intravenous aciclovir.

Progressive multifocal leukoencephalopathy

Progressive multifocal leukoencephalopathy (PML) is caused by reactivation of the polyomavirus JC, which is a common asymptomatic infection in childhood. Presentation is with development of multiple, progressive, neurological defects. CT scan shows multiple non-enhancing lesions. Brain biopsy may be required to exclude other treatable lesions. There is no specific treatment for PML.

Malignancy

Kaposi's sarcoma, non-Hodgkin's lymphoma and cervical carcinoma define the advanced clinical stages of HIV infection.

Kaposi's sarcoma occurs almost exclusively in homosexual males, suggesting that an additional sexually transmitted agent is important. Palpable, violaceous cutaneous nodules occur most commonly on the head and neck. Lesions also occur in other organs, including lungs and gastrointestinal tract. Radiotherapy can cause regression of local disease.

Non-Hodgkin's lymphoma often presents with widespread extranodal disease. Differentiation of central nervous system lymphoma from *Toxoplasma gondii* infection can be difficult and require brain biopsy.

Cervical carcinoma, abnormal cervical cytology and human papillomavirus infection are all more common in HIV-infected women, who should have cervical smears at least annually.

Primary treatment of HIV

The development of therapies for AIDS requires an understanding of how the HIV-1 virus integrates into the human genome, and how viral replication and viral gene expression are regulated (Figs. 21.1 and 21.2).

The proviral genome of HIV-1 is 9–10 kb long and has three main structural genes:

- The *gag* (group-specific antigen) gene encodes the core protein antigens of the virion (intact virus particle). These are formed as the cleaved products of a larger precursor protein.
- The *pol* (polymerase) gene encodes the viral reverse transcriptase, and also the IN protein required for integration of viral DNA into the host genome.
- The *env* gene encodes the two envelope glycoproteins, which are cleaved from a larger precursor.

When the HIV virion binds to a CD4 molecule on the cell surface, a conformational change occurs in the envelope glycoprotein, and the virus enters the cell via fusion of lipid bilayers at the cell surface. The uncoated core of the virion then uses its viral reverse transcriptase to transcribe one of the two identical

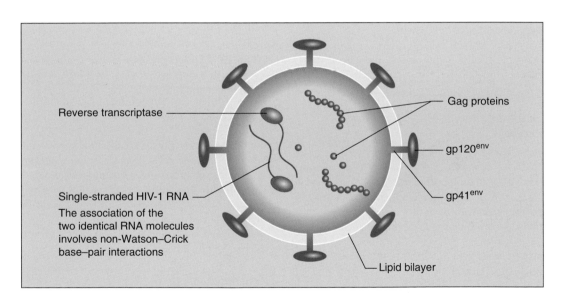

Figure 21.1 The structure of the HIV-1 virion. Source: Bradley, J.R., Johnson, D. and Rubenstein, D. (2001) *From Lecture Notes on Molecular Medicine*. Oxford: Wiley-Blackwell.

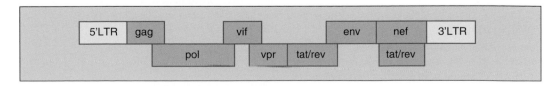

Figure 21.2 Representation of the HIV-1 genome. The 5′- and 3′- LTRs (long terminal repeats) contain regulatory sequences. Several genes overlap. Source: Bradley, J.R., Johnson, D. and Rubenstein, D. (2001) *From Lecture Notes on Molecular Medicine*. Oxford: Wiley-Blackwell.

strands of positive-sense RNA into DNA. This DNA is duplicated by a host cell DNA polymerase, and migrates to the nucleus where it is integrated at a random site into the genome. Transcription of the integrated viral DNA is regulated by both host factors (such as the DNA-binding protein NFκB), and viral regulatory proteins such as the tat and rev proteins. Virally encoded proteins are processed and assembled in the cytoplasm, and then bud from the cell surface as new infectious virions.

Anti-retroviral therapy (ART)

Several sites in the viral life cycle have been targeted, and effective treatment requires combination therapy.

WHO guidelines (Consolidated guidelines on the use of antiretroviral drugs for treating and preventing HIV infection; http://www.who.int/hiv/pub/arv/arv-2016/en/, June 2016) recommend that ART should be initiated in all children, adolescents and adults (including pregnant and breastfeeding women) living with HIV, regardless of WHO clinical stage and at any CD4 cell count.

First-line ART for adults usually consists of two nucleoside reverse-transcriptase inhibitors (NRTIs) plus a non-nucleoside reverse-transcriptase inhibitor (NNRTI) or an integrase inhibitor (INSTI)

Nucleoside reverse transcriptase inhibitors (NRTIs)

Zidovudine (AZT) was the first anti-HIV drug to be introduced. It is a nucleoside analogue which binds preferentially to viral reverse transcriptase compared to human DNA polymerase. Other NRTIs include didanosine (ddI), dideoxycytosine (ddC; zalcitabine), abacavir, lamivudine, stavudine, tenofovir and emtricitabine.

Non-nucleoside reverse transcriptase inhibitors (NNRTIs)

Efavirenz, etravirine, nevirapine, and rilpivirine are NNRTIs. Most share a conformation that allows them to interact with a hydrophobic site on reverse transcriptase. They are highly selective for HIV1 and do not inhibit HIV2.

Protease inhibitors

Ritonavir, indinavir, amprenavir, lopinavir, atavanavir, nelfinavir, tipranavir and saquinavir prevent viral maturation. Fosamprenavir is a pro-drug of amprenavir. Gastrointestinal side effects are common (nausea, diarrhoea, abdominal pain, vomiting). Protease inhibitors are associated with lipodystrophy, hyperlipidaemia, insulin resistance and hyperglycaemia.

Pre-exposure prophylaxis (PrEP)

Truvada (emtricitabine/tenofovir) is licensed by the European Medicines Agency for pre-exposure prophylaxis (PrEP) in combination with safer sex practices to reduce the risk of sexually-acquired human immunodeficiency virus type 1 (HIV-1) infection in adults at high risk.

Infectious mononucleosis (glandular fever)

Infectious mononucleosis is a common disease of the young, usually transmitted by saliva, with an excellent prognosis, It is caused by the Epstein–Barr virus (a herpes virus). Seroprevalence is >90% in adults.

Clinical presentation

Malaise, fever, sore throat, muscle and joint aches. Examination reveals a tonsillar exudate and palatal petechiae with generalised lymphadenopathy and splenomegaly. A macular–papular rash is common and more frequent if ampicillin is given for the sore throat. Mesenteric adenitis with appendicitis may occur.

Investigation

There is a leucocytosis with an absolute and relative (>50% of total white cells) increase in mononuclear cells. Patients with infectious mononucleosis produce IgM antibodies that bind to and agglutinate red cells from other species, giving rise to a positive Paul-Bunnell or monospot test.

Thrombocytopenia and abnormal liver function tests are common but rarely severe.

Complications

Tonsillar enlargement may be severe and prevent swallowing of saliva and even threaten airway obstruction. Rare complications include splenic rupture, autoimmune haemolytic anaemia, encephalitis, transverse myelitis, Bell's palsy and Guillain–Barrée syndrome. Lethargy may last for several months.

Differential diagnosis

The disease may be confused with:

- acute tonsillitis
- infections that produce a similar rash, e.g. measles, rubella

- infections that produce similar malaise and lymphadenopathy, e.g. toxoplasmosis, brucellosis, tuberculosis
- lymphomas and leukaemias
- HIV infection
- drug hypersensitivity
- acute appendicitis.

NB: Diphtheria should not be forgotten.

Treatment

Usually rest, aspirin gargles and anaesthetic lozenges for the sore throat are sufficient. If the tonsillar enlargement is great and swallowing is difficult or the airway threatened (anginose glandular fever – usually with severe general symptoms), a short course of steroids (prednisolone 40 mg/day for 5–10 days) rapidly reduces the symptoms.

Tuberculosis

Tuberculosis most commonly causes pulmonary disease (Chapter 11) but can affect any site, including the central nervous system (Chapter 15). In the UK it is a statutory requirement to notify all cases of tuberculosis, and this initiates contact tracing if appropriate. National Institute for Health and Clinical Excellence (NICE) guidelines (https://www.nice.org.uk/guidance/ng33) recommend a 6-month short-course regimen (Table 21.7), with four drugs in the initial phase, should be used for all forms of tuberculosis, except where there is central nervous system involvement, in children and adults. Drug-resistant tuberculosis is increasing and it is vital to confirm bacteriological diagnosis and drug susceptibility whenever possible. Treatment of drug-resistant tuberculosis, and in particular multidrug-resistance, requires specialist expertise and close collaboration with *Mycobacterium* reference laboratories.

Chronic fatigue syndrome

A report of the joint working group of the Royal Colleges of Physicians, Psychiatrists and General Practitioners used this term to describe the syndrome characterised by a minimum of 6 months of severe physical and mental fatigue and fatigability, made worse by minor exertion. The term myalgic encephalomyelitis (ME) was first used in 1955 to describe an unexplained illness in the staff of the Royal Free Hospital.

There is no convincing evidence that common viral infections are a risk factor for chronic fatigue syndrome, with the exception of the fatigue that follows less than 10% of Epstein–Barr virus infections.

Investigation

Criteria for the diagnosis of chronic fatigue syndrome have been described (see Box 21.1). No laboratory tests can confirm the diagnosis. The following should be performed to exclude other causes of fatigue:

- full blood count, erythrocyte sedimentation rate
- creatinine and electrolytes, liver function test, C-reactive protein, glucose

Table 21.7 Treatment of tuberculosis

	Initial phase	Months	Continuation phase	Months
Active TB without central nervous system involvement	I, R, P, E	2	I, R	4
Active TB with central nervous system involvement	I, R, P, E	2	I, R	10

I, isoniazid; R, rifampicin; P, pyrazinamide; E, ethambutol. Pyridoxine should be given with isoniazid.
Liver function tests (LFTs) should be checked before starting therapy. Transient asymptomatic increases in serum transaminases are very common after starting treatment. Discontinuation is not indicated unless there are symptoms of hepatitis (anorexia, vomiting, hepatomegaly) or jaundice.

Box 21.1 Criteria for the diagnosis of chronic fatigue syndrome

The **Centers for Disease Control** in Atlanta produced the CDC-1994 criteria for chronic fatigue syndrome (*Annals of Internal Medicine* 1994; **121**: 953–959):

1. Clinically evaluated unexplained persistent or relapsing fatigue that is not:
   - of new onset
   - the result of ongoing exertion
   - substantially alleviated by rest, and
   - results in substantial reduction in previous levels of occupational, educational, social or personal activities.

2. With four or more of the following symptoms, concurrently present for 6 months:
   - impaired memory or concentration
   - sore throat
   - tender cervical or axillary lymph nodes
   - muscle pain
   - multi-joint pain
   - new headaches
   - unrefreshing sleep
   - post-exertion malaise.

- thyroid and adrenal function
- creatine kinase
- urinalysis for protein and sugar.

Management

A gradual planned increase in exercise is the main objective. Cognitive behaviour therapy helps achieve this in some patients. NICE guidelines highlight the importance of shared decision-making between the patient and healthcare professional, with provision of advice on sleep management, introduction of physical and cognitive activities with rest periods, and relaxation techniques. (http://www.nice.org.uk/nicemedia/pdf/CG53FullGuidance.pdf).

22

Toxicology

Poisoning is one of the commonest medical emergencies and accounts for approximately 5–10% of all acute medical admissions in the UK. Table 22.1 lists the most frequently encountered causes, but is not exhaustive, and the clinician must keep an open mind when poisoning is suspected as patients may take/be exposed to a diverse array of toxic substances (with considerable variation from country to country). Accidental poisoning is common in children and drugs are best kept in child-proof containers out of their reach.

Deliberate self-administration of drugs/substances with a view to causing harm or even death presents a major challenge not only in terms of dealing with the physical consequences of exposure to one or more toxins, but also with respect to addressing underlying psychosocial issues. Clinicians involved in the management of these complex cases need to adopt a holistic approach – ensuring that the patient comes to no/minimal physical harm is only the first step in management, and additional psychological/ongoing support to minimise the risk of further similar episodes is almost always required.

Not all episodes of poisoning are immediately self-evident, and it is important to keep an open mind when assessing patients for whom the immediate cause of their presentation is unclear. Clues that should alert you to a possible case of poisoning include: current/past history of depression/psychiatric illness; previous history of overdose/self-harm; history of excess alcohol consumption; social isolation/difficulties; needle marks; empty packets of drugs brought in by relatives/paramedics; admission from a workplace/environment where potential toxins are present.

Clinical presentation

Many patients who take drug overdoses are still conscious when seen and will often state which tablets they have taken and/or bring the bottle(s)/packet(s) with them. If unconscious, then other causes of coma must also be considered even if an overdose is suspected, e.g. is the patient known to have diabetes (exclude hypoglycaemia) or be steroid-dependent (check for steroid card or alert bracelet)? Is there any evidence of a head injury? Relatives or friends may know whether the patient is currently under active medical treatment. Patients often take more than one drug and very often alcohol in addition.

As always, a good history and careful physical examination are central both to establishing the extent to which the patient has suffered adverse effects in cases of known poisoning and to providing clues as to possible aetiological factors in suspected cases or where the agent is unknown. Figure 22.1 correlates clinical findings with specific poisons, although it is important to note that in the early stages clinical signs may be limited, while mixed overdoses can be associated with overlapping features.

Typical features of commonly encountered drug overdoses involving prescription/over-the-counter (OTC) medications are shown in Table 22.2, and those resulting from use of 'recreational' drugs and/or alcohol/ethanol in Table 22.3.

Clinical Medicine Lecture Notes, Eighth Edition. John R. Bradley, Mark Gurnell, and Diana F. Wood.
© 2019 John Wiley & Sons Ltd. Published 2019 by John Wiley & Sons Ltd.

Table 22.1 Common causes of poisoning in the UK

Class/agent	Example(s)
Alcohol	
Analgesics	Paracetamol (acetaminophen), aspirin and other NSAIDs (e.g. ibuprofen)
Antidepressants	Tricyclic antidepressants, selective serotonin reuptake inhibitors
Carbon monoxide	
Drugs of misuse	Amfetamines, cocaine, opioids
Solvents	Glue, lighter fuel

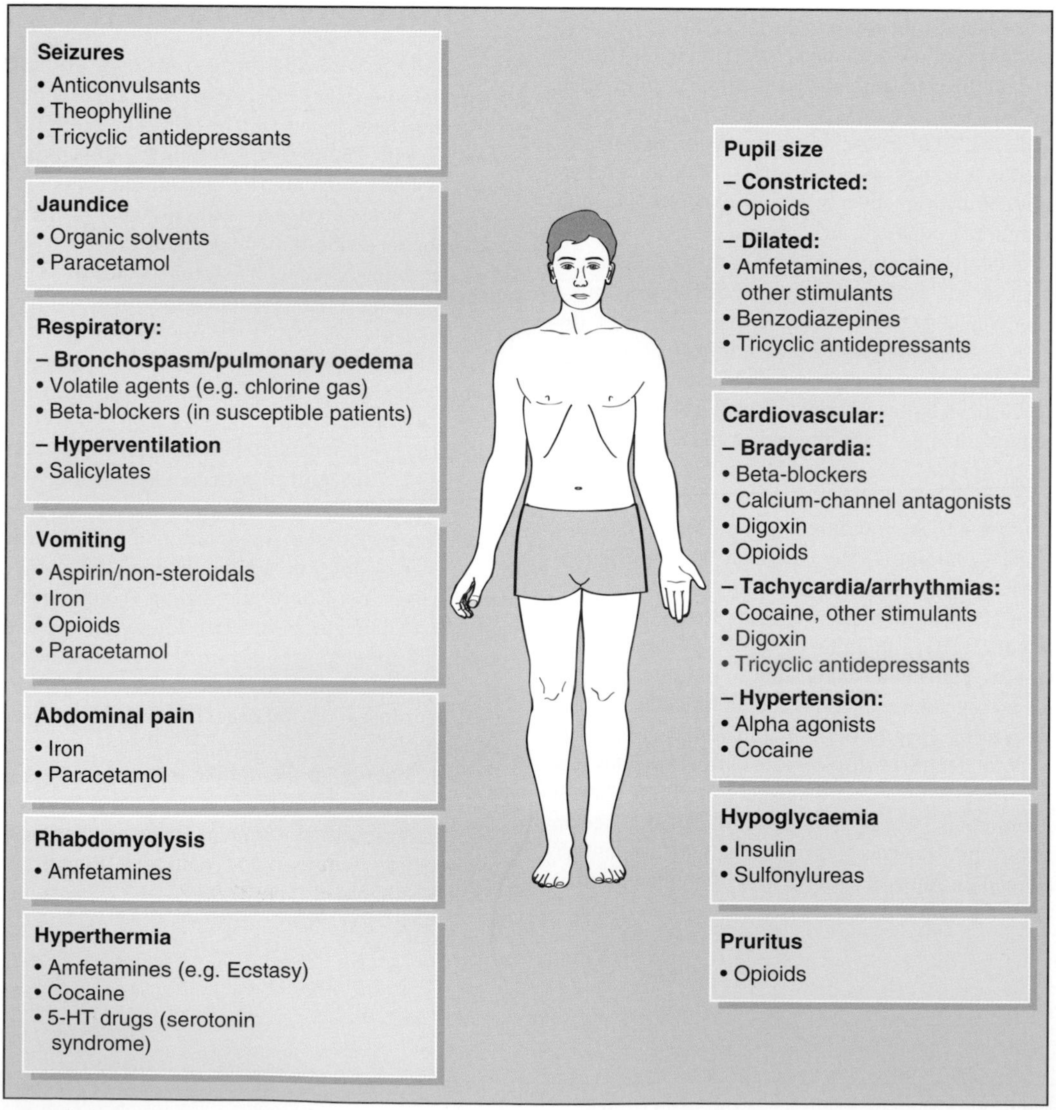

Seizures
- Anticonvulsants
- Theophylline
- Tricyclic antidepressants

Jaundice
- Organic solvents
- Paracetamol

Respiratory:
- **Bronchospasm/pulmonary oedema**
- Volatile agents (e.g. chlorine gas)
- Beta-blockers (in susceptible patients)
- **Hyperventilation**
- Salicylates

Vomiting
- Aspirin/non-steroidals
- Iron
- Opioids
- Paracetamol

Abdominal pain
- Iron
- Paracetamol

Rhabdomyolysis
- Amfetamines

Hyperthermia
- Amfetamines (e.g. Ecstasy)
- Cocaine
- 5-HT drugs (serotonin syndrome)

Pupil size
- **Constricted:**
- Opioids
- **Dilated:**
- Amfetamines, cocaine, other stimulants
- Benzodiazepines
- Tricyclic antidepressants

Cardiovascular:
- **Bradycardia:**
- Beta-blockers
- Calcium-channel antagonists
- Digoxin
- Opioids
- **Tachycardia/arrhythmias:**
- Cocaine, other stimulants
- Digoxin
- Tricyclic antidepressants
- **Hypertension:**
- Alpha agonists
- Cocaine

Hypoglycaemia
- Insulin
- Sulfonylureas

Pruritus
- Opioids

Figure 22.1 Clinical clues to poisoning with specific drugs/agents.

Table 22.2 Clinical features and specific investigations/management for overdoses involving prescription/over-the-counter drugs

Drug	Clinical features	Specific investigations	Specific management
Aspirin	• Hyperventilation, tinnitus/deafness, sweating, vasodilatation, abdominal pain • Complex acid–base disturbances (e.g. respiratory alkalosis with metabolic acidosis) • Seizures/coma in severe cases	• Plasma salicylate level (repeated measurements may be needed as absorption can be slow); generally the clinical severity of poisoning is low at concentrations <500 mg/l (3.6 mmol/l) unless there is evidence of metabolic acidosis (note: correlation is less reliable in the young or elderly): severe salicylate poisoning occurs with levels >700 mg/l (5.1 mmol/l)	• Activated charcoal if presenting within 1 h of ingestion of ≥125 mg/kg body weight • Consider alkaline diuresis with sodium bicarbonate if clinical condition dictates or plasma salicylate level >500 mg/l • Haemodialysis is the treatment of choice for severe salicylate poisoning
Benzodiazepines	• Drowsiness • Ataxia, dysarthria, confusion • Mild hypotension and respiratory depression • Increased toxicity when combined with other drugs/alcohol	• ABGs (including pH) • Measurement of plasma drug levels is of little clinical use • Consider oxygen saturation monitoring if concerns regarding respiratory depression	• Activated charcoal if presenting within 1 h of ingestion providing patient is alert and airway protected • The benzodiazepine antagonist flumazenil should **not** be routinely used, and must be **avoided** in those with a history of seizures or if there is concomitant ingestion of tricyclic antidepressants (lowers seizure and arrhythmia thresholds)
Beta-blockers	• Bradycardia, hypotension • Bronchospasm or heart failure in susceptible individuals • Seizures and coma may occur with some agents, e.g. propranolol	• Measurement of plasma drug levels is of little clinical use	• Cardiac monitoring • Atropine to correct bradycardia/hypotension • Glucagon infusion may be beneficial in refractory/severe cases • Isoprenaline or transvenous pacing may be used to increase heart rate
Calcium channel blockers	• Nausea, vomiting, dizziness, agitation • Hypotension • Confusion, coma and metabolic acidosis in more severe cases • Bradycardia/arrhythmias with diltiazem and verapamil	• Measurement of plasma drug levels is of little clinical use	• Activated charcoal if presenting within 1 h of ingestion – repeated doses may be considered if a modified release preparation is involved • Cardiac monitoring • Atropine may be used to correct bradycardia • NPIS should be consulted over choice of inotrope in cases of refractory hypotension • Calcium chloride or calcium gluconate may be tried in severe poisoning

(Continued)

Table 22.2 (*Continued*)

Drug	Clinical features	Specific investigations	Specific management
Digoxin	• Gastrointestinal upset (nausea, vomiting, diarrhoea) • Altered colour vision • Arrhythmias	• Plasma digoxin level does not indicate toxicity reliably, but values >1.5 mcg/l are associated with rising likelihood of toxicity • CE (check particularly for hypokalaemia)	• Cardiac monitoring • Correct hypokalaemia • Consider use of digoxin-specific antibody fragments (Digibind®) in severe poisoning
Iron salts	• Gastrointestinal upset (abdominal pain, nausea, vomiting, diarrhoea, haematemesis and rectal bleeding) • Hypotension • Metabolic acidosis, hepatic failure and coma in more severe cases	• Measurement of serum iron level as an emergency	• Advice regarding gastric lavage should be sought from NPIS if presenting within 1 h of ingestion • Desferrioxamine (do not delay treatment while awaiting serum iron level)
Lithium	• Apathy and restlessness are early features • Nausea, vomiting, diarrhoea • Ataxia, weakness, dysarthria, muscle twitching, tremor • Seizures, coma, renal failure in more severe cases	• Measurement of serum lithium levels provides an indication of severity of overdose (although in acute overdose higher serum concentrations may be present without features of toxicity) • CE, calcium	• Advice regarding gastric lavage should be sought from NPIS if presenting within 1 h of ingestion • Consider haemodialysis in more severe cases
Non-steroidal anti-inflammatory drugs (NSAIDs)	• Gastrointestinal upset (abdominal pain, vomiting, diarrhoea); occasionally tinnitus and headache • Seizures (particularly with mefanamic acid) • Renal failure, acidosis, coma in more severe cases	• Measurement of plasma drug levels is of little clinical use • FBC, CE, LFTs, ± ABGs (including pH)	• Activated charcoal if presenting within 1 h of ingestion of ≥100 mg/kg body weight of ibuprofen or ≥10 tablets of other NSAIDs • Proton-pump inhibitors may ameliorate gastric irritation
Opioids	• Small or pin-point pupils • Depressed respiration • Reduced conscious level • Needle marks • Marked hypoventilation, hypotension, non-cardiogenic pulmonary oedema, hypothermia and coma occur in more severe cases and may lead to death	• Plasma paracetamol level – consider possible overdose with combination analgesics (e.g. co-codamol)	• High-dependency monitoring of respiratory status and respiratory support • Naloxone (opioid antagonist) is effective in reversing respiratory depression and coma, but has a short half-life and repeated doses/infusion are often required, especially when long-acting opioids (e.g. methadone) have been ingested

	Clinical features	Investigations	Management
Paracetamol (acetaminophen)	• Initial asymptomatic latent phase of variable duration • Followed by nausea/vomiting, jaundice, hepatic tenderness • Hepatic failure • Renal failure (less common) but may occur independently of liver toxicity	• Plasma paracetamol level (interpret with respect to timing of overdose – see Fig. 22.2); in staggered overdoses levels are not reliable and treatment should be instituted without delay • In those presenting late check CE, LFTs, INR, ABGs	• Activated charcoal if presenting within 1 h of ingestion of ≥150 mg/kg body weight (≥75 mg/kg if considered high risk – see Fig. 22.2) or >12 g in total (whichever is the smaller) • N-acetylcysteine infusion (most effective if given within 8 h of ingestion); decision to treat is based on single plasma paracetamol level taken at not <4 h after ingestion (see Fig. 22.2) • Contact NPIS if presenting >8 h post-ingestion (or staggered overdose) and commence N-acetylcysteine immediately (do not wait for blood level) • Liver transplantation should be considered in those who present with liver failure
Selective serotonin reuptake inhibitors	• Nausea, vomiting, diarrhoea, agitation, tremor • Drowsiness, tachycardia • Seizures • Rarely 'serotonin syndrome' – marked neuropsychiatric effects, neuromuscular hyperactivity, autonomic instability, hyperthermia, rhabdomyolysis	• Routine measurement of plasma drug levels is not indicated • No specific investigations in less severe cases • In more severe cases investigations are directed by presentation	• Activated charcoal if presenting within 1 h of ingestion
Tricyclic antidepressants	• Anticholinergic effects: dry mouth/skin, blurred vision/dilated pupils, tachycardia, urinary retention • Seizures, depressed respiration, reduced consciousness, coma, arrhythmias, hypotension • Metabolic acidosis	• Routine measurement of plasma drug levels is not indicated • CE (+ calcium and magnesium if ECG abnormalities); ABGs (including pH) • ECG: prolongation of QRS interval (>140 ms), SVT, VT/VF	• Activated charcoal if presenting within 1 h of ingestion • Cardiac monitoring • Correct electrolyte abnormalities, hypoxia and acidosis • Avoid anti-arrhythmic drugs (proarrhythmogenic in this setting) • Sodium bicarbonate (50 ml of 8.4% – repeated as necessary) for those with QRS prolongation, arrhythmias or hypotension; consider transvenous pacing wire if recurrent arrhythmias

ABGs, arterial blood gases; CE, creatinine and electrolytes; ECG, electrocardiogram; FBC, full blood count; INR, international normalised ratio; LFTs, liver function tests; NPIS, National Poisons Information Service; PT, prothrombin time; SVT, supraventricular tachycardia; VT/VF, ventricular tachycardia/fibrillation.

Table 22.3 Clinical features and specific investigations/management for overdoses involving alcohol and other 'recreational' drugs

Drug	Clinical features	Specific investigations	Specific management
Alcohol/ ethanol	• Impaired coordination/reactions • Dysarthria, ataxia, diplopia, tachycardia, sweating • Drowsiness, coma, hypothermia, hypoglycaemia, seizures, metabolic acidosis, respiratory arrest	• Breath/blood alcohol level • CE, glucose • ABGs	• Monitor respiratory status/protect airway • Correct hypovolaemia and hypoglycaemia • Benzodiazepines if recurrent/prolonged seizures • Haemodialysis in cases of severe poisoning
Amfetamines	• Wakefulness, excessive activity, agitation, paranoia, hallucinations	• CE, LFTs, CK, glucose, FBC • ECG	• Close monitoring of temperature and blood pressure
Ecstasy (MDMA)	• Nausea, trismus (jaw-clenching), dilated pupils, blurred vision, sweating, hyper-reflexia • Hypertension • Exhaustion, seizures, coma, hyperthermia • As per other amfetamines • Dehydration • May also cause severe reactions even at previously tolerated doses: delirium, coma, seizures, arrhythmias, hyperthermia, rhabdomyolysis, renal/ hepatic failure, ARDS, DIC • Hyponatraemia (excess water ingestion × increased ADH secretion) • Rarely may cause 'serotonin syndrome'		• Active cooling if pyrexial • Benzodiazepines for excessive agitation or seizures • Contact NPIS for advice on management of hypertension
Cannabis	• Low doses: conjunctival injection, drowsiness, tachycardia, slurred speech and ataxia • High doses: anxiety confusion, paranoid psychosis	• Although cannabinoid metabolites can be detected in urine, levels do not correlate well with toxicity	• Reassurance suffices in most cases of psychosis • Diazepam may be used for sedation

Cocaine/ crack cocaine	• Euphoria, agitation, aggression, hallucinations • Dilated pupils, sweating, pyrexia, nausea, vomiting • Tachycardia, hypertension • Seizures • Arrhythmias, hypertensive crisis, myocardial infarct and cerebrovascular accident (vasospasm), hyperpyrexia	• Cocaine can be detected in urine • ECG	• Activated charcoal if presenting within 1 h of oral ingestion • Cardiac monitoring • Close monitoring of temperature and blood pressure • Active cooling if pyrexial • Arrhythmias: correct electrolyte disturbances; consider verapamil for SVT; avoid beta-blockers (unopposed alpha-agonist activity) and other antiarrhythmic drugs • Cerebrovascular/myocardial ischaemia/infarction – seek expert help to confirm secondary to vasospasm (avoid thrombolysis); control blood pressure; symptom control • Benzodiazepines for seizures

ABGs, arterial blood gases; ADH, antidiuretic hormone; ARDS, adult respiratory distress syndrome; CE, creatinine and electrolytes; CK, creatine kinase; DIC, disseminated intravascular coagulation; ECG, electrocardiogram; FBC, full blood count; LFTs, liver function tests; MDMA, 3,4-methylenedioxymethamfetamine; NPIS, National Poisons Information Service.

Management

General measures

All patients with suspected poisoning should be admitted to hospital for further assessment/monitoring. Symptomatic treatment and supportive measures will suffice in most cases, but specific antidotes may be required.

Begin with an assessment of:

- A - Airway
- B - Breathing
- C - Circulation
- D - Disability
- E - Exposure

Cardiorespiratory dysfunction

Ventilatory support and optimisation of cardiac function/blood pressure should be provided where necessary in accordance with standard management guidelines/protocols for patients with cardiorespiratory depression. Patients with a reduced conscious level must be monitored in a high-dependency/intensive care setting.

Nausea/vomiting

Vomiting is a common side effect of poisoning and usually responds to anti-emetics.

Agitation

Simple reassurance and support and nursing in a quiet environment will suffice in most cases. Always exclude other possible treatable causes (e.g. hypoxia, hypotension, hypoglycaemia) before considering the use of sedatives. Where required, short-acting agents (e.g. diazepam) are preferred with appropriate monitoring.

Seizures

Single short-lived convulsions do not require treatment – but check that there is no other reversible cause (e.g. hypoglycaemia, electrolyte disturbance). Persistent or recurrent seizures should be treated with lorazepam or diazepam and the patient transferred to a high-dependency/intensive care setting.

Temperature dysregulation

Hypothermia may develop in any patient with a reduced conscious level, especially if cold-exposed. Active warming measures can be used to raise the temperature in a controlled manner, with cardiac monitoring for arrhythmias.

Hyperthermia may occur in patients taking CNS stimulants. Removal of excess clothing, use of a fan and sponging with tepid water may help. In cases of severe hyperthermia check with the National Poisons Information Service (see later) for advice on specific measures.

Psychiatric assessment

Once the physical consequences of poisoning have been prevented/treated, formal psychiatric evaluation is required in all cases of suspected self-harm. For patients deemed to be at high risk of further self-harm/suicidal intent, consider special (one-to-one) nursing while medical management is completed and psychiatric review awaited.

Specific measures

UK National Poisons Information Service and TOXBASE®

Specialist information and advice on the management of suspected/confirmed cases of poisoning is available 24 h a day from the UK National Poisons Information Service (NPIS; www.npis.org). If in doubt, seek early help. TOXBASE is the primary clinical toxicology database of NPIS and is available online to registered users at www.toxbase.org. It provides a wealth of information about diagnosis, investigation and treatment of patients who have been exposed to drugs, household products and industrial/agricultural chemicals.

Preventing absorption and enhancing elimination of ingested toxins

Gastric lavage

This is rarely required and is of limited value if performed more than 1 h after ingestion. Its use should be reserved for substances that cannot be effectively removed by other means (e.g. iron, lithium), and only if a life-threatening amount has been ingested within the previous hour. It must only be undertaken if the airway is adequately protected/secured, and should not be used if a corrosive substance has been swallowed. It is advisable to check with NPIS/TOXBASE if considering gastric lavage.

Activated charcoal

Given by mouth, activated charcoal (50 g in an adolescent/adult; children 1 g/kg) can bind many drugs/poisons in the gastrointestinal tract, thereby reducing their absorption. It should be given as soon as possible and confers benefits up to 1 h after ingestion, and occasionally longer if dealing with modified release preparations. Repeated doses may be required for certain toxins whose elimination is aided even after they have been absorbed (e.g. carbamazepine, quinine, theophylline).

Certain substances (acids, alkalis, metals/metallic salts (e.g. mercury, iron, lithium, methanol, ethylene glycol) are not bound by activated charcoal – if in doubt, check with NPIS/TOXBASE.

Alkaline diuresis and dialysis

Alkalinisation of the urine (pH 7.5–8.5) may aid elimination of salicylates. It should be undertaken in a high-dependency/intensive care setting.

Haemodialysis is generally reserved for patients who have ingested significant amounts of a toxin with a low volume of distribution/weak protein binding, e.g. salicylates, lithium, methanol, ethylene glycol.

Specific toxins

Specific antidotes are available for a small number of toxins and can be life-saving (e.g. *N*-acetylcysteine in paracetamol overdose) (Fig. 22.2). In addition, complications associated with certain poisons benefit from targeted therapies (e.g. use of sodium bicarbonate to treat arrhythmias caused by tricyclic antidepressant overdose), while in other cases avoidance of certain classes of drug is recommended to avoid exacerbating the situation (e.g. anti-arrhythmics in tricyclic antidepressant overdose). Tables 22.2 and 22.3 outline specific investigations and management measures for poisoning associated with prescription/over-the-counter medications (Table 22.2) and alcohol/'recreational' drugs (Table 22.3). For more detailed information on a broader range of toxins consult NPIS/TOXBASE.

Carbon monoxide poisoning

Carbon monoxide (CO) is a colourless, odourless, non-irritant gas; poisoning is usually due to inhalation of smoke, car exhaust or fumes from incomplete burning of gas fires/cookers, as occurs with blocked flues or when combustion occurs in a confined space. CO reduces the oxygen-carrying capacity of blood by binding to haemoglobin to form carboxyhaemoglobin (COHb) and dramatically reduces tissue oxygen delivery.

Clinical features vary from headache, nausea and vomiting with low level exposure, through drowsiness, hyperventilation and ataxia, to seizures, coma and death after exposure to high concentrations. Cerebral oedema is common and focal neurological signs may be present. If the patient survives the acute episode, neurological sequelae including tremor, memory impairment, personality change and visual loss may ensue, while other patients develop marked Parkinsonian features.

A high index of clinical suspicion is required; demonstration of an elevated COHb concentration in blood confirms the diagnosis but does not accurately predict prognosis, as treatment (O_2 therapy) prior to hospital admission can result in lower measured levels. Arterial blood gases should be checked and ECG monitoring performed.

Removal from the source of exposure is a critical first step in the management of suspected CO poisoning. In addition to basic life-support measures, high flow oxygen (e.g. 15 l/min via a tightly fitting face mask) should be delivered without delay and the patient transferred urgently to hospital for further assessment. Continued/prolonged oxygen therapy is often required until COHb levels fall to <5% (normal values range from 3–5% in non-smokers, up to 10% in smokers).

NB: Standard pulse oximetry is unreliable in CO poisoning as COHb is mistaken for oxyhaemoglobin. A specific pulse CO-oximeter may be used instead.

The role of hyperbaric oxygen in the treatment of CO poisoning remains controversial and all cases being considered for this should be discussed with NPIS. Cerebral oedema is treated along conventional lines.

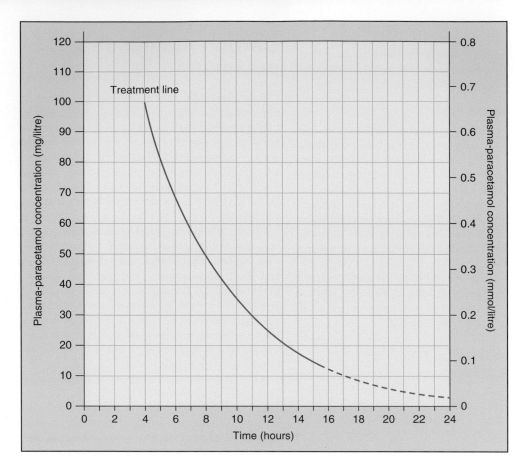

Figure 22.2 Algorithm for management of paracetamol overdose. Source: University of Wales College of Medicine Therapeutics and Toxicology Centre. Reproduced with permission.

S1 UNITS CONVERSION TABLE

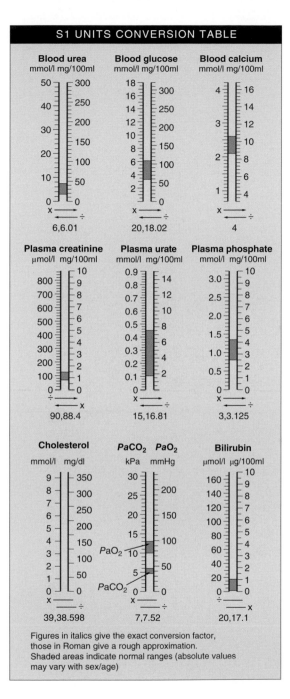

Blood urea
mmol/l mg/100ml

6,6.01

Blood glucose
mmol/l mg/100ml

20,18.02

Blood calcium
mmol/l mg/100ml

4

Plasma creatinine
µmol/l mg/100ml

90,88.4

Plasma urate
mmol/l mg/100ml

15,16.81

Plasma phosphate
mmol/l mg/100ml

3,3.125

Cholesterol
mmol/l mg/dl

39,38.598

PaCO₂ *PaO₂*
kPa mmHg

PaO_2

$PaCO_2$

7,7.52

Bilirubin
µmol/l µg/100ml

20,17.1

Figures in italics give the exact conversion factor,
those in Roman give a rough approximation.
Shaded areas indicate normal ranges (absolute values
may vary with sex/age)

Index